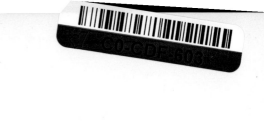

Electrodermal Activity
in Psychological Research

CONTRIBUTORS

GORDON H. BARLAND

M. J. CHRISTIE

M. E. DAWSON

SHEILA R. DEITZ

W. W. GRINGS

CYNTHIA L. JANES

EDWARD S. KATKIN

H. D. KIMMEL

KAROL L. KUMPFER

WILLIAM F. PROKASY

DAVID C. RASKIN

GARY E. SCHWARTZ

DAVID SHAPIRO

JOHN A. STERN

P. H. VENABLES

Electrodermal Activity
in Psychological Research

Edited by

WILLIAM F. PROKASY / DAVID C. RASKIN

Department of Psychology
University of Utah
Salt Lake City, Utah

ACADEMIC PRESS New York and London   1973

A Subsidiary of Harcourt Brace Jovanovich, Publishers

ACADEMIC PRESS, INC.
111 Fifth Avenue, New York, New York 10003

United Kingdom Edition published by
ACADEMIC PRESS, INC. (LONDON) LTD.
24/28 Oval Road, London NW1

Library of Congress Cataloging in Publication Data

Prokasy, William Frederick, DATE
    Electrodermal activity in psychological research.

    Includes bibliographies.
    1.   Galvanic skin response.   I.   Raskin, David C.,
joint author.   II.   Title.   [DNLM: 1.   Galvanic
skin response.   2.   Psychophysiology. WL106 P964e 1973]
QP372.P78   612'.83   72-12195
ISBN 0–12–565950–4

Contents

List of Contributors   ix

Preface   xi

Chapter 1. **Mechanisms, Instrumentation, Recording Techniques, and Quantification of Responses**

P. H. Venables and M. J. Christie

I.	Introduction	2
II.	Terminology	4
III.	Characteristics of Observed Electrodermal Phenomena	7
IV.	Mechanisms	10
V.	Measurement	48
VI.	Summary: "What Can Be Inferred from Measures of Electrodermal Activity?	99
	Appendix I: Recommended Circuits for Skin Conductance Measurement	101
	Appendix II: Construction of Electrodes	106
	Appendix III: Recommended Electrode Placements	108
	General References	109
	References	109

Chapter 2. **Attention and Arousal**

David C. Raskin

I.	Introduction	125
II.	Theories of Attention and Arousal	126
III.	Dependent Variables and Theoretical Concepts	131
IV.	Issues in Research	137
	References	150

Chapter 3. **Classical Conditioning**

William F. Prokasy and Karol L. Kumpfer

I.	Introduction	157
II.	Methodology	158

III.   Independent Variable Manipulations   173
IV.   Concluding Comments   194
       References   196

Chapter 4.   Complex Variables in Conditioning

W. W. Grings and M. E. Dawson

   I.   Introduction   204
  II.   Compound Signal Conditioning   204
 III.   Semantic Conditioning and Generalization   213
  IV.   Electrodermal Conditioning and the Unconditioned Response 221
   V.   Effects of Instructional Variables on Electrodermal Conditioning 228
  VI.   Individual Difference Factors   241
        References   245

Chapter 5.   Instrumental Conditioning

H. D. Kimmel

   I.   Background and Definitions   255
  II.   Literature Review   258
 III.   Summary and Theoretical Implications   276
        References   280

Chapter 6.   Personality and Psychopathology

John A. Stern and Cynthia L. Janes

    I.   Introduction   284
   II.   Schizophrenia   284
  III.   Depression   295
   IV.   Psychopathy   299
    V.   Mental Retardation   301
   VI.   Central Nervous System Damage   316
  VII.   Anxiety   322
 VIII.   Introversion–Extroversion   333
         References   337

Chapter 7.   Systematic Desensitization

Edward S. Katkin and Sheila R. Deitz

   I.   Introduction   347
  II.   Mechanisms Underlying Desensitization Therapy and Their Relationship to Electrodermal Activity   349

III. Empirical Findings and Their Relationship to Theory   353
IV. Summary   369
      References   372

Chapter 8. Social Psychophysiology

Gary E. Schwartz and David Shapiro

  I. Introduction   377
 II. Attitudes   383
III. Empathy   390
 IV. Small Groups and Social Interaction   397
  V. Cross-Cultural and Ethnic Differences   407
 VI. Summary and Conclusions   410
      References   413

Chapter 9. Detection of Deception

Gordon H. Barland and David C. Raskin

  I. Introduction   418
 II. Methodology   421
III. Theories of Lie Detection   445
 IV. Major Problems Requiring Research   447
  V. Countermeasures and Counter-Countermeasures   456
 VI. Summary and Conclusions   470
      References   471

AUTHOR INDEX   479
SUBJECT INDEX   495

List of Contributors

Numbers in parentheses indicate the pages on which the authors' contributions begin.

GORDON H. BARLAND (417), Department of Psychology, University of Utah, Salt Lake City, Utah

M. J. CHRISTIE (1), Department of Psychology, Birkbeck College, University of London, London, England

M. E. DAWSON (203), Gateways Hospital, Los Angeles, California

SHEILA R. DEITZ (347), Department of Psychology, State University of New York at Buffalo, Buffalo, New York

W. W. GRINGS (203), Department of Psychology, University of Southern California, Los Angeles, California

CYNTHIA L. JANES (283), Department of Child Psychiatry, Washington University School of Medicine, St. Louis, Missouri

EDWARD S. KATKIN (347), Department of Psychology, State University of New York at Buffalo, Buffalo, New York

H. D. KIMMEL (255), Department of Psychology, University of South Florida, Tampa, Florida

KAROL L. KUMPFER (157), Department of Psychology, Oberlin College, Oberlin, Ohio*

WILLIAM F. PROKASY (157), Department of Psychology, University of Utah, Salt Lake City, Utah

DAVID C. RASKIN (125, 417), Department of Psychology, University of Utah, Salt Lake City, Utah

* Present address: Department of Long-Range Planning, University of Utah, Salt Lake City, Utah.

GARY E. SCHWARTZ (377), Department of Psychology and Social Relations, Harvard University, Cambridge, Massachusetts

DAVID SHAPIRO (377), Harvard Medical School, Department of Psychiatry, Massachusetts Mental Health Center, Boston, Massachusetts

JOHN A. STERN (283), Department of Psychology, Washington University, St. Louis, Missouri

P. H. VENABLES (1), Department of Psychology, Birkbeck College, University of London, London, England.

Preface

The general purpose of this book is to summarize in a single source the information on electrodermal activity from many of the areas in which it has been employed: the methodological problems with its use are discussed, and much of what has been learned about human beings with that measure is described.

The book differs from most in one important respect. Rather than concentrating on a limited range of psychological concepts with a diversity of measurement techniques, it concentrates on a single measure as used in a variety of laboratory and field contexts. Since electrodermal activity is used so widely as a dependent variable in basic psychophysiological research, conditioning, psychopathology, therapy settings, efforts at detection of deception, and in social psychological research, that substantial differences of opinion exist as to its value in any given context, for example, as an indicator of emotion, and since there is no single reference source on its extensive use, the choice of this measure as a focus for the present work seemed reasonable.

The organization of this volume is generally from the molecular to the molar in sequence of chapters, from basic to applied research, and from the more elementary to the more complex independent variable manipulation. Chapter 1, by Venables and Christie, constitutes a rather complete treatment of terminology, recording and measuring techniques, electronic circuits, and current theories of the physiological mechanisms of electrodermal responding. In an effort to bring some standardization into the literature, the notation employed by Venables and Christie was adopted in the succeeding chapters.

In Chapter 2, Raskin provides an account of theories of attention and arousal, and describes the indices of electrodermal activity and their relationships to those theories. Some basic research issues in the area are reviewed and summarized.

Chapters 3 and 4 are concerned primarily with classical conditioning. In the former, Prokasy and Kumpfer deal with the more familiar independent variable manipulations. Half of their chapter is devoted to the problems of measurement and control, and the remaining half constitutes a review of the effects of various independent variable manipulations on simple and differential conditioning performance. In the following chapter, Grings and Dawson have selected a number of the more prominent complex conditioning contexts for discussion, including complex stimuli (such as compound and semantic stimuli), the effects of the conditioned stimulus–unconditioned stimulus relationship on the unconditioned response, and individual differences as related to personality variables.

In Chapter 5, Kimmel reviews the literature of instrumental conditioning of electrodermal activity with emphasis on some of the problems of controls. He concludes that the best evidence for instrumental conditioning has been found with unsignalled reward and punishment.

The use of electrodermal measures in research on personality and pathological states is the subject of Chapter 6. Stern and Janes discuss its use with schizophrenics, retardates, depressives, psychotherapy, CNS damage, anxiety, and introversion–extroversion. Some possible future directions of research are also mentioned.

Katkin and Deitz discuss the presumed mechanisms underlying systematic desensitization and the relationship of those mechanisms to electrodermal activity. Chapter 7 also includes a review of the literature and closes with the conclusion that electrodermal activity is a useful measure to assess outcome but is not particularly helpful in elucidating the underlying processes.

In Chapter 8, Schwartz and Shapiro discuss several widely divergent areas of social psychological research in which electrodermal activity has been employed as a dependent variable. Those include such areas as attitude, empathy, small groups, and social interactions. Their review illustrates how some of the older paradigms have been used in new ways. For example, classical conditioning is used to analyze cognitive processes functioning in a social setting.

In the concluding chapter on the detection of deception, Barland and Raskin bring together in a single review both the laboratory and field techniques and the results of investigations in an attempt to evaluate the scientific basis for the application of the paradigm to field situations of lie detection. They also discuss some of the problems encountered in the field use of detection of deception techniques, and they point to areas which require additional research.

Susan Massey and Margaret Sullivan contributed to this volume through their help in correspondence, typing, and general organization of time and effort. We would like to take this occasion to express our thanks to them, as their efforts certainly reduced the number of complications which otherwise we would have encountered.

CHAPTER 1

Mechanisms, Instrumentation, Recording Techniques, and Quantification of Responses

P. H. VENABLES

M. J. CHRISTIE

Department of Psychology
Birkbeck College
University of London
London, England

I.	Introduction	2
II.	Terminology	4
	A. Introduction	4
	B. Older Terminology	5
	C. Proposals of the Society for Psychophysiological Research	5
	D. Proposals of Venables and Martin	6
	E. Present Proposals	6
III.	Characteristics of Observed Electrodermal Phenomena	7
	A. Conventions of Write-Out	7
	B. Expected Values	8
	C. Other Points to Note	9
IV.	Mechanisms	10
	A. Overview	10
	B. Peripheral Mechanisms	13
	C. Hormonal Mechanisms	22
	D. Central Mechanisms	28
	E. Models and Mechanisms of Electrical Functioning of the Skin	36
V.	Measurement	48
	A. The Subject and the Environment	48
	B. Equipment	63
	C. Procedure and General Methodology	81
	D. Data Collection	89
VI.	Summary "What Can Be Inferred from Measures of Electrodermal Activity?"	99
	Appendix I: Recommended Circuits for Skin Conductance Measurement	101
	Appendix II: Construction of Electrodes	106
	Appendix III: Recommended Electrode Placements	108
	General References	109
	References	109

1

I. Introduction

Psychologists have used measurements of electrodermal activity since the turn of the century; there have been periods of study and development, and periods of stagnation. Much of the stagnation has been the consequence of disappointing, equivocal, or unrepeatable results, owing at least in part to the use of inadequate or ill-understood techniques.

There has been a recrudescence of interest in the subject during the past 20 years, reflecting growth and development of the discipline of psychophysiology. Along with this interest has arisen an awareness of the need for adequate techniques which are based upon an understanding of the mechanisms underlying electrodermal activity.

Although considerable progress has been made, and despite the developments subsequent to methodological reviews of 5 years ago (Edelberg, 1967; Venables & Martin, 1967a), there remain areas of unknown territory: methods and techniques proposed in this chapter, therefore, reflect the present state of the art, and though some recommendations are based upon well-established findings, others are judgments made from the best evidence currently available. Because of this there must be some personal biases involved, and there may be variations among the methods and techniques used in this and in subsequent chapters. Also, a terminology is advocated which, although it is increasingly accepted, departs from earlier tradition. Thus, tolerance may be required of the reader, when, for example, elimination of the hallowed term "GSR" (galvanic skin response) is advocated. It is hoped that the newer terminology provides less equivocal information about the particular electrodermal phenomenon being measured.

In writing a chapter such as this a dilemma arises immediately. There are a small number of workers in electrodermal activity who are intimately concerned with the minutiae of the mechanisms involved in producing electrical activity of the skin. On the other hand, there are a far larger number of workers whose interest is centered around electrodermal activity as an aspect of behavior that can be readily measured and quantified. It is more for this latter, wider group of readers that this chapter is intended. While it is the purpose of the chapter to reinforce the idea that reliable measurement cannot take place without adequate knowledge of the characteristics of the mechanisms involved, it is not intended to go into such detail about mechanisms that the general reader will be confused. However, while it may be legitimate to condition electrodermal activity in the same way as another piece of behavior may be conditioned, without any attention necessarily being paid to the underlying physiology, the position changes somewhat as soon as level of skin conductance is used as an index of arousal. The implication of underlying physiology in such a usage demands that the peripheral and central mechanisms be understood.

An attempt has been made to write the section on methodology at two levels; some material is a counsel of perfection for those who have facilities, time, opportunity, and finances. It is, however, only too obvious that compromises have to be made, and, therefore, acceptable falls from grace will also be discussed. Additionally, an attempt has been made to write for two levels of expertise and what we hope is clear and simple "cookbook" material has been included among more sophisticated exposition.

For a reader who is relatively unfamiliar with electrodermal phenomena, a helpful introduction is provided by Lykken (1968); his chapter discusses electrodermal phenomena within the wider context of neuropsychology and psychophysiology. More specialized treatment of electrodermal mechanisms has recently become available (Edelberg, 1971), and up-to-date discussion of measurement and mechanisms is to be found in Fowles (1973), and in Grings (1973). There are general reviews of methodology in two handbooks of psychophysiological methods (Edelberg, 1967; Venables & Martin, 1967a), and specialized reviews of specific aspects of electrodermal mechanisms have appeared at various times. Thus, Bloch's publication (1952) is concerned with the methods and conditions for recording electrodermal activity as a measure of psychological state, whereas Wang's two-part review (1957–1958) is described as being from the standpoint of reflex physiology and is particularly concerned with animal experiments on the central control of electrodermal phenomena. Insofar as most applications of electrodermal measurement have man as the subject, the review of Sourek (1965) is particularly important, as he is concerned with verifying by neurosurgical operations some of the new knowledge gained in experiments on animals. This appears to be the only major review of work on central mechanisms in man. In contrast, Montagu and Coles (1966) examine specifically the peripheral aspects of the electrodermal response, restricting the account to resistance/conductance phenomena, and focusing on the role of sweat glands in the generation of these. Martin and Venables (1966) provide a review of both central and peripheral mechanisms, and consider the possible role of nonsudorific factors; they report findings from both animal and human studies. Wilcott (1967) is concerned particularly with peripheral factors affecting arousal sweating (sweating to nonthermal stimuli) and with their relation to electrodermal phenomena; Fowles and Venables (1970) also consider the significance of two specific peripheral factors, poral closure, which accompanies hydration of the horny layer of the skin, and the active transport of sodium out of sweat in the ducts and through the ductal wall (see Fig. 2, page 13).

This brief introduction may have indicated the possible range of electrodermal phenomena and their underlying mechanisms. It is hoped that some justification has been provided for advocacy of precision in terminology, as described in the next section.

II.   Terminology

A.   Introduction

Throughout the history of electrodermal measurement two different types of techniques have been in common use (Neumann & Blanton, 1970). In one, a current is passed through the skin from an external source, and resistance to its passage is measured; this procedure is called *exosomatic*. In the second, so-called *endosomatic* method, no current is externally imposed and the only source of electrical activity is the skin itself and its interaction with the electrode–electrolyte system which serves to connect the body surface with the appropriate measuring apparatus (see Section V).

Two forms of exosomatic measurement have been used at one time or another. By far the most common, following the original work of Féré (1888), has involved the passage of a direct current through the skin, typically from some convenient source such as a dry cell or a battery of cells, and the skin and underlying tissue has been treated as though it was made up only of elements acting effectively as resistors. From time to time the use of this method has been questioned and an alternating source has been used to provide the imposed current. Two considerations underlie this use of an alternating source, both of which are probably of doubtful relevance. The first concerns the possible polarization of electrodes when using a direct current for more than a very short time. This polarization, owing to the use of inadequate electrode techniques, had the effect of the development of an artifactual apparent resistance which could not be distinguished from the wanted value of the resistance of the skin. The use of an alternating current source was intended to minimize the effect of such polarization. It is a problem which has, however, been minimized by the use of silver–silver chloride electrodes and appropriate electrode media (see Section V.B). The second consideration, suggesting the use of an alternating current source, was that it made possible the measurement of the capacitative component which is present as a parameter in the electrical activity of skin [see, for instance, the models reviewed by Landis (1932)]. However, it has not been shown that skin capacitance is an independent factor having any psychological relevance. There exists some controversy as to whether the capacitance in the skin is a true capacitance which does not change in value with the frequency of the impressed current, or whether it is a polarization capacitance which does. In any case, its measurement is a matter of some difficulty and its independence from the mechanisms responsible for skin conductance is doubtful (see Section IV.E.2). Furthermore, the use of an alternating source of impressed current necessitates consideration of a further parameter, namely, frequency. The general finding (for example, Montagu, 1964) of a near unity correlation between ac and dc methods of measurement at low frequencies (for example, 60 Hz) suggests that the use of ac is an unnecessary complication, while the occurrence of little electrical skin activity above 1000 Hz precludes measurement at this point.

B. Older Terminology

A wide variety of terms has been used to designate the electrical activity of the skin; perhaps the most widely employed is the term GSR. Unfortunately, it has been used to cover several aspects of electrical activity of the skin, and is thus ambiguous. Its correct usage is to designate the phasic response of exosomatically measured activity, that is, the skin resistance or conductance response. Sometimes, however, it has been used to indicate the skin potential response. Other well-used terms are PGR (psychogalvanic response) and EDR (electrodermal response), the latter sometimes made less ambiguous by the additional letter EDR(F) indicating the electrodermal response of Féré, that is, the skin resistance response, and EDR(T) the electrodermal response of Tarchanoff, that is, the skin potential response. There is thus apparent need for a more adequate terminology and labeling system to show whether responses or levels of activity are indicated, and whether or not resistance, conductance, or potential are being measured.

C. Proposals of the Society for Psychophysiological Research

In 1967 suggestions of a nomenclature committee of the Society for Psychophysiological Research were put forward (Brown, 1967). In these it was suggested that SCR, SRR, and SPR should be used to indicate skin conductance response, skin resistance response, and skin potential response respectively, while the letters, SC, SR, and SP should indicate levels of activity of the appropriate variables. Additionally, if alternating current measures were used, then SZ and SZR would indicate skin impedance level and skin impedance response, or if analogously with conductance, admittance is used as the reciprocal of impedance, then the terms SY and SYR would be employed. In 1970, Ax, the editor of the journal *Psychophysiology*, proposed further standardization by the elimination of the terms "skin resistance level" and "response," and the use of conductance only, as the measure of exosomatic activity (see Section IV.B for the rationale for the use of conductance).

D. Proposals of Venables and Martin[1]

While agreeing in general with the proposals of the Society for Psychophysiological Research, Venables and Martin suggested the use of the terms SCL, SRL, and SPL to indicate skin conductance level, skin resistance level, and skin potential level. This eliminates any ambiguity in designating tonic levels of activity and leaves the terms SC, SR, and SP for general usage. Thus, a description in the "Apparatus" section of a paper might read, "skin conductance (SC) was measured by a constant voltage system. Skin conductance levels (SCL) were measurable within a range of 1–50 μmho, and skin conductance responses (SCR) with a maximum sensitivity of .05 μmho per centimeter." Again, by extension of the Society for Psychophysiological Research proposals, SZL and SYL would be used for skin impedance level and skin admittance level.

E. Present Proposals

The case for exosomatic measurement in terms of conductance and not resistance is convincing (see Sections IV.B, and V.B and D). Therefore, it is proposed that the terms SCR, skin conductance response; SCL, skin conductance level; and SC, skin conductance (in a general context), should be generally employed for exosomatic measurement. In a similar fashion, where potential is measured, it is proposed that the terms SPR, skin potential response; SPL, skin potential level; SP, skin potential (in a general context), should be used. One ambiguity remains. The skin potential response, SPR, is classically biphasic with the first component negative and the second component positive going. Uniphasic negative and positive waveforms are reported, and triphasic

[1] From Venables and Martin (1967a).

forms are sometimes seen. In the present state of knowledge a clear description of the phenomena recorded is required. Thus, such a statement as, "the mean amplitude of the initial negative component of the SPR was 1 mV," provides the necessary information. Earlier suggestions to label the initial negative phase the *a* wave, and the second positive wave the *b* wave, are prone to ambiguity, especially when uniphasic positive responses are reported.

Difficulty sometimes arises when changes in tonic level occur as a result, for instance, of changing the nature of the experimental situation, when the change in level may be thought of as a response to the situational change. It is suggested that in these circumstances it is wise to talk of a change in SCL and to reserve the term SCR for those phasic changes having characteristic latency and shape criteria (see Section V).

Statistical considerations sometimes necessitate a transformation of the data collected in conductance or potential units. Thus, log skin conductance response (log SCR) is commonly used, and range correction (Lykken & Venables, 1971; Lykken, Rose, Luther, & Maley, 1966) has been advocated, giving rise to the terms ϕ_{SCR} and ϕ_{SPR}. Further consideration of the use of such methods is to be found in Section V.D.

III Characteristics of Observed Electrodermal Phenomena

This section indicates the characteristic parameters of the electrodermal activity which the reader is likely to record.

A. Conventions of Write-Out

Over the past 50 years there has been considerable disagreement about the directions in which psychophysiological activity should be recorded. There is a body of tradition among neurophysiologists that data should be recorded "negative up," and this has had influence in the newer discipline of psychophysiology. However, there would seem to be some logical basis for proposals which can be put forward in the light of present practice. In the case of exosomatic activity, the whole of this chapter emphasizes the use of conductance measures. If these are both recorded and presented on graphs in the "increasing conductance up" convention, then what may be loosely called increases in arousal or activation are indexed by increases in conductance, both from the point of view of tonic (SCL) and phasic (SCR) measures. Given that conductance is measured upward, it would be illogical to measure SPL as anything other than "negative up" (negativity being referred to as that of the active palmar electrode with respect to an indifferent reference electrode on the arm). Thus, for most of the time simultaneous recordings of SCL and SPL will move in the same direction. It then follows that the primary negative component of SPR will move in the upward direction and will thus move in the same direction as a SCR with which it will be approximately synchronized.

While what has been suggested is to be generally recommended, it may be necessary, if the data are to be recorded on magnetic tape for later analysis, to alter these conventions (see Section V.D.I.a). Aspects of major interest, for example, SCRs and the negative component of SPR, should be recorded so that they are positive-going on the magnetic tape because dropout artifacts, from which they may be distinguished, are normally negative-going.

B. Expected Values

1. Skin Conductance Level (SCL)

Values will depend upon the size of electrode used and should be quoted in micromhos per square centimeter (see Section V.D.2). With $1/cm^2$ electrodes and bipolar placement, the range of expected values will be most likely from 2 to 100 μmho/cm^2, with most values falling in the range 5–20 μmho/cm^2 (see, for example, Ax & Bamford, 1968; Campos & Johnson, 1967; Johnson & Campos, 1967; Johnson & Landon, 1965; Johnson, 1970; Kopacz & Smith, 1971; Kaplan, 1970; Lieblich, 1969).

2. Skin Potential Level (SPL)

Values will depend upon concentration of electrolyte used, but with .5% KCl as recommended (see Section V.B.5), values will range from $+10$ mV to -70 mV; exceptionally values of $+30$ mV may be recorded (see, for example, Ax & Bamford, 1968; Juniper & Dykman, 1967; O'Connell, Tursky, & Evans, 1967; Surwillo, 1969; Wyatt & Tursky, 1969).

3. Skin Conductance Response (SCR)

Examples of responses are shown in Fig. 1. As with SCL, values will depend upon the area of the electrodes used. The range of expected response amplitude is from .01 μmho to 5 μmho/cm^2, latencies will be from 1.3 to 2.5 sec (see, for example, Mefferd, Sadler, & Wieland, 1969;

Surwillo, 1967). Time to peak response is usually less than 1 sec and half recovery time $(t/2)$ (see Section V.D.2) will range from 1 to 10 sec. [If recovery rate is measured in terms of the time constant (tc) then $tc/(t/2) = 1.43$ (Edelberg, 1970).]

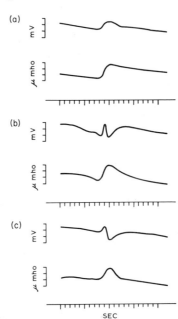

Fig. 1. Selected skin potential (upper tracing) and skin conductance (lower tracing) responses. For SPRs negativity is recorded upward. In (a), a uniphasic negative SPR is shown, accompanied by an SCR with a slow recovery. In (b), a biphasic SPR is shown, where the positive-going component is small, and is accompanied by an SCR having a moderate recovery rate. In (c) is a fully biphasic SPR, accompanied by an SCR with a very fast recovery rate.

4. SKIN POTENTIAL RESPONSE (SPR)

Examples of responses are shown in Fig. 1. As suggested in Section V.D.2, measurement of the real amplitudes of the SPR is not feasible. The actual recorded amplitudes of SPR will probably be in the following ranges: initial negative component up to 2 mV, secondary positive component up to 4 mV.

The latency of the initial negative component will be similar to that of the SCR.

C. Other Points to Note

1. SIMULTANEOUS RECORDING OF SCR AND SPR

As will be seen from Fig. 1, there is often a coincidence of long recovery limbs of SCRs with uniphasic negative SPRs and short recovery limbs of SCRs with biphasic SPRs.

2.   NONSPECIFIC FLUCTUATIONS

The presence or absence of nonspecific, spontaneous, or unelicited electrodermal activity depends on two factors. The first is that it really is spontaneous, and not elicited by extraneous stimuli, coughs, sighs, etc. The second is that its minimum value is defined. This will depend upon the amplification of the system involved in relation to the noise pickup of this system. Minimum values in practice are probably in the region of 0.01 μmho for spontaneous SCRs.

It should be noted that there is evidence that spontaneous fluctuations may, in some circumstances, have characteristics which distinguish them from typical electrodermal responses. Atypical responses have been reported as being present during stage 3 sleep (Johnson & Lubin, 1966), noted by us in two sleep records, and reported by Rickles and Day (1968) as being obtained from nonpalmar sites. The circumstances in which atypical responses are recorded, that is, in states of low arousal, or from sites having few eccrine sweat glands, suggest that such spontaneous fluctuations may be reflecting a mechanism other than secretory or reabsorptive function of sweat glands. It is possible that the atypical EDRs are observable only when sweat glands are relatively quiescent, or few in number.

IV.   Mechanisms

A.   Overview

Early work on the mechanisms of electrodermal activity has been most completely reviewed by Neumann and Blanton (1970) and reviews by Landis and De Wicke (1929) and Landis (1932) will enable the reader to extend his knowledge of the history of the subject from the end of Neumann and Blanton's review until the present period.

One name in particular links early pioneering days with contemporary research. In 1927 Darrow had already published a summary of his work in the field, and in 1970 an issue of *Psychophysiology* carried "The peripheral mechanism of the galvanic skin response" by Darrow and Gullickson. Darrow's writings would seem to exemplify the fact that much of the spade work had already been done by the late 1920s, and yet the field still contains unanswered questions of detail.

In 1950, in a period of disenchantment, McCleary published, "The nature of the galvanic skin response," in which one could read "the GSR has not lived up to its expectation" and that "there is the basic question about the GSR. *What is it?* What are the physiological changes that give rise to it? [p. 98]." So McCleary settled to the task of reviewing the physiological basis of the EDR as it appeared at midcentury, presenting three viewpoints: the muscular theory, which met an early end, the vascular theory, and the secretory one.

Sommer, in 1902, had suggested that the change in SR seen in response to stimulation was the result of involuntary muscular activity, but French (1944) recorded EDR and finger tremor simultaneously; the latter had a markedly shorter latency and a faster recovery time. This fact fitted the evidence that EDR is an autonomic response with slower rate of conduction associated with autonomic pathways, and together with the dearth of positive evidence from the muscular theory, led to its abandonment.

There remained the vascular and secretory theories, the former being attributed to Féré (1888), the latter to Tarchonoff (1889, 1890). One ingenious version of the vascular theory was suggested by McDowell (1933). He argued that the resistance of the blood was higher than that of extracellular fluid (ECF), and that in consequence, when vasoconstriction diminished the blood content of the skin, there was a fall in resistance. Two versions of the secretory theory are presented. One, which is rejected by McLeary, is that an increase in the amount of sweat in and on the skin increases conductivity and thus lowers resistance to impressed current. The alternative explanation is that a presecretory change in sweat glands may increase the permeability of the cell membranes involved in conducting pathways. Later consideration of these alternatives in Section IV shows that both survive to the present day.

McLeary drew attention to Hemphill's (1942) work on skin hydration. Hemphill suggested that the water content of the skin was relevant to the level of recorded skin resistance, and his careful methodology remains as an example for the present day. McLeary also covers topics such as drug studies, the effects of atropine and pilocarpine, anatomical evidence for the link between low skin resistance and high sweat gland density, Darrow's suggestion that the EDR is part of a preparatory response (1936), and an examination of the extent of knowledge about the nervous control of electrodermal responses.

McLeary's review concludes with his judgment that, at that time, the EDR had not lived up to earlier expectations of it. He suggested that although there was certainty that the sympathetic chain and its postganglionic fibers are the final common pathway of the reflex, and that the premotor cortex is involved, the subcortical pathways "caused more trouble." This was in spite of an extensive review of the neural mechanisms controlling the palmar galvanic skin reflex and palmar sweating by Darrow in 1937, much of which accords with our present-day knowledge of this area as outlined in Section IV.B.

In the face of the pessimism left by McCleary's paper, it might reasonably be imagined that the years between 1950 and the present day would see a gradual decline of interest in the use of the EDR. However, Lykken and Venables in 1971 wrote that "it continues stoutly to provide useful data in spite of being abused by measurement techniques which range from the arbitrary to the positively weird [p. 656]."

The present work on electrodermal activity exemplifies much that has been present since the turn of the century, but there has perhaps been a broadening of the base against which it can be seen. Darrow's view of physiological determination was that a relatively simple model incorporating eccrine sweat glands and their associated epidermal tissues could be used to explain the apparent complexity of electrodermal phenomena. When the sweat ducts are full, he argues, these provide a low resistance pathway to deeper parts of the gland, and when empty, surface recording then reflects electrical changes in the epidermis (Darrow, 1964; Darrow & Gullickson, 1970).

Concern with the extent of epidermal contributions to electrodermal phenomena is seen in the work of Edelberg and of Wilcott. Both, however, view the epidermal mechanism as being more actively involved than is implied by Darrow's model (Edelberg, 1970; Wilcott, 1966). Edelberg in particular emphasizes the role of superficial layers in regulating the hydration of the skin and argues the close relation between electrodermal phenomena and the operation of such regulating mechanisms (Edelberg, 1968). Other workers concerned with the role of hydration include Fowles and Venables (1970); Juniper, Blanton, and Dykman (1967); and Shimizu, Tajimi, Watanabe, and Niimi (1969). Niimi has also presented some treatment of a related topic, namely the relevance of ionic concentrations in the generation of electrodermal potentials (Niimi, Yamazake, & Watanabe, 1968). These workers, however, were concerned only with the external ionic concentrations in the electrolyte material used at the electrode–skin interfaces. Further examination of the role of electrolyte concentrations has examined the suggested significance (Venables, 1963a; Martin & Venables, 1966) of internal ionic concentrations (Christie & Venables, 1971a, b, c, d). These authors have suggested that the basal skin potential level (see Sections II and IV.E.5), recordable from related subjects in whom there is minimal palmar sweat gland activity, may be largely determined by the concentration gradient between the external and epidermal sources of electrolyte. The epidermal source of electrolyte is not known, but may not be so much within the sweat glands as in the intercellular spaces of the horny layer. Work has, however, been directed toward examining the significance of eccrine sweat concentrations for electrodermal measurement. Johnson and Landon (1965) suggested that racial differences might exist, and Fowles and Venables (1968, 1970) postulated a generation of negative potential by sodium reabsorption in the sweat gland duct.

Consideration of mechanisms relevant to electrodermal phenomena is, for convenience, divided into peripheral, central, and hormonal aspects. Hormonal influences may, however, operate at both central and peripheral sites.

B.   *Peripheral Mechanisms*

1.   INTRODUCTION

Peripheral mechanisms have been investigated since the earliest days of electrodermal history. Neumann and Blanton (1970) have described the elegant experiments of Herman and Luchsinger (1878) on sweat gland contributions, and there is now developing interest in nonsudorific factors. Figure 2 shows schematically the structures probably implicated in the generation of electrodermal activity, involving eccrine sweat glands, associated epidermal tissue, and extracellular fluids.

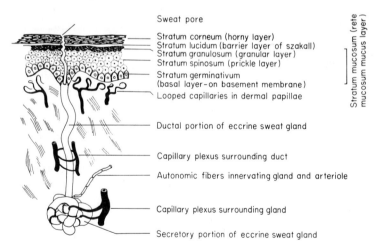

Fig. 2. Semischematic presentation of a section of the palmar skin showing an eccrine sweat gland and epidermal structures concerned in electrodermal activity.

It might, perhaps, be argued that in order to use electrodermal measures as a tool in psychological research there is no need for concern with the mechanisms underlying such phenomena. It is suggested, how-

ever, that knowledge of underlying physiology is essential for the awareness of potential error, and for development of the usefulness of electrodermal measures.

It is proposed, therefore, to present a brief account of selected aspects
of skin structure and function; the account is in no way comprehensive,
but focuses on those aspects which have particular relevance for electrodermal phenomena. Such "relevance" ranges from established and long-
standing findings to speculative observations made in the growing points
of electrodermal research.

2. THE SKIN: STRUCTURE AND FUNCTION

The material presented here has been selected from a range of sources:
brief but useful accounts of the skin can be found in two of the newer
introductions to physiology, namely, Green (1972) and Passmore and
Robson (1968). The American Physiological Association's Handbook of
Physiology (Vol. 4, *Adaptation to the Environment*) includes a chapter
on the skin viewed as an organ of adaptation (Yoshimura, 1964). A
concise and valuable description of the structure of skin is available
in Carleton and Short's (1954) volume of *Shafer's Essentials of Histology*, and there is a classic account of the physiology and biochemistry
of skin in Rothman (1954). Rothman also edited *The Human Integument*
(1959), in which Greisemer's account of the movement of matter through
the epidermis is relevant to electrodermatologists; this topic is also considered by Tregear (1966) in the general context of the physical function
of the skin. Montagna has been associated with a number of volumes
as author or editor (1962; Montagna & Lobitz 1964), including a series
of Advances in Biology of the Skin, which has treatment of circulatory
aspects (Montagna & Ellis, 1961), innervation (1960), and eccrine sweating (Montagna, Ellis, & Silver, 1962). A classic account of sweat glands
is that of Kuno (1956); Weiner and Hellman published their review of
this topic in 1960; sweat glands are included in Schwartz's treatment of
extrarenal handling of minerals (1960); and Thaysen considers such
exocrine handling of the alkali metals (1960).

In an attempt to systematize the present account of selected aspects
of the skin, a general account of its function is included, and is followed
by specific attention to the epidermis, and to the eccrine sweat gland
at palmar or plantar sites.

In all animals the skin is an envelope and a sense organ. In lower
forms of life its functions include respiration, alimentation, and excretion;
with ascent through the phylogenetic scale, however, these functions
become less important as skin permeability decreases. In higher animals
the skin has become a selective barrier that generally prevents entry

of foreign matter, and selectively facilitates passage of materials from the bloodstream to the exterior. Such passage may be via the sweat glands for water and solutes, and via the epidermis for water vapor. This latter passage is termed transepidermal water loss (TEWL); it is probably a passive process, may be reduced in states of dehydration, and the direction of movement can be reversed if the ambient vapor pressure is high, that is, there can be uptake of water by the epidermis.

The water content of the epidermis probably contributes to the maintenance of skin pliability and resilience; one of its sources is blood plasma in the capillary networks at the dermal surface. Cannon (1939) is credited with the theory of "storage by innundation"; when blood volume is inadequate, water passes back through the permeable walls of the dermal capillaries, and the skin thus acts as a mobile reservoir. The amount of water stored in the skin is to some extent determined by the integument's fat content.

The relation between skin hydration and maintenance of flexibility has been noted: this quality is, however, less necessary in the skin of palm and sole, the horny layer of which is specially adapted for weight-bearing and friction, has a thickness of 600 μ as compared with 15 μ in other areas, and is also more permeable. The skin is thus seen to be an envelope and a protection: the human skin has a unique quality in that its horny layer has developed to replace the protective layer of hair or fur present in nonhuman organisms. It is an adaptive organ aiding the maintenance of water balance, and is, in homeotherms, a means of maintaining constant body temperature. In man such maintenance is accomplished largely by adjustment of external heat loss, heat production being possible only by shivering. Control of heat loss involves two interrelated mechanisms, namely the adjustment of skin temperature by changes in the amount of blood flowing through it, and variation in the extent of heat loss resulting from evaporation with variation in the production of eccrine sweat. This thermoregulatory function of eccrine sweat glands is normally seen at palmar and plantar sites only when ambient temperatures exceed some 30°C. These sweat glands show a greater response when the adequate stimulus originates from brain centers other than thermoregulatory ones, that is, from psychic stimulation, producing arousal sweating (Wilcott, 1967). (See Section IV.D for details of the central factors in palmar sweating.)

Returning to the role of the blood supply in regulating skin temperatures, such regulation operates within the zone of vasomotor control, as, for example, in the case of a subject being at rest and lightly clothed in an ambient temperature of 25–31°C. In such conditions, if there is need for heat loss from the body, cutaneous vasodilation increases the flow of blood at the surface, and subsequent heat loss by the processes of radiation, conduction, and convection. For heat conservation, reflex mechanisms induce vasoconstriction and a fall in skin temperature, there being an increase in the thickness of the "shell" interposed between the heat source of internal body core and potential heat loss at the body surface.

When the need for heat loss exceeds the capacity of the vasodilatory mechanism, when cutaneous blood flow and skin temperature have attained their maxima (for example, at 31–32°C), then eccrine sweating and evaporative heat loss are increased. Temperature control is then within the zone of evaporative regulation.

The thermoregulatory activity of eccrine sweat glands is controlled by centers in the anterior hypothalamus; skin temperature influences these, but the critical elevation of skin temperature at which sweating increases varies with the physiological condition of the subject, and with the ambient climate. There are also seasonal differences in the reaction of eccrine sweat glands to a thermal stimulus; in summer the latency of the reflex is shorter and the rate of sweating increased. Kuno (1956) attributed such seasonal changes to changes in the excitability of the sweating center (acclimatization), but there may also be local changes in the sudorific response (training). Another seasonal change is seen in the differential lowering of temperature at various skin sites when there are decreases in environmental temperature, trunk site temperatures remaining relatively constant, in contrast to temperature changes on the limbs.

Finally, brief mention should be made of the skin's role as a sense organ, being richly supplied with nerves and end organs. These are not shown in Fig. 2 which presents those structures which have been more directly implicated in the production of electrodermal phenomena, and which are described in the next section.

3. THE EPIDERMIS

The epidermis, as seen in Fig. 2, is a stratified epithelium, the three deeper layers of which (strata granulosum, spinosum, germinativum) are soft, protoplasmic, and form the stratum malpighii. The last-named is also known as the rete mucosum, or the mucus layer. The most superficial layer (stratum corneum, horny layer) is hard, and thickest on palmar and plantar surfaces as described in Section IV.B.2; on such surfaces it is also easiest to detect, immediately below the stratum corneum, the presence of the stratum lucidum, a layer that has been associated with the barrier function of the epidermis (Szakall, 1958). Below the stratum lucidum the epidermal cells are nucleated and alive;

above the stratum granulosum, however, "cells" are dead, and the superficial squames are continually being removed by abrasion. The epidermis is constantly being renewed by the process of mitosis and keratinization. Cell division takes place in the stratum germinativum, above which layer the cells are nonmitotic as they are pushed, by lower layers, outward to the stratum corneum and eventual loss from the skin surface. Such outward progress of epidermal cells (keratinization) is marked by changes in their structure and composition: cells of the stratum granulosum are filled with a material, eleiden, which becomes transformed into the keratin of more superficial strata. Keratin may thus be regarded as a metabolic end product of epidermal cells, and is a mixture of fibrous proteins.

Bullough and Lawrence (see, for example, Bullough, 1970) have investigated a homeostatic mechanism which ensures that cell production (mitosis) balances cell loss (keratinization): a chalone (kalōn = an internal secretion produced by a tissue to control, by inhibition, the rate of cell production in that same tissue) both preventing the entry of cells into their mitotic cycle in the basal layer, and the completion of keratinization with cell death at the bottom of the stratum corneum. The action of the epidermal chalone appears to be strengthened by adrenaline, the action of which is itself strengthened and prolonged by glucocorticoid. The rate of cell division is high in sleep and slow with muscular exercise; in stress the normal diurnal variation in mitosis may disappear, and cell division almost cease.

Mention was made earlier of the association of the barrier function of epidermis and the stratum lucidum; recent work is, however, tending to suggest that the barrier function may be associated with the whole of the stratum corneum. Thus, on the one hand, Malkinson and Rothman (1963) wrote that "the upper layers cannot be considered a barrier since they are composed of a coarse and porous framework of keratin fibres which are readily penetrated . . . [p. 97]," while Kligman describes work on the stratum corneum which has led him to *his* view of this epidermal layer. Kligman argues that the entire stratum corneum has barrier function, and that there is probably an inverted-U gradient of impermeability which is associated with a similar gradient of cell cohesiveness. Such cohesiveness, he suggests, is due to the presence of mucopolysaccharides as an "intercellular glue," and to the physical forces of cell shape and structure. Kligman argues that previous misconceptions about the stratum corneum may be attributed to customary histological techniques presenting a transverse section of the epidermis as "a loose desquamating layer of scales permeated by large spaces and cracks, a mortuary of dead cells falling apart from each other [Kligman, 1964, p. 388]." In contrast to this picture, Kligman and co-workers have found the stratum corneum to be a "tough, resilient membrane, a cellular fabric of hardy constitution, resembling to a surprising degree a fine sheet of semi-transparent plastic [p. 388]" allowing a rate of water diffusion not unlike that of intact skin, and being highly hygroscopic. Complementary statements from other dermatological workers suggest that, on the one hand, older dermatological findings may require reinterpretation in the light of recent work employing electron microscopy (Mercer, 1962), and on the other, that it is possible to extract from the mixture of proteins comprising epidermal keratin, one which will dry to a smooth, transparent, flexible membrane. This membrane, extracted by Crounse (1965), will limit water passage to a rate comparable with that of intact epidermis *in vitro*.

In the context of suggestions that the stratum corneum is more than a "mortuary of dead cells," it becomes appropriate to mention its intercellular fluid. Christie and Venables (1971d) have argued the possible significance, for basal SPL generation, of electrolyte concentrations in epidermal intercellular fluid. These concentrations are not known with any certainty (Greisemer, 1959), but the fluid is described by Kuno (1956) as originating from plasma sources in the superficial capillaries of the corium, and as the fluid moves upward to the intercellular spaces its electrolyte concentration is probably altered by, for example, adsorption onto mucopolysaccharides (Manery, 1961), addition of K^+ from keratinization products, or addition of either Na^+ or K^+ from sweat residues (Rothman, 1954). An attempt has been made to estimate the Na^+ and K^+ concentrations of horny layer intercellular fluid by analyzing palmar surface film collected when palmar sweat glands are quiescent (Bell, Christie, & Venables, 1973). Normative data from studies undertaken during summer and winter conditions are summarized in Christie and Venables (1971d), and the mean value for palmar surface K^+ (18.2 mEq/liter) agrees reasonably with the estimate of 16–17 mEq/liter as the concentration, or strictly the "activity," of the intercellular K^+ derived from use of the Nernst model and BSPL values (see Section IV.E).

In summary, then, it may be said that the epidermis has as a major function the protection of the organism; that, in the human, the development of a thicker stratum corneum compensates for the absence of a protective hairy covering, and that constant renewal of the outer protection is achieved by a precise homeostatic mechanism controlled by an epidermal chalone. Finally, another aspect of protection relates to the barrier function of the epidermis. This may be associated with certain properties of the stratum corneum rather than with the restriction of barrier activity to the stratum lucidum.

4. THE ECCRINE SWEAT GLANDS

The schematic presentation of human palmar skin in Fig. 2 includes an eccrine sweat gland, one of the epidermal derivatives which, like aprocrine glands, develops during fetal life. The classification of apocrine and eccrine was introduced by Schiefferdecker (1917, 1922) to describe different modes of secretion. Thus apocrine (secreted from) reflects the belief that part of the secretion process involves breakdown of secretory cells and the liberation of their contents into the lumen of the gland by a necrobiotic process. In contrast, eccrine (secreted out of) implies that fluid passes across an intact membrane from secretory cell into lumen. There is, however, some dispute about whether an apocrine process *is* involved in the functioning of apocrine glands (Weiner & Hellman, 1960), and recent literature tends to adopt the criterion of whether ducts open directly onto the skin surface (as in Fig. 2), or are associated with hair follicles (as for apocrine glands). Thus, Bligh (1967) uses the terminology atrichial (without hair) and epitrichial (by the hair), while Weiner and Hellman (1960) counsel retention of the terms eccrine and apocrine to describe these two types of simple exocrine gland.

The apocrine glands are of little apparent relevance for the electrodermatologist. They are not under nervous control, but secretion is stimulated by circulating adrenaline. Small amounts of fluid are secreted, in stress or with sexual stimulation, and the glands are associated with hair follicles in a number of specific sites such as the axillae and mons pubis. In contrast, eccrine sweat glands are distributed all over the body surface. Regional differences in distribution are given by Weiner and Hellman (1960) as palm and foot, not less than $2000/cm^2$; axillae, $200-300/cm^2$; trunk and extremities, $100-200/cm^2$. There are also reported racial differences in distribution, the Japanese having more eccrine sweat glands on extremities than do Europeans, and reported age and sex differences in distribution and activity (see Section V).

The palmer eccrine sweat glands develop in the fetus at $3\frac{1}{2}$ months, whereas those on other body sites do not become evident until the fifth month. The thermoregulatory role of eccrine sweat glands was described in Section IV.B.2, but it has been suggested (Darrow, 1933) that their role at palmar and plantar sites is associated primarily with grasping behavior rather than evaporative cooling. Eccrine glands in all locations do, however, have the capacity to respond to both psychic and thermal stimulation, but there are, as suggested in Section IV.B.2, regional differences in the thresholds of response to these forms of stimulation. Thus glands of palm and sole respond to psychic stimuli, but more intense and sustained thermal stimulation is needed to elicit a

response in these areas. Eccrine glands of the axillae and forehead oc-
cupy an intermediate position in that they will respond to moderate
levels of both psychic and thermal stimulation, while those of remaining
areas are primarily thermoregulatory. Psychic stimuli can, however, more
readily evoke generalized sweating in a warm environment, when they
are said to act synergistically with thermal stimuli (Kuno, 1956).

It can be seen in Fig. 2 that the coiled secretory portion of the eccrine
sweat gland is sited in the subdermis. It is therefore supplied by the
capillary network of that area with essential raw materials such as water,
electrolytes, and oxygen. During secretory activity the blood supply can
apparently be increased by local vasodilation; this results from the formation of bradykinin which is produced by the reaction of a proteo-
lytic enzyme released when gland activity begins, and tissue fluid
protein. Bradykinin has been said to increase sweat gland efficiency by
its vasodilatory property, thus resulting in an increased supply of raw
materials to the gland.

Innervation of eccrine sweat glands is solely via the sympathetic
branch of the autonomic nervous system, but the postganglionic synapse
is cholinergic, having acetylcholine, not noradrenaline, as the transmitter.
Sweat gland activity may be initiated nonneurogenically by intradermal
injections of acetylcholine (Chalmers & Keele, 1952) and cholinomimetics (Foster, 1971), but responses of eccrine sweat glands to such
stimulation, and indeed to thermal stimulation, disappear promptly after
glandular denervation. This is in contrast to Cannon's rule of denervation
sensitivity, and Rothman (1954) suggests that innervation serves to
maintain a glandular tonus, changes in which are seen after conditioning
or training of sweat glands.

In addition to the production of sweating by local treatment with
cholinomimetics, mention should be made of inhibition by local treatment with anticholinergic agents. Sweat glands have been inactivated
by topical applications of poldine methosulfate (Grice & Bettley, 1966)
and by iontophoresis of atropine and hyoscyamine (Lader, 1970; Lader
& Montagu, 1962; Venables & Martin, 1967b). Inhibition of eccrine
sweat gland activity has also been reported by Goodall (1970) with
a wide range of cholinergic blocking agents. Goodall also notes that
the sympathetic neurohormones, noradrenaline and adrenaline, can produce limited eccrine sweating but suggests that this adrenergic action
is on the ductal myoepithelium which by contraction expels the contents
of the sweat glands.

Having described on a more molar level what can be regarded as
prerequisites for eccrine sweat gland activity, it becomes more difficult
when one attempts to be precise about the secretory process itself taking

place in the coiled region of the gland to produce the primary secretion which enters the ductal portion. Thaysen (1960) reports Lundberg's electrophysiological studies (1955) of outward transport of electrolytes in acini of salivary glands in the cat. Thaysen's justification for extrapolation from salivary to sweat glands would be his argument that submaxillary and parotid glands, together with eccrine sweat glands, form his Type 1 group which is characterized by similarity of histological structure, and, more importantly in the present context, by similar handling of the Na^+ and K^+ ions in the primary secretion as it passes through the ductal portion of the gland (Thaysen, 1960). This handling involves the facultative reabsorption of Na^+, and the linked loss of K^+, by a limited maximal capacity process. Thus a characteristic feature of Type 1 handling of Na^+ is an increase in concentration with increases in flow rate. There appears to be a dearth of information on the Na^+ and K^+ concentration of the final fluid appearing at the sweat gland orifice of palmar eccrine glands (Weiner & Hellman, 1960). Figures of 5–100 mEq/liter for Na^+ and 1–15 mEq/liter for K^+ are of the order suggested.

Lundeberg's work showed that there was a polarized membrane implicated in the activity of the salivary gland, and evidence for active transport of electrolytes from plasma to the glandular lumen. In 1960 Thaysen concluded that "much work remains to be done before the outward transport of electrolytes and water in the glandular acini is clarified in detail [p. 428]." More recently Sato and Dobson have published a number of papers reporting their investigation of eccrine sweat gland activities, both secretive and reabsorptive (1970a, b, c). One of these studies (1970a) examined the secretory mechanism of monkey palmar eccrine sweat glands. Earlier work (Skou, 1965) has linked the enzyme $Na + K - ATPase$ with the active transport of cations across membranes. This enzyme is inhibited by ouabain, and intradermal ouabain inhibited both ductal reabsorption and secretion in sweat glands (Sato, Taylor, & Dobson, 1969). Sato and Dobson (1970a) reported that estimates of $Na + K - ATPase$ activity are similar in both secretory and reabsorptive areas of sweat glands. The authors, while emphasizing that secretory mechanisms are still controversial, interpret their results in terms of secretion of a primary product involving the active transport of Na^+ into the lumen, followed by a passive transport of water and chloride (Cl^-). After this, Na^+ is then actively reabsorbed into the ductal portion. Detailed accounts of ductal reabsorption and its possible relevance for electrodermatologists have recently been provided by Fowles and Venables (1970), Fowles (1973), and Grings (1973); it is examined in more detail in Section IV.E.

Progress of sweat up the ducts may be assisted by rhythmic contraction of myoepithelial fibers around the tubule, and a rhythmic rise and fall of the column of sweat can be observed within the duct of a resting gland. Sulzberger, Herrman, Keller and Pisha (1950) have suggested that the gland outlet is electrically negative in relation to its deeper portions, and argued that a potential gradient may be one of the factors promoting movement of water and electrolytes along the duct.

Thus in the eccrine sweat gland, the final product resulting from the primary secretion may reach the skin surface, and there add to hydration of the stratum corneum by overflowing onto this hygroscopic tissue. Or the product may never reach the surface, but be reabsorbed in the sweat duct. A complex set of factors, in addition to the intensity of stimulation, interacts to determine the extent of overflow or reabsorption. Some description of such factors will be introduced at relevant points in subsequent sections as, for example, Section IV.E.

C. Hormonal Mechanisms

It has previously been stated that evidence for the significance of physiological mechanisms in the context of electrodermal activity can range from established data collected during electrodermal investigations to extrapolations from findings in what are essentially physiological studies. Such findings are, however, of potential and possible relevance for electrodermatologists, suggesting areas in urgent need of research activity.

In consideration of hormonal influences we are, in the main, extrapolating from physiological sources, and suggesting *possible* relevance for electrodermal phenomena; such relevance is seen largely, in relation to sweat gland activity.

Our earlier consideration of eccrine sweat gland function was centered on response of the organ to stimulation received via the sympathetic branch of the autonomic nervous system. In this case stimulus and response were temporally close, and, further, it was possible to discuss functioning of the sweat gland in relative isolation from functioning of other organs. True, the remainder of the organism had to be taken into consideration in, for example, discussion of heat conservation; but, we would argue, consideration of cause and effect is infinitely more interrelated when one considers hormonal effects on sweat gland functioning. Such interrelations become evident if we now extend our preliminary treatment of heat conservation, and look at some aspects of the endocrine response to increases in environmental temperature. In 1968 Collins and Weiner provided a comprehensive review of current evidence concerning the pattern of endocrine adjustments to heat: if the sweat gland responses to heat, which were described in Section I.V.B.2, can be regarded as the immediate or primary response to heat, and mediated primarily by nervous influences, then the endocrine adjustments can be regarded as slower, secondary adaptation. Such adaptation implicates the extracellular fluid (ECF) compartment, its volume, and its electrolyte concentration, marked changes in which could occur after prolonged sweating if compensatory mechanisms were not brought into play. The *behavioral* significance of ECF electrolyte concentrations has been suggested by Venables (1970), who speculates on relations between K+, thresholds of neuron firing, and "noise" in the central nervous system. Thus in the face of the organism's urgent need to maintain the constancy of its electrolytes in the internal environment, there is a complex pattern of adjustment centered on the pituitary–adrenal axis, with regulatory roles for both pituitary and adrenal hormones in the maintenance of salt and water balance. Collins and Weiner (1968) present a wide range of evidence relating to hormonal effects on eccrine sweat gland function in both thermogenic and nonthermogenic sweating. We have selected from their review such material as appears particularly relevant for electrodermatologists; inevitably some of the data refer to eccrine sweat glands at other than palmar sites, but we are not aware of evidence of significant differences between palmar and nonpalmar sites in relation to the response to hormonal influences.

1. CATECHOLAMINES

We examine first the possible influence of adrenaline and noradrenaline. There appears to be no doubt that in man (Collins, Sargent, & Weiner, 1959; Weiner & Hellman, 1960) and cat (Foster, 1967) sweating by eccrine sweat glands is mediated through a cholinergic, sympathetic innervation as indicated in Section IV.B.4, yet, intradermal injections of both adrenaline and noradrenaline (Chalmers & Keele, 1952; Foster, Ginsburg, & Weiner, 1967) can evoke local sweating in man and in cat (Edison & Lloyd, 1970). This local effect is not blocked by atropine but *is* inhibited by catecholamine antagonists such as phentolamine (Foster *et al.*, 1967); this raises the question of possible adrenergic innervation of eccrine sweat glands. However, Chalmers and Keele (1952) had found that although the sweating provoked by intradermal adrenaline was not inhibited by atropine, thermal sweating was completely suppressed. They also found that antiadrenaline substances inhibited the adrenaline-induced but not the neurogenic sweating. This was confirmed by Foster *et al.* (1967), and Collins and Weiner (1968) conclude that there is evidence of the ability of circulating adrenaline to influence sweat gland activity in man. More recent work on the relation between adrenaline and eccrine sweat gland activity includes that of Warndoff and Neefs (1971) and Edison and Lloyd (1970). It appears possible that one effect of sympathomimetic agents on sweat glands may be, as previously suggested (Section IV.B.4), the result of stimulating the myoepithelia associated with the gland, thus causing a ductal contraction and expulsion of the contents (Goodall, 1970).

There has been continued interest in the possibility that eccrine sweating can be reduced by increases in circulating catecholamine concentrations (Darrow, 1937; Elliott, 1905; Foster, Ginsburg, & Weiner, 1970). Two workers concerned with investigation of effects on palmar eccrine sweat glands of the stress response in general, and catecholamine levels in particular (Harrison, 1964; Harrison & MacKinnon, 1966; MacKinnon, 1964; MacKinnon, 1969) have demonstrated an anhidrotic response to catecholamines, and argue the case for a central rather than a peripheral determinant of the phenomenon.

2. ANTIDIURETIC HORMONE (ADH)

We have argued the need to view hormonal effects on eccrine sweat glands within the wider context of a homeostatic organism maintaining the constancy of its internal environment; it becomes relevant at this point to consider the need for water conservation in relation to sweating. When water conservation is necessary, urine flow may be reduced, and antidiuretic hormone (ADH) is an essential factor, water reabsorption in the distal tubule and collecting ducts being a consequence of increased water permeability under the influence of ADH. There is some evidence of water reabsorption in the eccrine sweat duct (Weiner & Hellman, 1960; Fowles & Venables, 1970) though Collins and Weiner (1968) caution that evidence for the influence of ADH on eccrine ductal reabsorption is contradictory. Recently Quatrale and Speir (1970) described studies of antidiuretic activity in the eccrine sweat glands of the rat's foot pad. They examined the effects of ADH and of octapressin, and interpreted their data as evidence for a reduction in the magnitude and duration of the sweat response being due to antidiuretic rather than vasopressive activity. Quatrale and Speir (1970) suggest that their results for the rat agree in general with those of Fascio, Totel, and Johnson (1969) for the human.

It is of interest, in the context of psychophysiology, to note that, although ADH secretion is mainly responsive to the tonicity of plasma, discharge of ADH can be produced by emotional states such as fear of an impending procedure, e.g., venipuncture (Keele & Neil, 1971), or with sexual stimulation (Irvine, Cullen, Stewart, Ewart, & Baird, 1968).

Linking the effect of ADH on permeabilities of ductal tissue with the work of Edelberg on skin hydration, it becomes interesting to speculate on the extent to which ADH, discharged in heightened emotion, could contribute to the findings which he has reported (1966, 1970; see Section IV.E for discussion of the recovery limb of the SCR).

3. ADRENAL CORTICAL INFLUENCES

Perhaps the adrenal cortical influence that is of major contemporary interest in relation to eccrine sweating and electrodermatological phenomena is that of the mineralocorticoids. Thus, if Edelberg can be linked with the phenomenon of water reabsorption, the work of Fowles and Venables (1968, 1970) becomes relevant to consideration of sodium reabsorption, and its relation to measured palmar skin potential level. These workers argue that active transport of sodium in the eccrine sweat ducts can contribute to the negativity of recorded SPL.

Previous reference has been made to Thaysen's (1960) description of the Type 1 salivary and sweat gland, and the active process of Na^+ conservation which takes place in their ducts. Bush (1962) pointed out that there is a resemblance between renal tubules and such ducts, making it likely that there is a common intrinsic action of mineralocorticoids such as aldosterone on all these tissues. Much of the fundamental research has been carried out on the parotid gland of sheep (Denton, 1957, 1965), and relates a gradual loss of Na^+ via parotid fistula to the gradual increase in circulating aldosterone. As this most potent mineralocorticoid stimulates both reabsorption of sodium ions and complementary excretion of potassium, its effects can be seen as a fall in the Na/K ratios of transcellular fluids such as urine, sweat, and saliva. In Denton's 1965 study, as the loss of saliva from a parotid fistula depleted Na^+ stores and resulted in decreasing concentrations of blood Na^+, there was a progressive rise in circulating aldosterone levels. Renal conservation of Na^+, reflected in decreased urinary Na/K ratios, was commensurate with the increase in circulating aldosterone. Salivary Na/K ratios, however, began to decrease only when aldosterone secretion had increased two or threefold, and to the value of a previously determined threshold level of response for parotid salivary Na/K. Although when one turns to the more directly relevant question of relations in man between Na^+ deficiency resulting from sweating, levels of circulating aldosterone, and evidence of Na^+ conservation in eccrine ductal tissue, data similar to Denton's are not available, there is some indication of asynchrony between kidney and sweat gland response. Thus Collins (1966) showed a longer latency and relatively lower sensitivity of sweat glands compared with kidney tubules, suggesting that, like sheep parotid tissue, human sweat glands begin to conserve Na^+ only when aldosterone secretion has risen to a threshold value. Further, investigation of the effect of subcutaneous d-aldosterone on urine and sweat Na/K ratios showed that whereas the former fluid had lowered values within 2 hr, the latter exhibited such lowering only after some 6 hr. This longer latency, Collins and Weiner (1968) suggest, may be explained in terms of differences in the oxygen supply available at sweat gland and kidney sites. Thus, if active transport of Na^+ is dependent on aerobic metabolic pathways, and if the high concentration of lactate in sweat indicates an anaerobic component pathway in the gland's glycogen metabolism (Collins, Crockford, & Weiner, 1965), this suggests that oxygen supply to the sweat gland may be relatively low, and therefore conditions for the action of aldosterone would be relatively unfavorable.

Additional evidence for a direct effect of salt-active steroids in human sweat glands comes from investigations of the competitive aldosterone inhibitor spironolactone, and the increase in Na^+ concentrations of both thermal (Furman & Beer, 1963; Ladell & Shepherd, 1962; May, 1965) and nonthermal (Collins, 1966) sweat which result from its administration.

Thus, Collins concludes, there are good grounds for the belief that Na-retaining adrenal steroids, including aldosterone, actively control the concentrations of cations in sweat. The implications of this for electrodermatologists lie in suggestions that Na^+ reabsorption could increase the negativity of recorded SPL (Fowles and Venables, 1968, 1970), and that epidermal K^+ concentrations may be implicated in the generation of the low basal SPL recordable from relaxed human subjects (Christie & Venables, 1971d). Further, the latency of sweat gland response to aldosterone suggests that the effects on electrodermal phenomena of stimuli likely to induce increases in circulating aldosterone may not be seen for some hours; such stimuli include increases in the ambient temperature, the effects of which on basal SPL have been reported by Christie and Venables (1971c) and stress, as reported, for example, by Oken (1967). Further, the Na^+ retaining activity in eccrine sweat glands, as evidenced by reductions in the sweat Na/K ratio, may persist for some time after increases in aldosterone levels. Collins (1966) reported that it can be some 60 hr after aldosterone injection before sweat Na/K ratios return to normal. The implication of this for psychophysiologists can be stated in terms of the general difficulty in relating cause and effect when one is concerned with the slower-acting and more diffuse functioning of the endocrine rather than the nervous system. This then emphasizes the possibility that, for example, a stressor experienced by one's subject during the 24 hr preceding his appearance in the psychophysiological laboratory had influences on his endocrine balance, the aftereffects of which remain to modify his electrodermal activity in the recording situation.

Before leaving the topic of mineralocorticoid function, we should mention that, although aldosterone is the most potent material, other Na-retaining adrenal steroids may affect the eccrine sweat gland. O'Connor (1962) states that cortisol and cortisone could account for a sizable amount of Na-retaining activity. Thus an administration of ACTH, while having negligible effects on plasma aldosterone levels, could effect a threefold increase in plasma cortisol concentrations, and thus, because of its mineralocorticoid activity, increase the Na retaining activity of circulating adrenocortical hormones.

Further evidence of adrenocortical influences on sweat electrolyte concentrations comes from clinical sources: sweat Na^+ concentrations are abnormally high with the adrenal hypofunction of Addison's disease, low with the hyperfunction of Cushing's syndrome, and in primary or secondary aldosteronism (Conn, 1949; Koch, Elster, Heindorf, Crusius, Crössman, Angersbach, & Rick, 1963).

Finally, in relation to the interpretation of electrodermal data obtained from the cat, and from which extrapolations may be made to human phenomena, it should be noted that the cat sweat gland is unresponsive to aldosterone, has a ductal length which is, in contrast to man, short in relative total glandular length, produces sweat which is isosmotic or hypertonic in relation to plasma, and thus provides a range of evidence suggesting that there is no Na^+-retaining activity in the eccrine sweat duct of the cat's foot pad.

4. PROGESTERONE

The emphasis in Sections IV.C.2 and 3 has been on those hormonal factors which can modulate eccrine sweat gland activity to conserve water and electrolytes when, for example, increased sweat production during heat adaptation threatens the constancy of the internal environment. Considerably less is known, however, about the effects of sex hormones on eccrine sweat gland function, though suggestions have been made that this is an area requiring research (Christie & Venables, 1971d), especially in relation to significant sex differences in basal skin potential levels.

One hormone of particular significance is progesterone, and the findings of MacKinnon and co-workers strongly indicate its ability to decrease palmar eccrine sweat output. Thus there is a reduction in the palmar sweat count during the luteal phase of the menstrual cycle

(MacKinnon, 1954a) and after administration of progesterone (MacKinnon & Harrison, 1961). Administration of adrenocorticotropic hormone also results in an eventual decrease in palmar sweating (MacKinnon & Harrison, 1961), after some 5 hr. Progesterone itself depresses sweating after a 3-hr interval, and MacKinnon (1964) has argued that the longer latency required for ACTH to produce an effect reflects its role in stimulating the adrenal cortex which, in turn, then produces progesterone. It may be that the effect of progesterone is mediated through central nervous rather than peripheral mechanisms; there is, however, evidence for aldosterone-blocking activity of progesterone (Sharp & Leaf, 1966) which suggests that this potential local effect on eccrine sweating should not be totally ignored by electrodermatologists. Perhaps it may ultimately be possible to show that the central, anesthetic effects of progesterone are particularly relevant to electrodermal response characteristics, whereas local aldosterone-blocking functions affect measured skin potential levels.

D. Central Mechanisms

1. INTRODUCTION

Consideration of which central mechanisms are relevant to electrodermal activity depends on demonstration of the mechanisms thought to be responsible at the periphery. The most straightforward approach is to consider that the main interest is in the innervated control of peripheral sudorific mechanisms via sympathetic fibers, although, as shown in Section V.B.4, their final control is cholinergic. By adopting this criterion, the central mechanisms which are then relevant for consideration are those where workers have considered the neural control of sweating, or the neural control of electrodermal activity (although workers in this field have often taken the electrodermal activity as a convenient index of sudorific activity and not as activity of interest in its own right).

While the major part of the relevant material is thus concerned with the neural control of sweat production, it should not be forgotten that innervation of other peripheral mechanisms might be considered. While it was outlined in Section II that muscular and vascular factors had been shown not to be of prime importance in the production of electrodermal activity, their secondary role should not be entirely dismissed in view, for instance, of the role of ductal myoepithelium in the ejection of sweat gland contents (Bligh, 1967). (See Sections IV.B.4 and

IV.E.4.c.) Nor should the possibility suggested by Edelberg and Wright (1964) that there is innervation of the epidermis be ruled out. Nevertheless, in the absence of any definitive knowledge of the role of these secondary peripheral factors, it is difficult at this time to consider their central control.

An early review of the material in this area is that of Darrow (1937a). The other major reviews are those of Wang (1957, 1958, 1964). Later material is to be found in individual papers, and reflects general development in the understanding of brain mechanisms and in the techniques for their investigation. Thus, Darrow's review was written before the work of Moruzzi and Magoun (1949) which set in train a spate of investigation on the activity of the brain stem reticular system and its accompanying construct arousal. In a similar way, although Papez' famous monograph, which was published in 1937, could be seen as the start of work on the limbic system, the importance of the system did not become apparent until later, and the elicitation of electrodermal activity by stimulation of some limbic structures did not have the significance it has at present. There are a limited number of studies directly concerned with the effect of particular central mechanisms upon electrodermal activity. However, the amount of material concerned with higher nervous system activity which is of indirect importance is vast and is outside the range of this chapter. It is essential, therefore, that this restricted coverage of directly relevant material should be viewed with a background of this wider literature in mind. Most work on central mechanisms has been carried out on animals; however, Sourek (1965) presents an extensive review of data which gives insight into the control of electrodermal activity in man.

A most important point of technique to be considered in reviewing work on central determinants of electrodermal activity is the state of anesthesia of the animal on which the studies are carried out. For instance, most of the work reported by Wang was carried out on cats under heavy chloralose anesthesia. Under these conditions, with the activity of the cortex suppressed, a different pattern of hierarchical levels of control is achieved from that, for instance, reported by Bloch and Bonvallet (1959) who, with nonanesthetized animals, showed that cortical tonus has an effect on reticular control of electrodermal activity that was absent in Wang's experiments.

In Section IV.B.4 description of the innervation of the eccrine sweat glands solely by fibers from the sympathetic branch of the autonomic nervous system has been given. A once-common interpretation of this action of the sympathetic system as gross and nondifferentiated, leading to a too-close identification of electrical activity of the skin with other functions mediated by the sympathetic system is, however, erroneous. This sort of interpretation has been strenuously opposed by Miller (1969), and the independent nature of electrical activity of the skin is exemplified, by, for instance, comparing changes in it and heart rate in orienting and defensive reflexes, and in the low correlations usually reported between electrodermal indices and indices of other autonomic functions. Evidence suggests that although the final nervous pathway to the eccrine sweat glands is anatomically sympathetic, excitation of these glands is perhaps more usefully considered in some instances as functionally parasympathetic insofar, for instance, as peripheral activity may be excited by stimulation of the anterior rather than the posterior hypothalamus.

2. SPINAL LEVEL

Pools of sympathetic neurons controlling the sweat secretion of each limb are to be found, in animals, in the ipsilateral ventrolateral horn of the spinal cord at high thoracic level of the forelimbs, and thoracicolumbar level for the hind limbs (Patton, 1948). These four pools of spinal neurons are probably not structurally connected; they are normally under the control of higher centers and this control results in synchronized discharge at all four limbs. In man, data reviewed by Sourek (1965) suggest that the spinal pathways mediating electrodermal activity are in the anterolateral and dorsolateral quadrants.

In the spinal cat, spontaneous electrodermal activity in each limb is desynchronized; within each spinal pool individual neurons discharge spontaneously (Ladpli, 1962; Ladpli & Wang, 1960). Synchronized responses by all limbs in a cat with high spinal section can be achieved by afferent stimulation of sufficient strength, and the amplitude of the resulting response is higher than the intervening spontaneous discharge, suggesting that the spontaneous activity in each limb results from the discharge, in a nonsynchronized manner, of only a few of the neurons in the pool, while simultaneous activation of the pools by an adequate stimulus brings about a larger discharge.

3. THE VENTROMEDIAL, BULBAR, RETICULAR FORMATION

The evidence for the inhibitory effect of this structure on electrodermal activity is extensive. Wang (1958, p. 35) reports, "intercollicular decerebration—that is, removal of the forebrain, the interbrain, and the rostral half of the midbrain—causes a sharp fall in the intensity of the galvanic skin reflex, and it is abolished a short time after the operation." That is, an operation which allows the descending activity of the ventromedial reticular formation to appear, unmodified by any higher activity, shows that this activity is inhibitory. When the influence of this structure is eliminated by a lower spinal transection, the electrodermal activity then reappears as shown in the previous section. In an intact animal the inhibitory influence of the ventromedial reticular formation is overcome by the excitatory influences of other structures at a higher level. Thus, Wang and Brown (1956a, p. 450) showed that, "in a normal cat acute spinal transection removed excitatory influences and thus causes a decrease in the intensity of the galvanic skin reflex. In a decerebrate cat it removes inhibitory influences and thus releases the abolished galvanic skin reflex from inhibition resulting in its re-appearance." In cats heavily anesthetized with chloralose, Wang and Brown (1956b) were able to show that stimulation of the ventromedial reticular formation had a profound inhibitory effect, and that this structure had a lower threshold and greater inhibitory effect than the cerebellar anterior lobe and the frontal cerebral cortex which they also stimulated. Bloch and Bonvallet (1960a), however, emphasize the importance of the level of anesthesia in these experiments. They show that, "le puissant contrôle inhibiteur bulbaire ne peut être mis en évidence qu'après suppression ou dépression de l'influence prédominante des formations activatrices mésencéphaliques, dont l'activité a son tour ne peut être observée, a l'état pour qu'après suppression des décharges inhibitrices rétroactives corticifuges [1960a, p. 45]." They also go on to point out that the sensitivity to anesthesia is maximal at the cortical level and minimal at the bulbar level. It is possible therefore that Wang and Brown's finding of a smaller inhibitory effect of cortical stimulation was due to the greater effect of anesthesia at this level. Yokota, Sato, and Fujimori (1963a) were, however, able to show an inhibitory response from the bulbar reticular formation in cats immobilized with Flaxedil and not otherwise anesthetized.

4. THE RETICULAR ACTIVATING SYSTEM

Although in 1964 he said that the midbrain does not seem to play an important part in the control of sweating Wang (1957, 1958), reporting an unpublished experiment by himself and Brown, stated that stimulation of the reticular activity system by a weak current elicited no response, but augmented the response to peripheral stimulation. Stronger stimulation evoked a response and had a longer-lasting facilitatory effect. In the absence of more definite details of the experiment, it is necessary to consider this report in relation to the findings of Bloch and Bonvallet. In 1959, these workers showed that in a decorticate preparation stimulation of the mesencephalic reticular formation produced an immediate response and subsequently an augmentation of spontaneous fluctuations. In intact nonanesthetized animals, however, they showed that the response given to a somaesthetic stimulus was dependent upon the level of cortical activity. If the length of stimulation of the reticular formation was such as to bring about EEG signs of cortical alerting, then the SPR evoked by a cutaneous stimulus was depressed or supressed. They hypothesized that there is, "un contrôle inhibiteur corticifuge, dont l'efficacité est fonction du tonus corticale se surimpose au controle reticulaire [Bloch & Bonvallet, 1959, p. 406]."

In 1960 Bloch and Bonvallet (1960b) published a paper which helps to clarify the position. They make the point that the electrodermal response resulting from a short, weak, peripheral stimulus is mediated by the brief reticular activation which it provokes. They then examined the effect of direct brief stimulation of the reticular system and surrounding areas. (It must be assumed, following their 1959 paper, that they presume that the duration and intensity of their reticular stimulation is not sufficient to alter cortical tonus, as they have previously assumed that the corticofugal inhibitory effect is directly on the midbrain reticular formation.) They show that low-voltage, short-duration stimulation of the brain stem gives the same form of electrodermal response as is given normally by peripheral stimulation. They also show that the part of the brain stem which gives rise to these responses is the same part which gives EEG signs of wakefulness, and facilitates motor activity. Within this region, which extends between the bulbar area and the posterior hypothalamus, the threshold for eliciting electrodermal responses is uniform and low. Outside this region the threshold is much higher, and they were never able to evoke electrodermal responses from thalamic regions or the central gray matter. The only region outside the reticular formation which they explored, which had a low threshold for evoking electrodermal responses, was a limited area of the anterior hypothalamus. With lesions above the brain stem, the possibility of peripheral elicitation of electrodermal activity was maintained; with lesions below the brain stem reticular formation, thresholds for peripheral stimulation of electrodermal activity were greatly raised. However, it was possible to trigger an SPR from the lateral bulbar reticular formation, a fact which accords with the findings of Yokota et al. (1963a). Explanations of the equivocal reports of Wang and his colleagues, in relation to the midbrain reticular formation, is perhaps to be found in the fact that the doses of chloralose (35 mg/kg) which they typically employed in their experiments were shown by Bloch and Bonvallet to lower the activity of the brain-stem reticular system, and to bring about a massive increase in its threshold for stimulation. This level of anesthesia had no effect on the spinal animal. Bloch and Bonvallet (1960b, p. 26) conclude that

> . . . c'est par leur projections ascendantes activant le système réticulaire facilitateur que les afférences sensorielles déclenchent des reponses electrodermales. Il est très vraisemblable que c'est également par l'intermediare de ce systeme, active par des projections cortico-réticulaires, que sont déclenchés chez l'animal vigile les réponses électrodermale évoquées par des stimuli complexes dont l'éfficatité implique l'intervention du cortex cérébral.

5. THE LIMBIC SYSTEM

Data in this area are not very extensive, but that from animal work appears to be reasonably consistent. Sourek (1965) suggests, from limited data on man, that the limbic system (rhinencephalon) is involved in electrodermal activity. Yokota, Sato, and Fujimori (1963b) report an experiment on cats immobilized with Flaxedil and under artificial respiration. Peripheral stimulation to elicit a response was to the sciatic or peroneal nerve, and the role of stimulation of the hippocampus, fornix, amygdala, and preoptic area in producing facilitation or inhibition of response was examined. Stimulation of the hippocampus produced inhibition of SPR while stimulation of the fornix produce more marked inhibition of SPR and depression of SPL. Strong stimulation of the amygdala produced facilitation of SPR. Facilitation of SPR was also obtained with stimulation of the lateral preoptic area. Lang, Tuovinen, and Valleala (1964) investigated the effect of direct stimulation of the amygdala upon electrodermal activity in lightly anesthetized cats. Stimulation of the amygdala, of sufficient intensity to cause an afterdischarge, brought about an increase in SPL which matched in time the duration of the afterdischarge. Stimulation of the amygdala, of an intensity which was insufficient to cause an afterdischarge, resulted in a phasic SPR. Lang et al. (1964) suggest that the discharge of the amygdala does not produce a change in SPL directly, but that the brain stem reticular formation acts as a transmitting structure, a view which would accord with the position of Bloch and Bonvallet outlined in the previous section. In line with the general picture of the facilitatory role of the amygdala in regard to electrodermal activity, Bagshaw, Kimble, and Pribram (1965) showed that amygdalectomy in monkeys produced a marked diminution of SCR to tones (a finding replicated by Bagshaw & Benzies, 1968), while ablation of the hippocampus and inferotemporal cortex had no effect either or SCR on its habituation. In a parallel experiment on monkeys, Kimble, Bagshaw, and Pribram (1965) showed that lateral frontal cortical lesions depressed SCR while medial frontal-anterior cingulate lesions did not. Isamat (1961) explored a wide area of the medial wall of the cortex with stimulating electrodes, and showed that, "the region from which GSRs were more readily obtained includes the anterior limbic and the infralimbic areas of the cortex ahead of and behind the rostrum of the corpus callosum [p. 180]." Examination of Isamat's diagrams shows that he did not obtain responses from the area of the medial cortex where Kimble, Bagshaw, and Pribram showed no effect of lesions; there is thus no conflict between these two sets of results.

6. The Hypothalamus

Work directly concerned with the influence of the hypothalamus upon electrodermal activity does not appear to have been carried out recently in the context of contemporary neurophysiological investigation. The incidental report of Bloch and Bonvallet (1960b) that stimulation of the anterior hypothalamus gives rise to electrodermal activity is, however, in accord with much of the earlier work cited by Darrow (1937a) in support of the view that the anterior hypothalamus can be involved in the mediation of electrodermal activity. While at one time it was thought that the sweat glands of palmar and plantar surface were not involved in thermoregulatory activity, studies (e.g., Conklin, 1951; Maulsby & Edelberg, 1960; Wilcott, 1963) have now shown that there is, within certain temperature ranges, thermoregulatory activity at these areas. This would seem to make it more likely that the electrodermal activity which is seen as a result of stimulation of the anterior hypothalamus, in regions known to be involved in thermoregulation, is that which might be expected from the activation of palmar and plantar sweat glands in their thermoregulatory role. This may be too simple a point of view and does not do justice to the role of the hypothalamus as a mediator and coordinator of activity of other centers; it does, however, suggest a rather secondary role for the hypothalamus in the mediation of nonthermoregulatory electrodermal activity.

7. The Cortex

It is unrealistic to attempt to show any simple involvement of cortical areas in electrodermal activity. It seems best to see the cortex in its role as coordinator of lower activities and to give what must perforce be a cursory treatment of this most important eventual determinant of electrodermal activity.

Wang (1964) makes a powerful case for viewing the central mechanisms controlling electrodermal activity in terms of Fulton's (1926) principles of "long-circuiting"; that is, that unless otherwise prevented there is a tendency for electrodermal reflexes to involve control by the highest centers. If this is correct, then it will be expected that cortical regulation enters into much of the control of electrodermal activity normally recorded. It is perhaps worthwhile to view electrodermal activity in this context as a component of the orienting reflex, and following this to cite Luria and Homskaya (1970, pp. 304, 305) who say, "the efferent apparatus of the orienting reflex is located at the level of the reticular formation of the brain stem and of the non-specific thalamic system, while the afferent link of the orienting reflex is located at the level of the cortex of the large hemispheres," and later, "undoubtedly, the neo-cortex of the cerebral hemispheres and, above all, the cortex of the frontal lobes of the brain take part in the regulation of the orienting reflex." This point, concerning the essential role of the cortex in the regulation of electrodermal activity, is also made by Bloch and Bonvallet (1959), who emphasize the importance of not eliminating the activity of the cortex by deep anesthesia when investigating the activity of lower structures.

In the context of these more general remarks it is perhaps worth examining two points of particular interest. In his extensive review Darrow (1937a) covers a large amount of material, making the case for an association between motor and secretory activity; thus, for instance, lesions of the premotor area, which result in the loss of inhibitory control of motor movement, and in the condition of forced grasping, also involve the lack of inhibition of secretory activity, giving rise to profuse sweating. It is, in the context of the material, possible to see electrodermal activity associated with this regulation of the behavioral activity as a component of the total orienting reflex.

The other cortical area mentioned by Luria and Homskaya (1970) as being of major importance is that of the frontal lobes. They say, "thus the whole aggregate of facts . . . arrived at in experiments with animals as well as with man convince one that the neocortex of the frontal lobes of the brain belongs to the number of apparatuses taking part in the regulation of arousal processes and may be the highest form of this regulation [1970, p. 307]." Later they make the point that in patients with frontal lobe lesions, "there are observed substantial disturbances of the regulating effect of the speech system on the dynamics of the vegetative components of the orienting reflex [p. 318]." The importance of the lateral frontal cortex in particular is emphasized by the work of Kimble et al. (1965), who showed in lesions of this area in monkeys there were diminished SCRs to initial and novel presentations of stimuli, that is, stimuli which were distinguished from others as having different signal and hence meaningful value.

8. CONCLUSION

While this section has omitted reference to some of the central mechanisms covered by more complete reviews such as those by Wang (1957, 1958, 1964), a picture does emerge which supports Wang's general thesis of "a hierarchy of suprasegmental controls" which, following Fulton's (1926) long-circulating principles, are in the reverse order to that in which they have been presented. What follows from this is, it is hoped, a basis for examining some of the more conventional behavioral psychological concomitants of electrodermal activity, and the sorts of change in that activity which might be expected if the hierarchy of suprasegmental controls is disturbed.

What has been investigated most fully in any work on central mechanisms is their involvement in phasic electrodermal responses. How central activity may affect long-term tonic activity is a function of the extent to which this is a product of continued phasic interacting with hormonal determinants of peripheral function as previously outlined.

E. Models and Mechanisms of Electrical Functioning of the Skin

1. INTRODUCTION

There have, in general, been two approaches to the description of the electrical function of the skin; one, arising perhaps more from dermatological interests, views the skin as a "black box," and endeavors to describe its electrical characteristics by examining its behavior in relation to impressed electrical potentials having known parameters. This is a traditional method with which an attempt might be made to determine the electrical characteristics of any unknown object. The second type of approach, more emphasized by electrophysiologists, is to suggest what sort of a model, having as its elements the known physiological functions of elements of the skin, might account for known characteristics of electrodermal phenomena. These two approaches are by no means mutually exclusive and the findings of one illuminate the data of the other. Where perhaps the two approaches have different outcomes is that a description of the skin as a substance having electrical characteristics has tended to take the skin as a rather static unchanging tissue, but has given a full analysis in terms of its capacitative as well as its resistive elements. On the other hand, the second, more functional, approach has emphasized the resistive and potential source elements in the skin, and their dynamic interaction in response.

2. CAPACITANCE AND IMPEDANCE CHARACTERISTICS OF SKIN

Although there is a considerable body of early work in this field, recent authoritative statements by Edelberg (1971), Lykken (1971), and Tregear (1966) present most that is now known about these aspects of the skin.

That the skin has capacitance properties is indicated by the fact that its impedance decreases as the frequency of the imposed measuring current increases. This was demonstrated by Gildemesiter in 1915, who showed that the impedance offered to 5–6-kHz current was only 2 or 3% of that offered to dc. The controversy which has followed this fairly straightforward demonstration is centered around whether the capacitative element in the skin is a true capacitance, that is, its size is independent of frequency, or whether it is a polarization capacitance whose value changes with frequency. A true capacitance would be due to static dielectric properties of the skin, whereas the polarization capacitance is a function of ionic distribution following passage of current.

There is a parallel, but not identical, argument as to whether the resistive element in skin is a true ohmic resistance or is due to a counter electromotive force (emf) developed by passage of current.

At the present time, the simplest view of an electrical model of the skin is that shown in Fig. 3. This is the simple model used by Lykken (1971) and in essence by Tregear (1966), although the latter represents C as a polarization impedance.

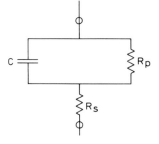

Fig. 3. Simple model of the skin. (Adapted from Lykken, 1971.)

Lykken argues that the equivalent skin current is dependent upon the type of system which is used in its measurement, and demonstrates that if the apparent capacitance of the circuit in Fig. 3 is measured with a bridge having parallel R and C elements, the capacitance will appear to be frequency dependent even when it is made up of "real elements" (i.e., hardware) and C is fixed. Following Hozawa (1928), Lykken (1971) employs the method of square wave analyses of skin impedance and provides evidence to suggest that C is in fact a true capacitance. More critical experimentation shows that two RC parallel elements in series with a resistive element provide a model which more closely represents the electrical characteristics of the skin. Indeed, a closer approximation to reality can probably be achieved with a large number of parallel RC elements in series with a series resistance, effectively parts of R_s, in between each RC element. This accords with the view of Tregear (1966) who suggests that each of the 10–100 cell laminae in the human stratum corneum behaves as a parallel RC element. Edelberg (1972 a), following these hypotheses, suggests that it is the small elements of series resistance between these laminae which can be changed by hydration. Lykken shows that the capacitative elements reside in the superficial layers of the stratum corneum, as the skin no longer behaves as though it has a capacitative element when the stratum corneum is removed by skin drilling. This drilling also effectively removes R_p. Further analysis suggests that R_s probably represents at least three anatomically distinct components of resistance located in the stratum corneum, the lower epidermis, and the body core. Although out of this particular context, it is interesting to note that Lykken's work at this time suggests that the source of tonic skin potential lies in the lower layers of the stratum corneum. Also, he suggests that, "to account for steady state phenomena as well, a fourth component is required [in addition to the three components of Fig. 3] consisting of a battery . . . which acts as though in series with the R–RC circuit [Lykken, 1971, p. 274]." Lykken's calculations suggest mean values of 13.2 kΩ/cm^2 for R_s of which only some 500 Ω/cm^2 lie in the deep tissues, and 187 kΩ/cm^2 for R_p for an unstimulated palmar site, Lykken, Miller, and Strahan (1968), using the square wave technique, suggest that during an SCR, R_s does not change but rather that according to McLendon and Hemingway (1930), there is a change in "polarization capacity," that is, in the present context a change in the parallel RC circuit. Lykken suggests that changes equivalent to an SCR can be obtained by changing only R_p in the RC circuit and doubts that others' claims that C changes during an SCR are correct. The constancy of C during an SCR is in accordance with the work of Montagu (1964) and Yokota and Fujimori (1962). Edelberg (1971) proposes that it is reasonable to suggest that if the capacitance of the skin is static it is necessary to question the idea that dc skin resistance is a counter emf "since membrane polarization would by its very nature be associated with polarization capacitance [p. 535]." At low currents the skin does, in fact, behave as though it were a true ohmic resistance (Edelberg, Greiner, & Burch, 1960). The discussion of this aspect of electrodermal activity is presented in greater detail in Section V.B.3.a(i) in the context of measurement by constant current or constant voltage methods.

3. Sweat Glands and Epidermis as Conductive Pathways

Montagu and Coles (1966) present an equivalent circuit of the skin, of which Fig. 4 is a modification. This is similar to Lykken's circuit shown in Fig. 3, but with the addition of r_1–r_n resistors in parallel,

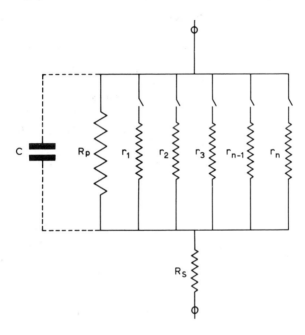

Fig. 4. Model of the skin. (Adapted from Montagu & Coles, 1966.)

themselves in parallel with R_p. These resistors r_1–r_n represent sweat ducts and are shown as capable of being switched in and out depending on whether or not they are active. In this figure, R_p continues to represent a resistance lying largely in the stratum corneum, while R_s represents a three-part pathway lying in the stratum corneum, the lower epidermis, and body core. Support for this model, having a conductive pathways sweat glands in parallel, is provided by the data of Thomas and Korr (1957) who were able to show a linear relationship between number of active sweat glands and conductance. These authors present a model almost identical to that of Fig. 4, omitting C, which for their analysis was irrelevant, and showing R_p as a variable resistor varying with surface moisture. Thomas and Korrs' measurements suggest values of from 3 to 20 MΩ for the resistance of single sweat glands, and a calculated value of from 3 to 10 MΩ for R_p, based upon the equation $G_t = G_p + G_g N$ $(G = I/R)$, where G_t is total conductance, G_p is the conductance of epidermal nonsudorific tissue, and $G_g N$ is the conductance of N individual sweat glands, each having a mean conductance of G_g. If no sweating is taking place, then G_t should equal G_p; measured values of R_p under these conditions were always higher than calculated values and ranged from 10 to 100 MΩ. Thomas and Korr, however, used dry electrodes, and these would thus be poor contact conditions in nonsudorific states. The values obtained by these authors using a 2.54-cm² electrode area are, however, much larger than those of Lykken (1971), suggesting 187 kΩ/cm² for R_p. This model in its simple form most conveniently accounts for differences in SCL by suggesting that this is a function of the number of active conducting sweat glands and of the state of the epidermal tissue. As already suggested, that part of R_s which lies in the epidermis is affected by hydration and decreases as the epidermis absorbs water. The work of Adams (1966) and Adams and Vaughan (1965) is concerned with the "hydraulic capacitance" of the epidermis. Their clearest demonstration is that when SR and evaporative water loss from the skin are measured at the same time, it can be shown that when sweat gland activity is increasing SR falls as evaporative water loss increases; however, when sweat gland activity decreases EWL decreases, but SR remains at a low level, suggesting that the water remaining in the epidermis is responsible for a low conductive pathway $R_s + R_p$. This accords with the earlier work of Thomas and Korr (1957) showing the direction of sweat gland activity was important in determining the extent of the epidermal component. Although in Fig. 4 the resistors representing the sweat glands are shown as having fixed values and capable of being switched in and out, there is evidence that the sweat gland may in fact act as a variable resistor. Lloyd (1960) presents a model of the sweat gland which suggests that it acts as a core conductor with the variable level of sweat in the gland effectively acting to short circuit the resistors representing the epidermal lining of the duct wall. Montagu and Coles (1968) also present an argument for the graded response of a sweat gland suggesting that the morphological unit, the sweat gland, is in fact formed of several physiological units, the secretory cells. Thus, although these cells may act in an all-or-none fashion as the resistors $r_1 - r_n$ in Fig. 4, the sweat gland itself may effectively act in a graded fashion.

The number of active sweat glands, and the extent of their activity, together with the hydration of the epidermis, due at least in part to reabsorption of water from sweat ducts, is able to provide a reasonable explanation for SCL. This viewpoint is consistent with findings that sympathetcomy and elimination of sweat gland activity by cholinergic blocking agents bring about marked decreases in SCL. However, this comparatively simple model for SCL has to be elaborated before it is able to encompass the phenomena of SCR and SPR.

4. MODELS OF SCR AND SPR

a. THE SITE OF RESPONSE MECHANISMS. Before going into detail concerning the mechanisms involved, it is important to reintroduce some of the phenomena of SCR and SPR which have to be explained and which present difficulties for a simple sweat gland and epidermal hydration mechanism, such as that which appears to afford an explanation for SCL. Skin potential responses, as shown in Section II.E, may be either uniphasic negative, biphasic (negative followed by positive), triphasic, or on occasions, uniphasic positive. Skin conductance responses, while simpler, being unidirectional, show marked differences in recovery rate. If SPR and SCR are recorded together, then slow recovery SCRs are usually accompanied by uniphasic negative SPRs while fast recovery SCRs are recorded in the presence of biphasic SPRs (see Fig. 1).

There is no doubt that sweat gland activity is responsible for phasic electrodermal activity insofar as SCRs and SPRs are eliminated after blocking of the cholinergically activated secretory mechanisms with atropine or hyoscymine (Lader & Montagu, 1962; Wilcott, 1964; Venables & Martin, 1967b). Responses are also absent in those persons suffering from a congenital absence of sweat glands (Richter, 1927; Wagner, 1952). However, a simple explanation in terms of depolarization of secretory cells, decrease in resistance due to duct filling, and lateral diffusion of water into the corneum, although providing a partial solution cannot encompass all the known phenomena of SCR and SPR.

Edelberg (1971), on the basis of a number of previous demonstrations (Edelberg, 1964, 1966; Edelberg & Wright, 1964), makes the case for an epidermal component in the determination of phasic electrodermal activity. These demonstrations include evidence of very similar SCRs from palmar and from dorsal sites, the former being accompanied by signs of sweat gland activity which are absent in the latter; the involvement of sweat gland activity is dependent uon the type of signal used to elicit the response. Evidence provided by Mordkoff, Edelberg, and Ustick (1967) suggests that the two types of effector response can apparently be separately conditioned. The difficulty with the idea of a separate epidermal mechanism is that the separate innervation of such a mechanism has not been demonstrated. Insofar as atropinization eliminates all signs of responding, if there is separate innervation it must be cholinergic.

Another important range of findings which point to an epidermal effector having membranelike properties is that of Edelberg et al. (1960) who show that the size of SRRs and SPRs is affected by use of different salts as external electrolytes. When different salts were used at anodal sites (at which the cations are carried into the skin) the amplitude of the SRR increases with the size of the hydrated cation in the order KCL, NaCl, LiCl, NH_4Cl, $CaCl_2$, $AlCl_3$. Edelberg (1971) and Fowles (1973) review the evidence on the sites accessible to such externally applied electrolytes and suggest that the sweat duct wall rather than the secretory portion of the duct is accessible, and that there is a major pathway for current through the duct wall and probably only a small proportion of the total current in the sweat gland passes down to the lower secretory portion. Further evidence for the importance of a relatively distal ductal mechanism being involved in electrodermal responses is provided by Shaver, Brusilow, and Cooke (1965) who showed that as a microelectrode was inserted into a sweat duct and potential responses recorded, these negative-going responses decreased in amplitude and reached zero as the tip of the electrode passed the stratum germinativum. When the epidermis had been dissected away, the lumen negative potential disappeared and even though the duct continued on stimulation to pour forth sweat, no potential could be measured. This and other evidence reviewed by Edelberg (1971) and Fowles (1973) makes a strong case for a mechanism in the ductal portion of the sweat gland to be heavily involved in electrodermal responding. Independently Lang (1967) has suggested that the SPR in cat is evidently a composite of the numerous potential events of a nonpropagated graded type which are produced by cells in the wall of the distal epidermal part of the sweat channel. Two notes of caution, however, need to be sounded. The first is that there is evidence that the sweat glands and ducts of the cat on which so much relevant work has been done are not wholly similar to those of man (see Section IV.B.4), and second, there is no evidence of direct innervation of the areas of the distal duct wall which have been just discussed as candidates for electrodermal response mechanisms. We must come to the conclusion that electrodermal activity as exhibited is the result of the operation of a chain of mechanisms, each being a necessary but not sufficient factor in the production of the response. Before examining further evidence, it is worthwhile introducing the model of electrodermal activity presented by Edelberg (1968) which has probably been the most influential in present-day thinking in the area.

b. The Model for "Biopotentials from the Skin Surface."[2] In 1966, Martin and Venables discussed the evidence for two sources of SP: first, a secretory potential in the sweat glands, and second, an epidermal membrane potential, the independence of which was demonstrated by the fact that an appreciable value of SPL remained after the elimination of sweat gland activity by iontophoresis of hyoscyamine (Venables & Martin, 1967b). Much of the discussion in the Martin and Venables' (1966) paper was based on ideas of Edelberg which had been presented in a paper in 1963. While the earlier models suggested a surface-positive sudorific potential, Edelberg's 1968 model, as shown in Fig. 5, is aligned

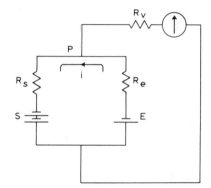

Fig. 5. Model of the skin. (From Edelberg, 1968.)

with a more consistent body of data, some of which has already been presented, suggesting that there is a lumen negative potential in the sweat duct. The importance of the 1968 model is that it suggests that it is necessary to take into account current pathways within the skin as explanatory mechanisms for some response phenomena. In the model (Fig. 5)

> the batteries S and E represent potentials across sweat gland membranes and epidermal membranes respectively. The combined internal and series resistance of each of these two elements is correspondingly denoted by R_s and R_e. These sources of potential are arranged in parallel, connected together on the tissue side by the highly conducting corium and on the surface by the electrode medium. The value of R_s depends upon the permeability of the sweat gland membrane and upon the height of the column of saline in the duct. The value of R_e is determined by the permeability

[2] From Edelberg (1968).

of a layer of cells in the epidermis and by the resistance of the corneum between the barrier layer and the surface. It is this last which is all important [Edelberg, 1968, p. 254].

In his latest paper explaining and extending his earlier presentation, Edelberg (1972a) gives a clear description of the working of the model. When sudomotor activity starts, R_s falls and as less potential is dropped across R_s, a negative SPR appears coincidental with an SCR. If then there is no further sweating, there will be slow lateral diffusion of sweat into the horny layer, giving a decrease in negativity (as R_e falls) and an SCR with a slow recovery phase. However, as many SPRs and SCRs have respectively biphasic wave forms and quick recovery phases, more passive diffusion of water into the corneum is not a sufficient explanation. In accord with the presentation in the previous section proposing the duct wall at the level of the stratum germinativum as a point of free passage for current, a rapid decrease in R_e can be shown to produce a sharply recovering SCR and an SPR with a positive secondary wave. Edelberg (1968) notes elements of similarity between his model and Darrow's (1964), who also stressed the influence of hydration on the level of measured potential. Darrow, however, did not include an epidermal source of potential. Independently, although drawing on some of Edelberg's earlier work, Lang (1968, p. 252) proposed a model somewhat similar to Edelberg's. He says, "we are inclined to assume that the negative phase of the endosomatic GSR is a composite potential which arises in a complex circuit of resistive elements and UPGs (unit potential generators—the effector cell groups in the walls of the distal epidermal part of the sweat channel) the latter being coupled in parallel to each other and in series with the surface electrode." Lang also discusses changes in the resistive elements as a result of hydration. Edelberg says little in the presentation of his model about the sources of potential, but rather concentrates on the role of changes in R_s and R_e in producing SCRs and SPRs; Fowles, however (Fowles & Venables, 1970; Fowles, 1973), has extended Edelberg's model to take account of potential sources.

c. FOWLES'S EXTENSION OF EDELBERG'S (1968) MODEL. Edelberg's (1968, 1972) explanation of the negative phase of the SPR and the SCR is in terms of duct filling and the reduction of R_s. Fowles and Venables (1970) suggest a direct source of negative potential in the sodium reabsorption mechanisms in the dermal portion of the human sweat duct. The most direct evidence for this mechanism is provided by Schultz, Ullrich, Frömter, Holzgreve, Frick, and Hegel (1965). Potentials of about 50 mV negative relative to interstitial fluid were found in the subepidermal portion of the duct. This was the case even when the secretory portion of the duct was filled with oil, ruling out the possibility that the potential came from the secretory coil. Inhibition of this dermal sodium pump mechanism by g-strophanthin (ouabain) reduced the potential in the duct and increased the NaCl concentration of the sweat (see Section V.B.4). It was shown earlier that the work of Shaver *et al.* (1965) indicated that no potentials in the duct were found below the level of the epidermis in cat. However, the cat differs from man in that it lacks the dermal duct sodium reabsorption system (Munger, 1961; Munger & Brusilow, 1961). In cat, therefore, there is the possibility that the potential shown as S in Edelberg's model is in the duct at the level of the epidermis, while this is at dermal level (or possibly both levels) in man. It is likely, therefore, that the negativity of the SPR is a function of both an increase in S and a fall in R_s due to duct filling. In both cases the existence of sweating is required.

Evidence that there are two ductal mechanisms in man is provided by Slegers (1967). The approach of this author is mathematical. He was able to show a double exponential plot of sodium concentration against perfusion time in normal subjects and a single exponential function in patients suffering from cystic fibrosis. He suggests that the overall activity of the gland fits best to a two-step reabsorption hypothesis in which sodium chloride is reabsorbed in the proximal (dermal) part of the duct while low sodium chloride concentrations will reach the distal part of the duct where sodium can be exchanged for potassium or hydrogen ions. In patients with cystic fibrosis the proximal process is thought to be defective. The evidence reviewed by Edelberg (1971), suggesting that there is a major pathway for current through the sweat duct wall at epidermal level is in accord with these data, suggesting a fairly unselective reabsorption mechanism at epidermal level. Fowles (1973) makes two suggestions for mechanisms which might trigger the response of the epidermal ductal mechanism. One is sodium concentration, the epidermal mechanism acting as a second line of defense for the dermal mechanism in high sweating rates. The second mechanism which he suggests is increase in lumenal hydrostatic pressure. It is known that sweat is reabsorbed in states of poral closure when, as a consequence, lumenal pressure is increased (Fowles & Venables, 1970), and that SCRs and positive SPRs may be elicited by applying pressure to the skin (Edelberg, 1971).

We may extend Fowles' thinking in this area by suggesting other mechanisms which might trigger the epidermal ductal hydrostatic pressure sensing mechanism. One possibility is that of ductal myoepithelial contraction (Bligh, 1967) which, as has been suggested (Goodall, 1970), has adrenergic innervation (see Section IV.B.4), and hence offers the possibility of independent sympathetic innervation which may be separately conditioned (Mordkoff, 1968) (see Section IV.E.4). A second more indirect suggestion is that a vasodilation response of the area under an electrode, occurring at a point shortly after sweat secretion could act in a similar way; thus, some of the earlier suggestions of the involvement of vascular or muscular mechanisms may have been partly correct. As, however, they are mechanisms which are secondary to sudorific activity, the elimination of this (Lader & Montagu, 1962) would eliminate any apparent role of these mechanisms. Fowles (1973) summarizes his modification of Edelberg's (1968) model by the presentation of a circuit which is reproduced in slightly modified form in Fig. 6. In this,

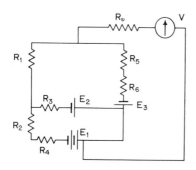

Fig. 6. Model of the skin. (From Fowles, 1973.)

E_1 is the potential generated by the sodium reabsorption mechanism in the duct wall at dermal level, and E_2 is the potential across the duct wall at epidermal level; both are lumen negative. E_3 is a potential involved in skin potential level measurements which will shortly be described. R_v is the internal resistance of the measuring device v. The resistances R_1–R_4 are identified as follows: R_1, resistance of the epidermal duct; R_3, resistance of the epidermal duct wall (associated with E_2); R_2, resistance of the dermal duct; R_4, the resistance of the dermal duct wall (associated with E_1); R_1 and R_2 are variable resistors associated with duct filling (cf. Lloyd, 1960, and Section IV.E.3). The major current pathway is along R_1 and R_3. R_5 represents the resistance of the stratum corneum and varies with hydration [the epidermal portion of R_s in Lykken's model (Fig. 3)]. R_6 represents a fairly fixed resistance across an epidermal barrier layer (possibly the stratum lucidum).

With minimal sudorific activity R_2 and probably R_1 are decreased, producing a slow recovery SCR; at the same time lumen sodium increases, and there is a consequent increase in E_1, producing a slow recovery negative SPR. Greater sudomotor activity further decreases R_1 and R_2, and may trigger the response of the epidermal duct wall, thus decreasing the value of R_3 and producing a small potential E_2. The epidermal ductal membrane response will produce a rapid recovery SCR and a positive SPR because of the stimulating effect on E_1. The model thus produces an association between slow recovery SCRs and uniphasic negative SPRs on the one hand, and fast recovery SCRs and biphasic SPRs which accords with observations (see Section IV). The model is also in accord with the findings reviewed by Martin and Venables (1966) showing the association of biphasic SPR with high negative SPLs. Our possible extension of the Fowles model, by suggesting an independent triggering of the epidermal ductal mechanism by adrenergic myoepithelial activity, also gives greater flexibility to the model and greater significance to the recovery phase of the SCR and positive wave of the SPR (Edelberg, 1970).

5. SKIN POTENTIAL LEVEL

In a series of studies Venables and Martin (1967b) blocked palmar sweat gland activity, using hyoscyamine iontophoresis, and demonstrated that recorded SPL after such treatment was still some 75% of the pretreatment value. It was suggested, therefore, that if 25% of the pretreatment SPL could be attributed to sudorific activity, the remaining portion might reflect the contribution from some form of epidermal mechanism. In 1966 Martin and Venables reviewed the mechanisms generating palmar SPL, and suggested that a semipermeable membrane, possibly at the level of the stratum lucidum, might, in association with body fluid electrolytes, be responsible for the production of a potential.

In a series of recent studies Christie and Venables (1971a, b, c, d) have investigated the mechanism involved in the generation of nonsudorific SPL, but instead of inactivating sweat glands by means of blocking agents, they adopted a procedure for attaining the relative quiescence of sweat glands characteristic of habituated subjects in unstimulating conditions (Christie & Venables, 1971a). Lykken, Rose, Luther, and Maley (1966) have reported that in relaxed subjects such as these there are individual differences in the lowest recordable SPL, which they were unwilling to attribute to individual differences in arousal. Thus it seemed possible, on the basis of the suggestions of Martin and Venables (1966), that individual differences in this low, nonsudorific potential, recorded when sweat glands were relatively quiescent, might reflect individual differences in tissue fluid electrolytes.

The series of studies investigating this low basal SPL (BSPL), using KCl as the external electrolyte (Venables & Sayer, 1963), with its concentration adjusted to match probable palmar surface values (Christie & Venables, 1971d), produced evidence that both individual differences in ECF K^+ concentrations in palmar tissue, and external K^+ concentrations in the electrolyte jelly, were significant parameters. Thus, for example, there was a significant inverse relation ($r = -0.70$, $p < 0.001$) between the amplitude of the electrocardiogram (ECG) T wave, which is itself related positively to plasma K^+ ($r = +0.68$, $p < 0.001$) (Papadimitriou, Roy, & Varkarakis, 1970) and BSPL (Christie and Venables, 1971b). Further, lowering in the negativity of BSPL was systematically associated with reductions in the concentration of the external KCl (Christie & Venables, 1971c). These authors suggested that findings such as this might be usefully explained by means of a Nernst equation model, where

$$\text{BSPL} = f \log \frac{\text{concentration } K^+ \text{ in external electrolyte}}{\text{concentration } K^+ \text{ in internal tissue fluid}}.$$

Initial studies with NaCl as the external electrolyte (Christie & Venables, 1971d) have suggested that the Nernst relation may possibly be relevant to the role of Na^+ in the generation of BSPL, i.e., with the recorded potential being a function of the concentration gradient existing between internal tissue Na^+ and the Na^+ in the external electrolyte.

This basal, electrolyte-determined value of SPL is the potential designated as E_3 in the Fowles model (Fig. 6). It is shown (Christie & Venables, 1971a) that there is a slow decline in SPL during rest. It is suggested that this decline is due to the diminution of sudorific involvement and hence of E_1 and E_2, the dermal and epidermal ductal potentials, leaving E_3 the "potassium potential," as the only factor in BSPL. At any level higher than BSPL, SPL is a complicated function of E_1, E_2, and E_3 in a circuit containing several resistive pathways representing either membranes or hydrated layers of corneum. It is thus to be expected that relationship to external variables will be somewhat limited and will depend heavily on a variety of factors, particularly those involved in the hydration of the corneum.

V. Measurement

A. The Subject and the Environment

1. INTRODUCTION

Under this broad, general heading an attempt will be made to focus on some specific aspects of subject and environment which merit consideration during planning of psychophysiological studies. Psychophysiological phenomena which appear from one experimenter's reports to be robust, healthy specimens, sometimes prove distinctly uncertain in the hands of another worker. In such situations it may be that the phenomena, though robust, has been totally buried by a mass of random variance, much of which might be avoided by prior attention to some aspects of subject and environment.

Consideration of subject variables requires looking at age, sex, race, and looking not only at effects of a variable *per se,* but also at possible interaction with experimenter characteristics. Further, it may be that there is need to standardize or control the behavior of one's subjects during a period immediately before they take part in an experiment, and it may also be advisable to standardize the amount of previous experience of the experimental environment and its procedures which subjects have had.

Consideration of the environment involves, on the one hand, attention to physical aspects such as temperature or humidity which could have direct effects on electrodermal phenomena, and consideration of its social aspects such as experimenter behavior and interactions with subjects, which could, via the intervening variable of their individual responses, have a range of indirect effects on electrodermal phenomena (see, for example, Hicks, 1970, 1971; Back, Wilson, Bogdonoff, & Troyer, 1969; Mason & Brady, 1965; Rosenthal, 1966).

2. Age, Sex, and Race

General reviews of the aging process and its possible significance within psychology have become available during recent years (for example, Welford & Birren, 1965; Talland, 1968). Examination of the age factor in relation to experimenter–subject interaction can be found in the work of Rosenthal (e.g., 1966), and dermatological literature provides some indications of those aspects of skin aging which could be of significance for electrodermatologists (e.g., a general account from Spencer & Kierland, 1970; decreases in epidermal keratinization and water content: Stoughton, 1962; atrophy of dermal papillae: Lorincz, 1960; reduced sweating: Strauss, Kligman, & Ponchi, 1962).

No attempt will be made here to examine the effects of age in relation to subject–experimenter interactions, and their possible significance for electrodermal recording within psychophysiology; the reader is referred to Rosenthal (1966) for some treatment of this. There is, however, as Brown (1966) suggests, little known about possible age differences in the emotional response to being a subject or experiencing experimental stress (Back & Bogdonoff, 1967). Some work has been undertaken to investigate age differences in electrodermal phenomena *per se,* notably from Surwillo (1965, 1969), Surwillo, and Quilter (1965), Shmavonian, Yarmat, and Cohen (1965), Shmavonian, Miller, and Cohen (1968), and their co-workers.

Surwillo undertook a study of 132 male subjects between the ages of 22 and 85; a number of reports describe various aspects of the findings obtained from monitoring some aspects of SP activity while the subjects carried out an hour's watchkeeping. Relevant findings were:

1. Older male subjects had fewer spontaneous SPRs during the period.
2. There was a low but significant inverse correlation ($r = -0.23$, $p < 0.02$) between age and SPL.
3. The distribution of SPL recorded during watchkeeping departed significantly from normal in the young male subjects.

Shmavonian and co-workers, examining age differences in conditioning, noted:

1. Aged males showed poorer conditioning of both SC and vasomotor responses (Shmavonian, *et al.*, 1965), but that there was evidence of significantly higher adrenaline metabolite excretion and of significantly more electroencephalogram (EEG) activity.
2. Aged males showed lower SCLs, and higher significant reductions in SCR amplitudes (Shmavonian *et al.*, 1968), as reported also by Botwinick and Kornetsky (1960).

The suggested interpretations of Shmavonian *et al.* (1965) are that both central and peripheral determinants of such phenomena require consideration; with regard to the former they cite Andrew (1956, p. 588), "nuclei of the hypothalamus show perhaps the most impressive and striking incidents of the specificity of age changes seen anywhere in the nervous system," and report Gellhorn, Nakao, and Redgate (1956) in saying that there is a diminution of the reflex involving the anterior (parasympathetic) division of the hypothalamus with age.

In relation to peripheral determinants of age differences in electrodermal activity, there are a number of relevant findings. MacKinnon (1954b) reported a reduction of palmar sweat counts with age in male subjects, and Juniper and Dykman (1967), in an examination of male, female, Negro, and Caucasian subjects, noted a similar reduction.

Shmavonian *et al.* (1968) suggest also the possible significance of sex hormones, citing the work of Baitsch (1954) who reported that although there is higher electrodermal responsivity and lower SRL in male subjects, these sex differences are not seen in prepubertal subjects. Effects of sex hormones could be central and/or peripheral; in relation to the latter they could exert an effect on sweat gland or associated epidermis. This possibility is not pursued here by consideration of electrodermatological work with prepubertal subjects, but the next section provides some coverage of sex differences in relation to the field.

Again, Rosenthal (1966) is suggested as a source of information on the potential complexities of sex differences in the social context of the psychological experiment, and no attempt will be made to consider here this aspect of the environment.

Turning, however, to questions of sex differences in electrodermal phenomena and their underlying physiological determinants, there has been, during the past decade, increasing attention paid both to sex differences in electrodermal phenomena as a source of variance, and to the precise nature of their underlying determinants. Even so, the summary provided by Bell (1971) in Table 1 suggests that there are experimenters

TABLE 1

SEX OF SUBJECTS AS REPORTED IN TWO PSYCHOLOGICAL JOURNALS (from Bell, 1971)

Subject information	Psychophysiology[a]	Journal of Experimental Psychology[b]
No sex stated (%)	14.3	3.6
Male and female (%)	24.2	71.1
All male (%)	54.5	19.3
All female (%)	7.0	6.0
Experiments with control for the menstrual cycle (%)	2.6	Not given

[a] Psychophysiology, 1964–1970, Vols. 1–6.
[b] Journal of Experimental Psychology, 1966–1967, Vols. 71–75 (after Schultz, 1969).

apparently happy to ignore the warning that "it would be grossly erroneous to mix men and women subjects where physiological measures are being obtained [Shmavonian et al., 1965, p. 241]." Even the more enlightened experimenters seem to opt for simplification by selecting the simpler male. There are, however, a number of relevant studies where comparisons have been made between electrodermal activity in male and female subjects. Kopacz and Smith (1971) investigated the effects of three levels of shock threat on the skin conductance of 30 male and 30 female subjects, and reported significant main and interaction effects for electrodermal levels and responses. Their introductory section includes a useful review of earlier work on sex differences in SC, and Kopacz and Smith conclude with a discussion of the possible significance of Broverman, Klaiber, Kobayashi, and Vogel (1968); these workers had suggested that a behaviorally relevant physiological sex difference of major significance could be the more potent activating effect of estrogen as compared with androgen. Hormonal effects have been tentatively suggested as a determinant of sex differences in basal skin potential level recorded with both NaCl and KCl as the external electrolytes (Christie & Venables, 1971d).

Shmavonian *et al.* (1965, 1968) reported sex differences in SCR conditioning, with males showing more rapid conditioning, slower extinction, and lower amplitude responses. Juniper and Dykman (1967) reported sweat counts to be higher in women; their discussion in this and in a later publication (Juniper, Blanton, & Dykman, 1967) introduced also the possible significance of nonsudorific mechanisms being determinants of some sex differences in electrodermal activity.

Turning now from consideration of differences in electrodermal activity betwen the sexes to examination of differences within female subjects which are associated with the menstrual cycle, there has been a development of interest in this rhythmic function, and growth of its status from a variable considered by only the more careful experimenters (Wenger, 1962) to a phenomenon of intrinsic research interest. Part of this development is attributable to the growing awarness of rhythmic functions of the living system (Wolf, 1962) and their significance for the behavioral sciences. Some further treatment of this general area can be found in Section V.A.4 and general treatment of the menstrual cycle is available in Dalton (1970). Redgrove (1971), within the context of biological rhythms and human performance, writes a chapter on menstrual cycles, and basic physiological texts (e.g., Green, 1972; Passmore & Robson, 1968) provide details of endocrine changes involving estrogen during the first (follicular) half and progesterone plus estrogen during the second (luteal) half of the cycle.

In contrast to the accumulation of data on endocrine aspects of the mentrual cycle, Wineman reports (1971) a dearth of evidence on autonomic function. This author reports her work with Wenger's measure of autonomic balance (Wenger, 1966). Earlier investigations had suggested that higher estrogen activity might be associated with lower levels of sympathetic nervous system (SNS) arousal. Haigh, Kitchin, and Pickford (1963) had suggested that peripheral vasodilation, observed after estrogen administration, paralleled the effect of sympathetic nervous system denervation, and Wieland, Cullen, and Wenger (1958) suggested that changes in autonomic balance as indicated by the measure of $\bar{A}$ could be interpreted in terms of an association below low sympathetic nervous system activity and high estrogen. Wineman (1971) confirmed this suggestion, showing $\bar{A}$ scores to be higher during menses, the follicular, and the ovulatory phases, and lowest during the luteal phase, that is, during the second half of the cycle when progesterone is secreted by the corpus luteum. Wineman concludes with a comment that the relationship between the endocrine system is far from simple. Attempts to examine this in finer detail, by focusing on either estrogen or progesterone, lead one even further from "simplicity." It would seem useful, however, to undertake the attempt, one justification being that female subjects may no longer be characterized by a textbook cycle; they may, instead, present a heterogenous population, part of which is taking steroidal contraceptives with a possibly wide range of doses, estrogen/progesterone ratios, and schedules. We are unaware, as yet, of studies relating electrodermal activity to steroidal contraceptive intake, but it may be that the evidence presented below in relation to some physiological effects of estrogen and progesterone may allow extrapolation to guide the electrodermatologist. Some details of synthetic steroids used in oral contraceptives, their ratios, and schedules, are available in sources such as Maas (1970), or Saunders (1970).

One relevant line of enquiry into possibly significant central and peripheral effects stems from the anesthetic action of progesterone. This was reported by Selye in 1941; reviews of its interactions with the central nervous system are given by Hamburg (1966) and Motta, Piva, and Martini (1970). These last-named cite a range of evidence that progesterone, its derivatives, and its metabolites, can exert hyperthermic effects, induce significant changes in the electrical activity of the brain as evaluated by both EEG and unit recording techniques, and influence the level and turnover of brain catecholamines. Kopell, Lunde, Clayton, Moos, and Hamburg (1969) reported a study of indices of arousal recorded through the menstrual cycle; they had equivocal findings with the elctrodermal measure of SPL, but, in contrast, Bell has reported changes in resting SPL such as increases in negativity at the ovulatory and premenstrual phases.

Bell interprets his findings in terms of the possible nonsudorific electrolyte determinant generating SPL; it may be that his choice of resting SPL was significant, and resulted in his recording predominantly basal SPLs (Christie & Venables, 1971a), which would appear to reflect tissue values of electrolytes (Christie & Venables, 1971d) rather than arousal. This is suggesting the significance of a peripheral rather than a central reflection of hormonal changes through the menstrual cycle, and their effects on electrodermal phenomena. MacKinnon (1954a) has also reported a peripheral reflection of progesterone activity in her data showing lowered palmar sweat counts during the luteal phase. MacKinnon (1964) and MacKinnon and Harrison (1961) have argued that the effect of progesterone on palmar sweating is mediated by a central nervous system response to the hormone; it remains possible, however, that some direct peripheral effect of progesterone on sweat gland function could also be implicated, perhaps in relation to aldosterone control of sweat sodium reabsorption.

Thus, like the effects of age, the sex variable is complex, implicating biosocial aspects of experimenter–subject interaction, hormonal and central nervous system relationships, and the modulating effect of the endocrine system on eccrine sweat glands. The final subsection considers briefly the topic of race and ethnic variables in relation to electrodermatology, and again there is the inevitable complex of social interactions, culturally determined sets and attitudes to being a subject for psychophysiologists, and possible racial differences in some physiological determinants. Again, Rosenthal (1966) is suggested as a source for discussion of major issues relating to the social aspects of the experimental environments. After citing some electrodermal literature he does, however, comment that "in general the effect of experimenter's race on subjects' physiological responses is poorly understood and, up to the present, little studied [Rosenthal, 1966, p. 59]." Another line of enquiry is that followed by Lazarus and co-workers (see Lazarus, 1966) into racial differences in the physiological response to stressors experienced by Japanese subjects in the experimental situation. Subsequent work has included investigation of racial differences in the response to psychological (Back et al., 1969) and physical stressors (Tursky & Sternbach, 1967). The first-named authors used the term "experimental stress" (Back & Bogdonoff, 1967) to describe the experience of entering and participating in an experiment, and have investigated autonomic nervous system responses of both Negro and Caucasian subjects when they were investigated together with friends or strangers. Tursky and Sternbach (1967) in this and an earlier publication (Sternbach & Tursky, 1965) investigated ethnic differences in the autonomic nervous system response to shock, postulating as a result of their findings intervening variables such as set and attitude, which were culturally determined, and which were influential in producing the differential responses of the autonomic nervous system in their range of subjects.

An interesting review of some relevant electrodermal literature is given by Kugelmass and Lieblich (1968) in a report of their work on Bedouin and town-dwelling Jews.

Finally, there has been continuing interest in possible racial differences in eccrine sweat gland function since the report of Johnson and Corah (1963); these workers showed Negro subjects to have significantly higher SRLs than Caucasian subjects. Initial suggestions were that the former group might have thicker stratum corneum, or fewer active palmar eccrine sweat glands. Johnson and Landon (1965) subsequently reported inability to demonstrate differences in palmar sweat glands, and suggested that differences in sweat electrolyte concentrations might be implicated. Malmo (1965), however, subsequently confirmed that his dark-skinned subjects had lower palmar SC (supporting the Johnson & Corah, 1963 report of higher SR), but he also demonstrated lower sweat counts in such subjects. Juniper and Dykman (1967) also reported that Negro males had fewer active sweat glands than Caucasian males of the same age range (40–60 years), and that Negro women of 20–39 years had fewer than Caucasian females of the same age range. So it remains that there are possible racial factors to trap the electrodermatologist; brief mention was made in Section IV that in a comparison of Japanese and European subjects it became apparent that there were race differences in the frequency of eccrine sweat glands on trunk and limbs, but it must have become apparent through this brief subsection that racial or ethnic differences between subjects are likely to be much more complexly determined, involving possible physiological determinants, and a range of biosocial interactions.

3. "Habituation," Control, and Comfort

One possible reduction of the complexity inherent in the biosocial interactions of the experimental environment is possible when a population of habituated subjects can be used. Obviously there are many experimental designs requiring naive subjects, but when it *is* feasible, work with an habituated group has a number of advantages. Thus, those features of experimental stress which originate from unfamiliarity with the environment, its procedures, and its personnel, can be eliminated after repeated testing of a subject. Additionally, such repeated testing allows the experimenter to become familiar with the subjects' characteristic physiological profiles, for example, his electrodermal levels recordable in specific experimental conditions, and with usual wave formations or amplitudes of response. Against such a familiar background the appearance of an atypical record stands out clearly, often providing valuable leads for future research. To optimize the value of habituated subjects, care should be taken to retain as unchanged as possible the physical characteristics of the experimental environment; at its simplest level this means retaining equipment and furniture in identical positions, but it is appropriate at this point to consider the more difficult question of maintaining constant heat, humidity, and noise levels. Ideally, temperature should be maintained within the physiological range of vasomotor control (see Section IV.B.2) at 20–30°C, with a tolerance

of $\pm1°C$. It should be remembered, however, that the optimal comfort
zone for a relatively active experimenter may be several degrees below
that for a subject required to be inactive for any length of time: it
is invaluable experience for a prospective experimenter to be a subject
in the conditions proposed for his study; Section V.C.1.h becomes relevant in this context. Too cool an experimental environment increases
the probability of having nonisothermal electrodes, as well as causing
discomfort in the subject, and possibly altering the characteristics of
electrodermal activity (Scholander, 1963; Surwillo, 1967). One simple
but effective way of increasing a subject's comfort is, when the nature
of the experimental procedures allow, by providing a light covering
which can be positioned over both hand and arm electrodes. Even in
summer a light sheet may be welcomed by subjects who are required
to be inactive, especially if they are exposed to air currents generated
by an air-conditiong system.

It is possibly a counsel of perfection to suggest that humidity should
also be controlled, but there is evidence of correlation between SCL
and relative humidity (Venables, 1955). In general, climatic factors can
present a range of problems (see Section V.A); often, though, one can
do little except be aware of their existence when designing studies
(Wenger & Cullen, 1962).

Random noise disturbance should be eliminated by soundproofing
plus reduction at source; suitable masking noise is worth considering,
and air-conditioning equipment can sometimes produce a convenient
masking hum.

Lighting should be given some attention, and if subjects are required
to relax completely, low-level illumination is preferable to total darkness.

It has been suggested that in order to optimize the value of work
with habituated subjects, one essential is to maintain a constant and
appropriate physical environment. This is, of course, not implying that
when nonhabituated subjects are being used one can abandon attempts
at environmental control. Similarly, it is suggested, now, that attempts
should be made also to standardize and control the social environment
insofar as it is possible to standardize and control the behavior of the
experimenter; such attempts are valuable for work with any human
(or for that matter, animal) subjects. It is well worth an experimenter's
effort to prepare as much as can possibly be done before the subject's
arrival: electrodes can be checked, filled with electrolyte, and attached
to suitable lengths of adhesive, then covered with small polystyrene
pots until required. Such preparations can be undertaken in the 30 min
or so before a subject arrives, during the time required for optimal
warmup of the polygraph. In this period, too, the experimenter can

check the details of his experimental procedure, so that when the subject does arrive subsequent operations are reduced to the minimum and are smooth, swift, and efficient.

It is appropriate, at this point, to consider what the subject does during the 30 min before his arrival: there are vast differences between subject A, who came, in freezing weather, on a motor bike, through city traffic, arrived late, and rushed upstairs at the last minute, and subject B, who followed the schedule in a handout which suggested that he spend the 30 min before the appointment (1) in quiet, nonactive ways, (2) within the college, (3) avoiding food, drink, and smoking, (4) in a moderate temperature, calling in at the lavatory on his way to the laboratory, and walking up the last flight of stairs. Wilder (1967) has argued the need to consider the effects on physiological measures of subjects' previous activities and it may be that many an otherwise robust phenomenon lies buried beneath variance introduced by A-type subjects! One obvious advantage of using experienced habituated subjects is the familiaity with an experimenter's requirements regarding preliminary controls, and it would seem that subjects with whom one has worked for a number of months or years are more likely to remember and adhere to requests about such requirements.

Obviously there is a limit to the restrictions one can reasonably ask of one's subject; one may not be able to standardize behavior for longer periods before recording, but it is often useful to have records of activities in, say, the 24 hr before testing. Information about sleep amounts, times and size of meals, minor illnesses, drug intake, and the like can often provide useful insights and suggestions for future work.

Following the line of thought from the subjects' time before he arrives into time after, the next section looks first at the question of suitable temporal intervals for recording, at problems associated with long sessions and protracted studies, in relation to levels of arousal, diurnal rhythms, and climatic effects.

4. Length of Record, Time of Day, and Season

Consideration of costs and payoffs is a valuable preliminary to planning the length of a psychophysiological recording session. There always exists the thought that, having enlisted and probably paid subjects, acquired equipment, controlled the environment and so on, then it makes sense to collect as much potentially useful data as possible in a session. Two "costs," however, merit some consideration, one being the effect of an overdemanding schedule on the efficiency and serenity of the experimenter, the other being the effects of overdemanding conditions on the subjects. An example of the latter is the effects of overlong sessions, with the possibilities of associated overload or understimulation. One might also predict interactions between over- or understimulation and personality variables. Thus, for example, Eysenck's predictions from his model of extroversion suggest that, because of more rapid development of reactive inhibition, extroverts would react differently from introverts (Eysenck, 1967).

On the basis of unpublished data we suggest that, for unstimulating conditions, 20 min appears to be an optimal testing period, but obviously it is impossible to generalize. What may be of value is to consider whether there are advantages in attempting to maintain relatively constant subjects' levels of arousal throughout a session by means of experimental activities such as watch-keeping (Surwillo, 1969) or threshold determinations (Venables, 1963b).

In relation to more protracted recording sessions, one must consider also the effect on skin of prolonged exposure to the external electrolyte. Unpublished data from 10 subjects have shown that, even within periods of less than an hour, there can be marked reductions in the amplitude of SPRs recorded from an old site, in contrast to simultaneous records obtained from a fresh one. These recordings were made using .5% KCl as the external electrolyte, and interpretations of the phenomenon center around hydration of the hygroscopic horny layer (Fowles & Venables, 1970), subsequent poral closure (Peiss, Randall, & Hertzman, 1956), and possible attenuation of electrical signals originating from sweat gland activity. There were no apparent effects of site "age" on BSPL, and there were noticeable intersubject differences on SPR amplitude. This latter was tentatively attributed to individual differences in the extent of epidermal hydration existing before electrode placement. One possible way of avoiding response amplitude reduction may be found by using the suggested glycol-based electrolyte of Edelberg (1967), but, as he notes, there is a general need for investigation of the effects on the electrodes and sites of prolonged wear.

It was suggested, in discussion of the menstrual cycle, that there had been a growth of interest in biological rhythms; there are, however, a relatively small number of data relating directly to rhythmic changes in electrodermal activity. Some of the reason for the dearth of data undoubtedly lies in the fact that it is laborious to collect, making great demands on both experimenter and subject. Conroy and Mills (1970), however, cite Sollberger, Apple, Greenway, King, Lindan, and Reswick (1965) as an example of the growing use of automated analysis, and telemetry, as aids for biological rhythm research.

Mills (1966) has noted that, in contrast to the concept of *la fixété du milieu interieur,* we are now urged to envisage a milieu which is constantly changing, with physiological processes oscillating within an approximately 24-hr period (Mills, 1968). Biological rhythms may, therefore, be designated as circadian (*circa dies*) after Halberg's usage (1959), indicating a period of approximately 24 hr (20–28). Alternatively, it is possible to use the term "diurnal" in its stricter sense to designate rhythms observed through a day (Conroy & Mills, 1970). This term is adopted here; the bulk of evidence presented will relate to experimenters' data from the working day (Gates, 1910). No attempt will be made to consider the extensive literature of sleep studies.

General treatment of biological rhythms is given by Mills (1966, 1968), Conroy and Mills (1970), Kleitman (1963), and Harker (1964). Sollberger (1965) is a useful source of references; Colquhoun (1971) has recently edited a collection of contributed chapters on biological rhythms and human performance; and Brožek published a review of literature relating to what he has termed "psychorhythmics" (1964). In 1962 Wolf edited symposium proceedings on rhythmic functions in the living system, and both Kleitman and Halberg made contributions to Flaherty's reports on the psychophysiology of space flight (1961).

Focusing now on relevant aspects of diurnal variation in electrodermal activity, there are some data from a handful of studies of SCL, a little material relating to spontaneous electrodermal responding, and one study reporting the direction of change in basal SPL. Reported diurnal variations in indices of general arousal have probable relevance, and it may be useful also to consider reported diurnal variation in body fluid electrolytes.

It can be concluded from Niimi's (1967) study of three subjects that SCL reaches a zenith between the hours of 1–3 p.m.; similar findings were reported by Waller (1919). Christie and Venables (1973) recorded simultaneously the diurnal variation in SC, heart rate (HR), oral temperature, and basal SPL. They reported that while SCL, heart rate, and oral temperature exhibited the reported zenith in 2 p.m. recording, the BSPL trend was a mirror image of this, exhibiting an early afternoon nadir. A trend similar to that of BSPL was noted in the data of Venables and Martin (1967b), obtained from recording at that level of skin potential which remains after hyoscyamine iontophoresis. The similarity between this posttreatment level and the basal SPL recordable when sweat glands are quiescent is described in Section V.E.5. Sollberger (1965) cites other work on SR, and Mills (1966) cites Rutenfranz's (1961) report that the diurnal variation in skin resistance is evident during the first week of life, being the only physiological function to establish rhythmic changes at that age.

The basic role of body temperature in determining changes in a range of physiological functions, and in human efficiency, has been emphasized by Kleitman (1963); Waller (1919) reported that his diurnal variation in SC approximated that of body temperature, and this was found by Christie and Venables (1973). It should, perhaps, be emphasized at this point that such evidence relates to core temperature, or rather such approximations to it as can be obtained from oral, rectal, tympanic, or transcutaneous probe values (Fox & Solman, 1970). In contrast to core temperature, finger temperature trends are a mirror-image, having a nadir and not a zenith in the afternoon (Mills, 1968). The relation between core (rectal) temperature and HR is given by Mills (1966) as 10–15 beats per minute increase for every °F rise in rectal temperature.

The suggested dependence of some physiological variation on body temperature is of particular interest in relation to consideration of "morning" and "evening" types (Kleitman, 1963), and their preferred times of day (Bakan, 1963). A posthumously published chapter by Blake (1971, p. 109) reports his work on temperament and time of day: concluding sentences report that introverts had relatively higher oral temperatures at 8:00 a.m. but that at 9:00 p.m. the reverse was true, and that "taken together the results described in this chapter therefore favor the view that introverts have higher arousal levels than extroverts in the morning, that there is a general increase in level of arousal in both 'types' throughout the day, and that the level of arousal increases at a greater rate in extroverts than in introverts."

It may be relevant to mention also at this point Scandinavian work on morning and evening types, in relation to adrenaline and its reported diurnal variation (Levi, 1966); such work includes that of Patkai (1970, 1971).

In relation to the possible interactions between temperament, preferred time of day, and electrodermal activity, Zuckerman, Persky, and Link (1969), in their report of sensory deprivation work, noted a significant interaction effect for time of day (morning and afternoon) and amounts of nonspecific GSRs.

Finally, there is some evidence that although diurnal variation in serum potassium has not been demonstrated (Pollard, 1964; Seamen, Engel, & Swank, 1965; Mills, 1966), there *is* a diurnal variation in urinary potassium (Lobban, 1965; Buchsbaum, & Harris, 1971), and in salivary Na/K ratios (de Traverse & Coquelet, 1952; Morris, 1963). As the trend for potassium in these transcellular fluids suggests that potassium levels are relatively high in the afternoon, and as this is the period when BSPL, recorded with external KCl reaches a nadir (Christie & Venables, 1973), this supports the view (see Section IV.E.5) that BSPL generation implicates tissue values of potassium. Further, the authors have suggested that, given the apparent relative constancy of serum potassium, and the apparent diurnal variation in an index of epidermal potassium, this supports the view of Yoshimura (1964) that the skin functions as a mobile reservoir of water and electrolytes acting as a buffer to defend the intravascular compartment (Christie & Venables, 1971d).

In conclusion, it might be said that an awareness of diurnal variation in relevant physiological functions, plus the possibility of complex interactions between temperament and time of day, make the task of designing psychophysiological studies even more demanding. We would, however, argue with Wieland and Mefferd (1970) that the effort is rewarding, when one's statistical error variance can be reduced by attention to time of day and to its effects on the human subject. Wieland and Mefferd's most comprehensive account of their carefully controlled 120-day study really says something about most of the topics with which Section V.A has been concerned, and is relevant to the last part, concerned with the effects of protracted studies. Two aspects of these will be considered briefly, namely the extent of possible change within subjects on whom repeated investigations are made during protracted temporal periods, and the possible effects on electrodermal measures of changes in climate during extended studies.

Wieland and Mefferd (1970) reported individual differences over a 4-month period during intensive investigation of three subjects. Skin response level (SRL) and SSR were included in their battery of physiological measures; autocorrelation techniques revealed the presence of systematic changes (cycles or trends) in all their measures. These authors concluded that intraindividual differences in such variables are nearly as large as interindividual differences, and cannot be explained as errors of measurement; they also cite their earlier work on controlled longitudinal studies (Mefferd, LaBrosse, Gawienowski, & Williams, 1958; Mefferd & Pokorny, 1967).

Two recent studies report longitudinal investigations of electrodermal activity, one of which (Obrist, 1963) introduces also the topic of differences which are possibly attributable to handedness.

Docter and Friedman (1966) investigated the 30-day stability of spontaneous electrodermal response in 23 male students recorded through a week, then recorded similarly after 30 days. There were significant correlations between measures taken 24 hr apart, as well as significant correlations between median weekly rates of spontaneous EDRs recorded with a 30-day interval between them. However, emission rates on comparable recording days when separated by the 30-day interval failed to manifest a significant relationship.

Obrist (1963) recorded, from five subjects, SRL and SRR simultaneously from both sides of the body over periods of 24–36 days. He noted that a lateral effect shifted during the course of the study, and Wyatt and Tursky (1969) reported that in one of their subjects there was a reversal noted for SPL. Although both right and left-handed groups had higher SPLs on their right side, it was noted that in one subject higher SPLs were initially found on the right side but began to be recorded from the left hand during subsequent investigation. Wyatt and Tursky (1969) also report findings from SRR recording, as did Culp and Edelberg (1966), who showed augmentation of response amplitude on the hand ipsilateral to another active member such as the foot. Varni, Doerr, and Franklin (1971) have investigated bilateral differences in skin resistance level and photoplethysmographic vasomotor measures. They reported that bilateral differences were not related to handedness.

Some work has been undertaken to investigate central determinants of hand differences in electrodermal activity (e.g., Parsons & Chandler, 1969; Holloway & Parsons, 1969). The picture, however, is not clear, and really it appears impossible to give any precise guidance with regard to electrode placement. Some suggestions have been made in Section V.C.1.b, and Christie and Venables (1972) give recommended finger sitings, but as so often happens, the individual experimenter probably has to make his own decision from what is basically relatively insufficient evidence.

Turning, finally, to the problem of climatic change as a variable in protracted studies, Wieland and Mefferd (1970) consider some aspects of this, citing Wenger (1943), Wenger and Cullen (1962), Mefferd (1959), and Hale, Ellis, and Van Fossan (1960). Wenger and Cullen (1962) noted that they were unable to replicate, in summer months, psychophysiological findings obtained in temperate periods; Christie and Venables (1971b) reported a similar inability to replicate, in summer months, findings on BSPL and ECG T-wave relationships. The latter authors suggested the significance, for both eccrine sweating and epidermal tissue electrolytes, of neuroendocrine responses to heat which involve the regulatory role of the pituitary-adrenal cortical axis. The pattern of activity involved in such regulation has been detailed by Collins and Weiner (1968); seasonal variations in catecholamine output have been reported by Johansson, Frankenhaeuser, and Lambert (1969); and Neumann (1968) has described seasonal changes in the relationship between palm and arm skin resistances.

In an attempt at summarizing this section (V.A), its message is probably that while the usefulness of electrodermal measures depends in a major way upon technical aspects of methodology as described in the following sections, subject, experimenter, and environmental variables require prior consideration. While one has frequently to say that there are no hard-and-fast rules, there is often sufficient suggestive evidence from related areas which permits an individual experimenter to make an appropriate decision for his own particular circumstances.

B. Equipment

1. INTRODUCTION

From a position, a decade or more ago, when it was common for workers in this field to use equipment built in their own laboratories, the movement is now toward a greater availability of suitable commercially manufactured apparatus with its advantages of standardization and greater reliability. In addition, it is now less common than it was to record only a single channel of electrodermal activity, and skin conductance, and skin potential measures are generally recorded alongside other psychophysiological variables. It is thus convenient to consider the equipment used for recording electrodermal variables in the light of the fact that a polygraph will usually be used. This means that in general the main amplifiers and recording pens will have characteristics common to all channels and it is necessary therefore to consider the details of the circuitry and equipment such as preamplifiers and electrodes which are particular to the recording of electrodermal activity. Some controversial principles of technique are now to some extent past history and it seems possible to propose in this section a simpler set of recommendations than would have been possible even 5 years ago. It is, however, still recognized that there is still probably insufficient knowledge of the electrical characteristics of the skin to enable absolutely definitive statements to be made about the requirements of ideal measuring devices, and what is presented is in the nature of a summary of the present state of the art. This is essentially a more definite set of recommendations than those which were made in two overviews published in 1967 by Edelberg and by Venables and Martin. Little of what is presented here is not given in these reviews; what does seem legitimate now is to make a definite choice of methods from among the alternatives which were proposed at that time.

2. THE POLYGRAPH

The usual recording chain when using a polygraph consists of transducers, in this case electrodes–preamplifiers–main amplifier–recording pens and other devices for the analysis of the data. As stated previously, the main amplifier and other associated recording equipment is in general common to all channels of psychophysiological measurement and is designed to have parameters which will cover a wide range of requirements.

It is usual for the main amplifier to be directly coupled, and for it to be capable of faithfully amplifying steady or slowly changing signals corresponding to SCL and SPL as well as those more rapid fluctuations in potential which correspond to SCRs and SPRs. Even these fluctuations are comparatively slow and the amplifier need only have an upper frequency response of 2 Hz (see Edelberg, 1967, p. 35) to be suitable for amplifying electrodermal activity. In general, main amplifiers will have a very much higher frequency response. A requirement of an upper frequency response of only 2 Hz, however, makes it perfectly legitimate to use 50- or 60-Hz notch filters to eliminate mains or line frequency interference. It is, however, preferable to use recording conditions which do not make the filtering necessary.

It is the function of the main amplifier to provide sufficient power to drive the pen or stylus of the recording system. While ink recording is probably the most common and cheapest method, the hot wire stylus writing on wax-coated paper has some advantages in spite of the considerably greater cost of the recording paper. These are rectilinear recording (that is, the trace moves in a straight line across the paper at right angles to the direction of paper travel), and additionally it obviates one of the perennial disadvantages of ink recording, that of pen blockage. Most ink recording methods use a rectilinear trace, the pen arm moving on the arc of a circle, and it is important to use recording paper prepared for use with the polygraph which has curvilinear marking so that the timing of components of SCRs and SPRs may be accurately undertaken. [Venables (1967) presents a fuller discussion of visual recording methods.] For most purposes when responses are being recorded, a paper speed of 25, 30 (the standard EEG speed), or 50 mm/sec is adequate; a much slower speed can of course be used when only changes in SCL or SPL are of interest.

With the recent growth in the computer analysis of psychophysiological variables, it is important that the main amplifier of the polygraph should have output facilities which provide a signal capable of feeding the analog-digital converter of the laboratory computer for direct on-line analysis of the signal, or, alternatively, an instrumentation tape recorder for intermediate storage before analysis. The usual output level required for feeding a computer or tape recorder and complying with IRIG standards is 1 V RMS (2.8 V peak to peak) from a low impedance source (e.g., 100 Ω).

This high-level source is also convenient if some form of signal conditioning is used as an aid to analysis, e.g., if the primary trace is differentiated to provide an easier means of measuring such variables as latency and recovery phase (see Section V.D.2.a).

3. PREAMPLIFIERS

Under this heading it is intended to include all that circuitry which intervenes between the electrodes and the main amplifier. Thus, such items as calibration sources, couplers and sources of backing off, bucking or supression voltages, temperature compensators, etc., as well as initial stages of amplification are covered.

a. SKIN CONDUCTANCE MEASUREMENT. It is unfortunate that none of the preamplifiers/couplers commercially available appear to fit the requirements which are demanded by a full analysis of the process of measurement of SC, and which are necessary if all characteristics of the SCR wave form are to be accurately measured.[3] It therefore becomes necessary to recommend circuitry which may be constructed in the laboratory which may form the initial stage of the recording chain. A complete circuit is shown in Appendix I. This is a practical version derived from the analysis of principles now to be discussed.

(i) *Constant-Voltage versus Constant-Current Systems.* One of the major points of issue in skin conductance methodology has been that concerning the use of constant-voltage or constant-current methods of measurement. The principle invoked in the measurement of skin resistance or conductance is that of Ohm's law. If this is written $R = V/I$, where R is the skin resistance, and I the current through the skin is held constant, then V, the potential difference between two electrodes placed on the skin surface, varies directly with the skin resistance R, provided that Ohm's law holds for the physiological electrochemical circuit involved. If, on the other hand, we write G (skin conductance) $= 1/R = I/V$ and we hold the voltage across the electrodes on the skin constant, then I, the current through the skin, varies directly as the conductance G of the circuit between the electrodes—again provided that Ohm's law holds. In the statement above, the terms "holding current constant," or "holding voltage constant," denote the use of circuitry which within limits automatically achieves this.

In fact, Ohm's law only holds when measuring exosomatic electrodermal activity over a limited range of conditions, and these are imperfectly understood. Until 1967 the definitive statement was that of Edelberg

[3] A coupler on the lines of that recommended in Appendix I is now available for use with Beckman Offner Dynagraphs.

et al. (1960), to the effect that Ohm's law was only operative in a linear fashion with current densities at the electrode of less than 10 $\mu A/cm^2$. (Current density is expressed as the amount of current flowing per unit electrode area.) Beyond this limit, with higher current densities, both SRL and SRR were shown to decrease substantially. This finding of the inverse relationship between current density and SR had been previously shown by Grings (1953). These findings provided support for the advocacy of constant current methodology and the use of circuitry devised to limited current density of 10 $\mu A/cm^2$ and to maintain it at that value. (Current density obviously depends upon the size of electrodes used, a point which will be considered at a later stage.) In contrast to the 1960 findings of Edelberg *et al.*, Edelberg (1967) reported an experiment in which a series of voltage–current curves was obtained from 40 subjects. It was shown that subjects with very low resistance levels could tolerate current densities as high as 75 $\mu A/cm^2$ before nonlinearity was apparent, whereas at very high resistance levels the voltage current relationship became nonlinear with densities as low as 4 $\mu A/cm^2$. An explanation which is consistent with these findings is that in a situation with high SRL, there are few sweat glands active and that these have to carry all the current. If, individually, these sweat glands have a low threshold for nonlinearity, then the overall threshold with high SRL will be low. On the other hand, when there is a low tonic SRL, the total current will divide proportionately over the large number of active sweat glands (these glands being effectively in parallel, see Section IV.E), and the total current density which may be used before the threshold of nonlinearity is reached may be considerably higher than in the high SRL case, although the electrode size in use is the same in both cases. With the constant current system, by definition, the same current will flow whether or not there are many or few active sweat glands. In low SRLs all the current will have to be passed by few glands which will exceed their threshold for nonlinearity. On the other hand, with a constant voltage system, the voltage across each sweat gland is independent of the number of active glands and the current through an individual gland remains the same, however many are active, provided the activity of that gland is constant.

In his 1967 experiment, Edelberg reported that the voltage–current curves for all records were linear below a voltage level of .8 V across a single site. This value was obtained with a briefly impressed voltage. If, however, the time of exposure was lengthened, there was a gradual decrease in apparent SRL. Insufficient work has been carried out to determine the extent of this time variant effect. Kryspin (1965), however, suggests that there is a double effect with apparent resistance decreasing not only with increasing time but also increasing voltage. Lykken (1971) also provides data which support Edelberg's (1967) conclusion that it is the applied voltage rather than the current density which determines the upper limit of the range in which the skin obeys Ohm's law. Edelberg (1967) suggests the adoption of a value of .5 V across a site as that which would avoid both time-variant and time-invariant nonlinearity. This proposal is supported by Lykken (1971) and Lykken and Venables (1971), and implies, of course, the adoption of a constant voltage system in place of the rather more frequently used constant current system. Without the advantage of the voltage–current curves of Edelberg (1967), Montagu and Coles (1966) also advocates the constant voltage method, and state that it seems to possess distinct advantages over the constant-current principle.

It has already been stated (see Section IV.E) that it is physiologically realistic to view the conducting pathways in palmar skin as being made up of sweat glands and an epidermal conducting pathway, connected at one end by the overlying electrode–electrolyte system, and at the other by the underlying dermal and other tissue, as resistors in parallel. Resistors in parallel add as their reciprocals; it is, however, more convenient to think of conductance as the reciprocal of resistance and conductances as directly additive. On that basis, having n more sweat glands active means that n more units of conductance may be added to the existing level (a view which makes clear the notion that changes in conductance may be independent of basal level, see Section V.D.2). It is thus physiologically more reasonable to measure exosomatic electrodermal activity in terms of conductance rather than resistance. On this basis it has been advocated for some time (e.g., Montagu & Coles, 1966) that resistance measurements should be converted to conductance units using tables of reciprocals. The adoption of constant voltage circuitry has the immediate advantage that recording is directly in terms of conductance and no potentially error-producing conversion has to be carried out. To understand further the principles underlying constant-current and constant-voltage methods, two simplified circuits are presented in Fig. 7 for comparative purposes.

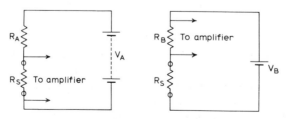

Fig. 7. Schematic circuits showing the principles of constant current (left) and constant voltage (right) methods of measuring skin conductance.

In the constant-current circuit (I) the value of R_A is high in comparison with the subject resistance R_S. With $R_A = 10$ MΩ and $V_A = V$, the current flowing in the circuit is 9.99 μA if the subject resistance R_S is at a very low value of 10 kΩ ($= 100$ μmho) and 9.75 μA if $R_S = 250$ kΩ ($= 4$ μmho). Thus, over the range of SRLs likely to be encountered in practice, simple choice of component values ensures a current variation of only 2.5%. The subject's resistance R_S is measured directly by measuring the potential difference across the electrodes arising from the passage of current ($V = IR$ where I is constant).

In the constant-voltage circuit (2) the value of R_B is low in comparison to the subject resistance, so that with the potential divider comprising R_B and R_S only a very small proportion of V_B appears across R_B, and the potential across the subject remains approximately constant and close to V_B whatever the current flow in the circuit. If we take the value for V_B of 0.5 V and $R_B = 100$ Ω, then the voltage across the subject varies from 0.4950 to 0.4998 V (i.e., 1%) as R_S varies from 10 kΩ to 250 kΩ, i.e., from 100 μmho to 4 μmho. The signal voltage appearing across R_B can, however, be considered rather small, 5.0 mV at 100 μmho and 0.2 mV at 4 μmho. It can be increased tenfold by increasing R_B to 1000 Ω. If this is done, however, the percentage variation in voltage with the same change in subject conductance as before is 8.6%. A larger signal can be obtained across R_B by doubling V_B. This, however, results in an increase in current through the 100 μmho subject of from 49.5 μA with $V_B = .5$ V; a figure within the linear range of voltage-current curves, to 99.0 μA, a value outside that range. The choice of value for R_B and V_B is clearly a matter of compromise and is limited by the level of amplification which is possible from succeeding stages in the polygraph. The practical circuit in the appendix adopts values of .5 for V_B and 200 Ω for R_B, giving a value of 100 μV per micromho (approximately) which is well within the capabilities of most modern polygraphs to enable a signal of 1 or 2 μmho per centimeter of pen deflection to be produced. A rough rule of thumb calculation for the value of the signal voltage obtained across R_B is that V_{sig} in μV/μmho $= V_B \times R_B$.

Another advantage of the constant voltage circuit is that the amplifier is always "looking at" a constant impedance source, and because this is low in relation to the normal input impedance of the amplifier, the latter will not provide a shunt pathway leading to error in measurement. In the constant current case the amplifier "looks at" a varying source, R_S, and under certain circumstances R_S may approach the input impedance of the amplifier in value resulting in error arising from a change in current through the subject by providing a shunt pathway. Edelberg (1967, p. 27) states that one of the advantages of the constant voltage system is that "the system in a sense is self correcting for peripheral effect of base level or response amplitude. Thus less gain change is required." This partly arises from the analysis earlier in this section showing that the addition of conductance units is independent of the level to which they are added. Lykken and Venables (1971), however, provide an analysis of a practical situation showing that to maintain a 1-μmho full-scale deflection as a subject's SCL changes from 10 to 5 μmho will require between 5 and 10 resettings of the suppression control, while with a constant current method 10 to 20 resettings will be required.

(ii) *The Problem of Measuring SCL and SCR Simultaneously.* Typically a subject may have an SCL of 20 μmho and a largest SCR on initial elicitation of the order of 1 μmho. Thus if the gain of the total recording system is set so that a full-scale deflection gives a reading of around 20 μmho, a change of 1 μmho is seen as an unreadably small deflection. Two solutions are available to suppress SCL and thereby enable the recording system to be operated with sufficient gain to allow a full-scale deflection for the largest SCR. These are (*a*) to record with a capacitatively coupled system which does not reproduce the voltage level across R_B in Fig. 7 corresponding to SCL but does allow the fluctuating potentials arising from SCRs to be recorded, or (*b*) to record with a directly coupled system but to suppress the voltage level corresponding to SCL by opposing it with a measured potential opposite in sign, that is, a backing off, bucking, or suppression voltage. There are advantages and disadvantages to both systems but the solution favored in this chapter is (*b*).

In the case of (*a*) no measure of SCL is possible unless some subsidiary steps are taken to provide a parallel measurement of this parameter. Systems are available (e.g., McGraw, Kleinman, Brown, & Korol, 1969) which provide a high-gain capacitatively coupled channel for measurement of SCR and a low-gain directly coupled channel for the measurement of SCL. With this solution either two channels are taken up on the polygraph or, as in the case of the circuit by McGraw *et al.* (1969), SCL is signaled by a voltage to frequency conversion circuit which presents "blips" on the SCR trace the frequency of which is linearly related to SCL. (It should be noted that this form of recording makes for difficulties if computer analysis of SCR is attempted.) The greatest difficulty with capacitatively coupled recording of SCR is, however, the possible distortion of the trace. Every capacitatively coupled system has a characteristic time constant; a system with a long time constant will reproduce slow changes in the signal. On the other hand, a short time constant will reduce and distort response to low frequency signals. Long and short time constants are long and short in relation to the characteristics of the signals involved. Edelberg (1967) recommends a time constant of at least 15 sec for the faithful reproduction of SCRs and even this may be somewhat short. If long recovery limbs (Edelberg, 1970) are of interest, their accurate measurement is important. The circuit as given by McGraw et al. (1969) has a time constant of 3 sec which, however, they say may be modified; a commercially available development of the McGraw et al. circuit has switched time constants of 1, 3, and 10 sec. Another attempted solution of the problem is that of Simons and Perez (1965) who present a circuit in which there is greater amplification of SCR than there is of SCL on the same trace. Unfortunately, the SCR is in effect amplified by a capacitatively coupled circuit and the whole system uses a constant current configuration.

Solution (b), using a suppression or backing off voltage, involves the insertion of a calibrated voltage between the signal resistor R_B in Fig. 7, and the following directly coupled amplifier. The operator thus notes on the recording chart the setting of the suppression control, which may be calibrated directly in micromhos, and the SCR appears as faithfully reproduced deviations about this line. As stated earlier, resetting this control is less frequent with a constant voltage device than with a constant current device. If it is undesirable that the setting be noted on the chart, it is an easy matter to reproduce the value of the setting control on a second channel or even with a voltage/frequency converter as used in connection with solution (a) above. In practice, little difficulty is found in the use of the simpler means of noting the setting on the chart. Where difficulty does arise, however, is if computer analysis of the trace is required. The computer may only be required to analyze SCRs without reference to SCL, in which case it must be told to ignore changes in the record brought about by resetting. If, however, SCL is to be taken into account in the analysis, then this must be signaled to the computer. At the moment, a solution which is simple and feasible is to type in the SCL values initially and at points through the record where a change is made unless these values are available separately on another channel of recording. The circuit provided in Appendix I employs direct coupling and a calibrated suppression control as suggested in this section.

Another form of constant voltage circuit is presented by Hagfors (1970) and has the same features of balancing SCL and showing SCR as a deviation around the set value of SCL. This circuit is shown in Fig. 8.

If $B_1 = B_2$, then the bridge will balance when $(I/R_S) + (I/R_{bal}) =$ (I/R_k), and no current will flow through input impedance of the amplifier R_{amp}. In conductance terms then $G_{subj} + G_{bal} = G_{cons}$, where $G_{subj} =$ SCL. Skin conductance responses are then shown as deviations from balance and can be subject to suitable levels of amplification. Another version of the Hagfors circuit is shown in Appendix I; it has the advantage of employing a low input impedance amplifier and is thus not subject to capacitative mains interference. Hagfors (1970) has reported that this form of circuit is most useful in group recording systems where there are extensive measuring leads likely to pick up hum.

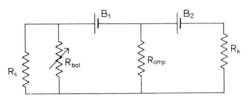

Fig. 8. Circuit for the measurement of skin conductance proposed by Hagfors (1970).

(iii) *ac versus dc Systems.* Thus far discussion has dealt exclusively with systems which involve the passage of direct current through the skin; on several occasions in the past the use of the passage of alternating current has been advocated. There are two main reasons for using ac: one is that it enables the investigation of capacitative elements in skin structure to be made; the second is the more practical one of attempting to combat polarization of electrodes caused by the passage of direct current. In relation to the first aspect McLendon and Hemingway (1930) and Lloyd (1960) provided evidence to suggest that mechanisms responsible for changes in skin conductance gave rise to parallel changes in capacitance and therefore that the independent status of capacitance was doubtful. Section IV.E.2 has presented discussion concerning the nature of skin capacitance. This is further emphasized by the work of Montagu (1964) reporting correlations of .99 between skin resistance and skin impedance measures using 60-Hz source. If then, the purpose of measurement of electrical activity of the skin is to provide indices of behavioral usefulness, there is possibly no reason to adopt the use of ac techniques on this account. This is not to deny the value of employing this methodology to investigate electrodermal mechanisms in their own right. The other point concerned with the polarization of electrodes is, however, more important in the use of electrodermal activity as a behavioral index. Edelberg (1967) suggests that skin impedance only behaves like skin resistance (in its role as a behavioral index) below about 200 Hz. Grings (1953) and Stephens (1961) provide data in accord with this. It is thus with passage of low frequency currents through the skin that we are concerned. The characteristics of electrodes are considered in a later section and although, for instance, the silver–silver chloride electrodes which are advocated there are generally excellent in use, it is virtually impossible to eliminate completely polarization caused by the passage of a direct current. Polarization may be defined as a counter electromotor force arising at the interface between the electrode and electrolyte which has the effect of reducing the current flow through the electrode and increasing the apparent resistance of the measuring circuit. While it would seem that the reversal of direction of current resulting from the use of ac might eliminate polarization, Lykken (1959) stated that this assumption did not hold for most metal–electrolyte combinations, nor within the range of frequencies in which SCR and SCL are observed. Subsequent work by Montagu and Coles (1968) suggested that this may not be so. They reported no detectable polarization with lead electrodes and the passage of 5-Hz currents as high as 2 mA for more than 1 hr. On this basis they advocate the use of a constant voltage system with a 5-Hz source of .1 V. The standard constant voltage circuit shown in Fig. 7 is applicable with V_B replaced by a source of ac. The voltage developed across R_B is rectified, smoothed, and then backed off by the insertion of a suppression voltage in the same manner as for the dc case. Edelberg (1967, Fig. 1.9, p. 32), is appropriate in this instance.

(iv) *Other Circuitry.* The discussion of units of measurement of exosomatic electrodermal activity will be taken up later. The use of log skin conductance has been advocated by some workers (Montagu & Coles, 1966). A circuit is available which provides a direct write-out in terms of log conductance (Kuechenmeister, 1970). Bearing in mind what has been said earlier in this section, it should, however, be noted that it uses the constant current principle.

(v) *Interference from Skin Potential.* At the same time as measuring exosomatic activity two electrodes on the skin surface may pick up endosomatic activity. In a constant voltage system the endosomatic potential will tend to divide in the circuit in the same manner as the battery voltage V_B (Fig. 7) and will thus contribute least to error of measurement if the signal resistor R_B is small in relation to R_S; the desirability of this has already been emphasized. The error introduced by SP is a function of its size relative to V_B and is an argument for keeping

V_B as large as possible consistent with maintaining the current through the skin within the limits described.

Interference from SP is no problem if an ac method of measurement is used and proposals have been made for simultaneous measurement of SC and SP through the same electrodes (Montagu, 1958; Tolles & Carberry, 1960). The most direct way of tackling interference from SP is, however, by the use of bipolar rather than unipolar placements of electrodes. The potential difference between two palmar sites tends to zero as does the change in that potential difference due to SPRs. If electrodes for measuring SCL and SCR are thus used with bipolar placement, the interference due to SP will be minimized, and in addition, as SC changes will take place under both sites rather than under one as in unipolar placement with one palmar and one inactive site, exosomatic activity will be maximized. The sites chosen should be those having most common SCR activity, that is, the fore and middle finger, or the ring and little finger or the corresponding palmar thenar or hypothenar palmar sites.

(vi) *Balanced versus Single-Ended Recording.* Normally the preamplifier and main amplifier recording chain of a polygraph employs differential amplifiers. With the use of these, neither input terminal is grounded and the in-phase rejection function of these amplifiers is operative. If, however, an SC measuring system is used in which one subject terminal is grounded, then not only does the in-phase rejection system become inoperative, but there is increased possibility of interference with other recording channels. Edelberg (1967, p. 37) represents an analysis of how this occurs. The circuits shown in Appendix I are not designed to work with one terminal grounded. A separate single ground or earth electrode will, however, normally be used (see Section V.C.1).

b. SKIN POTENTIAL MEASUREMENT. The concern here is to measure SPLs ranging in magnitude from 100 mV negative to about 30 mV positive at the palmar site with respect to an inactive forearm site. Varying about SPL are SPRs having negative and positive components with amplitudes up to 10 mV.

(i) *The Problem of Source and Amplifier Input Resistance.* For the purposes of measurement only, it is possible to represent skin potential as a voltage source in series with an internal or source resistance. When the skin is intact under both electrodes, this source resistance is of the order of 1 mΩ. The problem of measurement of SP is then an example of measurement of any potential from a high resistance source. If the input resistance of the measuring device is, for instance, equal to the source resistance of the skin potential, as it may well be using a standard polygraph preamplifier, then half the skin potential will be measured by the amplifier. This is because the source resistance and the input resistance of the amplifier may be considered to be a potentiometer divider which, with two equal resistances, divides the applied potential in half. There are two methods that change this state of affairs which are applied for other reasons. First, in order that a truly zero potential reference point may be produced against which to measure activity at the palmar site, the skin at another site, usually the forearm, is ruptured by skin drilling or sandpapering (see Section VI.C.2.a); this has the effect of reducing the source to 100 kΩ or less. This immediately has the effect of reducing the error of measurement from 50% as it was with intact skin to 10% (with a 1-MΩ input resistance amplifier). Second, the problem of measuring SPL and SPR is similar to that of measuring SCL and SCR in that there is a large, relatively invariant signal, with a small response signal imposed upon it. Again, the most common method of dealing with this situation is to oppose the SPL with an equal and opposite calibrated suppression or backing off voltage. The zero reading of the recording pen is then at the value of this backing-off voltage and the value of SPR, now recorded with an adequate gain, is measured as deviation from this voltage level. If the backing off is absolutely accurate and SPL is stable, then no current can flow in the circuit and the input resistance of the amplifier is effectively infinite. It may be calculated that even if the difference between the subjects and the backing off voltages rises as high as 5 mV, the effective input resistance of the circuit with an actual input resistance of 1 MΩ will be as high as 10 MΩ, and the error of measurement will fall to 1%. A formula for calculating the accuracy of measurement with various values of input resistance, source resistance, subject voltage, and backing off voltage is given by Venables and Martin (1967a, p. 88). Skin potential responses may of course be considered as mismatch voltage and will be inaccurately measured as a function of the lowness of the input resistance of the amplifier and the inaccuracy of backing off or voltage suppression.

In recent years, stable high input impedance preamplifiers have become available. These preamplifiers with field-effect transistor input stages have input impedance as high as 1000 MΩ, and with care they provide ideal means of measuring skin potentials. One point to which particular attention has to be paid when using these probes is in the adequate earthing of the subject. In the absence of a good earth or ground the high-impedance probe may measure the electrostatic charge on the subject which will vary in accordance with the type of clothing the subject is wearing and the dryness of his skin. Even with the use of a high input impedance probe, suppression of SPL is still a useful facility.

(ii) *Recording with Capacitatively Coupled Amplifiers.* As with SCR measurements, it is possible to measure SPRs by means of a capacitatively coupled amplifier. Here, as with SCR, the problem is that of the time constant available on the amplifier. There is a temptation to use an EEG preamplifier for SPR measurement. However, it is very rarely that a time constant as long as 15 sec will be available on such a preamplifier, nor is the input impedance usually high enough for the error caused by this factor to be acceptably reduced. It must be remembered that the EEG preamplifier is suitable for use with two abraded sites and hence a source impedance of around 5–10 kΩ; with one abraded site, as in SP measurement, source resistance rarely falls below 100 kΩ. On these counts either a circuit with voltage suppression or a very high input impedance probe is to be preferred.

(iii) *Voltage Suppression.* Practical voltage suppression, backing off or bucking cicuits are given in Edelberg (1967, Fig. 1.7, p. 30) and Venables and Martin (1967a, Fig. 2.7, p. 89). The Venables and Martin circuit provides a decade form of control, while the Edelberg circuit is suitable for accurate control if the 1-kΩ potentiometer is of the 10-turn type. It is useful to note that if the subject's terminals of an SP measuring system are short-circuited, the backing off voltage appears across the preamplifier and may be used for calibration.

(iv) *Temperature Compensation.* Differences in electrodermal activity due to changes in body temperature have been considered in Section V.A.3. Another point at which temperature differences have an effect is a purely electrothermal mechanism, and arises if the electrodes used in measurement are at different temperatures. Venables and Sayer (1963) examined the hand and forearm temperature of 26 subjects and found that while forearm temperature was remarkably constant over subjects (range 29.0–31.5°C), hand temperature ranged from 20.7 to 34.2°C. With Ag–AgCl electrodes and .5 g/100 ml KCl electrolyte, the potential produced by nonisothermal electrodes is about 450 μV/°C, the hotter electrode being positive. A mean error of some 2 mV might therefore be expected from this factor. The circuit shown in Fig. 9 may be used to eliminate automatically this source of error (Venables & Sayer, 1963). The thermistors, resistors with high temperature coefficient, Th_1 and Th_2 mounted in the same way as disk electrodes (see Section V.B.4) for built-in conjunction with the electrodes (see Miller, 1968) are placed alongside the hand and arm electrodes. They form two arms of a Wheatstone bridge and differences in temperature may be used to produce an out-of-balance voltage which may be adjusted to 450 $\mu V/^\circ C$. This voltage is inserted in series with the amplifier and backing off circuit and automatically compensates for the potential difference arising at the electrodes. The voltage–temperature relationship depends upon the nature and concentration of the electrolyte as well as the type of electrode used, and the operation of the compensation system should be determined empirically before use.

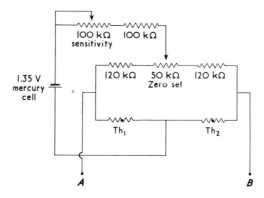

Fig. 9.   Circuit for compensating for potential produced by nonisothermal electrodes. (From Venables & Martin, 1967a, Fig. 2.5.)

4. ELECTRODES

a. BIAS AND POLARIZATION POTENTIALS.   Two characteristics of electrodes used in electrodermal measurement are (a) polarization potentials, and (b) bias potentials. The former is of major importance to conductance and the latter to potential measurement. Polarization potentials have already been considered in relation to the use of ac methods of measuring conductance. They are those potentials arising at the interface between electrode and electrolyte, due either to an energy barrier in the oxidation reduction interaction at the electrode surface, or to a limitation placed upon ion transfer by the rate of diffusion of ions to or from the interface (Hozawa, 1931), and result from a passage of current. The effect of polarization is the buildup of a counter emf which has the effect of an apparent increase in subject resistance. Bias potentials are a manifestation of the difference between electrodes such that their half-cell potentials with respect to the electrolyte are dissimilar. The bias potential is most easily measured by immersing a pair of electrodes in electrolyte of the concentration used in the electrode medium and measuring the potential with the same type of high impedance device as would be used to measure skin potential. It is usual for skin potential work to use electrode pairs having a bias potential of under 1 mV. More usually, pairs of electrodes with a bias of 100–250 μV may be used, thus making for only a small addition to percentage error in the total measurement procedure. Data are also available which show that electrode pairs with low bias potentials normally shown low drift of potentials with use. Polarization tendency is a characteristic which is independent of bias potential and must be tested for separately. Edelberg (1967, p. 7) presents several methods of testing for polarization; the simplest of these involves the knowledge of the characteristics of the electrolyte media used in measurement. As an example, the specific resistance of 0.1 N NaCl is about 100 Ω cm and thus if two electrodes each 1 cm^2 are placed in the solution 1 cm apart and a current of 10 μA passed through, then the predicted voltage across them will be 1 mV; deviation from this figure can be attributed to polarization. This polarization should be a small proportion of the imposed constant voltage, and should thus be not more than 5 mV if a figure of 1% error is to be maintained.

b. TYPES OF ELECTRODE. Examination of the available literature suggests that both bias and polarization potentials are lowest with reversible electrodes. These consist of a metal in contact with a solution of its own ions. Commonly used varieties in electrodermal research are Ag–AgCl and Zn–ZnSO$_4$. The latter is used with NaCl to form a liquid junction compatible with physiological salines. This has an additional error-producing interface between the ZnSO$_4$ and NaCl solutions. Using Zn–ZnCl$_2$ involves having zinc salts adjacent to the skin. Edelberg and Burch (1962) have reported an artificial potentiation of electrical activity of the skin by zinc salts. Both Edelberg (1967) and Venables and Martin (1967a), after considering a large amount of data, come to the conclusion that Ag–AgCl electrodes have many advantages and advocate their use. Grings (1973) and Lykken and Venables (1971) continue the advocacy of this type of electrode.

Three types of silver–silver chloride electrodes are commonly available; these are "disk," a silver disk with an electrolytic deposition of silver chloride on one surface (see Fig. 10); "sponge," a sponge of silver made by a thermal process and followed by an electrolytic deposition of silver chloride (see Fig. 11); and the "pellet," or sintered disk electrode in

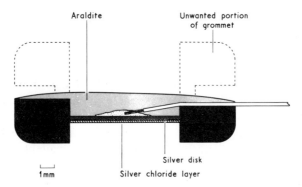

Fig. 10. Cross section of disk type silver–silver chloride electrode. (From Venables & Martin, 1967a, Fig. 2.9.)

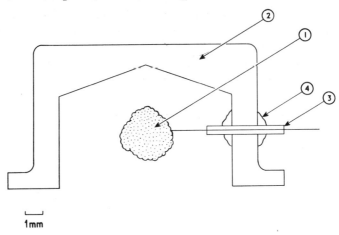

Fig. 11. Cross section of sponge type silver–silver chloride electrode: (1) Ag–AgCl sponge; (2) plastic "top-hat" electrode body; (3) silver lead wire; (4) resin cement. (From Venables & Martin, 1967a, Fig. 2.8.)

which the active element consists of a porous silver–silver chloride matrix. The first two types of electrode can be made in the laboratory, although the process of manufacture of the sponge electrode is tedious, and they can be bought commercially. If cost is a factor to be considered, the disk electrode is fairly cheap and straightforward to make; directions for its manufacture are given in Appendix II, or details of construction of a modified version by Miller (1968) can be followed. If facilities for making electrodes do not exist, however, it may be more satisfactory to buy electrodes, and in this case the pellet type is probably the best choice.

The disk type of electrode is sufficiently cheap to make to allow for the discarding of electrodes which do not meet criteria for low bias and polarization potentials when tested. With care in construction, bias potentials of 250 μV or less should be achievable and polarization potentials of 5 mV feasible. Manufacturers' figures for the pellet type of electrode are for bias potentials less than 250 μV and for polarization potentials as low as 5 μV. The development of polarization potentials may be minimized by using a large electrode to reduce current density. This is possible in the case of the forearm electrode if a unipolar method of recording is adopted for SC. If, however, the bipolar method as advocated here is used, electrode area is limited by the size of a relatively immobile site available on the palmar surface. Sponge electrodes have the advantage in this application in that the electrode itself inherently has a large area although the effective area in contact with the skin is limited by the opening of the "top hat" (see Fig. 11).

A fourth type of Ag–AgCl electrode is the silver cloth electrode advocated by Edelberg (1967, p. 13). This, like the sponge electrode, has a large surface area per unit of electrode site area and has been so satisfactory in use that Edelberg reported that he adopted it as the method of choice.

c. CARE OF ELECTRODES. (i) *Storage.* There is no unanimity of opinion about storage. It seems reasonable, and has proved so in practice, to store stocks of electrodes dry, but to allow them to soak for at least 24 hr in a solution of the electrolyte in which they are to be used before they are used for measurement. This allows adequate time for the electrolyte to penetrate into the interstices of porous or sponge electrodes.

(ii) *Shorting in Pairs or Groups.* Again, there is no unanimity of opinion on this procedure. With new electrodes there is probably some advantage in shorting them together during their first soakage so that currents generated by any local electrochemical reactions may be allowed to flow and equilibrium may be reached. Thereafter there seems to be little advantage in keeping electrodes shorted together.

(iii) *Cleaning.* In the case of disk electrodes particularly, it is very important not to rupture the silver chloride layer and expose the bright metal underneath. A large increase in bias potentials will result if this is done. Cleaning by a jet of water (e.g., via a polythene wash bottle) is all that is necessary, or desirable, although manufacturers of the pellet type of electrodes state that more vigorous cleaning with *nonmetallic* materials is allowable.

5. ELECTROLYTES

a. TYPES OF SALT. The electrolyte serves two purposes in electrodermal measurement. First it is the conductive medium in the interface
between electrode and skin, and second, in the case of skin potential
measurement, it is at least partly concerned with the generation of the
potential which is measured. It is important that it should be compatible
with the biological system with which it is in contact, and for that
reason either NaCl or KCl are the electrolytes of choice. Edelberg *et
al.* (1960) demonstrated potent effects of multivalent ions such as Ca^{2+},
Zn^{2+}, Al^{3+} on SCR activity and a lowering effect on SPL dependent
on the effective size of the ion. It is also important that the concentration
of the electrolyte used should not be markedly changed when it is contaminated by biological solutions such as sweat. On this basis Edelberg
(1967, p. 10) recommends the use of .05 M NaCl as an electrolyte.
Venables and Sayer (1963), employing the criterion of obtaining a wide
range of potentials which were of the same polarity (i.e., negative at the
palm) advocated the use of .5 g/100 ml KCl. (A .05 M solution of NaCl
contains approximately 2.39 g NaCl per 100 ml water while a .05 M
solution of KCl contains approximately .4 g KCl per 100 ml water.)
In practice, concentrations of either of these salts in the range specified
produce stable results. One theoretical reason for preferring KCl to NaCl
is that the ionic mobilities and temperature coefficients of these mobilities
for K^+ and Cl^- are approximately equal and should thus result in more
stable records in the case of SP measurement. In no case should commercial electrode jellies having near saturation concentrations of saline be
used for SP measurement and their use with SC measurement will result
in a continuous fall of SCL and SCR amplitude over time.

Finally, it should be noted that either NaCl or KCl are compatible
in use with Ag–AgCl electrodes.

b. ELECTROLYTE MEDIA. In the case of SP measurement, the effective
size of the electrode area is unimportant (see next section). In the
case of SC measurement, delineation of the effective electrode area is
of prime importance as SC measurements should be expressed in terms
of specific conductances (i.e., μmhos/cm^2). It is important, therefore,
to use an electrolyte–electrode system in which the area of contact
with the skin is stable and uniform. This is achieved partly by the
electrode mounting and method of attachment, but also partly by the
use of a viscous electrode medium.

Various thickening media may be used. Starch paste is prepared by
mixing 6 g/100 ml of electrolyte solution and bringing to the boil while

continuously stirring. After 30 sec the mixture is poured into containers and capped (Edelberg, 1967, p. 11). Agar-agar paste is made similarly with the use of 2 g agar-agar per 100 ml electrolyte. It must be stirred continuously while cooling, otherwise lumpiness will result [Venables & Martin, 1967a, p. 84]. Lykken has successfully used a commercial neutral ointment base as the viscous medium, but the electrochemical properties of the mixture have not been fully examined (Lykken & Venables, 1971). In no case should clay bases, such as kaolin or bentonite, be used because of their electrolyte content.

C. Procedure and General Methodology

1. Skin Conductance

a. Unipolar versus Bipolar Placement of Electrodes. By unipolar we mean the placement of the electrodes over one active site, i.e., a site showing electrodermal activity, and one inactive site, showing minimal activity or none (see Appendix III). The term bipolar implies placement over two active sites. There are several reasons for employing bipolar placement: (a) (as explained in Section III.B.3 and 5) bipolar placement minimizes interference of SC measurement by SP; (b) the use of two active sites means that changes in conductance are twice as large as with a single site; (c) there is no need for abrasion to achieve an inactive site, (d) with a constant voltage method of measurement, the voltage is divided approximately equally across the two sites and the figure for threshold for nonlinearity of .5 V *across a single site* recommended by Edelberg (1967) can therefore be doubled, thus allowing the use of a higher V_B (see Fig. 7) with consequent further improvement and size of signal and freedom from endosomatic contamination (see Section V.B.3). It is important that the two active sites should be on the same limb, otherwise heart artifact will be apparent. While bipolar placement appears to have the advantages outlined above, unipolar placement may be used if more convenient. This will particularly be the case if the subject has to indulge in some activity where hand movement artifact will be doubled by having two electrodes on the hands.

b. Sites and Preparation. Edelberg (1967, p. 15) presents a table showing the relative SCL and SCR of different parts of the body with respect to the commonly used palmar finger site. This table shows that the palmar surface of the hand has both higher SCR and SCL than the finger. He also draws attention to a particularly convenient site on the medial side of the foot over the abductor hallucis muscle adjacent to the plantar surface and midway between the first phalange and a point directly beneath the ankle. This has an SCL 1.26 times higher, and an SCR 1.70 times higher than the comparison site on the palmar finger surface.

For bipolar placement no preparation of the skin site is required other than washing. Although some authors recommend the use of a grease solvent such as acetone or ether prior to electrode placement, little effect can be noted. A fairly marked fall in conductance has, however, been noted with the use of soap and water. As some subjects will have washed their hands before coming to the laboratory, it is possibly advisable to standardize the procedure and ask all subjects to wash their hands before electrode application.

In the case of unipolar placement, it is necessary to achieve an inactive reference site. This is usually done by skin drilling (Shackel, 1959) or by sandpapering. Comparison of the two methods by Venables and Sayer (1963), with particular emphasis on SP measurement, suggested there was little difference between the two methods, and there is little doubt that sandpapering is less disturbing to most subjects. Drilling should be carried out with a dental burr drill; small battery-driven food or drink mixers provide suitable motive power. The criterion for depth of drilling is the achievement of a small shiny pit in the epidermis. Pasquale and Roveri (1971) propose the measurement of resistance at the drill point during drilling as a criterion for extent of abrasion. Sandpapering is normally carried out until a powdery dust of skin debris is formed in the case of dry skin, or a slight reddening is seen with moist skin. If abrasion is undesirable, as would be the case with young children, then sites of minimal electrodermal activity should be used as inactive sites. Edelberg (1967, p. 29) recommends the inner aspects of the ear lobe, a point over the ulnar bone and a point over the tibia. Of the three, the ear lobe site is most inactive, but may introduce EKG artifacts.

The side of the body to which electrodes are attached should be kept standard. The relation of electrodermal activity to handedness has been discussed in Section VI.A.

c. POLARITY. If a bipolar placement of electrodes as recommended above is used, then it does not matter in which direction the current flows between the two electrodes. However, this is important if a unipolar placement is adopted. Lykken et al. (1968) have reported an apparent SCL about 13% higher when the active site was positive than in the reverse condition. Their analysis of this finding suggests that this is due to the endogenous SPL either augmenting or reducing the applied voltage across the skin. In the case of bipolar placement with two active sites there should, however, be no difference in SPL between the two sites.

d. EARTHING OR GROUNDING. If bipolar placement, and an ungrounded circuit feeding a differential amplifier are used, then there may be no need to ground the subject specifically for the measurement of electrodermal activity. If hum artifact is a problem, then an earth electrode should be placed on an inactive site, abraded as detailed in the previous section, on the same side of the body as the active electrodes. It should be grounded to the earth terminal of the polygraph; If other psychophysiological measurements are carried out, it should be noted that there should only be one earth on the body; the placement of this will probably depend on the optimization of the weakest signal, which will almost certainly not be SCR or SPR.

e. EFFECTS OF ELECTRODE AREA. Blank and Finesinger (1946) showed that the effective electrode area was that area of the skin covered by electrode plus that covered by excess electrolyte or surface sweat. It is important therefore as conductance varies with effective electrode area to maintain that area constant throughout the experiment. It should be noted that the relative error due to seepage of electrolyte beyond the electrode depends on electrode size; 1 mm of seepage with a .5-cm diam electrode causes an area increase of 100%; the same amount of seepage with a 1.5-cm electrode will cause an increase in effective area of only 35%. Because of this and for other reasons already detailed, the size of electrode used should be the maximum compatible with the area of the hand available.

Various methods have been adopted for maintaining electrode area constant. In general, these may be divided into unmasked and masked techniques. In the former, the electrode itself has a defined rim as in the case of the disk electrode (see Fig. 10); it is applied fairly firmly and used with a viscous electrolyte. With this technique little seepage is observed and there is little indication of increase in electrode area. In the case of the marked site, some form of seal such as pressure-sensitive tape with a hole punched in it is applied to the site prior to electrode application. Another form of mask which has been used effectively is the corn plaster which in addition to acting as a mask also serves as an electrolyte chamber (Miller, 1968). Venables and Martin (1967a) expressed some doubt about the use of this technique as they observed a sudden breakdown of the adhesive surface of the pad and a rapid increase in electrode area after a time. More recently, double-sided adhesive disks have become available commercialy, and these serve both as mask and means of attachment. Provided that they are firmly fixed so that there is no seepage along palmar ridges under the adhesive, these appear to provide the ideal solution (see Day & Lippitt, 1964).

f. METHODS OF ATTACHMENT. The double-sided adhesive disk appears to be a method of choice, but otherwise attachment using plastic adhesive tape is satisfactory and provides a very firm attachment if a finger site is chosen. Zinc oxide tapes should not be used as these provide possible contamination of the electrode site. There is a danger when using a tape method of attachment round a finger that too great pressure will be put on the electrode area. Not only may blood flow be occluded, but changes in pressure may act to produce the local response of Ebbecke which may be mistaken for an SCR.

g. LONG-TERM RECORDING. The length of a recording session probably falls into three categories, "normal," that is, 15–60 min, "sleep," i.e., over a sleep period of 7–8 hr, and "long term," up to 10 or more days as in space programs. The problems imposed are quite different in each of these cases. Edelberg (1967, p. 39) discusses the last category fully and it will not be dealt with further here.

The problems involved otherwise are the possibility of skin irritation from contact with saline or with fixative, the possibility of the electrolyte drying out, and the effects of hydration of the skin. With the methods so far described, no problems of irritation or drying out should be encountered and the factor of hydration which remains is common both to normal and to sleep recording. Although there is work on the effect of hydration on skin potential (Fowles & Venables, 1970, 1971), there is no direct evidence of the effect of hydration due to electrolytes on skin conductance measurement. Fowles (1973) suggests that due to hydration of the corneum, an increase in SCL might be expected, while due to poral closure, a decrease in the sweat gland contribution might be expressed with a fall in SCL. Clearly, a ready extrapolation from these suggestions is not easy. It is, however, likely that poral closure will bring about a diminution in SCR amplitude, the sort of finding reported by Edelberg (1967) from empirical testing of the effects of long-term electrode attachment (see also Section V.A).

h. TEMPERATURE EFFECTS. The effect of laboratory temperature on comfort has already been discussed in a previous section (V.A); provided sufficient time is allowed for the subject to feel comfortably warm, no difficulties should be experienced. While the degree to which the subject is clothed, and the extent to which he is occupied in a task are obvious factors to be taken into account in adjusting environmental temperature, a room temperature of about 21–25°C is generally to be recommended. As stated earlier, in Section V.B.3.b(iv), hand temperature may vary from about 20–34°C and over this range, parameters of SCL and SCR may change markedly. Maulsby and Edelberg (1960) reported that SRL increased by about 3% for each drop in temperature of 1°C. Skin conductance response, however, shows a more complicated relation involving changes in amplitude with changes in temperature which then return to control level as temperature is stabilized. If, however, temperature falls below 20°C, SCR amplitude falls progressively and responses may disappear entirely. Changes in latency, time to peak amplitude, and length of the recovery limb are also shown, all times being extended as temperature falls (Floyd & Keele, 1936; Carmichael, Honeyman, Kolb, & Stewart, 1941; Smith, 1937).

i. INTERACTION WITH TWO OR MORE CHANNELS OF SC RECORDING. To investigate site differences in SCL and SCR, it is necessary to simultaneously record with two or more channels. Interaction between channels will be shown if they have common elements. It is usual in many polygraphs to use an internal power source for constant current or constant voltage which will then be common to all channels. To overcome this trouble, V_B (Fig. 7) should be an independent cell in each case and the circuit recommended in Appendix I incorporates this feature. Interaction may also be experienced if a single-sided method of recording is used with one side of the input earthed or grounded. For this reason bipolar recording is recommended.

2. SKIN POTENTIAL

a. SITES AND PREPARATION. As outlined in Section V.B.3.b(i), it is necessary to record skin potential in a unipolar fashion, one electrode being over an active and the other over an inactive neutral reference site. For the active site, a palmar or plantar placement is usually chosen; the palmar surfaces of the fingers tend to show a lower SPL (about 2 mV) than the palm proper. If the latter area is used, then the thenar or hypothenar eminences are suitable. On the foot, the site over the abductor hallucis muscle previously mentioned as being preferred for SC recording is also useful for SP, showing nearly palmar values of SPL and higher than palmar values of SPR. Whatever site is used should be chosen to avoid obvious cuts and skin blemishes which might disrupt the normal state of the skin under the electrode. Little effect can be shown by cleaning with grease solvents, but washing with soap and water has a marked effect and so should be adopted by all subjects to eliminate variance due to those subjects who come to the laboratory having, or not having, washed their hands. While no effects of grease solvents such as acetone or ether are apparent when used immediately before recording, chronic usage of these solvents does appear to lead to lower SPL, while subjects, such as butchers, who work in constant contact with fat tend to show higher then normal SPLs.

In the case of the inactive site, it is desirable to rupture the skin to achieve both a neutral reference site and to reduce source resistance. The methods of drilling and sandpapering have been already discussed in Section IV.C.1.b in relation to unipolar recording of skin potential. While drilling is probably easier and quicker, it is rather disturbing to some subjects, and equally good results may sometimes be achieved by sandpapering with the finer grade of "flour" paper. Montagu and Coles (1966) report variable results using sandpaper and suggest with Venables and Sayer (1963) that the only satisfactory method is to measure the resistance of the site. As it is not desirable to pass current through a site before measuring potential, an indirect method of measuring source resistance is necessary. The technique is as follows: the subject's SPL is accurately measured, a variable resistance is then placed across the subject's terminals and adjusted until the amplifier records exactly half that previously measured. In this condition half the SPL appears across the source resistance and half across the variable resistance. These two resistances must therefore be equal. If this value is 100 kΩ or less, abrasion may be considered to be adequate. It should be noted that this relationship only holds if the input resistance of the amplifier is effectively infinite. If a high input impedance probe is used, the measurement will be satisfactory; if not, the backing off in measurement of both potentials must be accurately carried out. An inactive site on the forearm is most convenient; experience has shown that a site two-thirds of the distance from wrist to elbow on the volar surface, avoiding blemishes and underlying blood vessels, gives satisfactory artifact-free recording (see Appendix III).

There is no effect of electrode size on SP measurement and hence it is not necessary to take quite the same precautions to restrict effective electrode area as there is with SC recording. Nevertheless, the same electrodes and methods of attachment may be used and a standardized procedure for all electrodermal recording is advocated.

b. EARTHING OR GROUNDING. As SP should be recorded with a differential amplifier, with neither electrode grounded, in-phase rejection of unwanted signals should be good. However, the use of a nonabraded, and hence high resistance, active site will cause some imbalance. It may be necessary, therefore, to earth or ground the subject with a separate electrode. If other channels of psychophysiological recording are made, only one ground electrode should be used.

c. TEMPERATURE EFFECTS. The elimination of artifacts due to the use of nonthermal electrodes has already been mentioned (Section V.B.3). Nevertheless, overall skin temperature is of importance. If, as suggested in Section V.B, at least one factor involved in the production of SPL is a membrane or liquid junction system, then it is probable that a temperature effect of some 200 $\mu V/°$ might be expected over the range of skin temperatures likely to be encountered. As with SCR, the latency and form of SPR is temperature dependent (see Yokota, Takahashi, Kondo, & Fujimori, 1959). Because of these effects, it may be thought desirable to monitor skin temperature. Suitable methods are discussed by Trolander (1967).

3. THE RECORDING OF SP AND SC AT THE SAME TIME

If the methods advocated above for the recording of SC and SP are used, little difficulty should be experienced in recording SC and SP at the same time. If it is convenient to use separate hands, then the possibility of interaction is minimized.

Montagu (1964) showed that it was possible to measure exosomatic and endosomatic activity simultaneously through the same electrode by using an ac measurement of conductance (strictly admittance). In this instance he used a 60-Hz source for admittance measurement, but there is no reason to believe that the 4-Hz ac that he and Coles (1968) later advocated would not provide similar results. Edelberg (1967, p. 42) gives further details of a similar method.

It is possible also to measure SC using SPL as the source of current. The principle involved is that used in measuring source resistance of SPL described above (Section IV.C.2.a). It was shown there that the shunt resistance across the subject's terminals which caused the measured SPL to drop by one half was equal to the source or internal resistance. Edelberg (1967) shows that any shunt may be used to calculate the internal resistance by the following equation:

$$R_i = \frac{V_o - V_s}{V_s} \times R_s,$$

where R_i = internal resistance, R_s = shunt resistance, V_o is the measured potential in absence of the shunt, and V_s is the potential with the shunt in circuit. Again, it is important that a high impedance method of measurement of SPL be used. Lykken *et al.* (1968) similarly have shown the possibility of such a method, and in a comparison of SCL measured in this way and SCL measured by the standard constant voltage method, have shown a high correlation ($r = .997$) between the two measures across subjects and a median correlation of .93 for data obtained within subjects.

4. SC AND SP: INTERFERENCE WITH AND FROM OTHER CHANNELS

Theoretically and in practice there should be no interference between channels of a polygraph if these involve direct connections between differential amplifiers and pairs of electrodes having equal tissue resistances underneath them, neither of them being grounded. It is in departures from this ideal state that interferring factors arise. In the case of skin conductance, out-of-balance conditions tend to be set up by the flow of exosomatic current. However, provided that the whole SC circuit is free-floating and uses separate batteries, no difficulty should be experienced, although switching artifacts on other channels may occur when the SC channel is switched on. Similarly, switching in and out of suppression or backing off voltages in SC and SP channels may cause artifacts until balance is achieved.

Probably the most likely artifact in multichannel recording is likely to occur from the EKG. This of course occurs if recording of SP or SC is made with electrodes on opposite hands, but a much more intractable problem occurs in channels with electrodes on limbs and the single earth electrode on the head, or in channels with electrodes on the head with the earth electrode on the arm. Artifacts are more likely to appear in any channel when out-of-balance electrode contacts with the skin are present, and on the whole it can be said that good techniques throughout will minimize interference.

5. MOVEMENT ARTIFACTS

Movement artifacts occur when there is change in the intimacy of contact between electrode and skin. It is important in order to minimize this, to ensure that the cup of the electrode is completely filled, that no air space is left, and that the attachment of the electrode to the skin is intimate. To achieve the last condition, it is important to choose sites where the skin under the electrode does not move with muscular activity or with the pulse of blood flow. Finger sites are to be recommended as well as the thenar or hypothenar eminence, in contrast, for instance, to the·center of the palm where the electrode may easily lose contact with the skin. A compromise must, however, be achieved between a firm and a tight method of attachment; with the latter even a slight movement may cause a pressure response (Ebbecke response) having some features which make it difficult to distinguish it from a normal SCR. Edelberg (1967) recommends splinting the hand or finger if movement artifacts are a problem and also placing the electrodes on the nonpreferred hand which is less used for both intentional and spontaneous movements.

Movement artifacts are also caused by the movement of the limb and attached electrode leads through a magnetic field. Elimination of this sort of artifact demands foresight in planning a laboratory and its setting as far as possible away from such things as elevators, centrifuges, and refrigerators with motors having a large magnetic field. However, in the absence of ability to remove these sources of interference, reorientation of the subject may often result in a large improvement.

D. Data Collection

1. SUBSIDIARY APPARATUS

a. TAPE RECORDERS. Even in these days of more sophisticated methodology, it is probably still good advice to recommend that a paper record of electrodermal activity be taken as a routine procedure in order that it may be annotated with range changes, changes in suppression voltage, the existence of loud extraneous noises, restlessness of the subject, and the like, in addition to providing an opportunity to monitor artifacts. However, the tedium of scoring large numbers of records of electrodermal activity may now be relieved by the use of a laboratory computer. It is often more convenient to store the data on magnetic tape prior to computer analysis rather than to take up real time on the computer by using it on-line.

The requirements of a suitable tape recorder are that it should be able to reproduce low-frequency signals from dc to a few hertz (5 Hz might be considered a maximum). This normally presupposes the use of an FM (frequency modulation) system, although other forms of modulation are possible but not in common use. It is necessary to have a low impedance output from the polygraph to feed into the tape recorder and if one is not available then additional circuitry may be necessary to provide this. Even if only one channel of electrodermal activity is measured, a second tape recorder channel is usually required on which signals, temporally related to the stimuli presented to the subject, may be recorded in order that time parameters of responses may be measured. It is important that these signals should be of a form capable of providing an accurate identifiable trigger for a computer. Artifacts such as pinholes or dropouts caused by defects in the coating of the magnetic tape generally produce a negative-going spike. It is important, therefore, to ensure that any trigger signal recorded on the tape should be positive-going and the program written to work with these only. The recording of electrodermal activity itself should be made with care so as not to overload the channel; it is always possible, within limits, to amplify a recording that is of an inadequate level, but it is impossible to deal with large signals that exceed the recording level of this system. One very valuable advantage of an instrumentation tape recorder is that the original record may be made at a very low speed (particularly in the case of electrodermal data which do not demand high frequency response); playback into the computer may then be at a faster speed, thus saving computer time. However, care should be taken over two points; it is important to check that the integrity of the trigger signal is maintained at higher tape speeds, and also that when interstimulus intervals are considered in time, sufficient time elapses between the responses resulting from these stimuli for the necessary computer operations to take place.

b. COMPUTERS. Practical use of computers to analyze electrodermal records demands that these records be broken up into sections of time. If the SCR to a definable stimulus is being analyzed, then the section of time for analysis may be identified in relation to that stimulus. If, however, spontaneous SCRs are being measured, then sections of time will have to be defined arbitrarily. In the first case of elicited response, the section of time must be long enough to include the whole of the response and should thus be about 20 sec as a minimum. If, in addition, a period of prestimulus record is to be analyzed, then say 25 sec of record will be the period which is analyzed. If the program demands that these data be written out on tape for later analysis, this process might take about 5 sec, thus making a total period of 30 sec which is to be considered as the intertrial period. If, to save computer time, periods of tape-recorded record are fed in at faster than real time speeds, then it may be necessary (if possible) to stop and start the tape recorder with computer control while the computer "dumps" digitized data.

Input of electrodermal data to the computer, either directly or via an instrumentation tape recorder, necessitates analog to digital conversion, and this process places limits on the signal which can be dealt with. Digitization of the analog signal depends on the design of the

A–D converter. A typical model might, however, deal with a ± 1 V signal in units of 4 mV, giving an accuracy of 2%. This accuracy will only hold, however, if the signal occupies the full scale of ± 1 V. It is important, therefore, to work with signals which closely approach, but do not exceed, this value. It must also be recognized that with this typical A–D converter the signal which does not exceed ± 2 mV will not be quantized. These limitations necessitate accurate work by the electrodermatologist to ensure that the signal with which he is working falls within the ± 2 mV to ± 1 V range. Care should be taken to consult the manuals of the A–D converter so that those figures similar to these typical ones are be determined before use. One major problem with the use of computers in the analysis of electrodermal data is that of telling the computer about changes in backing off or changes in gain. One way of dealing with the problem might be to record one channel of low gain, giving a record of SCL or SPL and one channel at high gain giving a record of SCR or SPR, or, alternatively, to feed into the computer via a subsidiary circuit the setting of the backing off control. In practice, however, it is possible to tell the computer about intertrial gain and backing off changes when the whole record has been fed in, these changes having been noted on the polygraph record (or separately) at the time of the recording.

c. TELEMETRY. In contrast to ECG and EEG, few attempts appear to have been made to telemeter electrodermal data. In part this is owing to the existence of marked movement artifacts when recording from the ambulant subject, and in part the difficulty in accurate telemetry of dc data. The simplest form of telemetry which would be suitable for use with electrodermal data codes the dc and low-frequency data in terms of a signal whose frequency varies with the voltage level of the electrodermal input—exactly in the same way in which frequency modulation of the signal is employed for instrumentation tape recording. This signal may then be sent by radio or telephone to a receiver where it is demodulated for analysis. The accuracy of the signal frequency transmitted in relation to the amplitude of the electrodermal signal is dependent upon the stability of the oscillator used in the telemetry transmitter. There is an incompatibility between the requirements of small size of the portable transmitter and the stability of the transmitter. One way, however, in which a practical system may be achieved is by arranging for the subject's terminals to be short circuited periodically (e.g., by a small clockwork mechanism or by respiration; see Wolff, 1967) so that a reference value may be transmitted for comparison with the signal value of any stimulus.

d. Group Studies. Hagfors (1970) has presented details of work with group registration of skin conductance measures. No fundamental modification of circuitry for measurement of skin conductance using constant voltage methodology is required for group registration, as parallel connection of subjects can be viewed as analogous to sweat glands in parallel. Because subjects are connected in parallel, an open circuit connection on one subject does not give rise to artifactual recording of the remainder. The circuit (shown in Appendix I) recommended by Hagfors (1970) is particularly suitable for group work because its basically simple and low resistance design helps to eliminate capacitative interference which is possible when there are long trailing leads, which are unavoidable in group work. Another suitable circuit is provided by Edelberg (1967, p. 44). Hagfors (1970) uses two similar channels of recording, with his group divided into two halves; by this means either one channel may be seen as a replication of the other, or alternatively the division of the group may be by subject characteristics so that the group differences immediately become apparent. Similar end results may be obtained if the data obtained from subjects exposed to an absolutely identical series of stimuli are subsequently combined by computer techniques. The insights into group differences produced by these means may give rise to essential analyses which might not otherwise have been contemplated.

2. Treatment of Data

a. Skin Conductance. (i) *Amplitude Measurement.* The case for direct measurement of exosomatic electrodermal activity in terms of conductance by the constant voltage method has been strongly advocated in earlier sections (IV.E and V.B) Data will thus be obtained in micromhos; however, since conductance varies directly with electrode area, all measurements should be reported as specific conductances, that is, as micromhos per square centimeter. If a bipolar placement is used as suggested in Section V.C.1.a, and each electrode is applied to an intact skin area of equal size, then the effective electrode area for reporting specific conductance will be half that under a single electrode. Thus if two 1-cm^2 electrodes produce a measured conductance of 10 μmho, the specific conductance is $10/.5 = 20$ μmho/cm^2. Or, putting it another way, this is the conductance which would be obtained if only one single skin area of 1-cm^2 area were used. If a unipolar arrangement is employed, then the effective electrode area is that area of intact skin under the active electrode as it may be assumed for the purposes of measurement that the drilled reference site has a conductance of hundreds of micromhos. Consequently the measured conductance is divided by the area of the single active electrode.

Apart from the physiological reality of measuring exosomatic activity in terms of conductance, several other advantages accrue. Lykken and Venables (1971) show, for instance, that when skin conductance is measured as advocated in Section V.B.3.a(ii), with SCR measured at a high gain and the conductance due to SCL being suppressed by a backing off control, then the number of resettings of that control will be about half of those required when using a constant current measuring equivalent values of SRR directly and suppressing value of SRL.

A most dramatic demonstration of the relative stability of SCR measurements (hence not requiring range, or gain change resettings) is given by Lader (1970) who presents data showing decline in responses measured in conductance and resistance units as a result of atropinization. In the case of the conductance data the decline is orderly while the SRRs vary wildly before reaching an eventual zero value. In view of what has been discussed earlier (Section V.D.1) about the necessity not to exceed full-scale deflection when using tape recorders and computers, the comparative ease with which this may be achieved when using conductance measures speaks for itself. If the only apparatus which is available does use a constant current method and the primary data are in terms of resistance, then these data may of course be transformed into conductance units using tables of reciprocals. For those workers more used to thinking in terms of resistance measurement, some marked values are worth remembering. For instance, about the lowest SRL obtainable, 10 kΩ, is equivalent to 100 μmho, an average SRL of 50 kΩ is equivalent to 20 μmho, and a large SRL of 250 kΩ is equivalent to 4 μmho.

Over the years, measurement in terms of log skin conductance has been suggested. In the present state of knowledge there seems to be no particular physiological reason for using this measurement as there is for preferring skin conductance to skin resistance. This being so, the only reason for transforming data to log skin conductance measures seems to be to obtain a more normal distribution of data for statistical purposes. In most cases SC data appear to be fairly normally distributed, and in view of the general robustness of normal parametric statistics, transformation usually appears to be unnecessary.

Following a suggestion first made by Paintal (1951), Lykken and his colleagues (Lykken *et al.*, 1966) have put forward a strong case for expressing a subject's skin conductance (or indeed any psychophysiological measure) in terms of his range of values on that variable. Lykken *et al.* (1968) report, for instance, that the minimum SCL shown by one subject after 30 min of rest was nearly twice as high as the maximum shown by another subject while blowing up a balloon to bursting. It would not be sensible to suggest that the first subject was more aroused then the second, hence the evident requirement to express each subject's conductance values in terms of his own maximum–minimum scale. The formula for achieving this when measuring skin conductance level is given by Lykken *et al.* (1966) and is

$$\phi_{\mathrm{SCL}_x} = \frac{\mathrm{SCL}_x - \mathrm{SCL}_{\min}}{\mathrm{SCL}_{\max} - \mathrm{SCL}_{\min}}.$$

In this, SCL_x refers to SCL measured on the particular occasion of interest. However, while the principle is appropriate and easy to state, putting it into practice is less easy as it involves obtaining values of $\mathrm{SCL}_{\min}$ and $\mathrm{SCL}_{\max}$. Lykken has found that the procedure of blowing up a balloon until it bursts is reasonably effective for producing a maximum value, but obtaining a minimum value does present problems. One possible criterion is to use the occasion at which BSPL (basal skin potential level) is obtained (see Section V.E.5, and Christie & Venables, 1971a) as a reference time for the measurement of simultaneously recorded SCL. (The time of BSPL is easy to measure as it is at a point of inflexion in the fall of SPL as the subject relaxes, after which a rise in SP is seen.) At this time no (or minimal) sudorific activity is present. Originally, Lykken and his colleagues suggested that SCRs should be corrected in the same way as SCLs by dividing the measured SCR by the same denominator as that in the formula above. However, as Lykken and Venables (1971) point out, this procedure assumes that the mechanisms underlying SCL and SCR are identical, and as outlined in Section IV this view is untenable. Because of this, Lykken and Venables (1971) advocate the correction of an SCR by dividing it by the maximum SCR value obtained by the subject at some other time during the session; hence

$$\phi_{\mathrm{SCR}_x} = \frac{\mathrm{SCR}_x}{\mathrm{SCR}_{\max}}.$$

Because there is no need to measure $\mathrm{SCR}_{\min}$ which is clearly zero and $\mathrm{SCR}_{\max}$ is not so difficult to obtain, the use of range correction for responses is easier than for levels. The inclusion of one loud noise, a shock or a deep breath during the session will probably elicit a maximal response and even the first stimulus of a series of orienting tones frequently produces the maximum response obtained during the session. It has been found in practice that SCRs corrected for range by $\mathrm{SCR}_{\max}$, and SCRs corrected by the use of SCL range, only correlate by about .60, so that the two methods evidently produce different results. It should be noted that both these range correction methods result in data values between 0 and 1.

(ii) *Latency Measurement.* The measurement of latency of SCR from a paper record is a matter of compromise of two conflicting requirements. First in order to measure latency accurately it appears to be necessary to use a fast paper speed. Unfortunately when this is done the slope of the leading edge of the SCR is so shallow as to present difficulty in the clear identification of the point of inflection. Because of this, it is probably not possible to measure latency from a primary paper record with an accuracy of better than 1/10 sec. By differentiating the primary wave form, the point of rate of change of slope may be more accurately determined. However, if better accuracy is required, the use of a computer with a program that effectively differentiates the primary wave form and identifies the point of change of rate is to be recommended. In addition, hardware circuitry is available which differentiates the primary input, identifies the point of inflexion, and uses this and the stimulus input time to operate a conventional timing circuit (Brooke & Hill, 1970).

(iii) *Measurement of the Recovery Phase.* The recovery limb of the SCR has as a first approximation, an exponential form (Darrow, 1937b) and as such its rate constant, or in reciprocal terms its time constant, is independent of amplitude. Thus mathematically, as well as for physiological reasons, there is reason to think of the recovery phase as having status independent of the amplitude of the reponse. This is in contrast to the onset phase where the slope has been shown (Edelberg, 1967, p. 36) to be closely related to the amplitude of the SCR. Edelberg (1970) advocates two methods for quantifying recovery phase. One is the "half-time" measure, that is, the time taken to 50% recovery (which is linearly related to the time constant defined as the time taken to 63% recovery). It is most easily measured by the use of a transparent overlay scale as described by Edelberg (1970, p. 529). The scale consists of a set of horizontal parallel lines crossed by a single vertical line. The central horizontal line is longer than the rest and contains a metric scale on the right-hand side of its intersection with the vertical line, this intersection having zero value. The scale is moved up and down until the central horizontal line is midway between the onset and peak values of the response. This distance for the vertical line (at peak response) to the point of intersection of the central parallel line with the recovery phase may then be measured. This method can, of course, only be used with responses which recover at least 50% before a second response occurs.

The half-time measure is more appropriate for use with curvilinear recordings when the vertical line on the template may be made curvilinear; correction for curvilinearity of recording is more difficult with the curve-matching procedure and Edelberg recommends that the method is restricted to rectilinear recordings or to the middle third of the curvilinear scale. Interrater reliability checks carried out on the more subjective curve-matching procedure indicated that the method was very reliable (Kendall's $W = .93$). There was a close relationship between independent scoring of the same responses by the half-time and curve-marking procedures ($r = .94$).

More automatic methods are discussed by Edelberg in an unpublished paper. These are based on consideration of the exponential form of the recovery phase. When C is a value of conductance, then $dC/dt = kC$, where k is the rate constant of the change in conductance and t ($= 1/k$) is the time constant (measured by the curve-matching procedure, or by the half-time measure which is equal to $.7t$). From the above equation $k = -C/C'$ where C' is the slope of C or its first derivative. From this k can be derived by taking the slope and amplitude at any point on the exponential position of the recovery limb—that is, beyond the inflection point after the peak of the response. The amplitude at this point is, however, highly related to peak amplitude which may be more objectively measured. Peak amplitude is, as mentioned above, in turn closely related to the maximum value of the first derivative of the onset limb. It can also be shown that C' may be measured by the maximum value of the first derivative of the recovery limb. Using a differentiating circuit, these two values may be obtained and k the rate constant measured. In practice, when using a differentiating circuit it is necessary to use a top-cut filter set at about 2 Hz with a steep rolloff in order to eliminate noise which is exaggerated by the differentiating circuit. The principles described can be used in computer programs written to give measure of recovery rate.

b. SKIN POTENTIAL. (i) *Measurement of SPR.* Skin potential responses may be commonly uniphasic negative and biphasic with initial negative and secondary positive components; and less commonly uniphasic positive and negative, positive, negative triphasic. About the only aspect that can be unequivocally measured is the latency of the first response using the methods which are appropriate for latency of SCR. In the case of the amplitude of the negative wave this is frequently attenuated by the onset of the after-coming positive wave and even when the wave form appears to be uniphasic negative it is impossible to say how much of this is attenuated by a positive-going process which is, however, of insufficient size to drive the wave form in a positive direction. The amplitude of the positive phase is more likely to be uncontaminated as it is possible that the negative process is completed by the time the peak of the positive response is reached. The latency of the positive phase may only be estimated by extrapolation of the onset limb of that phase to that value of SCL before the response complex started. There seems to be little basis for using as a measure of amplitude the difference in potential between the peaks of the negative and positive component. As a tool for behavioral use it seems preferable to suggest that if it is necessary to measure responses, then SCR presents fewer problems. If, however, there is need to indicate certain aspects of the electrodermal process, then concurrent recording of SCR and SPR has much to commend it. The coincidence of fast recovery limb of the SCR and the positive component of SPR is an example of such usefulness.

(ii) *Measurement of SPL.* A minimum value of SPL (basal SPL: BSPL) is obtained in a resting subject with minimal sudorific activity, and may be either positive or negative at the palmar site with respect to an indifferent reference electrode. It is obtained usually after 5–20 min (mean time = 12 min) and appears as a minimum point of inflection after which the record becomes progressively more negative. Maximum SPL does not universally appear to be obtained in conditions which it would be thought produced the highest arousal. Lykken *et al.* (1968) report that balloon stress which brought about an increase in SCL, brought about a decrease in SPL. There thus appear to be opposing processes around the maximum and minimum values of SPL which give rise to recordings that are nonlinear functions of either rising or falling arousal as indexed by SCL. Care should thus be taken to examine fully the total record from which any measure of SPL is taken.

There seems to be no case for treating endosomatic activity in units of measurement other than millivolts. Data from Shapiro and Leiderman (1964) suggest that a normal distribution of values is obtained, although this may not be the case in low levels of activity where some subjects are without sudorific activity and have achieved BSPL, others also still exhibiting sudorific activity and have higher SPLs because of lack of habituation.

c. The "Law of Initial Value." There is hardly any topic in the psychophysiological literature that has engendered more controversy than the "law of initial value," that is, that the size of a response is related to the level from which it starts.

There are at least three aspects to the problem. One is concerned with "apparent law of initial value" and is dependent upon the choice of units for the measurement of electrodermal activity. The second, related to the first in practice, but not in logic, is the statistical "necessity" to eliminate a relationship between response amplitude and tonic level so that the responses of subjects having different levels may be compared. The third consideration has nothing necessarily to do with the first two but asks the question "is it reasonable, physiologically, to expect that there should be a relation between response size and tonic level?" This question, too, bifurcates and requires consideration of the idea that response amplitude may be limited by some ceiling value above which the peripheral process cannot rise, or alternatively that there is some opposing (central) processes which limits extent of responding.

In the last case the balanced operation of a doubly innervated system is presupposed, thus the expectation that the doubly innervated cardiac system exhibits the law of initial value is confirmed in practice. In the case of electrodermal activity there is no evidence of antagonistic double innervation at the periphery. There may, however, be the possibility of ceiling effects. There are, for instance, finite numbers of sweat glands and finite extent of hydratable tissue under an electrode, so that a ceiling effect is to be expected in skin conductance measurement. Similarly, the extent of membrane and electrolyte pump processes is limited so that in potential measurement a ceiling effect is to be anticipated. Ceiling effects do not, however, automatically give rise to the law of initial value (LIV) phenomenon, and the controversy centers more around the statistical and artifactual nature of the problem.

Throughout the chapter the use of skin conductance has been advocated; one of the consequences of this is to remove an artifactual source of LIV. Skin conductance units are additive and the size of response due to adding a conductance unit (say another parallel sweat gland pathway) does not depend upon the existing level of conductance ($G_3 = G_1 + G_2$, where G_3 is the new value of skin conductance arising from an addition of a value G_2 to an existing SCL, G_1). If, however, the same operation is performed in resistance terms, the extent of the response is dependent upon the level of resistance before the response $[(1/R_3) = (1/R_1) + (1/R_2)$ or $R_3 = (R_1 R_2 / (R_1 + R_2))$; where R_3 is the new value of skin resistance arising from the addition of a value R_2 to an existing SRL, R_2; R_3 is clearly a function of $R_1]$. Much of the search which went on in the 1950s for a unit of response measurement which was independent of tonic level and which empirically rejected resistance in favor of conductance need have looked no further than the mathematics involved.

Lykken and Venables (1971) examine a further determinant of phasic-tonic correlation. From the material already reviewed in Section IV, and discussed in Section V.D.a (i), it is evident that there are wide individual differences in range of SCL. Momentary skin conductance as measured will, it is suggested, be some function of the product of central excitation (y) and some peripheral reactivity (z), that is, SC = $f(y \times z)$. If there is a linear relation between SC and central excitation, then $SC_i = K + y_i z$ where SC_i and y_i represent skin conductance and central excitation at the ith occasion in time. If central excitation increases and there is a phasic change in SC_i to SC_j, then SCR = $SC_j - SC_i = Z(y_j - y_i)$. (The assumption is made of an independence of z and y which is probably incorrect, but the example serves to illustrate the point.) If z remains constant, then within individuals SCR and SCL will not be correlated, but if z differs between subjects, between subject correlations will be inflated by this factor. The range correction methods described in Section V.D.2.a(i) result in a reduction in the importance of this factor by eliminating the effect of differences in z. Whatever relation now remains between SCR and SCL is a "real" relationship which it may not be sensible to neglect. There is every possibility of a physiological reason why tonic and phasic measures should be related. This relation need not, however, be artifactually inflated by the choice of units or methods employed in analysis. Hord, Johnson, and Lubin (1964) provide data which support the analysis above showing that LIV is not found with electrodermal data measured in conductance terms. They do, however (but unfortunately for the wrong reasons), suggest that LIV is apparent with resistance measurements. Skin potential measurement has not generated the degree of controversy in relation to LIV which skin conductance measurement has. Bearing in mind the difficulty in measuring SPR which has just been described, the most important question is whether change in SPL is related to the SPL from which the change is made. Shapiro and Leiderman (1964) provide data which show that SPL change is not related to SPL. In general, therefore, there would seem to be no reason to apply methods for "undoing" LIV when electrodermal data are involved. If, however, on examination relations do exist between change scores and initial and final values of the variables, analysis of covariance should be used provided *that the assumptions underlying it are not violated* (Benjamin, 1967).

VI. Summary: "What Can Be Inferred from Measures of Electrodermal Activity?"

If the methods of measurement and the experimental controls which have been used are inadequate, the answer to the question in the summary title could very well be "nothing but error variance." However, assuming that a reliable and stable measure has been obtained, there is a legitimate case for considering electrodermal activity to be a piece of behavior, albeit covert, in its own right. Phasic activity may, therefore, be used, for example, as a response which may be conditioned without considering the physiological substratum which underlies it.

There tends, however, to be a practical, if not a logical difficulty in staying strictly at this level of analysis if some knowledge of underlying physiology is required for correct methods of measurement to be applied. In contrast to this strictly behavioral approach, this chapter has adopted the viewpoint that electrodermal activity may be considered as an index of something else; but even after all the data presented in Section IV have been digested, it is not all that easy to say what. One clear aspect of the analysis is that there are a number of measures that can be derived from electrodermal recording, and it is necessary to separate these before further statements can be attempted.

In Section III four basic measures were outlined; these were SCL, SPL, SCR, and SPR.

On the face of it, the simplest measure is probably SCL, which may be viewed as a continuum reflecting the number of active sweat glands, and to some extent their immediately past activity in hydrating the corneum.

In the case of SPL, it has been suggested (see Section IV.E.5) that this electrical measure may reflect two aspects of physiological activity. At low levels of SPL (or BSPL if the lowest possible level achievable, with no evident sudorific activity, is reached) the main determinants would seem to be ionic concentrations of potassium or sodium in the epidermis. At higher levels, in the presence of sudorific activity, SPL is probably largely determined by the extent of sodium pumping in the lumen of the sweat ducts, and by the hydration of the elements acting as short-circuit pathways to those voltage sources (see Section IV.E); there is thus one continuous measure acting as an index for two separate mechanisms.

In the case of SCR, three measures are commonly used: these are latency, amplitude, and recovery rate; there does not seem to be any case for considering latency as an independent measure (see Section VI.D.2.a); however, recent work using recovery rate (Edelberg, 1972b; Furedy, 1972; Lockhart, 1972) suggests the value of this measure as an index of activity which is independent from other aspects of the SCR. The most difficult measure to quantify, as has already been stated (Section VI.D.2.b), is SPR, and it is probably worth considering only its latency, and the presence or absence of negative, positive, and possibly second negative components; their quantification, however, is uncertain. In the case of both response measures, and it is most unusual not to find both appearing coincidentally, the frequency of their appearance, either elicited or unelicited has been used.

Appendix I: Recommended Circuits for Skin Conductance Measurement

A. Circuit Developed from the Principles Embodied in Fig. 7 and Section VI.B.3

The circuit to be described embodies the constant voltage method of measurement of skin conductance, together with the suppression method of dealing with SCL advocated in Section VI. It is a development of the circuits presented in Lykken (1968) and Lykken and Venables (1971). The circuit will work conveniently with any polygraph which has a dc preamplifier having adequate sensitivity. If reference is made to Fig. 7 R_B in that circuit is R_{11} in the present circuit with a value of 200 Ω and V_B in that figure is the potential appearing across R_{10} which is adjusted to be 0.5 V. Following the analysis of the principles involved, which were outlined in Section IV.B.3.a(i), the potential developed across the output terminals (SW5 in the operate position) will be 100 μV per μmho. With a dc preamplifier having a maximum sensitivity of 10 μV/cm, a sensitivity of .1 μmho/cm will then be achievable.

1. Description of Circuit

The complete circuit is shown in Fig. 12 and the external appearance of a version made up on a Beckman-Offner Type 9801 blank coupler chassis is shown in Fig. 13. Component values are given in Table 2.

The output connections shown on the RH side of Fig. 12 are for general use; for connection to pins 2 and 3 of a standard Grass input plug connector; and to the rear plug connections on the Beckman-Offner coupler. Two mercury cells are incorporated, the left-hand one in conjunction with the potential divider R_9 and R_{10} provides the "constant" voltage source V_B (see Fig. 7). The right-hand cell in conjunction with R_{14}, R_{15}, and R_{16} supplies the suppression voltage to oppose that voltage arising across R_{11} (R_B) which is proportional to SCL. Both cells are switched on by the operation of the relay from the low-voltage dc source provided by the polygraph and are thus automatically disconnected when the polygraph is switched off. If such a source is not available

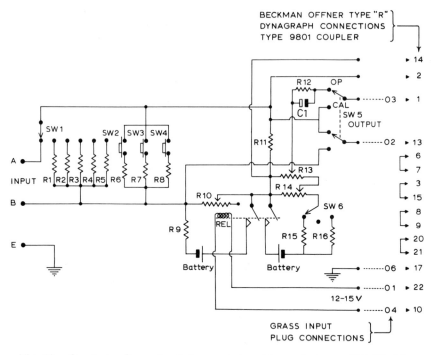

Fig. 12. Constant voltage circuit for measuring skin conductance. (Modified from Lykken, 1968.)

TABLE 2

VALUES OF COMPONENTS IN CIRCUIT SHOWN IN FIG. 12

R1	50 kΩ	±1%	R9	120 Ω	
R2	100 kΩ	±1%	R10	200 Ω	Trim pot
R3	200 kΩ	±1%	R11	200 Ω	±1%
R4	500 kΩ	±1%	R12	10 Ω	±1%
R5	1 MΩ	±1%	R13	500 Ω	10 Turn pot
R6	200 kΩ	±1%	R14	200 Ω	Trim pot
R7	500 kΩ	±1%	R15	10 kΩ	±1%
R8	2 MΩ	±1%	R16	100 kΩ	±1%

Batt.	1.35 V mercury cell
Cl.	500 μF 3 V
SW1	Input selector Subj — 20–10–5–2–1 μmho
SW2	Min push "5 μmho"
SW3	Min push "2 μmho"
SW4	Min push ".5 μmho"
SW5	DPDT Min "Cal-Operate"
SW6	SPDT Center off Supp range 10–100
Rel	DPST Reed

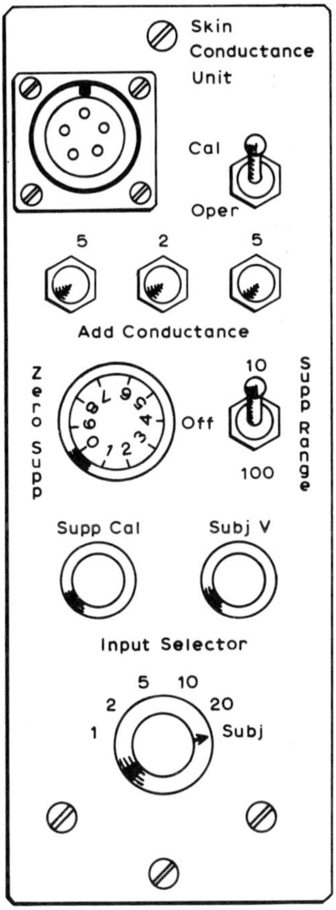

Fig. 13. Layout of panel for constant voltage skin conductance circuit (Fig. 12).

then the relay should be replaced by a double pole switch. Switch 1 is used to connect either the subject, or one of a set of dummy subjects across the input; this is the input selection switch in Fig. 13. Additionally SW_2, SW_3, and SW_4, the "add conductance" press buttons, may be used to check calibration when actually running a subject by adding either .5, 2, or 5 μmho to whatever conductance is being measured. Switch 5 in the CAL position switches the potential across R_{10}, the "constant voltage," across the input terminals of the preamplifier. By this means the polygraph may be used to check that this constant voltage is in fact .5 V (some preamplifiers are not able to cope with a signal as large as this and the voltage may have to be checked externally). This voltage may be adjusted by R_{10}; "Subj V" in Fig. 13. Switch 5 in the operate position connects the input of the polygraph across R_{11}, the "signal" resistor Switch 6 ("Supp range" in Fig. 13) determines the

range of suppression control available by R_{13} ("zero suppression" the
ten-turn potentiometer in Fig. 13). Calibration of this control is by R_{14},
the "Supp cal" control in Fig. 13.

2. OPERATION

N.B. It is most important that any backing off, or balance voltage
control *on the preamplifier* should be set at zero; otherwise false readings
will be obtained.

CALIBRATION OF SENSITIVITY
1. Set input selector to "subj"—open circuit.
2. Set supp range to "off."
3. Set Cal-Operate switch to "Cal."
4. Set polygraph to measure .5 V or, if this is not possible, use digital
   voltmeter or oscilloscope to measure .5 V.
5. Adjust "Subj V" control to obtain .5 V.

Alternative method and/or check for Steps 1–5:

6. Set Cal-Operate switch to "Oper."
7. Set input selector to 10 μmho.
8. Set suppression range switch to "off."
9. Set polygraph to measure 1 mV/cm.
10. Adjust "Subj V" to obtain 1-cm deflection.
11. Check that other values give appropriate deflections, e.g., that
    20 μmho produces a 2-cm deflection.
12. Set input selector switch to 1 μmho and polygraph to read 100
    μV (.1 mV) per centimeter. Check that 1-cm deflection is ob-
    tained. Pressing the .5-μmho "add conductance" button should
    produce an additional .5-cm deflection.

CALIBRATION OF SUPPRESSION
The "zero suppression" control may be set so that an appropriate
range of expected values of SCL may be suppressed. The procedure
to be described is for one (out of many) setting of the range of suppression. The example in this instance is to cover a range of 50 μmho
on the ten-turn zero-suppression potentiometer, so that each turn will
correspond to 5 μmho, and each dial figure to .5 μmho.

13. Set Cal-Operate switch to oper.
14. Set input-selection switch to 20 μmho.
15. Set polygraph to read 1 mV/cm; a 2-cm deflection should be
    obtained.

16. Set supp-range switch to 100.
17. Turn zero suppression potentiometer four turns (i.e., to correspond to 20 μmho when 10 turns = 50 μmho).
18. Turn "supp cal" control until zero deflection is obtained.
19. Check calibration by switching input selection to 10 when two turns of the zero suppression potentiometer should zero the pen.

Note that the suppression control is independent of the sensitivity of the amplifier.

To demonstrate this:

20. Turn input selector to 20 μmho, turn zero suppression potentiometer four turns; pen should zero.
21. Set gain of polygraph to 100 μV/cm. Pen should remain on zero.
22. Press 2 μmho "add conductance"; a 2-cm deflection should be obtained. Note that this is equivalent to having an SCL of 20 μmho and an SCR of 2 μmho.

OPERATION
23. Set polygraph sensitivity to 5 mV/cm; the system is now operating at 50 μmho/cm.
24. Set input selector switch to Subj; read subject's SCL.
25. If in the range 0–50 μmho, operate zero suppression control to zero pen; note value on this control.
    (If not in the range 0–50, steps 13–19 will need to be repeated to obtain a suppression range of say 0–100 μmho. Experience will determine this range which will depend upon the type of subject and situation employed.)
26. Increase gain of polygraph to 100 μV/cm which is equal to a sensitivity of 1 μmho/cm. Increase or decrease gain as appropriate to obtain an SCR which occupies about 75% of the full-scale deflection.

B. Circuit Proposed by Hagfors[4]

The circuit shown in Fig. 14, with the values of components shown in Table 3, is a practical version of that shown in Fig. 8.

Hagfors states that this circuit is very suitable for use with low input impedance operational amplifiers and that because of the general simplicity of its construction and low input impedance, it works well when

[4] From Hagfors (1970).

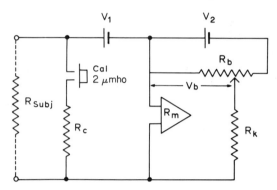

Fig. 14. Constant-voltage circuit for measuring skin conductance, suitable for use with group studies. (After Hagfors, 1970.)

TABLE 3

VALUES OF COMPONENTS IN CIRCUIT SHOWN IN FIG. 14

R_C	.5 MΩ
R_B	1 kΩ 10-turn pot
R_K	10 kΩ
R_M	Operational amplifier with approx. 100-Ω input impedance
V_1 and V_2	1.35-V mercury cells

used with groups of subjects connected in parallel (see Section VI.D.4) where there is a large likelihood of hum pickup from trailing leads.

With 1.35-V mercury cells at V_1 and V_2, .675 V appears across each site and bipolar recording is thus necessary.

In operation, the current flow through R_{subj} and R_M produces a potential difference across R_M, and equal and opposite potential is produced by the current flow through R_L and R_M due to a proportion of the voltage V_2 appearing across R_B (= V_B).

R_B is initially calibrated by the use of dummy subject resistors placed across the input and the setting of R_B then acts as suppression control to eliminate SCL. The sensitivity of the amplifiers following R_M are adjusted to provide suitable deflections corresponding to SCR, which can be checked by the switching in of the 2-μmho calibrating resistor R_C.

Appendix II: Construction of Electrodes

The method proposed here is for the construction of the silver–silver chloride electrodes, shown in Fig. 10; it is essentially the same as that given in Venables and Sayer (1963) and Venables and Martin (1967a). Details of construction of a modified form of this type of electrode are given in Miller (1968). No constructional details are given for the sponge type of electrodes, which are difficult to make in the average psychological laboratory and also are commercially available. Should details of construction of sponge electrodes be required, they are obtainable in Venables and Martin (1967a, pp. 94–95).

Construction of Ag–AgCl Disk Electrodes

A size which has been found suitable for skin potential measurement is given first, with a size suitable for SC measurement second.

1. Cut disks 5/16 ($\frac{1}{2}$) in. in diameter from 0.020-in. thick 99.99% pure soft silver sheet. This is most easily accomplished in a miniature press.
2. Wash disks for 10 min in 2 N HCl to remove any trace of iron left by the cutting process.
3. Wash in distilled water and lay on filter paper.
4. Solder a lead, for example, 7/0.004 8-in. tinned copper wire, P.V.C. insulated to one face of disk, *great care being taken not to let the solder run to edge of disk.* Scrape off excess flux and wash in methylated spirit to dissolve any remaining flux.
5. Set silver disk in rubber ring of appropriate size (halves of electric wiring grommets are convenient).
6. Drop resin cement (Araldite) into the back of the ring until a slightly convex surface is obtained.
7. Electrolytically etch the silver surface by making the disk the anode in an electroplating cell using a silver nitrate solution with a silver cathode. A current of 1 A is passed until it is seen that the top layer of silver is removed and a grayish white crystalline surface revealed.
8. Wash electrodes in distilled water and place in .5 g/100 ml KCl or NaCl solution.
9. Chloride a batch of six electrodes by making them the anodes in a fresh KCl or NaCl solution. Use a silver cathode and a current of .5 mA (1.25 mA) per electrode for 1 hr.
10. Wash electrodes in distilled water and place with leads shorted together in a fresh KCl or NaCl solution to age for a day.
11. Reject electrodes showing a potential difference between a pair of greater than 100 μV when taken off short circuit. Reject those having a potential difference of greater than 100 μV after being open circuited for 1 hr.

Appendix III: Recommended Electrode Placements

Figure 15 shows the sites referred to in Sections VI.C.1 and 2. For skin conductance measurement, a bipolar placement is recommended. The sites shown on the medial phalanges of the fingers avoid the greater

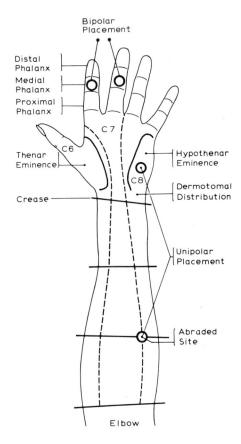

Fig. 15. Recommended placements of electrodes for measuring SC and SP.

incidence of cuts on the distal phalanges. The two electrodes should be placed on either the second and third fingers or the fourth and fifth fingers and not on other pairs of fingers which cross the dermatomal distribution. The pattern of activity is slightly different between dermatomes, and a cross dermatomal placement will thus not avoid the interference of SCR from SPR which is otherwise one of its valuable features.

For skin potential measurement a unipolar placement is essential. One inactive reference electrode should be placed on an abraded site on the forearm and the other active electrode on the palm, while a site on the hypothenar eminence as shown in Fig. 15 is very suitable. A site on the fingers can equally well be used.

Acknowledgments

We would like to thank the following people for their invaluable help in the preparation of this chapter: Reg. Hayes, for drawing Fig. 2; Chris Cromarty, for the preparation of the remainder of the figures; Ron Shaw and Brian Aviss, for technical help in the preparation of circuits; Dr. Edna Lawrence, for advice on the physiology of the skin; and particularly Mrs. Patricia Caple for the preparation of the typescript. The chapter was written while in receipt of a grant from the Social Science Research Council.

General References

Readers who are unfamiliar with the electrical concepts used in this chapter may find the following recommended texts on basic electrical knowledge useful:

Grob, B. *Basic Electronics.* New York: McGraw-Hill, 1965.

Malmstadt, H. V., Enke, C. G., & Toren, E. C. *Electronics for Scientists.* New York: Benjamin, 1963.

Margerison, J. H., Binnie, C. D., & Venables, P. H. Basic physical principles. Chapter 1. In P. H. Venables & I. Martin (Eds.), *A manual of psychophysiological methods.* Chapter 1. Amsterdam: North-Holland Publ. 1967.

Sidowski, J. B., & Smith, M. J. Basic instrumentation. In J. B. Sidowiski, *Experimental Methods and Instrumentation in Psychology.* Chapter 2. New York: McGraw-Hill, 1966.

Whitfield, I. C. *An introduction to electronics for physiological workers.* London: Macmillan, 1960.

Worcester, R. *Electronics.* London: Hamlyn, 1969.

References

Adams, T. Characteristics of eccrine sweat gland activity in the footpad of the cat. *Journal of Applied Physiology,* 1966, 21, 1004–1012.

Adams, T., & Vaughan, J. A. Human eccrine sweat gland activity and palmar electrical skin resistance. *Journal of Applied Physiology,* 1965, 20, 980–983.

Andrew, W. Structural alterations with aging in the nervous system. *Journal of Chronic Diseasess* 1956, 3, 575–596.

Ax, A. F. Editorial. *Psychophysiology,* 1970, 7, 1–2.

Ax, A. F., & Bamford, J. L. Validation of a psychophysiological test of aptitude for learning social motives. *Psychophysiology,* 1968, 5, 316–332.

Back, K. W., & Bogdonoff, M. D. Buffer conditions in experimental stress. *Behavioral Science,* 1967, 12, 384–390.

Back, K. W., Wilson, S. R., Bogdonoff, M. D., & Troyer, W. G. Racial environment, cohesion, conformity, and stress. *Journal of Psychosomatic Research,* 1969, **13,** 27–36.

Bagshaw, M. H., & Benzies, S. Multiple measures of the orienting reaction and their dissociation after amygdalectomy in monkeys. *Experimental Neurology,* 1968, **20,** 175–187.

Bagshaw, M. H., Kimble, D. P., & Pribram, K. H. The GSR of monkeys during orienting and habituation and after ablation of the amygdala, hippocampus, and inferotemporal cortex. *Neuropsychologia,* 1965, **3,** 111–119.

Baitsch, H. Uber geschlechts und seitendifferenzen im "Niveau"—elektrodermatogramm. *Confine Neurologica,* 1954, **14,** 88–100.

Bakan, P. Time-of-day preference, vigilance and extraversion-introversion. In D. N. Buckner & J. M. McGrath (Eds.), *Vigilance: A symposium.* New York: McGraw-Hill, 1963.

Bell, B. Personal communication, 1971.

Bell, B., Christie, M. J., & Venables, P. H. Menstrual cycle variation in epidermal potassium. In preparation, 1973.

Benjamin, L. S. Facts and artifacts in using analysis of covariance to "undo" the Law of Initial Values. *Psychophysiology,* 1967, **4,** 187–206.

Blake, M. J. F. Temperament and time of day. In W. P. Colquhoun (Ed.), *Biological rhythms and human performance.* London: Academic Press, 1971.

Blank, I. H., & Finesinger, J. E. Electrical resistance of the skin. *Archives of Neurological Psychiatry,* 1946, **56,** 544–557.

Bligh, J. A thesis concerning the processes of secretion and discharge of sweat. *Environmental Research,* 1967, **1,** 28–45.

Bloch, V. Nouveaux aspects de la méthode psychogalvanique ou électrodermogaphique (E.D.G.) comme critère des tensions affectives. *Année Psychologique,* 1952, **52,** 329–362.

Bloch, V., & Bonvallet, M. Contrôle cortico-reticulaire de l'activité électrodermale, (réponse psychogalvanique.) *Journal de Physiologie* (Paris), 1959, **51,** 405–406.

Bloch, V., & Bonvallet, M. Le contrôle inhibiteur bulbaire des réponses électrodermales. *Comptes Rendues de la Société de Biologie.* 1960, **154,** 42–45. (a)

Bloch, V., & Bonvallet, M. Le déclenchement des résponses électrodermales à partir du système réticulaire facilitateur. *Journal de Physiologie,* 1960, **52,** 25–26. (b)

Botwinick, J., & Kornetsky, C. Age differences in the acquisition and extinction of the GSR. *Journal of Gerontology,* 1960, **15,** 83–84.

Brooke, G., & Hill, G. B. A comparison of two tranquillisers using the Synaptic Latency Meter (a new technique.) *World Medical Instrumentation,* February, 1970.

Broverman, D. M., Klaiber, E. L., Kobayashi, Y., & Vogel, W. Roles of activation and inhibition in sex differences in cognitive abilities. *Psychological Review,* 1968, **75,** 23–50.

Brown, C. C. Psychophysiology at an interface. *Psychophysiology,* 1966, **3,** 1–7.

Brown, C. C. A proposed standard nomenclature for psychophysiological measures. *Psychophysiology,* 1967, **4,** 260–264.

Brožek, J. Psychorhythmics: A special review. *Psychophysiology,* 1964, **1,** 127–141.

Buchsbaum, M., & Harris, E. K. Diurnal variation in serum and urine electrolytes. *Journal of Applied Physiology,* 1971, **30,** 27–35.

Bullough, W. S. The rejuvenation of the skin. *Journal of the Society of Cosmetic Chemists,* 1970, 31, 503–520.

Bush, I. E. Chemical and biological factors in the activity of adrenocortical steroids. *Pharmacological Reviews,* 1962, 14, 317–445.

Campos, J. J., & Johnson, H. J. Affect, verbalization and direct fractionation of autonomic responses. *Psychophysiology,* 1967, 3, 285–290.

Cannon, W. B. *The wisdom of the body.* London: Kegan Paul, 1939.

Carleton, H. M., & Short, R. H. D. *Schafer's essentials of histology.* New York: Longmans, Green, 1954.

Carmichael, E. A., Honeyman, W. H., Kolb, L. C. & Stewart, W. K. A physiological study of the skin resistance response in man. *Journal of Physiology* (London), 1941, 99, 329–337.

Chalmers, T. M., & Keele, C. A. The nervous and chemical control of sweating. *British Journal of Dermatology,* 1952, 64, 43–54.

Christie, M. J., & Venables, P. H. Characteristics of palmar skin potential and conductance in relaxed human subjects. *Psychophysiology,* 1971, 8, 523–532. (a)

Christie, M. J., & Venables, P. H. Basal palmar skin potential and the electrocardiogram T-wave. *Psychophysiology,* 1971, 8, 779–786. (b)

Christie, M. J., & Venables, P. H. Effects on "basal" skin potential level of varying the concentration of an external electrolyte. *Journal of Psychosomatic Research,* 1971, 15, 343–348. (c)

Christie, M. J., & Venables, P. H. Sodium and potassium electrolytes and "basal" skin potential levels in male and female subjects. *Japanese Journal of Physiology,* 1971, 21, 659–668. (d)

Christie, M. J., & Venables, P. H. Site, state, and subject characteristics of palmar skin potential levels. *Psychophysiology,* 1972, 9, 645–649.

Christie, M. J., & Venables, P. H. Diurnal variation in "basal" skin potential level. In preparation, 1973.

Collins, K. J. The action of exogenous aldosterone on the secretion and composition of drug-induced sweat. *Clinical Science,* 1966, 30, 207–221.

Collins, K. J., & Weiner, J. S. Endocrinological aspects of exposure to high environmental temperatures. *Physiological Reviews,* 1968, 4, 785–839.

Collins, K. J., Crockford, G. W., & Weiner, J. S. Sweat gland training by drugs and thermal stress. *Archives of Environmental Health,* 1965, 11, 407–422.

Collins, K. J., Sargent, J. F., & Weiner, J. S. Excitation and depression of eccrine sweat glands by acetylcholine, acetyl-β-methylcholine, and adrenaline. *Journal of Physiology* (London), 1959, 148, 592–614.

Colquhoun, W. P. (Ed.), *Biological rhythms and human performance.* London: Academic Press, 1971.

Conklin, J. E. Three factors affecting the general level of electrical skin resistance. *American Journal of Psychology,* 1951, 64, 78–86.

Conn, J. W. The mechanism of acclimatization to heat. *Advances in Internal Medicine,* 1949, 3, 373–393.

Conroy, R., & Mills, J. *Human circadian rhythms.* London: Churchill, 1970.

Crounse, R. G. Keratin and the barrier. *Archives on Environmental Health,* 1965, 11, 522–528.

Culp, W. C., & Edelberg, R. Regional response specificity in the electrodermal reflex. *Perceptual and Motor Skills,* 1966, 23, 623–627.

Dalton, K. *The menstrual cycle.* Harmondsworth: Penguin Books, 1970.

Darrow, C. W. Sensory, secretory, and electrical changes in the skin following bodily excitation. *Journal of Experimental Psychology*, 1927, **10**, 197–225.

Darrow, C. W. The functional significance of the galvanic skin reflex and perspiration on the backs and palms of the hands. *Psychological Bulletin*, 1933, **30**, 712.

Darrow, C. W. The galvanic skin reflex (sweating) and blood pressure as preparatory and facilitative functions. *Psychological Bulletin*, 1936, **33**, 73–94.

Darrow, C. W. Neural mechanisms controlling the palmar galvanic skin reflex and palmar sweating. *Archives of Neurological Psychiatry*, 1937, **37**, 641–663. (a)

Darrow, C. W. The equation of the galvanic skin reflex curve. I. The dynamics of reaction in relation to excitation "background." *Journal of General Psychology*, 1937, **16**, 285–309. (b)

Darrow, C. W. The rationale for treating the change in galvanic skin response as a change in conductance. *Psychophysiology*, 1964, **1**, 31–38.

Darrow, C. W., & Gullickson, G. R. The peripheral mechanism of the galvanic skin response. *Psychophysiology*, 1970, **6**, 597–600.

Day, J. L., & Lippitt, M. W. A long-term electrode system for electrocardiography and impedance pneumography. *Psychophysiology*, 1964, **1**, 174–182.

Denton, D. A. The study of sheep with permanent unilateral parotid fistulae. *Quarterly Journal of Experimental Physiology*, 1957, **42**, 72–95.

Denton, D. A. Evolutionary aspects of the emergence of aldosterone secretion and salt appetite. *Physiological Reviews*, 1965, **45**, 245–295.

de Traverse, P. M., & Coquelet, M-L. Variations nychthémérales du rapport sodium/potassium dans la saline et l'urine. *Biologie Comptes Rendus*, 1952, **146**, 1099–1102.

Docter, R. F., & Friedman, L. F. Thirty-day stability of spontaneous galvanic skin responses in man. *Psychophysiology*, 1966, **2**, 311–315.

Edelberg, R. Electrophysiologic characteristics and interpretation of skin potentials. USAF School of Aerospace Medicine Technical Documentary Report, No. SAM-TDR-63-95, 1963.

Edelberg, R. Independence of galvanic skin response amplitude and sweat production. *Journal of Investigative Dermatology*, 1964, **42**, 443–448.

Edelberg, R. Response of cutaneous water barrier to ideational stimulation. *Journal of Comparative and Physiological Psychology*, 1966, **61**, 28–33.

Edelberg, R. Electrical properties of the skin. In C. C. Brown (Ed.), *Methods in psychophysiology*. Baltimore, Maryland: Williams & Wilkins, 1967.

Edelberg, R. Biopotentials from the skin surface: The hydration effect. In W. Fedor (Ed.), *Bioelectrodes. Annals of the New York Academy of Sciences*, 1968, **148**, 252–262.

Edelberg, R. The information content of the recovery limb of the electrodermal response. *Psychophysiology*, 1970, **6**, 527–539.

Edelberg, R. Electrical properties of the skin. In H. R. Elden (Ed.), *A treatise on skin*. Vol. I. New York: Wiley, 1971.

Edelberg, R. The electrodermal system. In N. S. Greenfield & R. A. Sternbach (Eds.), *Handbook of psychophysiology*. New York: Holt, 1972. (a)

Edelberg, R. Electrodermal recovery rate, goal-orientation and aversion. *Psychophysiology*, 1972, **9**, 512–520. (b)

Edelberg, R., & Burch, N. R. Skin resistance and galvanic skin response. *Archives of General Psychiatry*, 1962, **7**, 163–169.

Edelberg, R., & Wright, D. J. Two galvanic skin response effector organs and their stimulus specificity. *Psychophysiology*, 1964, **1**, 39–47.

Edelberg, R., Greiner, T., & Burch, N. R. Some membrane properties of the effector in the galvanic skin response. *Journal of Applied Physiology*, 1960, **15**, 691–696.

Edison, A. E. U., & Lloyd, D. P. C. Action of adrenaline on sweat glands and sudomotor transmission. *Journal of Physiology*, 1970, **210**, 164–165P.

Eliott, T. R. The action of adrenaline. *Journal of Physiology* (London), 1905, **32**, 401–466.

Eysenck, H. J. *The biological bases of personality.* Springfield, Illinois: Thomas, 1967.

Fascio, J. C., Totel, G. L., & Johnson, R. E. Antidiuretic hormone and human eccrine sweating. *Journal of Applied Physiology*, 1969, **27**, 303–307.

Féré, C. Note sur des modifications de la résistance électrique sous l'influence des excitations sensorielles et des émotions. *Comptes Rendus Société de Biologie*, 1888 (Ser. 9), **5**, 217–219.

Flaherty, B. (Ed.), *Psychophysiological aspects of space flight.* London and New York: Oxford Univ. Press, 1961.

Floyd, W. F., & Keele, C. A. Further observations of changes of potential and E.M.F. recorded from the human skin. *Journal of Physiology* (London), 1936, **86**, 23–25P.

Foster, K. G. Effects of bretylium, guanethidine, and bethanidine on the cat's sweat pad glands. *Journal of Physiology* (London), 1967, **190**, 21P.

Foster, K. G. Factors affecting the quantitative response of human eccrine sweat glands to intradermal injections of acetylcholine and methacholine. *Journal of Physiology* (London), 1971, **213**, 277–290.

Foster, K. G., Ginsburg, J., & Weiner, J. S. Adrenaline and sweating in man. *Journal of Physiology* (London), 1967, **191**, 131–132P.

Foster, K. G., Ginsburg, J., & Weiner, J. S. Role of circulating catecholamines in human eccrine sweat gland control. *Clinical Science*, 1970, **39**, 823–832.

Fowles, D. C. Mechanisms of electrodermal activity. In R. F. Thompson & M. M. Patterson (Eds.), *Methods in physiological psychology.* Vol. 1: *Bioelectric recording techniques,* Part C, *Receptor and effector processes.* New York: Academic Press, 1973.

Fowles, D. C., & Venables, P. H. Endocrine factors in palmar skin potential. *Psychonomic Science*, 1968, **10**, 387–388.

Fowles, D. C., & Venables, P. H. The effects of epidermal hydration and sodium reabsorption on palmar skin potential. *Psychological Bulletin*, 1970, **73**, 363–378.

Fowles, D. C., & Venables, P. H. The reduction of palmar skin potential by epidermal hydration. *Psychophysiology*, 1971, **7**, 254–261.

Fox, R. H., & Solman, A. J. A new technique for monitoring deep body temperature in man from the intact skin surface. *Journal of Physiology*, 1970, **212**, 8–10P.

French, J. W. A comparison of finger tremor with the galvanic skin reflex impulse. *Journal of Experimental Psychology*, 1944, **34**, 494–505.

Fulton, J. F. *Muscular contraction and the reflex control of movement.* Baltimore, Maryland: Williams & Wilkins, 1926.

Furedy, J. F. Electrodermal recovery time as a suprasensitive autonomic index of anticipated intensity of threatened shock. *Psychophysiology*, 1972, **9**, 281–282.

Furman, K. I., & Beer, G. Dynamic changes in sweat electrolyte composition induced by heat stress as an indication of acclimatization and aldosterone activity. *Clinical Science*, 1963, **24**, 7–12.

Gates, A. I. *Diurnal variation in memory and attention.* Berkeley, California: University of California Publications in Psychology I, 1910.

Gellhorn, E., Nakao, H., & Redgate, E. S. The influence of lesions in the anterior and posterior hypothalamus on tonic and phasic autonomic reactions. *Journal of Physiology*, 1956, **131**, 402–423.

Goodall, McC. Innervation and inhibition of eccrine and apocrine sweating in man. *Journal of Clinical Pharmacology*, 1970, **10**, 235–246.

Green, J. H. *An introduction to human physiology*. London and New York: Oxford Univ. Press, 1972.

Greisemer, R. D. Protection against the transfer of matter through the skin. In S. Rothman (Ed.), *The human integument*. Washington, D.C.: Amer. Assoc. Advan. Sci., 1959.

Grice, K. A., & Bettley, F. R. Inhibition of sweating by poldine methosulphate (Nacton). *British Journal of Dermatology*, 1966, **78**, 453–464.

Grings, W. W. Methodological considerations underlying electrodermal measurement. *Journal of Psychology*, 1953, **35**, 271–282.

Grings, W. W. Recording of electrodermal phenomena. In R. F. Thompson and M. M. Patterson (Eds.), *Methods in physiological psychology*. Vol. I: *Bioelectric recording techniques*, Part C: *Receptor and effector processes*. New York: Academic Press, 1973.

Hagfors, C. The galvanic skin response and its application to the group registration of psychophysiological processes. *Jyväskylä Studies in Education, Psychology, and social Research*, 1970, **23**. Jyväskylä: Jyväskylän Yliopisto.

Haigh, A. L., Kitchin, A. H., & Pickford, M. The effect of oxytocin on hand blood flow following the administration of an oestrogen and isopredaline. *Journal of Physiology*, 1963, **169**, 161–166.

Halberg, F. Physiologic 24-hour periodicity: general and procedural considerations with reference to the adrenal cycle. *Zeitschrift für Vitamin-Hormon-und Fermentforschung*, 1959, **10**, 225–296.

Hale, H. B., Ellis, J. P., Jr., & Van Fossan, D. P. Seasonal variation in human amino acid excretion. *Journal of Applied Physiology*, 1960, **15**, 121–124.

Hamburg, D. Effects of progesterone on behavior. *Research Publications of the Association for Research in Nervous and Mental Disease*, 1966, **43**, 251–265.

Harker, J. E. *The physiology of diurnal rhythms*. London and New York: Cambridge Univ. Press, 1964.

Harrison, J. The behaviour of the palmar sweat glands in stress. *Journal of Psychosomatic Research*, 1964, **8**, 187–191.

Harrison, J., & MacKinnon, P. C. B. Physiological role of the adrenal medulla in palmar anhidrotic response to stress. *Journal of Physiology*, 1966, **21**, 88–92.

Hemphill, R. E. Electrical resistance of the skin. *Journal of Mental Science*, 1942, **88**, 285–305.

Herman, L., & Luchsinger, B. Über die Secretionsströme der Haut bei der Katz. *Pflügers Archiv für die gesammte Physiologie*, 1878, **17**, 310–319.

Hicks, R. G. Experimenter effects on the physiological experiment. *Psychophysiology*, 1970, **7**, 10–17.

Hicks, R. G. Converging operations in the psychological experiment. *Psychophysiology*, 1971, **8**, 93–101.

Holloway, F. A., & Parsons, O. A. Unilateral brain damage and bilateral skin conductance levels in humans. *Psychophysiology*, 1969, **6**, 138–148.

Hord, D. J., Johnson, L. C., & Lubin, A. Differential effect of the Law of Initial Value (LIV) on autonomic variables. *Psychophysiology*, 1964, **1**, 79–87.

Hozawa, S. Studien über die Polarisation der Haut. *Pflügers Archiv für die gesammte Physiologie*, 1928, **219**, 111–158.

Hozawa, S. Zur Theorie über die Polarisation und die Diffusionkapazität lebender Zellen, insobesondere der Haut. *Zeitschrift für Biologie*, 1931, **91**, 297–314.

Irvine, W. J., Cullen, D. R., Stewart, A. G., Ewart, R. L., & Baird, J. D. The endocrine system. In R. Passmore & J. S. Robson (Eds.), *A companion to medical studies*. Vol. I: *Anataomy, biochemistry, physiology and related subjects.* Oxford: Blackwell, 1968.

Isamat, F. Galvanic skin responses from stimulation of limbic cortex. *Journal of Neurophysiology*, 1961, 4, 176–181.

Johansson, G., Frankenhaeuser, M., & Lambert, W. W. Seasonal variations in catecholamine output. *Perceptual and Motor Skills*, 1969, **28**, 677–678.

Johnson, H. J., & Campos, J. J. The effect of cognitive tasks and verbalization instructions on heart rate and skin conductance. *Psychophysiology*, 1967, 4, 143–150.

Johnson, L. C. A psychophysiology for all states. *Psychophysiology*, 1970, 6, 501–515.

Johnson, L. C., & Corah, N. L. Racial differences in skin resistance. *Science*, 1963, 139, 766–767.

Johnson, L. C., & Landon, M. M. Eccrine sweat gland activity and racial differences in resting skin conductance. *Psychophysiology*, 1965, 1, 322–329.

Johnson, L. C., & Lubin, A. Spontaneous electrodermal activity during waking and sleeping. *Psychophysiology*, 1966, 3, 8–17.

Juniper, K., & Dykman, R. A. Skin resistance, sweat-gland counts, salivary flow, and gastric secretion: Age, race, and sex differences, and intercorrelations. *Psychophysiology*, 1967, 4, 216–222.

Juniper, K., Blanton, D. E., & Dykman, R. A. Palmar skin resistance and sweat-gland counts in drug and non-drug states. *Psychophysiology*, 1967, 4, 231–243.

Kaplan, B. E. Psychophysiological and cognitive development in children. *Psychophysiology*, 1970, 7, 18–26.

Keele, C. A., & Neil, E. *Samson Wright's applied physiology.* London: Oxford Univ. Press, 1971.

Kimble, D. P., Bagshaw, M. H., & Pribram, K. H. The GSR of monkeys during orienting and habituation after selective partial ablations of the cingulate and frontal cortex. *Neuropsychologia*, 1965, 3, 121–128.

Kleitman, N. *Sleep and wakefulness.* Chicago, Illinois: Univ. of Chicago Press, 1963.

Kligman, A. M. The biology of the stratum corneum. In W. Montagna & W. C. Lobitz, Jr. (Eds.), *The epidermis.* New York: Academic Press, 1964.

Koch, E., Elster, M., Heindorf, M., Crusius, P., Crössmann, H. C., Angersbach, P., & Rick, W. The effect of aldosterone on sweat gland. In H. Nowakowski (Ed.), *Aldosteron.* Berlin and New York: Springer-Verlag, 1963.

Kopacz, F. M., & Smith, B. D. Sex differences in skin conductance measures as a function of shock threat. *Psychophysiology*, 1971, 8, 293–303.

Kopell, B., Lunde, D., Clayton, R., Moos, R., & Hamburg, D. Variations in some measures of arousal during the normal menstrual cycle. *Journal of Nervous and Mental Disease*, 1969, **148**, 180–187.

Kryspin, J. The phoreographical determination of the electrical properties of human skin. *Journal of Investigative Dermatology*, 1965, **44**, 227–229.

Kuechenmeister, C. A. Instrument for direct read-out of log conductance ($\log 1/R$) measures of the galvanic skin response. *Psychophysiology*, 1970, 7, 128–134.

Kugelmass, S., & Lieblich, I. Relation between ethnic origin and GSR reactivity in psychophysiological detection. *Journal of Applied Psychology*, 1968, **52**, 158–162.

Kuno, Y. *Human perspiration*. Springfield, Illinois: Thomas, 1956.

Ladell, W. S. S., & Shephard, R. J. Aldosterone inhibition and acclimatization to heat. *Journal of Physiology* (London), 1962, **160**, 16–20P.

Lader, M. H. The unit of quantification of the GSR. *Journal of Psychosomatic Research*, 1970, **14**, 109–110.

Lader, M. H., & Montagu, J. D. The psycho-galvanic reflex: a pharmacological study of the peripheral mechanism. *Journal of Neurological and Neurosurgical Psychiatry*, 1962, **25**, 126–133.

Ladpli, R. Galvanic skin reactions of chronic spinal cats. *American Journal of Physical Medicine*, 1962, **41**, 15–22.

Ladpli, R., & Wang, G. H. Spontaneous variations of skin potentials in footpads of normal, striatal and spinal cats. *Journal of Neurophysiology*, 1960, **23**, 448–452.

Landis, C. Electrical phenomena of the skin. *Psychological Bulletin*, 1932, **29**, 693–752.

Landis, C., & DeWicke, H. M. The electrical phenomena of the skin. *Psychological Bulletin*, 1929, **26**, 64–119.

Lang, A. H. Skin DC potentials and the endosomatic galvanic skin reaction in the cat. *Acta Physiologica Scandinavica*, 1967, **69**, 230–241.

Lang, A. H. On the physiological significance of the amplitude of the endosomatic galvanic skin reaction (GSR) in the cat. *Acta Physiologica Scandinavica*, 1968, **73**, 151–160.

Lang, A. H., Tuovinen, T., & Valleala, P. Amygdaloid after-discharge and galvanic skin response. *Electroencephalography and Clinical Neurophysiology*, 1964, **16**, 366–374.

Lazarus, R. S. *Psychological stress and the coping process*. New York: McGraw-Hill, 1966.

Levi, L. Physical and mental stress reactions during experimental conditions simulating combat. *Försvarmedicin*, 1966, **2**, 3–8.

Lieblich, I. Manipulation of contrast between differential GSR responses through the use of ordered tasks of information detection. *Psychophysiology*, 1969, **6**, 70–77.

Lloyd, D. P. C. Electrical impedance changes of the cat's foot pad in relation to sweat secretion and reabsorption. *Journal of General Physiology*, 1960, **43**, 713–722.

Lobban, M. C. Time, light, and diurnal rhythms. In O. G. Edholm & A. L. Bacharach (Eds.), *The physiology of human survival*. London and New York: Academic Press, 1965.

Lockhart, R. A. Interrelations between amplitude, latency, rise time, and the Edelberg recovery measure of the galvanic skin response. *Psychophysiology*, 1972, **9**, 437–442.

Lorincz, A. A. Physiology of aging skin. *Illinois Medical Journal*, 1960, **117**, 59–62.

Lundberg, A. Electrophysiology of the submaxillary gland of the cat. *Acta Physiologica Scandinavica*, 1955, **35**, 1–25.

Luria, A. R., & Homskaya, E. D. Frontal lobes and the regulation of arousal processes. In D. I. Mostofsky (Ed.), *Attention: Contemporary theory and analysis*. New York: Appleton, 1970.

Lykken, D. T. Properties of electrodes used in electrodermal measurements. *Journal of Comparative and Physiological Psychology*, 1959, **52**, 629–634.

Lykken, D. T. Neuropsychology and psychophysiology in personality research. In E. F. Borgatta & W. L. Lambert (Eds.), *Handbook of personality theory and research*. Chicago, Illinois: Rand McNally, 1968.

Lykken, D. T. Square wave analysis of skin impedance. *Psychophysiology*, 1971, **7**, 262–275.

Lykken, D. T., & Venables, P. H. Direct measurement of skin conductance: A proposal for standardization. *Psychophysiology*, 1971, **8**, 656–672.

Lykken, D. T., Miller, R. D., & Strahan, R. F. Some properties of skin conductance and potential. *Psychophysiology*, 1968, **5**, 253–268.

Lykken, D. T., Rose, R., Luther, B., & Maley, M. Correcting psychophysiological measures for individual differences in range. *Psychological Bulletin*, 1966, **66**, 481–484.

Maas, J. M. The oral contraceptives: their composition, properties, selection and performance. *Clinical Medicine*, 1970, **77**, 14–27.

MacKinnon, P. C. B. Variations in the number of active digital sweat glands during the human menstrual cycle. *Journal of Obstetrics and Gynecology of the British Empire*, 1954, **61**, 390–393. (a)

MacKinnon, P. C. B. Variations with age in the number of active palmar digital sweat glands. *Journal of Neurological and Neurosurgical Psychiatry*, 1954, **17**, 124–126. (b)

MacKinnon, P. C. B. Hormonal control of the reaction of the palmar sweat index to emotional stress. *Journal of Psychosomatic Research*, 1964, **8**, 193–196.

MacKinnon, P. C. B. The palmar anhidrotic response to stress in schizophrenic patients and in control groups. *Journal of Psychiatric Research*, 1969, **7**, 1–8.

MacKinnon, P. C. B., & Harrison, J. The influence of hormones associated with the pituitary-adrenal and sexual-cycle activity on palmar sweating. *Journal of Endocrinology*, 1961, **23**, 217–225.

Malkinson, F. D., & Rothman, S. Percutaneous absorption. In J. Jadassohn (Ed.), *Handbuch der Haut- und Geschlect skrankheiten, normale und pathologische Physiologie der Haut*. Vol. 8, Part 3. Berlin and New York: Springer-Verlag, 1963. Pp. 90–156.

Malmo, R. B. Finger-sweat prints in the differentiation of low and high incentive. *Psychophysiology*, 1965, **1**, 231–240.

Manery, J. F. Minerals in nonosseous connective tissue. In C. L. Comar & F. Bronner (Eds.), *Mineral metabolism—an advanced treatise*. New York: Academic Press, 1961.

Martin, I., & Venables, P. H. Mechanisms of palmar skin resistance and skin potential. *Psychological Bulletin*, 1966, **65**, 347–357.

Mason, J. W., & Brady, J. V. The sensitivity of psychoendocrine systems to social and physical environment. In P. H. Leiderman & D. Shapiro (Eds.), *Psychobiological approaches to social behavior*. London: Tavistock, 1965.

Maulsby, R. L., & Edelberg, R. The inter-relationship between the galvanic skin response, basal resistance and temperature. *Journal of Comparative and Physiological Psychology*, 1960, **53**, 475–479.

May, C. D. Electrolyte excretion by sweat glands and kidneys. *American Journal of Diseases of Children*, 1965, **109**, 2–8.

McCleary, R. A. The nature of the galvanic skin response. *Psychological Bulletin,* 1950, **47**, 97–117.

McDowell, R. J. The physiology of the psychogalvanic reflex. *Quarterly Journal of Experimental Physiology,* 1933, **23**, 277–285.

McGraw, E. R., Kleinman, K. M., Brown, M. L., & Korol, B. An accurate one channel basal level/response signal separation for skin resistance incorporating pulse coding of the basal level. *Psychophysiology,* 1969, **6**, 209–213.

McLendon, J. F., & Hemingway, A. The psychogalvanic reflex as related to the polarization capacity of the skin. *American Journal of Physiology,* 1930, **94**, 77–83.

Mefferd, R. B., Jr. Adaptive changes to moderate seasonal heat in humans. *Journal of Applied Physiology,* 1959, **14**, 995–996.

Mefferd, R. B., Jr., & Pokorny, A. D. Individual variability reexamined with standard clinical measures. *American Journal of Clinical Pathology,* 1967, **48**, 228–331.

Mefferd, R. B., Jr., LaBrosse, E. H., Gawienowski, A. M., & Williams, R. J. Influence of chlorpromazine on certain biochemical variables of chronic male schizophrenics. *Journal of Nervous and Mental Disease,* 1958, **127**, 167–179.

Mefferd, R. B., Sadler, T. G., & Wieland, B. A. Physiological responses to mild heteromodal stimulation. *Psychophysiology,* 1969, **6**, 186–196.

Mercer, E. H. *Keratin and keratinization.* Oxford: Pergamon, 1962.

Miller, N. E. Learning of visceral and glandular responses. *Science,* 1969, **163**, 434–445.

Miller, R. D. Silver–silver chloride electrodermal electrodes. *Psychophysiology,* 1968, **5**, 92–96.

Mills, J. N. Human circadian rhythms. *Physiological Reviews,* 1966, **46**, 128–171.

Mills, J. N. Circadian rhythms. In R. Passmore & J. S. Robson (Eds.), *A companion to medical studies.* Vol. I: Anatomy, biochemistry, physiology and related subjects. Oxford: Blackwell, 1968.

Montagna, W. (Ed.) Advances in biology of skin. Vol. I: *Cutaneous Innervation.* New York: Pergamon, 1960.

Montagna, W. *The structure and function of the skin.* New York: Academic Press, 1962.

Montagna, W., & Ellis, R. A. (Eds.) *Advances in biology of skin.* Vol. II: *Cutaneous blood vessels and circulation.* New York: Academic Press, 1961.

Montagna, W., Ellis, R. A., & Silver, A. F. (Eds.) *Advances in biology of skin.* Vol. III: *The eccrine sweat glands.* New York: Pergamon, 1962.

Montagna, W., & Lobitz, W. C. *The epidermis.* New York: Academic Press, 1964.

Montagu, J. D. The psycho-galvanic reflex. A comparison of AC skin resistance and skin potential changes. *Journal of Neurological and Neurosurgical Psychiatry,* 1958, **21**, 119–128.

Montagu, J. D. The psycho-galvanic reflex: a comparison of dc and ac methods of measurement. *Journal of Psychosomatic Research,* 1964, **8**, 49–65.

Montagu, J. D., & Coles, E. M. Mechanism and measurement of the galvanic skin response. *Psychological Bulletin,* 1966, **65**, 261–279.

Montagu, J. D., & Coles, E. M. Mechanism and measurement of the galvanic skin response: An addendum. *Psychological Bulletin,* 1968, **69**, 74–76.

Mordkoff, A. M. Palmar-dorsal skin conductance differences during classical conditioning. *Psychophysiology,* 1968, **5**, 61–66.

Mordkoff, A. M., Edelberg, R., & Ustick, M. The differential conditionability of two components of the skin conductance response. *Psychophysiology*, 1967, **4**, 40–47.

Morris, G. C. R. Factors determining sodium and potassium concentrations of saliva with speᶜial reference to aldosterone. Unpublished M.D. Thesis, University of Oxford, 1963.

Moruzzi, G., & Magoun, H. W. Brain stem reticular formation and activation of the EEG. *Electroencephalography and Clinical Neurophysiology*, 1949, **1**, 455–473.

Motta, M., Piva, F., & Martini, L. Effects of progesterone on the central nervous system. *Bulletin of the Swiss Academy of Medical Sciences*, 1970, **25**, 408–418.

Munger, B. L. The ultrastructure and histophysiology of human eccrine sweat glands. *Journal of Biophysical and Biochemical Cytology*, 1961, **11**, 383–402.

Munger, B. L., & Brusilow, S. W. An electron microscopic study of eccrine sweat glands of the cat foot and toe pads: evidence for ductal reabsorption in the human. *Journal of Biophysical and Biochemical Cytology*, 1961, **11**, 403–417.

Neumann, E. Thermal changes in palmar skin resistance patterns. *Psychophysiology*, 1968, **5**, 103–111.

Neumann, E., & Blanton, R. The early history of electrodermal research. *Psychophysiology*, 1970, **6**, 453–475.

Niimi, Y. The studies on electrical skin conductance and galvanic skin reflex by exosomatic method. *Bulletin of the Graduate Division of Literature of Waseda University*, 1967, **13**, 1–19.

Niimi, Y., Yamazaki, K., & Watanabe, T. Pseudoeffects of external electrolyte on measured skin potential levels. *Psychophysiology*, 1968, **5**, 188–191.

Obrist, P. A. Skin resistance levels and galvanic skin response: Unilateral differences. *Science*, 1963, **139**, 227–228.

O'Connell, D. N., Tursky, B., & Evans, F. J. Normality of distribution of resting palmar skin potential. *Psychophysiology*, 1967, **4**, 151–160.

O'Connor, W. J. *Renal function*. London: Arnold, 1962.

Oken, D. The psychophysiology and psychoendocrinology of stress and emotion. In M. H. Appley & R. Trumbull (Eds.), *Psychological stress*. New York: Appleton, 1967.

Paintal, A. S. A comparison of galvanic skin responses of normals and neurotics. *Journal of Experimental Psychology*, 1951, **41**, 425–428.

Papadimitriou, M., Roy, R. R., & Varkarakis, M. Electrocardiographic changes and plasma potassium levels in patients on regular dialysis. *British Medical Journal*, 1970, **2**, 268–269.

Papez, J. W. A proposed mechanism of emotion. *Archives of Neurology and Psychiatry*, 1937, **38**, 87–109.

Parsons, O. A., & Chandler, P. J. Electrodermal indicants of arousal in brain damage: cross-validated findings. *Psychophysiology*, 1969, **5**, 644–659.

Pasquali, E., & Roveri, R. Measurement of electrical skin resistance during skin drilling. *Psychophysiology*, 1971, **8**, 236–238.

Passmore, R., & Robson, J. S. (Eds.) *A companion to medical studies*. Volume I: *Anatomy, biochemistry, physiology, and related subjects*. Oxford: Blackwell, 1968.

Patkai, P. Diurnal differences between habitual morning workers and evening workers in some psychological and physiological functions. *Reports from the Psychological Laboratories of the University of Stockholm*, 1970, No. 311.

Patkai, P. Inter-individual differences in diurnal variations in alertness, performance, and adrenalin excretion. *Acta Physiologica Scandinavica*, 1971, **81**, 35–46.

Patton, H. D. Secretory innervation of the cat's foot pad. *Journal of Neurophysiology*, 1948, **11**, 211–227.

Peiss, C., Randall, W. D., & Hertzman, A. B. Hydration of the skin and its effect on sweating and evaporative water loss. *Journal of Investigative Dermatology*, 1956, **26**, 459–470.

Pollard, A. C. The quantitative changes which occur throughout the day in some commonly determined plasma constituents. *Technicon 3rd Symposium on Automation in Analytical Chemistry*, London, 1964.

Quatrale, R. P., & Speir, E. H. The effect of ADH on eccrine sweating in the rat. *Journal of Investigative Dermatology*, 1970, **55**, 344–349.

Redgrove, J. A. Menstrual cycles. In W. P. Colquhoun (Ed.), *Biological rhythms and human performance*. Chap. 6. London: Academic Press, 1971.

Richter, C. P. A study of the electrical skin resistance and the psychogalvanic reflex in a case of unilateral sweating. *Brain*, 1927, **50**, 216–235.

Rickles, W. H., & Day, J. L. Electrodermal activity in non-palmar skin sites. *Psychophysiology*, 1968, **4**, 421–435.

Rosenthal, R. *Experimenter effects in behavioral research*. New York: Appleton, 1966.

Rothman, S. *Physiology and biochemistry of the skin*. Chicago, Illinois: Univ. of Chicago Press, 1954.

Rothman, S. (Ed.) *The human integument*. Washington D.C.: Amer. Assoc. Advan. Sci., 1959.

Rutenfranz, J. The development of circadian system functions during infancy and childhood. In *Circadian systems* (39th Ross Conference on Pediatric Research.) Ohio: Ross Laboratories, 1961. 38–41.

Sato, K., & Dobson, R. L. Enzymatic basis for the active transport of sodium in the duct and secretory portion of the eccrine sweat gland. *Journal of Investigative Dermatology*, 1970, **55**, 53–56. (a)

Sato, K., & Dobson, R. L. Regional and individual variations in the function of the human eccrine sweat gland. *Journal of Investigative Dermatology*, 1970, **54**, 443–449. (b)

Sato, K., & Dobson, R. L. The effect of intracutaneous d-aldosterone and hydrocortisone on human eccrine sweat gland function. *Journal of Investigative Dermatology*, 1970, **54**, 450–462. (c)

Sato, K., Taylor, J. R., & Dobson, R. L. The effect of ouabain on eccrine sweat gland function. *Journal of Investigative Dermatology*, 1969, **33**, 275–280.

Saunders, F. J. Endocrine properties and mechanism of action of oral contraceptives. *Federation Proceedings*, 1970, **29**, 1211–1219.

Schiefferdecker, P. Die Hautdrüsen des Menschen und der Säugetiere, ihre biologische und rassenanatomische Bedeutung, sowie die Muscularis sexualis. *Biologische Zentralblatt*, 1917, **37**, 534–562.

Schiefferdecker, P. Die Hautdrüsen des Menschen und der Säugetiere, ihre biologische und rassenanotomische Bedeutung, sowie die Muscularis sexualis. *Zoologica Stuttgart*, 1922, **27**, 1–154.

Scholander, T. Some measures of electrodermal activity and their relationships as affected by varied temperatures. *Journal of Psychosomatic Research*, 1963, **7**, 151–158.

Schultz, D. P. The human subject in psychological research. *Psychological Bulletin,* 1969, **72,** 214–228.

Schultz, I., Ullrich, K. J., Frömter, E., Holzgreve, H., Frick, A., & Hegel, U. Mikropunktion und elektrische Potentialmessung an Schweißdrüsen des Menschen. *Pflügers Archiv für die gesamte Physiologie,* 1965, **284,** 360–372.

Schwartz, I. L. Extrarenal regulation with special reference to the sweat glands. In C. L. Comar & F. Bronner (Eds.), *Mineral metabolism—an advanced treatise.* Vol. I: Principles, processes, and systems. New York: Academic Press, 1960.

Seaman, G. F., Engel, R., & Swank, R. L. Circadian periodicity in some physico-chemical parameters of circulating blood. *Nature,* 1965, **207,** 833–835.

Selye, H. Anaesthetic effect of steroid hormones. *Proceedings of the Society for Experimental and Biological Medicine,* 1941, **46,** 116–121.

Shackel, B. Skin drilling: A method of diminishing galvanic skin potentials. *American Journal of Psychology,* 1959, **72,** 114–121.

Shapiro, D., & Leiderman, P. H. Studies on the galvanic skin potential level: some statistical properties. *Journal of Psychosomatic Research,* 1964, **7,** 269–275.

Sharp, G. W. G., & Leaf, A. Studies on the mode of action of aldosterone. *Recent Progress in Hormone Research,* 1966, **22,** 431–466.

Shaver, B. A., Brusilow, S. W., & Cooke, R. E. Electrophysiology of the sweat glands: Intradermal potential changes during secretion. *Bulletin of the Johns Hopkins Hospital,* 1965, **116,** 100–109.

Shimizu, K., Tajimi, T., Watanabe, T., & Niimi, Y. Effects of external electrolyte concentration on both skin potential level and reflex: successful observation. *Japanese Psychological Research,* 1969, **11,** 32–36.

Shmavonian, B. M., Yarmat, A. J., & Cohen, S. I. Relationships between the autonomic nervous system and central nervous system in age differences in behavior. In A. T. Welford & J. E. Birren (Eds.), *Behavior aging and the nervous system.* Springfield, Illinois: Thomas, 1965.

Shmavonian, B. M., Miller, L. H., & Cohen, S. I. Differences among age and sex groups in electrodermal conditioning. *Psychophysiology,* 1968, **5,** 119–131.

Simons, D. G., & Perez, R. E. The B/GSR module: A combined recording to present base skin resistance and galvanic skin reflex activity patterns. *Psychophysiology,* 1965, **2,** 116–124.

Skou, J. C. Enzymatic basis for active transport of Na^+ and K^+ across cell membrane. *Physiological Reviews,* 1965, **45,** 596–617.

Slegers, J. F. G. A mathematical approach to the two-step reabsorption hypothesis. *Modern Problems in Pediatrics,* 1967, **10,** 74–88.

Smith, C. E. The effect of changes in temperature and humidity of the air on the apparent skin resistance. *Journal of Psychology,* 1937, **3,** 325–331.

Sollberger, A. *Biological rhythm research.* Amsterdam: Elsevier, 1965.

Sollberger, A., Apple, H. P., Greenway, R. M., King, P. H., Lindan, O., & Reswick, J. B. Automation in biological rhythm research with special reference to studies on homo. In H. von Mayersbach (Ed.), *The cellular aspects of biological rhythms.* Berlin and New York: Springer-Verlag, 1965.

Sommer, R. Zur Messung electromotorischer Vorgänge an den Fingern. *Beiträge zur Psychologische Klinik,* 1902, **1,** Heft 3.

Sourek, K. *The nervous control of skin potentials in man.* Praha: Nakladatelství Československé Akademie Věd, 1965.

Spencer, S. K., & Kierland, R. R. The aging skin: Problems and their causes. *Geriatrics*, 1970, **25**, 81–89.

Stephens, W. G. A critical survey of the relationship between the output impedance and performance of medical stimulators. In *Proceedings of the 3rd International Conference of Medical Electronics*. London: International Federation for Medical Electronics, 1961.

Sternbach, R. A., & Tursky, B. Ethnic differences among housewives in psychophysical and skin potential responses to electric shock. *Psychophysiology*, 1965, **1**, 241–246.

Stoughton, R. B. Physiological changes from maturity through senescence. *Journal of the American Medical Association*, 1962, **179**, 636–638.

Strauss, J. S., Kligman, A. M., & Ponchi, P. E. The effect of androgens and estrogens on human sebaceous glands. *Journal of Investigative Dermatology*, 1962, **39**, 139–155.

Sulzberger, M. B., Herrman, F., Keller, R., & Pisha, B. V. Studies on sweating. III. Experimental factors influencing the function of the sweat ducts: A preliminary report. *Journal of Investigative Dermatology*, 1950, **14**, 91–109.

Surwillo, W. W. Level of skin potential in healthy males and the influence of age. *Journal of Gerontology*, 1965, **20**, 519–521.

Surwillo, W. W. The influence of some psychological factors on latency of the galvanic skin reflex. *Psychophysiology*, 1967, **4**, 223–228.

Surwillo, W. W. Statistical distribution of volar skin potential level in attention and the effects of age. *Psychophysiology*, 1969, **6**, 13–16.

Surwillo, W. W., & Quilter, R. E. The relation of frequency of spontaneous skin potential responses to vigilance and age. *Psychophysiology*, 1965, **1**, 272–276.

Szakall, A. Experimentalle Daten zur Klärung der Funktion der Wasserbarriere in der Epidermis des lebenden Menschen. *Berufsdermatosen*, 1958, **6**, 171–192.

Talland, G. A. (Ed.) *Human aging and behavior.* New York: Academic Press, 1968.

Tarchanoff, J. Décharges électriques dans la peau de l'homme sous l'influence de l'excitation des organes des sens et de différentes formes d'activité psychique. *Comptes Rendus Société de Biologie*, 1889 (Ser. 9), **41**, 447–451.

Tarchanoff, J. Über de galvanischen Erscheinungen an der Haut des Menschen bei Reizung der Sinnesorgane und bei verschiedenen Formen der psychischen Tätigkeit. *Pflügers Archiv für die gesamte Physiologie*, 1890, **46**, 46–55.

Thaysen, J. H. Handling of alkali metals by exocrine glands other than the kidney. In O. Eichler & A. Farah (Eds.), *Handbuch der experimentellen Pharmokologie*. Berlin and New York: Springer-Verlag, 1960.

Thomas, P. E., & Korr, I. M. Relationship between sweat gland activity and electrical resistance of the skin. *Journal of Applied Physiology*, 1957, **10**, 505–510.

Tolles, W. E., & Carberry, W. J. The measurement of tissue resistance in psychophysiological problems. In *Proceedings of the 2nd International Conference on Medical Electronics, Paris*. London: Iliffe, 1960.

Tregear, R. T. *Physical functions of the skin.* London and New York: Academic Press, 1966.

Trolander, H. W. The measurement of biological temperatures. In C. C. Brown (Ed.), *Methods in psychophysiology*. Baltimore, Maryland: Williams & Wilkins, 1967.

Tursky, B., & Sternbach, R. A. Further physiological correlates of ethnic differences in responses to shock. *Psychophysiology*, 1967, **4**, 67–74.

Varni, J. G., Doerr, H. O., & Franklin, J. R. Bilateral differences in skin resistance and vasomotor activity. *Psychophysiology*, 1971, 8, 390–400.

Venables, P. H. The relationship between PGR scores and temperature and humidity. *Quarterly Journal of Experimental Psychology*, 1955, 7, 12–18.

Venables, P. H. Amplitude of the electrocardiogram and level of skin potential. *Perceptual and Motor Skills*, 1963, 17, 54. (a)

Venables, P. H. The relationship between level of skin potential and fusion of paired light flashes in schizophrenic and normal subjects. *Journal of Psychiatric Research*, 1963, 1, 279–287. (b)

Venables, P. H. Visual recording methods. In P. H. Venables and I. Martin (Eds.), *A manual of psychophysiological methods*. Amsterdam: North-Holland, 1967.

Venables, P. H. Electrolytes and behaviour in man. In R. Porter & J. Birch (Eds.), *Chemical influences on behaviour*. London: Churchill, 1970.

Venables, P. H., & Martin, I. Skin resistance and skin potential. In P. H. Venables & I. Martin (Eds.), *A manual of psychophysiological methods*. Amsterdam: North-Holland Publ., 1967. (a)

Venables, P. H., & Martin, I. The relation of palmar sweat gland activity to level of skin potential and conductance. *Psychophysiology*, 1967, 3, 302–311. (b)

Venables, P. H., & Sayer, E. On the measurement of the level of skin potential. *British Journal of Psychology*, 1963, 54, 251–260.

Wagner, H. N. Electrical skin resistance studies in two persons with congenital absence of sweat glands. *Archives of Dermatology and Syphilology*, 1952, 65, 543–548.

Waller, A. D. Concerning emotive phenomena—Part II. Periodic variations of conductance of the palm of the human hand. *Proceedings of the Royal Society*, B, 1919, 91, 17–31.

Wang, G. H. The galvanic skin reflex. A review of old and recent works from a physiologic point of view. Part I. *American Journal of Physical Medicine*, 1957, 36, 295–320.

Wang, G. H. The galvanic skin reflex. A review of old and recent works from a physiologic point of view. Part II. *American Journal of Physical Medicine*, 1958, 37, 35–37.

Wang, G. H. *Neural control of sweating*. Madison: Univ. of Wisconsin Press, 1964.

Wang, G. H., & Brown, V. W. Changes in galvanic skin reflex after acute spinal transection in normal and decerebrate cats. *Journal of Neurophysiology*, 1956, 19, 446–451. (a)

Wang, G. H., & Brown, V. W. Suprasegmental inhibition of an autonomic reflex. *Journal of Neurophysiology*, 1956, 19, 564–572. (b)

Warndoff, J. A., & Neefs, J. A quantitative measurement of sweat production after local injection of adrenalin. *Journal of Investigative Dermatology*, 1971, 56, 384–386.

Weiner, J. S., & Hellman, K. The sweat glands. *Biological Reviews*, 1960. 35, 141–186.

Welford, A. T., & J. E. Birren (Eds.) *Behavior, aging, and the nervous system*. Springfield, Illinois: Thomas, 1965.

Wenger, M. A. Seasonal variations in some physiological variables. *Journal of Laboratory and Clinical Methods*, 1943, 5, 148–153.

Wenger, M. A. (with T. D. Cullen). Some problems in psychophysiological research. In R. Roessler & N. S. Greenfield (Eds.), *Physiological correlates of psychological disorder*. Madison: Univ. of Wisconsin Press, 1962.

Wenger, M. A. Studies of autonomic balance: A summary. *Psychophysiology*, 1966, 2, 173–186.

Wieland, B. A., & Mefferd, R. B. Systematic changes in levels of physiological activity during a four-month period. *Psychophysiology*, 1970, 6, 669–689.

Wieland, B. A., Cullen, T. D., & Wenger, M. A. Day to day stability of autonomic balance. Paper presented at a meeting of the Western Psychological Association, Monterey, California, 1958.

Wilcott, R. C. Effects of high environmental temperature on sweating and skin resistance. *Journal of Comparative and Physiological Psychology*, 1963, 56, 778–782.

Wilcott, R. C. The partial independence of skin potential and skin resistance from sweating. *Psychophysiology*, 1964, 1, 55–72.

Wilcott, R. C. Adaptive value of arousal sweating and epidermal mechanism related to skin potential and skin resistance. *Psychophysiology*, 1966, 2, 249–261.

Wilcott, R. C. Arousal, sweating and electrodermal phenomena. *Psychological Bulletin*, 1967, 67, 58–72.

Wilder, J. *Stimulus and response: The law of initial value.* Bristol: Wright, 1967.

Wineman, E. W. Autonomic balance changes during the human menstrual cycle. *Psychophysiology*, 1971, 8, 1–6.

Wolf, W. (Ed.) Rhythmic functions in the living system. *Annals of the New York Academy of Sciences*, 1962, 98, 753–1326.

Wolff, H. S. Telemetry of psychophysiological variables. In P. H. Venables & I. Martin (Eds.), *A manual of psychophysiological methods.* Amsterdam: North-Holland, 1967.

Wyatt, R., & Tursky, B. Skin potential levels in right- and left-handed males. *Psychophysiology*, 1969, 6, 133–137.

Yokota, T., & Fujimori, B. Impedance change of the skin during the galvanic skin reflex. *Japanese Journal of Physiology*, 1962, 12, 200–209.

Yokota, T., Sato, A., & Fujimori, B. Analysis of inhibitory influence of bulbar reticular formation upon sudomotor activity. *Japanese Journal of Physiology*, 1963, 13, 145–154. (a)

Yokota, T., Sato, A., & Fujimori, B. Inhibition of sympathetic activity by stimulation of limbic system. *Japanese Journal of Physiology*, 1963, 13, 137–143. (b)

Yokota, T., Takahashi, T., Kondo, M., & Fujimori, B. Studies on the diphasic wave form of the galvanic skin reflex. *Electroencephalography and Clinical Neurophysiology*, 1959, 11, 687–696.

Yoshimura, H. Organ systems in adaptation: The skin. In D. B. Dill (Ed.), *Adaptation to the environment.* A. P. S. Handbook of Physiology, Section 4. Baltimore, Maryland: Williams & Wilkins, 1964.

Zuckerman, M., Persky, H., & Link, K. E. The influence of set and diurnal factors on autonomic responses to sensory deprivation. *Psychophysiology*, 1969, 5, 612–624.

CHAPTER 2

Attention and Arousal

DAVID C. RASKIN

Department of Psychology
University of Utah
Salt Lake City, Utah

I.	Introduction	125
II.	Theories of Attention and Arousal	126
	A. Early History	126
	B. Arousal Theory	126
	C. Orienting Reflex Theory	127
	D. Habituation and Sensitization Theory	129
	E. Multiprocess Theory	130
III.	Dependent Variables and Theoretical Concepts	131
	A. Tonic Levels	131
	B. Phasic Responses	132
	C. Recovery Rates	134
	D. Nonspecific Responses	136
IV.	Issues in Research	137
	A. Stimulus Intensity and Repetitions	137
	B. Stimulus Quality	140
	C. Stimulus Change	141
	D. Instructions and Tasks	143
	E. Vigilance	145
	F. Learning and Memory	146
	G. Individual Differences	148
	References	150

I. Introduction

The general aim of this chapter is to discuss the use of measures of electrodermal activity (EDA) in relation to the theoretical concepts of attention and arousal. The presentation consists of three major sections. First, there is a brief history of the use of measures of EDA

125

as indicators of attention and arousal, followed by a more detailed description of the major contemporary theories of those processes. The second section deals with a more detailed analysis of the relationships between various measures of EDA and the theoretical concepts described in the first section. The remainder of the chapter is devoted to a variety of research problems in which measures of EDA have been employed to investigate many of the propositions and concepts developed in the various theoretical approaches to attention and arousal.

II. Theories of Attention and Arousal

A. Early History

Work on the psychological significance of EDA and its relation to arousal seems to have begun with the work of Féré (1888). He was interested in the effects of sensory and emotional stimuli on the development of "psychic energy" and developed a very early statement of a simple arousal theory (Neumann & Blanton, 1970). Féré measured skin resistance responses (SRRs) and demonstrated that sensory or emotional stimulation was accompanied by a decrease in skin resistance (SR). The report by Féré represents what appears to be the first attempt to use EDA as an index of an important psychological construct.

Since the work of Féré, a considerable effort has been devoted to studying the numerous facets of EDA in attempts to develop indices of a variety of theoretical concepts of significance to psychology. During the same period, a large body of literature has developed which has used those indices in studying the effects of experimental variables in an attempt to answer some of the questions generated from psychological theorizing. A description of some of those theories is necessary to understand the thrust of current electrodermal research.

B. Arousal Theory

After a long period of neglect, the early work of Féré led to what is known today as arousal or activation theory. This approach has developed from the work of a number of investigators (e.g., Duffy, 1962; Freeman, 1948; Hebb, 1955; Lindsley, 1951; Malmo, 1959). Duffy took the position that the general level of energy mobilization is a major aspect of what has been historically labeled as emotion. She pointed to skin conductance level (SCL) as an indicator of the level of energy mobilization (Duffy & Lacey, 1946).

The term energy mobilization was soon replaced by the term activation, which was put forth by Lindsley (1951). According to Schlosberg (1954), the term "activation" is preferable and embodies an increase in both activity and reactivity. Schlosberg went on to make a strong argument in favor of utilizing SCL as opposed to skin conductance responses (SCRs) as the best index of activation, citing the work of Duffy and Lacey (1946), Freeman (1940), and work from his own laboratory (Schlosberg & Stanley, 1953). He also pointed out that there was considerable indication that there is a curvilinear relationship between activation and behavioral efficiency which is manifested in the form of an inverted U function.

The concept of the inverted U function has been elaborated by Hebb (1955) and Malmo (1958), and Malmo has also supported the position that tonic measures such as SCL are the best indices of activation or general arousal. A great deal of the significance of that approach is derived from the work of Lindsley (1951, 1960), who has shown that activation or arousal is related to activity in the brain stem reticular formation and is manifested by increased frequency and decreased amplitude of EEG activity. Sharpless and Jasper (1956) have pointed out that the lower portions of the reticular formation are responsible for the longer-lasting changes in the level of reactivity, whereas the upper portions of the reticular formation seem to subserve attentive processes which are of briefer duration.

C. Orienting Reflex Theory

The distinction made by Sharpless and Jasper leads to a consideration of the relatively short-term or phasic responses such as SCRs which play a prominent role in theories of the orienting (OR) and defensive reflexes (DR). The concept of the OR was originally described by Pavlov (1927) as the investigatory or "what-is-it" reflex. Subsequent investigations were carried out by Sokolov (1960, 1963), who has developed a fairly detailed and very influential theory of receptivity to stimuli and information processing based upon the occurrence of ORs and DRs.

According to Sokolov, there are two types of generalized responses which are elicited by a wide variety of stimuli. One of these is the OR which is a generalized response to mild or moderately intense or novel stimuli, and habituates upon repetition of the stimuli. That response is characterized by a complex pattern of skeletal and physiological changes and includes changes in skin conductance (SC) as well as other autonomic and electroencephalographic (EEG) responses. The reader is referred to Lynn (1966) or Raskin, Kotses, and Bever (1969) for a more detailed description of the various indices of the OR. Sokolov has taken the position that the OR functions to produce heightened sensitivity to environmental stimulation and results in increased intake and processing of information.

In contrast to the OR, the DR is evoked by intense or noxious stimulation and is extremely resistant to habituation. Its function is to protect the organism by attenuating the perceptual effects of such stimulation. Using only measures of EDA, the occurrence of a DR is somewhat difficult to differentiate from an OR. However, some attempts have been made to use SCR (Raskin et al., 1969; Zimny & Kienstra, 1967) and skin potential response (SPR) (Raskin et al., 1969) to differentiate DRs from ORs. Recently, Edelberg (1972b) has suggested that measures of electrodermal recovery rate may distinguish defensive responses from goal-directed behavior.

Another important distinction described by Sokolov is that of tonic and phasic ORs. That distinction is based on the temporal characteristics of the response. Phasic ORs are characterized by a rapid response which shows a quick return to prestimulus levels, whereas tonic ORs persist for a longer time in the form of altered sensitivity to stimulation. The two types of ORs may be distinguished on the basis of EDA, with SCR or SPR indicative of a phasic OR and the slower changes in SCL and skin potential level (SPL) providing evidence of the occurrence of a tonic OR. Sokolov goes on to say that the tonic and phasic ORs are strongly interrelated. He states that "the complex of the orientation reflex, aiming at an increased state of preparedness of the whole body, and at better perception of the stimulus is, in fact, a combination of the two types of reflexes, tonic and phasic, which remain intimately interwoven [1963, p. 118]."

Sokolov has proposed a neuronal model to explain the habituation and dishabituation of the OR. The first time that a stimulus is presented, it is novel and evokes an OR. As the stimulus is repeated, a neuronal model of the stimulus is built up in the cortex. As the model begins to encode all of the properties of that stimulus, e.g., intensity, temporal, qualitative characteristics, it begins to inhibit the occurrence of the OR by preventing collaterals from the sensory pathways from stimulating the reticular formation. When the model completely matches the stimulus input, there is complete inhibition of the input to the reticular formation, and the OR shows complete habituation.

If any characteristic of the stimulus is changed, there will be a mismatch between the stimulus and the neuronal model, the inhibition of the reticular formation will not be generated, and the OR will be reinstated. Those properties of the modeling system provide the possibility of studying perceptual capacities of subjects without the use of overt responses and also provide a means of exploring gradients of generalization along physical stimulus dimensions (Corman, 1967).

Another way in which the magnitude of ORs and their rate of habituation may be altered is that of providing a stimulus with signal value. That may be accomplished by pairing a stimulus with an important event such as an intense or noxious stimulus, or by instructing the S to make a particular response (e.g., motor reaction, verbal association) whenever the stimulus occurs. Those procedures produce an enhancement of the OR to the stimulus and prevent the OR from habituating upon repeated presentations of the stimulus (Maltzman & Raskin, 1965; Sokolov, 1963). Thus, the effects of instructions given to the subject or the task required of him (Maltzman & Raskin, 1965) may be studied by using the amount or rate of habituation of EDRs. Also, phenomena such as semantic generalization (Raskin, 1969) may be studied by similar techniques (see Chapter 4 for a more detailed treatment of semantic generalization).

Maltzman and Raskin (1965) have extended Sokolov's theory to an exploration of the relationships between individual differences in ORs and the phenomena of conditioning and complex processes. They have identified the OR with the traditional concept of attention. On the basis of their findings they have concluded that the amplitude of electrodermal ORs may be interpreted as a stable individual difference parameter which can be used to predict such diverse phenomena as the magnitude of semantic conditioning and generalization (Raskin, 1969), rates of verbal learning (Belloni, 1964), and performance in a vigilance task (Krupski, Raskin, & Bakan, 1971).

D. Habituation and Sensitization Theory

Another theory that deals extensively with the problem of habituation has been proposed by Thompson (Groves & Thompson, 1970; Thompson & Spencer, 1966). He also employs a state concept called sensitization which is similar to the arousal notion put forward by Malmo. Thus, Thompson's formulation is a dual process theory which posits a stimulus–response (S–R) pathway through the central nervous system in order to explain the response decrements labeled habituation. The concept of sensitization, which refers to the general level of excitation or arousal, is introduced to explain the recurrence of the previously habituated response which results from changes in the stimulus.

In Thompson's theory, habituation resulting from repeated presentations of a stimulus is a decremental process which occurs in the interneurons of the central nervous system. It is a relatively stable process and represents a fundamental type of learning. Sensitization is an incremental process which also occurs in the central nervous system. However, it represents a temporary increase in responsiveness and is used to account for both the increment in response amplitude often observed following the first few presentations of a stimulus and the temporary return of a previously habituated response following an alteration in the parameters of the stimulus.

The two processes of habituation and sensitization are said to occur and develop independently; however, they do interact to yield the final behavioral outcome. That interaction is comparable to Sokolov's statement of the interaction between phasic and tonic ORs, which may be seen as analogous to Thompson's constructs of habituation and sensitization.

E. Multiprocess Theory

All of the foregoing theoretical approaches employ a concept of arousal which is a unitary state variable and, therefore, should be manifested by generalized increases in activity in the central nervous system and autonomic nervous system. Such a formulation in terms of the unity of the arousal state has been questioned by Lacey (1967) and Routtenberg (1968).

Lacey has based his criticisms upon data obtained from psychophysiological experiments with human Ss (Lacey, 1959; Lacey, Kagan, Lacey, & Moss, 1963). Those studies demonstrate that activity in some systems innervated by the autonomic nervous system may increase, whereas other systems innervated by the autonomic nervous system may show simultaneous decreases in activity. Lacey has labeled this phenomenon directional fractionation and has shown that its occurrence depends upon the nature of the task required of the S. Those findings have been challenged by some (Johnson & Campos, 1967) and confirmed by others (Porges & Raskin, 1969). Thus, there is evidence of a patterning of autonomic nervous system activity which varies in characteristic ways as a function of the stimulus conditions and the task required of the S. That patterning of autonomic nervous system activity has been termed situational stereotypy by Lacey (1967). Lacey has bolstered his attack upon the unitary arousal concept by drawing heavily on data from animal studies which show evidence of dissociation of central nervous system, autonomic nervous system, and behavioral indices of arousal.

In an attempt to resolve some of the difficulties apparent in the unidimensional concept of arousal, Routtenberg (1968) has proposed a dual process theory of arousal which involves the reticular activating system and the limbic system. According to Routtenberg's formulation, there are two mutually inhibitory systems which account for the arousal phenomena. Whereas the reticular activating system is described as responding to high intensity stimulation which produces heightened reactivity of the organism, the limbic system responds to less intense stimulation by prolonging its effects, facilitating information processing. The similarity between Routtenberg's formulation and Sokolov's concepts of the DR and OR has been noted by Graham and Jackson (1970).

III. Dependent Variables and Theoretical Concepts

There are a number of dependent variables which can be obtained from recordings of EDA. These are generally described as basal level (SRL, SCL, SPL), amplitude and latency of specific responses (SRR, SCR, SPR), frequency of nonspecific responses (SRR, SCR, SPR), and recovery time and recovery rate of SCR.

The different measures of EDA have been used for a variety of purposes including (1) indices of the level of tonic arousal, (2) the general level of alertness or attentiveness of the S, (3) the impact of different types and intensities of stimulation, (4) the rate and amount of habituation of responses as a function of different stimulus conditions, (5) a means of differentiating ORs and DRs, (6) assessing individual differences in responsiveness, attentiveness, conditioning, and anxiety, and (7) the investigation of differences among diagnostic categories. In this section some of those uses of EDA will be described in relation to various theoretical concepts.

A. Tonic Levels

The use of tonic levels such as SRL, SCL, and SPL as indices of the general level of arousal or activation has a long history which goes back to the work of Féré (1888). Since that time there have been numerous reports relating SRL, SCL, and SPL to arousal. Early studies by Waller and Wechsler (cited by Woodworth & Schlosberg, 1954) showed that during waking hours the cycle of activation in man is accompanied by changes in SCL, beginning with low levels in the morning, reaching a maximum at midday, and declining in the evening. Those results suggest that variations in alertness or energy mobilization may be indicated by changes in SCL.

The relationship between SCL and energy mobilization has been further developed by Duffy (Duffy, 1962; Duffy & Lacey, 1946) and Malmo (1959). Duffy and Lacey presented the S with a threshold determination task in which she was asked to tap her foot whenever she detected the tone. Their results showed that SCL decreased during the 2.5-min rest period, increased at the onset of the series of trials on each of the three days, and decreased during the course of each session and across the three sessions. The findings were interpreted as indicating that SCL varies directly with the task demands placed on the S.

Malmo also described levels of activation in terms of variations in SCL. His findings (Malmo, 1958, 1959) supplemented the earlier work on variations in SCL over the course of the day. He extended those data by demonstrating that SCL falls progressively during a night's sleep, dropping from an average of approximately 75 μmho at 11 p.m. to approximately 25 μmho by 8 a.m. the next morning (Malmo, 1958). In addition, he demonstrated that sleep deprivation during a prolonged vigil produced increases in SCL which were accompanied by increased EEG activation, as shown by decreased occurrence of alpha waves.

The foregoing studies make a strong case for the proposition that SCL is a good indicator of the general level of activation or arousal. That position, which has been strongly endorsed by Freeman (1948), Schlosberg (1954), and Malmo (1962), provides a solid basis for its current usage as a measure of the level of activation. That position has been confirmed by more recent evidence (Raskin et al., 1969).

The other measure of EDA which has been employed as an index of the level of activation or arousal is SPL. Liederman and Shapiro (1964) recorded SPL during different stimulus conditions. They reported that SPL was low during sleep, intermediate during a monotonous learning task, and high during the presentation of electric shock, noises, and air puffs, and during sensory deprivation. They concluded that SPL is a simple, objective technique for measuring various states of behavioral activation. In a more recent study, Raskin et al. (1969) measured several autonomic responses to different intensities of auditory stimulation. Using different groups of Ss they reported that as the intensity of white noise increased from 40 dB to 120 dB, there was a monotonic increase in the negativity of SPL. Those results lend further support to the conclusion that the SPL provides an index of autonomic arousal.

B. Phasic Responses

In general, the amplitude of SRRs, SCRs, and SPRs have been the most popular measures of EDA. Since Féré (1888) reported the first attempts to measure the SRR elicited by sensory stimuli, hundreds of experiments have employed phasic electrodermal responses (EDRs) as dependent variables. Such studies have included investigations of variations in parameters of simple stimuli (e.g., Davis, Buchwald, & Frankmann, 1955; Raskin et al., 1969), measures of anxiety (e.g., Martin, 1961), and individual differences in attention (Maltzman & Raskin, 1965). A comprehensive review of the early literature is provided by Woodworth and Schlosberg (1954), and specific topics will be dealt with in greater detail in later portions of this chapter.

One of the major questions which has been raised deals with the problem of what the phasic EDR actually indicates. Some writers have assumed that the phasic EDR is a measure of emotion or anxiety (see Martin, 1961), whereas Soviet investigators (e.g., Sokolov, 1963) and other American investigators (Maltzman & Raskin, 1965) have taken the position that such responses are more indicative of processes which have been traditionally labeled attention or orienting reflexes.

Recent evidence seems to favor the hypothesis that phasic responses accompany a wider range of psychological processes than can be subsumed under the label of anxiety or emotion. For example, Raskin (1969) reported that there was no relationship between amplitude of SCR evoked by a 1-sec presentation of 110-dB white noise and anxiety as measured by the Manifest Anxiety Scale. However, individual differences as measured by the amplitude of SCR evoked by the noise showed strong effects which were consistent with an attentional interpretation of the evoked SCR. In addition, the amplitude of SCRs and anxiety scores showed quite different relationships to other dependent variables studied in that experiment. Roessler, Burch, and Childers (1967) also failed to find any correlations between amplitude of SRRs evoked by varying intensities of auditory and visual stimuli and five different measures of anxiety. Using repeated presentations of a 1-kHz tone at 90 dB, Koepke and Pribram (1966) failed to find any significant correlation between manifest anxiety and magnitude of first SRR, number of trials to habituation of the SRR, SRL, and number of spontaneous SRRs. The reader is referred to Chapter 6 for a more complete review of the literature dealing with anxiety and EDRs.

In an attempt to answer directly the question of whether EDRs indicate emotion or attention, Flanagan (1967) obtained measures of amplitude of SCR and ratings of emotional reactions and "attention-getting" value of photographic stimuli. He found average correlations of +.64 between magnitude of SCR and attention scale values and average correlations of +.32 between magnitude of SCR and emotion scale values. Since the correlations with attention were significantly higher, Flanagan concluded that an attention interpretation of SCR is preferable to one based upon emotion.

For many years the bulk of the studies involving measures of EDA employed measures of SR or SC. However, there has been a resurgence of interest in the SPR, which was first reported by Tarchanoff (1889). A major reason for the lack of studies employing the SPR is the difficulty posed by the complex wave form of the SPR as compared to the simpler wave form of the SRR.

One of the first studies to deal with the problem of interpretation of the wave form of the SPR was reported by Forbes and Bolles (1936). Based on SPRs to a variety of stimuli such as electric shock, sudden loud shouts, a door slam, a gunshot, emotional words, and mental arithmetic, they reported that the negative wave of the SPR occurred in response to innocuous stimuli, whereas the positive wave was present during startle, mental effort, apprehension, and emotional reactions. Those findings have been confirmed by more recent investigators (Uno & Grings, 1965; Wilcott, Darrow, & Siegel, 1957; Yokota, Takahashi, Kondo, & Fujimori, 1959). An additional study by Burstein, Fenz, Bergeron, and Epstein (1965) concluded that the positive wave of the SPR reflects more intense arousal than does the presence of only the negative wave, and Raskin et al. (1969) associated the positive wave of the SPR with the occurrence of a DR and the negative wave with the occurrence of an OR.

C. Recovery Rates

In the past few years Edelberg (1970, 1972b) has reported that the rate at which the SCR recovers to prestimulus levels may be a useful index of psychological processes. The first use of that type of measure was reported by Freeman and Katzoff (1942). They developed the recovery quotient which was defined as the percent recovery of SR reached after 5 min following stimulation. The recovery quotient was described by them as an index of the capacity of the central nervous system to recover from a disturbance and was typically applied to responses of long duration.

In a series of recent experiments, Edelberg (1970, 1972a, b) has studied the information content of the recovery limb of the SCR. His first experiment (Edelberg, 1970) investigated the speed of recovery of the SCR as a function of different stimulus conditions. He showed that SCRs to nonsignal tones and light flashes recovered more slowly than did responses to the same tones and flashes which had been given

signal properties in reaction-time and perceptual tasks. The recovery
time was also decreased for responses which occurred in a guessing
game as compared to responses which occurred during a rest period.
In addition, Edelberg reported that positive SPRs were associated with
faster recovery rates. All of the findings were interpreted as demonstrating that steeper recovery slopes of the SCR are associated with goal-
directed behavior and represent the activity of a sweat reabsorption
mechanism which serves an adaptive function during such behavior.

In his second experiment, Edelberg (1972b) extended his results
to cover the effects of task complexity and aversive stimulation. He
reported that recovery rate was slowed during a painful cold-pressor
test and by warnings of electric shock during a reaction-time task. Those
results were interpreted as indicating that defensive reactions produced
by aversive stimulation are accompanied by a retardation of the recovery
rate of EDRs. Edelberg also reported that across a variety of conditions
individuals showed relatively stable recovery rates with respect to their
rank order in the group of Ss, and that Ss with shorter recovery times
tended to make fewer errors in a backward counting task. Since recovery
rates seemed to increase with task complexity and faster recovery was
associated with better performance, it seems reasonable to accept Edelberg's conclusion that speed of recovery represents an index of goal
orientation. Also, the identification of a slowing of recovery rate with
the occurrence of a defensive reaction is supported by the fact that
inhibition of sweat reabsorption leaves the skin more moist and less
susceptible to mechanical injury.

In his latest report, Edelberg (1972a) further investigated the relationship between slow electrodermal recovery rate and defensive behavior.
Using a word association task, he demonstrated that recovery rates of
responses to disturbing words such as *afraid, death, divorce,* and *electro-
cution* were reliably slower than recovery rates of responses to bland
words such as *apple, coffee, table,* and *tree.* He then speculated that
anxious individuals who perceive the world as vaguely threatening might
show slower electrodermal recovery rates than nonanxious individuals.
The Spielberger Anxiety Test was administered to 22 Ss, and the results
showed that there was a correlation of −.46 between the Spielberger
Trait Anxiety Quotient and recovery rate. From those data Edelberg concluded that the slower recovery rates observed in response to aversive
psychological stimuli and among relatively more anxious individuals support the interpretation that the retardation of electrodermal recovery
rate is an indicator of the occurrence of defensive reactions to both
mechanical and psychological threats.

D. Nonspecific Responses

Electrodermal responses that occur in the absence of a specific exteroceptive stimulus have been referred to as spontaneous or nonspecific
responses (Burch & Greiner, 1960; Lacey & Lacey, 1958). Burch and
Greiner investigated the relationship between level of arousal and different types of SRRs. They distinguished between specific SRRs which
are responses to a particular stimulus such as an electric shock and
spontaneous or nonspecific SRRs which are not related to a well-defined
stimulus. In order to study the relationship between level of arousal
and those two types of SRRs, they administered drugs which changed
the general level of arousal. They found that increasing dosages of Pento-
thal decreased the number of nonspecific SRRs, whereas increasing doses
of Metrazol increased the number of nonspecific SRRs. Thus, they demonstrated a monotonic relationship between the level of arousal and
the number of nonspecific SRRs. The finding that the number of nonspecific SRRs was positively correlated with EEG desynchrony supported that conclusion and Burch and Greiner's use of nonspecific SRRs
as an index of alertness.

In contrast to the results obtained with nonspecific SRRs, specific
SRRs evoked by electric shock stimuli seemed to show a nonmonotonic
relationship to arousal. That relationship was expressed in the form of
the frequently described inverted U function (Hebb, 1955; Stennett,
1957). Other evidence is consistent with that finding. Silverman, Cohen,
and Shmavonian (1959) reported a similar finding and concluded that
there is an inverse relationship between SRL and nonspecific SRRs.

The use of nonspecific SRRs as an index of alertness is supported
by the findings of Koepke and Pribram (1966). In reporting that a
higher rate of nonspecific SRRs is related to lower SRL, they stated
that "spontaneous activity in skin resistance is closely related to repetitive
orienting such that greater spontaneous activity implies a greater likelihood of continued orienting [p. 447]." Those theoretical statements
are supported by the data reported by Surwillo and Quilter (1965)
using a vigilance task. They found that significantly more nonspecific
SPRs preceded the occurrence of detected signals as compared to non-
detected signals, and they concluded that vigilance performance can
be partially predicted from the rate of nonspecific SPRs.

The notion that nonspecific EDRs can be used to index the entire
continuum of alertness has been challenged by Johnson and Lubin
(1966). They measured nonspecific SPRs and SRRs during wakefulness
and sleep. They reported that nonspecific SRRs were significantly more
frequent during stage 3 and 4 sleep than during the waking state, and

there were no significant differences between the waking state and stages 1, 2, and 1-rapid eye movement (REM) sleep. For nonspecific SPRs stages 2 and 3–4 sleep showed more SPRs than the waking state. In addition, they found no reliable correlations between rates of nonspecific EDRs during waking as compared to sleeping. Johnson and Lubin concluded that spontaneous EDRs have different meaning during sleep as compared to wakefulness and the physiological mechanisms and psychological relevance of nonspecific EDRs differ in the two states. Thus, nonspecific EDRs cannot be used as an index of level of alertness along the entire arousal continuum.

IV. Issues in Research

A. Stimulus Intensity and Repetitions

Since the topic of habituation of EDRs has been recently reviewed in an excellent paper by Graham (1973), it seems unnecessary to duplicate that effort. Therefore, this section will present some illustrative findings, discuss some of the interrelationships between various measures of EDA, and provide some data which may be useful for other applications.

Although measures of EDA have a long history of use in a variety of areas of investigation, and a large number of dependent measures have been utilized as indices of a number of processes, there have been relatively few attempts to examine the effects of variations in stimulus parameters on several simultaneous measures of EDA.

Uno and Grings (1965) conducted a study in which they presented a series of 2-sec noise stimuli at 60, 70, 80, 90, and 100 dB in a within-subjects design. All Ss received five presentations of each intensity, and they measured magnitude, latency, and recruitment time of SCRs and SPRs. They reported that both magnitude and recruitment time of SCR and SPR increased monotonically with increasing stimulus intensity, whereas latency of SCR and SPR decreased as stimulus intensity increased. Also, the number of diphasic SPRs increased with increases in stimulus intensity. In general, stimulus repetitions produced decrements in the magnitude of SCRs and SPRs, although there were occasional reversals across five repetitions and some lack of regularity in the ordering as a function of stimulus intensity. Those inconsistencies may have been due to procedures of presenting all five levels of stimulus intensity to the same Ss and the small number of presentations of each stimulus.

In an attempt to rectify some of the problems inherent in previous studies and also to relate EDRs to the concepts of OR and DR, Raskin *et al.* (1969) conducted an experiment which utilized a wider range of stimulus intensities and a between-Ss design. Different groups of Ss each received 30 presentations of .5 sec or 2.0 sec of white noise at one intensity (40, 60, 80, 100, or 120 dB). In addition to measuring SCRs and positive and negative components of SPR, they investigated the course of tonic levels of arousal by measuring SCL and SPL at the time of presentation of each of the 30 stimuli. Thus, the effects of stimuli selected to produce ORs or DRs could be examined in terms of phasic responses to successive stimuli and also in terms of longer-lasting changes in tonic levels.

The effects of stimulus intensity and repetition on magnitude of SCRs are presented in Fig. 1. Although initial stimulations were associated with only small differences in magnitude of SCR as a function of stimulus intensity, repetitions of stimuli produced differential rates of habituation as a function of stimulus intensity. As the initial ORs to the novel stimulation habituated, SCRs reached relatively stable levels which were directly related to stimulus intensity. It should be noted that SCRs to the 120-dB stimulus showed very little habituation.

A similar analysis of SPR data was made by Raskin and co-workers, and the results are shown in Fig. 2. They scored positive and negative components of SPR separately in an attempt to provide an index of

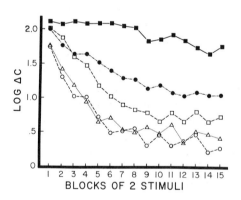

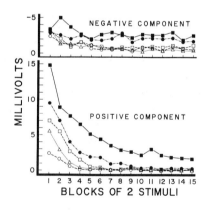

Fig. 1. Mean SCRs to the different stimulus intensities as a function of successive stimulations: (■) 120 dB; (●) 100 dB; (□) 80 dB; (△) 60 dB; (○) 40 dB. (From Raskin, Kotses, & Bever, 1969.)

Fig. 2. Mean negative and positive components of the SPRs to the different stimulus intensities as a function of successive stimulations (decibel values as in Fig. 1). (From Raskin, Kotses, & Bever, 1969).

ORs and DRs. Drawing inferences from previous reports in the literature (Forbes & Bolles, 1936; Yokota *et al.*, 1959), they hypothesized that the negative wave of the SPR represents the OR and the positive wave represents the DR. The data presented in Fig. 2 seem to lend some support to that speculation. In response to the initial stimulus presentations, the negative wave of the SPR provided no differentiation as a function of stimulus intensity. However, repeated stimulations produced stable magnitudes of responding which were relatively large for the two highest stimulus intensities and were very small for the three lowest intensities. The positive waves of the SPR showed marked initial differences in magnitude as a function of stimulus intensity, and repeated stimulation produced habituation to a zero level of response magnitude at all intensities except 120 dB.

Raskin and co-workers interpreted their data as providing evidence for the use of the negative wave of the SPR as an indicator of the occurrence of an OR and the positive wave as an indicator of a DR. However, they did point out that their interpretations were complicated by the possibility that a startle reflex and a specific acoustic reflex may have contributed to the results. Also, recent investigations of the relationship between recovery rate of the SCR and the occurrence of the positive wave of the SPR (Edelberg, 1970) call into question the interpretation of the positive wave of the SPR as an index of the DR. Edelberg reported that positive SPRs were associated with faster recovery rates than were negative SPRs. Since Edelberg's most recent study (1972a) reports that recovery rate is slowed down by aversive stimulation (the cold-pressor test, threat of electric shock, and emotionally disturbing words) and speeded up by goal-directed behavior (reaction-time task, mirror tracing, counting backward by 7s); additional questions arise concerning the proper interpretation of the positive wave of the SPR.

Raskin and co-workers also reported data on tonic levels of SPL and SCL during the course of stimulation. Those measurements were taken at the time of onset of each stimulus and are shown in Figs. 3 and 4. For both tonic measures of SPL and SCL the highest intensity of stimulation produced results which were different from those which occurred with all other intensities of stimulations. After the first few stimuli, SPL showed general decreases in magnitude at all stimulus intensities except 120 dB, which produced little change in SPL with an interstimulus interval of 45 sec and an increase in SPL when the interstimulus interval was 15 sec. The measures of SCL also showed differences between the 120-dB stimulus and all of the other intensities. Following the initial stimulations, SCL remained relatively constant or decreased with all levels of stimulus intensity except 120 dB, which produced a continual increase in SCL throughout the course of stimulations. The results of measures of tonic levels were used to support their conclusion that DRs are accompanied by persistent increases or stable, high levels of SCL and SPL, whereas ORs are accompanied by generally decreasing tonic levels of EDA.

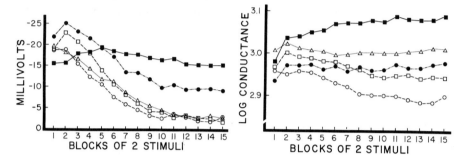

Fig. 3.   Mean SPL measured at the onset of successive stimuli (decibel values as in Fig. 1). (From Raskin, Kotses, & Bever, 1969).

Fig. 4.   Mean SCL measured at the onset of successive stimuli (decibel values as in Fig. 1). (From Raskin, Kotses, & Bever, 1969.)

B.   Stimulus Quality

In addition to using the traditional simple stimuli such as tones, noises, electric shock, lights, etc., some studies have employed stimuli designed to vary affective and motivational factors. For example, Fisher and Fisher (1969) presented Ss with different concentrations of gustatory stimuli which varied along hedonic dimensions from positive (sucrose) to neutral (water) to negative (quinine). The number of trials required to habituate the SRR was greater for the bitter quinine than for the other two stimuli. The authors concluded that the slower habituation of SRR to the quinine demonstrated a maintenance of the OR, since bitter substances are often toxic and the S is sensitized to the potential trauma. However, the results may also be interpreted as demonstrating that a DR was evoked by the noxious quinine stimulus since almost half of the Ss presented with the higher concentrations of quinine failed to meet the habituation criterion within the 25 trials presented.

Complex visual stimuli were employed by Hare, Wood, Britain, and Shadman (1970). They presented to male Ss a series of slides depicting homicides, nude females, and ordinary objects, and they reported that all three types of stimuli produced SCRs which habituated with repeated stimulation. Surprisingly, there were no differences in magnitude of SCR as a function of stimulus type, and all stimuli produced ORs as indicated by simultaneous occurrence of heart rate deceleration.

Berlyne and his associates (Berlyne, 1961; Berlyne, Craw, Salapatek, & Lewis, 1963) have varied stimulus qualities such as conflict, uncertainty, complexity, and incongruity. Their results have shown that many of those variables produce increases in frequency and amplitude of EDRs.

C. Stimulus Change

It was pointed out earlier that Sokolov's model states that any alterations in stimulus quality, intensity, or temporal characteristics provide conditions for reinstatement of the OR. Since Graham (in press) has thoroughly reviewed that literature, this section will merely summarize some of the major findings with respect to alterations in stimulus parameters. It is important to note that the recovery of ORs as a result of stimulus alterations may be a useful technique for assessing discriminative and attentional capacities in cases where standard laboratory techniques are not suitable for the S population. Thus, nonverbal Ss (neonates or infants), mentally retarded Ss, and psychotics may be studied by utilizing such techniques since verbal responses and compliance with complex instructions are not required of the Ss.

The manipulation of stimulus quality by changing the modality of the stimulus leads to an increase in SPRs (Forbes & Bolles, 1936). Houck and Mefferd (1969) reported that previously habituated SRRs were reinstated by a change from visual to auditory stimuli or vice versa, but there was no reinstatement of ORs produced by intramodal changes. Zimny and Kienstra (1967) reported that when a tone was interpolated among a series of electric shocks, the magnitude of SCR to the tone was greater than the SCR to the preceding shock, whereas a similar increase in SCR was not found when the tone had been preceded by a series of shocks and tones. The latter study demonstrates that in some situations the stimulus novelty may be a more potent determiner of magnitude of EDR than the noxious quality of the stimulus.

A number of other manipulations of stimulus properties have produced reinstatement of previously habituated EDRs. For example, Koepke and Pribram (1966) produced recovery of the SRR by alteration of the duration of the stimulus, and Kirk (1969) reported an increase in SCR as a result of unexpectedly reducing the interval between successive presentations of electric shock. That increase in magnitude of SCR cannot be attributed solely to the shorter interstimulus interval since Raskin *et al.* (1969) have shown that shorter interstimulus intervals lead to a reduction in magnitude of SCR.

The extent to which the S expects the stimulus to occur at a particular time certainly affects the EDR evoked by that stimulus. For example, Berlyne (1961) showed that changing the order of nonnovel visual stimuli produced increases in the magnitude of SCRs. Using a semantic conditioning paradigm, Raskin (1969) reported that the presentation of a noise unconditioned stimulus (UCS) following a word which had not previously been presented resulted in an increase in the magnitude of SCR which was evoked by noise. Also, omission of an expected stimulus or stimulus component has been demonstrated to produce EDRs (Allen, Hill, & Wickens, 1963; Badia & Defran, 1970).

Another set of experiments has produced positive results with variations of stimulus quality within a given stimulus modality. Thus, Williams (1963) and Corman (1967) produced gradients of EDRs as a function of amount of change in the pitch of a stimulus. Gabriel and Ball (1970) reported changes in the magnitude of SRR as a result of changing the specific location where a tactile stimulus was applied to the hand.

A number of variations in stimulus parameters were incorporated into a study by Zimny and Schwabe (1966) which was designed to test eight predictions derived from Sokolov's theory. They interpolated either a 1000-Hz or a 4000-Hz test stimulus four times throughout a series of 32 presentations of a standard 500-Hz tone. Seven of the eight predictions from Sokolov's theory were confirmed, including the prediction that the SRR to the test stimuli would be larger than the SRR to the standard stimulus and the prediction that the greater the difference between the test stimulus and the standard stimulus, the greater the dishabituation of the SRR to the standard stimulus which followed the test stimulus. They failed to confirm the prediction that the 4000-Hz test stimulus would evoke a larger SRR than the 1000-Hz stimulus.

However, other studies have shown that amplitude of EDR is related to the amount of stimulus change. Grim and White (1965) used colored lights, and they found that larger changes in the color of the lights produced larger EDRs. Also, Kimmel (1960) reported increased amplitude of SCR for larger changes in the intensity of an auditory stimulus, even when the change was in the direction of decreasing stimulus intensity.

The effects of changing stimuli and the maintenance of novelty may be extended to applications involving classical conditioning of EDRs. In a recent conditioning experiment Corah and Tomkiewicz (1971) replaced the usual aversive UCS with a series of stimuli which were designed to be novel and therefore evoke a stable level of EDR. The UCSs consisted of a series of slides which had been rated by female judges as above average on the Potency scale of the Semantic Differential and away from the mean on the Evaluative scale. The stimuli depicted objects described as a blue psychedelic face, a couple making love, a frog eating worms, a sign saying "You are ugly," etc. By pairing the CS+ with a different slide on each of the conditioning trials, the experimenters were able to produce reliable discrimination conditioning in the amplitude of SCR. It should be pointed out that the conditioning produced by that procedure was somewhat weaker than that usually obtained in EDR conditioning. That result may have been because EDRs to the UCSs were also smaller than those usually obtained with an aversive UCS.

D. Instructions and Tasks

In addition to the characteristics inherent in the stimuli presented to the S, the occurrence and resistance to habituation of EDRs are strongly influenced by the instructions given to Ss, the tasks required of them, and their expectations in the situation. Those variables are related to the concept of signal value described earlier and also to the perceptual disparity response. Signal value is usually established by instructing the S to perform a response or task whenever a particular stimulus event occurs, whereas perceptual disparity responses refer to the augmented EDRs which occur when "the receipt of stimulation is not in accord with past experience [Grings, 1960, p. 244]."

An example of the perceptual disparity response phenomenon was reported by Grings (1960). After Ss had learned that moving a lever in one direction turned on a tone and moving it in the other direction turned on a light, the outcomes were reversed. Those latter disparity trials produced reliable increases in the magnitude of the SCRs evoked by the same stimuli. Thus, if the occurrence of a familiar stimulus violated S's expectations established by previous experience, then the EDR to that stimulus was increased. Further studies reported by Grings (1960, 1965) demonstrated that the amount of that increase in SCR is a function of the strength of S's set or expectation.

Instructions and tasks were reported by Maltzman and Raskin (1965) to produce strong effects. They instructed different groups of Ss to engage in one of four different activities every time a particular stimulus word occurred in a long series of words presented orally. The four different instructions required Ss to press a foot pedal, implicitly associate to the word, implicitly count the number of occurrences of the word, or merely listen to the words. The magnitude of the SCRs which occurred to the critical stimulus word was largest for the overt motor response condition, next largest in the implicit association and counting conditions, and smallest in the listening condition. Also, they reported that the same ordering of magnitude of SCRs appeared in the responses to the list of habituation words which was presented prior to any occurrences of the word to which the Ss had been instructed to respond.

On the basis of those results, Maltzman and Raskin concluded that the different instructions resulted in differentially larger ORs in the conditions which imposed greater task demands on the Ss. Since the increase in magnitude of SCRs occurred before Ss actually began to perform the responses, that augmentation of ORs was interpreted as a response to an increase in signal value of the stimuli rather than being a result of the amount of motor activity. That interpretation is given support by the results of a study reported by Johnson and Campos (1967) in which Ss who were required to make an overt verbal response following the presentation of a stimulus produced larger changes in SCRs than Ss who were not required to verbalize overtly.

In order to separate the effects of response execution *per se* from the effects of the amount of signal value produced by varying response requirements, Germana (1968a) required Ss to withhold responses for 10 sec following stimulus presentation. In the first of a series of three experiments he varied the response requirements by asking Ss to read aloud only the even numbers when numbers from one to eight were visually presented. He reported that the numbers to which Ss were instructed to respond produced larger SCRs. In the second experiment Germana investigated the effects of amount of change in the required response by varying the number of finger movements Ss were required to make following the presentation of a visual stimulus. He found that magnitude of SCRs increased as a direct function of amount of change in response requirements. In the final experiment, Germana varied the amount of response information which S was required to encode. The findings indicated that magnitude of SCRs increased as a function of the number of alternatives from which S could choose his verbal response. Thus, Germana's experiments demonstrated that the characteristics of response or no response, amount of response change, and amount of information in the response alternatives all act to increase the magnitude of ORs evoked by the signal for performance of the response.

In a theoretical article, Bernstein (1969) raised a question concerning the necessary conditions for the evocation of an OR. Frequently his Ss reported awareness of changes in illumination of a visual stimulus without manifesting an accompanying EDR. Bernstein concluded that the OR is not an automatic accompaniment to perceptible stimulus novelty. He proposed a two-stage model in which stimulus change represents the first stage and signal value of the information represents the second stage. On the basis of his results, he proposed that ORs will follow stimulus change only if S judges the stimuli to be of some significance.

Bernstein's position is supported by the research of Harding and Punzo (1971), who demonstrated that the type of response (attentional or overt motor response) and the amount of response uncertainty both contribute to the SCL and the resistance to habituation of SCRs. Stimuli which required only an attentional response produced no systematic changes in SCR and SCL, whereas those requiring an overt motor response produced SCRs and SCL which were maintained at higher levels when response uncertainty was increased.

E. Vigilance

Measures of EDA have also been utilized in attempts to further our understanding of the dynamics of vigilance performance. For example, Ross, Dardano, and Hackman (1959) and Dardano (1962) have reported that generally high SCL is associated with little or no decrement in detection performance over time. Andreassi (1966) reported that faster reaction times in an auditory monitoring task were related to higher SCL. Thus, general level of arousal as indicated by high levels of skin conductance appears to be associated with better performance in the vigilance situation.

In addition to tonic levels of SC, other studies have shown that phasic EDA is related to vigilance performance. Surwillo and Quilter (1965) counted the number of nonspecific SPRs which Ss produced during the 18-sec period preceding the occurrence of a signal. They found that Ss produced significantly more SPRs during periods preceding signals which were detected as compared to signals which were not detected.

In a subsequent study, Krupski et al. (1971) investigated the relationship between EDA and overt commission errors. They measured the amplitude of SCRs which occurred when Ss correctly detected the occurrence of an auditory signal. The results indicated that Ss who produced larger amplitudes of SCR when they detected a signal produced fewer detection responses in the absence of signals. Since amplitude of SCRs was obtained only from trials where a detection response occurred, the difference in amplitude of SCR between Ss with high and low rates of commission errors was independent of any effects associated with the presence or absence of the detection response. The conclusion that Ss who produced large-amplitude SCRs manifested higher levels of attention and, therefore, better vigilance performance was also supported by the finding that Ss who showed large initial ORs (as indicated by the amplitude of SCR to the first stimulus presentation) made significantly fewer errors of commission.

F. Learning and Memory

One of the earliest investigations of the relationship between EDA and learning was conducted by Brown (1937) using a standard serial verbal learning procedure. He found that there was a strong, positive correlation between the magnitude of SRRs to the items and the order of learning of the items. He also reported that SRRs were generally larger to items prior to the point at which they were learned. Thus, larger SRRs were associated with the learning process rather than with simply making the correct verbal response.

A subsequent study reported by Kintsch (1965) employing a paired-associates learning task demonstrated that the amplitude of SRRs to a stimulus increases up to the point of the last error, and then declines after learning has been completed. The results obtained by Brown (1937) and Kintsch might be interpreted as indicating that ORs are evoked by the task demands placed upon the subject; and when the level of performance reaches that required by the situation, the OR begins to habituate.

Germana (1968b) pointed out that the above studies included no attempts to separate the activational responses which occur to the different components of a learning trial. Thus, EDRs which occur to the stimulus member of a pair are combined with the EDRs associated with the overt response required of the S. Therefore, Germana (1964) employed a concept-formation task in which Ss were instructed to withhold their response to the stimulus until an interval of time had elapsed. Using that procedure, he reported that the SCRs to the stimulus showed the characteristic increase followed by a decrease in amplitude, whereas the SCRs concurrent with the overt responses did not show a similar pattern. Thus, the phenomenon which Germana (1968b) describes as "activational peaking" occurs as a result of S's preparation to respond, and the SCRs begin to diminish as learning enables the S to respond with little preparatory effort.

A number of experiments have investigated the relationship between EDA and subsequent recall. Berry (1962) presented Ss with a paired-associates learning task and measured SCL during the course of learning and subsequent recall. He reported that intermediate levels of skin conductance during the first minute of the learning session were associated with better recall performance, and a similar relationship was found for SCL during the first minute of the recall period. He interpreted his results as supporting the concept of the inverted-U function relating arousal to performance.

A series of experiments at Michigan (Kleinsmith & Kaplan, 1963, 1964; Walker & Tarte, 1963) explored the relationship between the arousal associated with a stimulus and the extent to which that stimulus will be remembered. The general method of those experiments was to choose items to be learned which would produce either low or high arousal as measured by the amplitude of SRRs evoked by the items. Thus, Kleinsmith and Kaplan (1963) paired the words *kiss, rape, vomit, exam, dance, money, love,* and *swim* with the digits 2 through 9, and Ss were given one presentation of each stimulus word followed by the word paired with the numerical response. The amplitude of SRR to each stimulus word was measured, and the eight stimulus words were then ranked on the basis of SRR amplitude. The results indicated that words which produced higher arousal as measured by SRR amplitude were associated with poorer short-term recall (2 min) and better long-term recall (1 week).

Similar results were reported by Walker and Tarte (1963) and Kleinsmith and Kaplan (1964) and were explained in terms of a theory of memory which utilizes the concepts of perseverative consolidation, action decrement, and arousal. According to that theory, high arousal during learning will result in higher intensities of trace activity which produces an inhibition against early recall but results in greater ultimate memory. However, the whole series of experiments is open to the criticism that the effects of arousal may be totally confounded with idiosyncratic stimulus characteristics. Thus, the fact that the word *rape* produces a large SRR does not guarantee that memory for that item is related only to the level of arousal induced by its presentation. Certainly, the prior associations and meanings of the word *rape* differ appreciably from those associated with the word *swim*, and it is impossible to determine the specific factors that account for differences in recall of the two items. A better procedure would be to manipulate arousal independently of the meaning of the stimulus items and then test for learning and recall. Berlyne and his associates (Berlyne, Borsa, Craw, Gelman, & Mandell, 1965; Berlyne, Borsa, Hamacher, & Koenig, 1966) used such a procedure which involved the manipulation of arousal by the presentation of white noise at different intensities and different times during learning and recall. Their results were in general agreement with the results of the Michigan studies. Unfortunately, the studies by Berlyne and his associates did not include measures of EDA, and the relationship between arousal and memory requires additional study.

G. Individual Differences

Historically, most approaches to the relationship between attention, arousal, and performance have dealt with the problem without much emphasis on individual differences. However, in the past 15 years, there has been an increase in interest in exploring individual differences in autonomic activity and their relation to performance in a variety of situations. One major line of investigation was initiated by John Lacey and his co-workers (Lacey, 1959; Lacey, Kagan, Lacey, & Moss, 1963; Lacey & Lacey, 1958). That approach has focused on the relationships between individual differences in rate of nonspecific EDRs, performance in a variety of situations, and measures of personality variables.

A second approach to the study of individual differences in EDA was derived from Sokolov's (1963) model of ORs and DRs and is exemplified by the work of Maltzman and Raskin (1965). Their approach involves the use of an index of individual OR amplitude as a means of predicting performance in situations such as semantic conditioning and generalization of SCRs (Raskin, 1969) and EEG alpha blocking (Gould, Lodwig, Raskin, Watts, & Maltzman, 1966), verbal learning (Belloni, 1964), and verbal conditioning (Smith, 1966). The general procedure is to obtain a measure of the OR for each S by measuring the amplitude of SCR to the first stimulus or first UCS presented to the S and then assessing the degree of relationship between individual differences in the amplitude of ORs and performance.

Lacey and Lacey (1958) reported that the rate of nonspecific SRRs is a reliable individual characteristic. They counted the number of nonspecific SRRs during a rest period and during the performance of different tasks and the presentation of electric shock. They found that there were high correlations across time and conditions, and they concluded that autonomic lability is a stable, individual characteristic. In a second part of the study, Lacey and Lacey showed that electrodermal "labiles" (Ss above the median in number of nonspecific SRRs during rest) had faster reaction times and made more errors than did the "stabile" Ss.

A number of studies have assessed the stability of electrodermal lability. Test-retest reliabilities of the resting rate of nonspecific EDRs have been reported to range between .54–.89 within a 48-hr period (Doctor & Friedman, 1966; Johnson, 1963; Lacey & Lacey, 1958) and to be .62 and .50 for a 1-month (Doctor & Friedman, 1966) and 1-year interval (Dykman, Ackerman, Galbrecht, & Reese, 1963). Thus, electrodermal lability appears to be a relatively stable characteristic and also seems to be relatively independent of amplitude of SCR evoked by a specific stimulus (e.g., Koepke & Pribram, 1966; Lacey & Lacey, 1958). However, Crider and Lunn (1971) reported that speed of habituation of SPRs to repetitions of a tone showed greater stability ($r = .70$) over a 7-day period than did nonspecific SPRs ($r = .54$). Since the rate of nonspecific SPRs was highly correlated with speed of habituation ($r = .75$), they suggested that the two measures can be used relatively interchangeably as indices of electrodermal lability. Their data also indicated that electrodermal lability is negatively correlated with measures of extraversion and impulsivity and is unrelated to neuroticism.

A subsequent report by Crider (1972) demonstrated that electrodermal labiles (as measured by speed of habituation of SPRs to tones on two different occasions) show superior performance in an auditory vigilance task. Further analysis based on signal detection principles led Crider to conclude that electrodermal labiles do not differ from stabiles in any cognitive capacity but do show differences in levels of motivation and arousal. This position differs from the attentional capacity interpretation of electrodermal arousal put forth by Maltzman and Raskin (1965) and supported by the results obtained by Krupski et al. (1971) using the same vigilance task. Those findings indicated that Ss who produced larger ORs (as measured by the SCR to the first stimulus presented) showed lower rates of commission errors. Also, their data showed an indication that higher levels of SCL may be associated with lower rates of commission errors. That result is not in agreement with Crider's interpretation that electrodermal lability is an index of higher tonic arousal which may manifest itself in terms of relative indifference to commission errors. It may be that electrodermal lability, as measured by speed of habituation of EDRs or rate of nonspecific EDRs, is an individual characteristic which differs from that which is measured by the amplitude of EDRs evoked by a specific stimulus.

The data reported on the relationships between individual differences in electrodermal ORs and performance (e.g., Belloni, 1964; Maltzman & Raskin, 1965; Raskin, 1969) seem to indicate that individual differences in amplitude of electrodermal ORs are related to individual differences in attentional and learning capacities. For example, Raskin (1969) reported that Ss who produced larger SCRs to the first presentation of the UCS in a semantic conditioning experiment attained higher levels of semantic conditioning of SCRs, showed more evidence of semantic generalization of SCRs, and were better able to verbalize the contingencies in the experiment. Thus, high-OR Ss showed higher levels of responding in electrodermal systems and also showed greater awareness of stimulus relationships.

Those results were extended in an experiment reported by Belloni (1964). She utilized Ss who had participated in a previous experiment and on whom measures of electrodermal ORs had been obtained. They were then divided into low-OR and high-OR groups and asked to learn lists of paired associates. Belloni found that for male Ss, high ORs were associated with faster response speed on difficult items and fewer trials required to reach the criterion of learning. Significant results were not obtained with female Ss. Thus, the results for male Ss indicated that amplitude of electrodermal ORs is related to performance in paired-associates learning in a way which is predicted by the attentional–perceptual capacity interpretation of ORs.

Subsequent studies of electrodermal ORs have confirmed that interpretation. Gould *et al.* (1966) reported that individual differences in SCR measures of OR were related to semantic conditioning and generalization of EEG alpha blocking. High-OR Ss not only showed higher levels of semantic conditioning and generalization of alpha blocking, but they were also better able to verbalize the stimulus contingencies. Thus, electrodermal ORs showed reliable relationships to the amount of conditioning manifested in a CNS measure and also shown by a cognitive response. Those findings were further supported by the results of a verbal conditioning experiment (Smith, 1966). He reported that Ss who showed relatively large electrodermal ORs to the first verbal reinforcement in a verbal conditioning procedure produced approximately 50% more correct identifications of the stimulus contingencies.

The evidence available on individual differences in electrodermal activity seems to lead to two different interpretations. The data on electrodermal lability seem to argue for a motivational or arousal interpretation of individual differences. However, the research which has utilized measures of amplitude of SCRs evoked by specific stimuli appears to support an interpretation of individual differences in attention-learning capacities. Perhaps these different interpretations accurately reflect differences in the process underlying the phenomena of nonspecific changes as compared to specific responses. Obviously, the issue is far from settled. However, the data presented in subsequent chapters may help to shed some light on those issues.

References

Allen, C. K., Hill, F. A., & Wickens, D. D. The orienting reflex as a function of the interstimulus interval of compound stimuli. *Journal of Experimental Psychology*, 1963, **65**, 309–316.

Andreassi, J. L. Skin conductance and reaction-time in a continuous auditory monitoring task. *American Journal of Psychology,* 1966, **79,** 470–474.

Badia, P., & Defran, R. H. Orienting responses and GSR conditioning: A dilemma. *Psychological Review,* 1970, **77,** 171–181.

Belloni, M. L. The relationship of the orienting reaction and manifest anxiety to paired-associate learning. Unpublished doctoral dissertation. University of California, Los Angeles, 1964.

Berlyne, D. E. Conflict and the orientation reaction. *Journal of Experimental Psychology,* 1961, **62,** 476–483.

Berlyne, D. E., Borsa, D. M., Hamacher, J. H., & Koenig, I. D. V. Paired-associate learning and the timing of arousal. *Journal of Experimental Psychology,* 1966, **72,** 1–6.

Berlyne, D. E., Craw, M. A., Salapatek, P. H., & Lewis, J. L. Novelty, complexity, incongruity, extrinsic motivation, and the GSR. *Journal of Experimental Psychology,* 1963, **66,** 560–567.

Berlyne, D. E., Borsa, D. M., Craw, M. A., Gelman, R. S., & Mandell, E. E. Effects of stimulus complexity and induced arousal on paired-associate learning. *Journal of Verbal Learning and Verbal Behavior,* 1965, **4,** 291–299.

Bernstein, A. S. To what does the orienting response respond? *Psychophysiology,* 1969, **6,** 338–351.

Berry, R. N., Skin conductance levels and verbal recall. *Journal of Experimental Psychology,* 1962, **63,** 275–277.

Brown, C. H. The relation of magnitude of galvanic skin responses and resistance levels to the rate of learning. *Journal of Experimental Psychology,* 1937, **20,** 262–278.

Burch, N. R., & Greiner, T. H. A bioelectric scale of human alertness: Concurrent recordings of the EEG and GSR. *Psychiatric Research Reports,* 1960, **12,** 183–193.

Burstein, K. R., Fenz, W. D., Bergeron, J., & Epstein, S. A comparison of skin resistance measures of emotional responsivity. *Psychophysiology,* 1965, **2,** 14–24.

Corah, N. L., & Tomkiewicz, R. L. Classical conditioning of the electrodermal response with novel stimuli. *Psychophysiology,* 1971, **8,** 143–148.

Corman, C. D. Stimulus generalization of habituation of the galvanic skin response. *Journal of Experimental Psychology,* 1967, **74,** 236–240.

Crider, A. Electrodermal lability and vigilance performance. *Psychophysiology,* 1972, **9,** 268. (Abstract)

Crider, A., & Lunn, R. Electrodermal lability as a personality dimension. *Journal of Experimental Research in Personality,* 1971, **5,** 145–150.

Dardano, J. E. Relationships of intermittent noise, intersignal interval, and skin conductance to vigilance behavior. *Journal of Applied Psychology,* 1962, **46,** 106–114.

Davis, R. C., Buchwald, A. M., & Frankmann, R. W. Autonomic and muscular responses and their relation to simple stimuli. *Psychological Monographs,* 1955, **69,** 1–71.

Docter, R. F., & Friedman, L. F. Thirty-day stability of spontaneous galvanic skin responses in man. *Psychophysiology,* 1966, **2,** 311–315.

Duffy, E. *Activation and behavior.* New York: Wiley, 1962.

Duffy, E., & Lacey, O. L. Adaptation in energy mobilization: Changes in general level of palmar skin conductance. *Journal of Experimental Psychology,* 1946, **36,** 437–452.

Dykman, R. A., Ackerman, P. T., Galbrecht, C. R., & Reese, W. G. Physiological reactivity to different stressors and methods of evaluation. *Psychosomatic Medicine,* 1963, **25**, 37–59.

Edelberg, R. The information content of the recovery limb of the electrodermal response. *Psychophysiology,* 1970, **6**, 527–539.

Edelberg, R. The relation of slow electrodermal recovery rate to protective behavior. *Psychophysiology,* 1972, **9**, 275. (Abstract) (a)

Edelberg, R. Electrodermal recovery rate, goal orientation, and aversion. *Psychophysiology,* 1972, **9**, 512–520. (b)

Féré, C. Note sur les modifications de la résistance électrique sous l' influence des excitations sensorielles et des émotions. *Comptes Rendus Société de Biologie,* 1888 (Ser. 9), **5**, 217–219.

Fisher, G. L., & Fisher, B. E. Differential rates of GSR habituation to pleasant and unpleasant sapid stimuli. *Journal of Experimental Psychology,* 1969, **82**, 339–343.

Flanagan, J. Galvanic skin response: Emotion of attention. *Proceedings of the American Psychological Association,* 1967, **2**, 7–8.

Forbes, T. W., & Bolles, M. Correlation of the response potentials of the skin with "exciting" and non-"exciting" stimuli. *Journal of Psychology,* 1936, **2**, 273–285.

Freeman, G. L. The relationship between performance level and bodily activity. *Journal of Experimental Psychology,* 1940, **26**, 602–608.

Freeman, G. L. *The energetics of human behavior.* Ithaca, New York: Cornell Univ. Press, 1948.

Freeman, G. L., & Katzoff, E. T. Methodological evaluation of the galvanic skin response, with special reference to the formula for R.Q. (recovery quotient). *Journal of Experimental Psychology,* 1942, **31**, 239–248.

Gabriel, M., & Ball, T. S. Plethysmographic and GSR responses to single versus double-simultaneous novel tactile stimuli. *Journal of Experimental Psychology,* 1970, **85**, 368–373.

Germana, J. Autonomic correlates of acquisition and extinction. Unpublished master's thesis, Rutgers University, 1964.

Germana, J. Response characteristics and the orienting reflex. *Journal of Experimental Psychology,* 1968, **78**, 610–616. (a)

Germana, J. Psychophysiological correlates of conditioned response formation. *Psychological Bulletin,* 1968, **70**, 105–114. (b)

Gould, J., Lodwig, A., Raskin, D. C., Watts, W., & Maltzman, I. The orienting reflex and semantic conditioning and generalization of the galvanic skin response and alpha blocking. Paper presented at the Western Psychological Association, Long Beach, California, 1966.

Graham, F. K. Habituation and dishabituation of responses innervated by the autonomic nervous system. In H. V. S. Peeke & M. J. Herz (Eds.), *Habituation.* Vol. 1: *Behavioral studies.* New York: Academic Press, 1973.

Graham, F. K., & Jackson, J. C. Arousal systems and infant heart rate responses. In L. P. Lipsitt & H. W. Reese (Eds.), *Advances in Child Development and Behavior,* 1970, **5**, 59–117.

Grim, P. F., & White, S. H. Effects of stimulus change upon the GSR and reaction time. *Journal of Experimental Psychology,* 1965, **69**, 276–281.

Grings, W. W. Preparatory set variables in the classical conditioning of autonomic responses. *Psychological Review,* 1960, **67**, 243–252.

Grings, W. W. Verbal–perceptual factors in the conditioning of autonomic responses. In W. F. Prokasy (Ed.), *Classical conditioning.* New York: Appleton, 1965.

Groves, P. M., & Thompson, R. F. Habituation: A dual process theory. *Psychological Review,* 1970, **77,** 419–450.

Harding, G., & Punzo, F. Response uncertainty and skin conductance. *Journal of Experimental Psychology,* 1971, **88,** 265–272.

Hare, R., Wood, K., Britain, S., & Shadman, J. Autonomic responses to affective visual stimulation. *Psychophysiology,* 1970, **7,** 408–418.

Hebb, D. O. Drives and the C. N. S. (conceptual nervous system). *Psychological Review,* 1955, **62,** 243–254.

Houck, R. L., & Mefferd, R. B. Generalization of GSR habituation to mild intramodel stimuli. *Psychophysiology,* 1969, **6,** 202–206.

Johnson, H. J., & Campos, J. J. The effect of cognitive tasks and verbalization instructions on heart rate and skin conductance. *Psychophysiology,* 1967, **4,** 143–150.

Johnson, L. C. Some attributes of spontaneous autonomic activity. *Journal of Comparative and Physiological Psychology,* 1963, **56,** 415–422.

Johnson, L. C., & Lubin, A. Spontaneous electrodermal activity during waking and sleeping. *Psychophysiology,* 1966, **3,** 8–17.

Kimmel, H. D. The relationship between direction and amount of stimulus change and amount of perceptual disparity. *Journal of Experimental Psychology,* 1960, **59,** 68–72.

Kintsch, W. Habituation of the orienting reflex during paired-associate learning before and after learning has taken place. *Journal of Mathematical Psychology,* 1965, **2,** 330–341.

Kirk, W. E. UCR diminution in temporal conditioning and habituation. Paper presented at the Midwestern Psychological Association, Chicago, Illinois, 1969.

Kleinsmith, L. J., & Kaplan, S. Paired-associate learning as a function of arousal and interpolated interval. *Journal of Experimental Psychology,* 1963, **65,** 190–193.

Kleinsmith, L. J., & Kaplan, S. Interaction of arousal and recall interval in nonsense syllable paired-associate learning. *Journal of Experimental Psychology,* 1964, **67,** 124–126.

Koepke, J. E., & Pribram, K. H. Habituation of GSR as a function of stimulus duration and spontaneous activity. *Journal of Comparative and Physiological Psychology,* 1966, **61,** 442–448.

Krupski, A., Raskin, D. C., & Bakan, P. Physiological and personality correlates of commission errors in an auditory vigilance task. *Psychophysiology,* 1971, **8,** 304–311.

Lacey, J. I. Psychophysiological approaches to the evaluation of psychotherapeutic process and outcome. In E. A. Rubinstein & M. B. Parloff (Eds.), *Research in psychotherapy.* Washington, D.C.: Amer. Psych. Assoc., 1959. Pp. 179–208.

Lacey, J. I. Somatic response patterning and stress: Some revisions of activation theory. In M. H. Appley & R. Trumbull (Eds.), *Psychological stress: Issues in research.* New York: Appleton, 1967. Pp. 14–44.

Lacey, J. I., & Lacey, B. C. The relationship of resting autonomic activity to motor impulsivity. In *The brain and human behavior* (Proceedings of the Association for Research in Nervous and Mental Disease). Baltimore, Maryland: Williams & Wilkins, 1958. Pp. 144–209.

Lacey, J. I., Kagan, J., Lacey, B. C., & Moss, H. A. The visceral level: Situational determinants and behavioral correlates of autonomic response patterns. In

P. H. Knapp (Ed.), *Expression of the emotions of man.* New York: International Univ. Press, 1963. Pp. 161–196.

Liederman, P. H., & Shapiro, D. Studies on the galvanic skin potential level: Some behavioral correlates. *Journal of Psychosomatic Research,* 1964, **7,** 277–281.

Lindsley, D. B. Emotion. In S. S. Stevens (Ed.), *Handbook of experimental psychology.* New York: Wiley, 1951. Pp. 473–516.

Lindsley, D. B. Attention, consciousness, sleep and wakefulness. In J. Field, H. W. Magoun, & E. V. Hall (Eds.), *Handbook of physiology,* Section 1, Vol. III. Washington, D.C.: Amer. Physiol. Soc., 1960. Pp. 1553–1593.

Lynn, R. *Attention, arousal, and the orientation reaction.* Oxford: Pergamon, 1966.

Malmo, R. B. Measurement of drive: An unsolved problem in psychology. In M. R. Jones (Ed.), *Nebraska symposium on motivation.* Lincoln: Univ. of Nebraska Press, 1958. Pp. 229–265.

Malmo, R. B. Activation: A neurophysiological dimension. *Psychological Review,* 1959, **66,** 367–386.

Malmo, R. B. Activation. In A. J. Bachrach (Ed.), *Experimental foundations of clinical psychology.* New York: Basic Books, 1962. Pp. 386–422.

Maltzman, I., & Raskin, D. C. Effects of individual differences in the orienting reflex on conditioning and complex processes. *Journal of Experimental Research in Personality,* 1965, **1,** 1–16.

Martin, B. The assessment of anxiety by physiological behavioral measures. *Psychological Bulletin,* 1961, **58,** 234–255.

Neumann, E., & Blanton, R. The early history of electrodermal research. *Psychophysiology,* 1970, **6,** 453–475.

Pavlov, I. P. *Conditioned reflexes.* London and New York: Oxford Univ. Press (Clarendon), 1927.

Porges, S. W., & Raskin, D. C. Respiratory and heart rate components of attention. *Journal of Experimental Psychology,* 1969, **81,** 497–503.

Raskin, D. C. Semantic conditioning and generalization of autonomic responses. *Journal of Experimental Psychology,* 1969, **79,** 69–76.

Raskin, D. C., Kotses, H., & Bever, J. Autonomic indicators of orienting and defensive reflexes. *Journal of Experimental Psychology,* 1969, **80,** 423–433.

Roessler, R., Burch, N. R., & Childers, H. E. Personality and arousal correlates of specific galvanic skin responses. *Psychophysiology,* 1967, **3,** 115–130.

Ross, S., Dardano, J., & Hackman, R. Conductance levels during vigilance task performance. *Journal of Applied Psychology,* 1959, **43,** 65–69.

Routtenberg, A. The two arousal hypothesis: Reticular formation and limbic system. *Psychological Review,* 1968, **75,** 51–80.

Schlosberg, H. Three dimensions of emotion. *Psychological Review,* 1954, **61,** 81–88.

Schlosberg, H., & Stanley, W. C. A simple test of the normality of twenty-four distributions of electrical skin resistance. *Science,* 1953, **117,** 35–37.

Sharpless, S., & Jasper, H. Habituation of the arousal reaction. *Brain,* 1956, **79,** 655–680.

Silverman, A. J., Cohen, S. I., & Shmavonian, B. H. Investigation of psychophysiologic relationships with skin resistance measures. *Journal of Psychosomatic Research,* 1959, **4,** 65–87.

Smith, M. J. Variables influencing the orienting reflex, reinforcement and verbalization in verbal conditioning. Unpublished doctoral dissertation, University of California, Los Angeles, 1966.

Sokolov, E. N. Neuronal models and the orienting reflex. In M. A. B. Brazier

(Ed.), *The central nervous system and behavior,* New York: Josiah Macey, Jr. Foundation, 1960. Pp. 187–276.

Sokolov, E. N. *Perception and the conditioned reflex.* New York: Pergamon, 1963.

Stennett, R. G. The relationship of performance level to level of arousal. *Journal of Experimental Psychology,* 1957, **54,** 54–61.

Surwillo, W. W., & Quilter, R. E. The relation of frequency of spontaneous skin potential responses to vigilance and age. *Psychophysiology,* 1965, **1,** 272–276.

Tarchanoff, J. Décharges électriques dons la peau de l'homme sous l'influence de l'excitation des organes des sens et de différentes formes d'activité psychique. *Comptes Rendus Société de Biologie,* 1889 (Ser. 9), **41,** 447–451.

Thompson, R. F., & Spencer, W. A. Habituation: A model phenomenon for the study of neuronal substrates of behavior. *Psychological Review,* 1966, **73,** 16–43.

Uno, T., & Grings, W. W. Autonomic components of orienting behavior. *Psychophysiology,* 1965, **1,** 311–321.

Walker, L., & Tarte, R. D. Memory storage as a function of arousal and time with homogeneous and heterogeneous lists. *Journal of Verbal Learning and Verbal Behavior,* 1963, **2,** 113–119.

Wilcott, R. C., Darrow, C. W., & Siegel, A. Uniphasic and diphasic wave forms of the skin potential response. *Journal of Comparative and Physiological Psychology,* 1957, **50,** 217–219.

Williams, J. A. Novelty, GSR, and stimulus generalization. *Canadian Journal of Psychology,* 1963, **17,** 52–61.

Woodworth, R. S., & Schlosberg, H. *Experimental psychology.* New York: Holt, 1954.

Yokota, T., Takahashi, T., Kondo, M., & Fujimori, B. Studies on the diphasic wave form of the galvanic skin reflex. *Electroencephalogram and Clinical Neurophysiology,* 1959, **11,** 687–696.

Zimny, G. H., & Kienstra, R. A. Orienting and defensive responses to electric shock. *Psychophysiology,* 1967, **3,** 351–362.

Zimny, G. H., & Schwabe, L. W. Stimulus change and habituation of the orienting response. *Psychophysiology,* 1966, **2,** 103–115.

CHAPTER 3

Classical Conditioning

WILLIAM F. PROKASY

Department of Psychology
University of Utah
Salt Lake City, Utah

KAROL L. KUMPFER[1]

Department of Psychology
Oberlin College
Oberlin, Ohio

I.   Introduction 157
II. Methodology 158
     A. Response Measurement 158
     B. Response Form 162
     C. Controls 166
     D. Habituation and Conditioning 172
III. Independent Variable Manipulations 173
     A. Acquisition 174
     B. Interstimulus Interval 176
     C. Reinforcement Schedules 181
     D. Backward Conditioning 184
     E. Distributional Phenomena 186
     F. Conditioned Stimulus 186
     G. Trace versus Delay 189
     H. Stimulus Generalization 190
     I. Unconditioned Stimulus 192
IV. Concluding Comments 194
     References 196

I.   Introduction

This chapter will be concerned exclusively with what we have learned about how the electrodermal response (EDR) modifies as a consequence

[1] Present address: Department of Long-Range Planning, University of Utah, Salt Lake City, Utah.

of a contingency between conditioned stimulus (CS) and unconditioned stimulus (UCS). The basic paradigm is that of simple (single-cue) and differential (multiple-cue) conditioning, and in which the CSs are, in general, tones, lights, etc. More complex conditioned stimuli are considered in Chapter 4.

This chapter will have two major sections. The first section will emphasize problems of control and measurement, and the second will be a survey of the effects of the major independent variable manipulations which have been employed in EDR conditioning. Because so little has been done with the skin potential response (SPR) within a conditioning framework, the treatment will be principally of the exosomatic measures of skin conductance and resistance levels, SCL and SRL, respectively, and of skin conductance and resistance change, SCR and SRR, respectively.

II. Methodology

In spite of the fact that the conditioned EDR has been an object of study for about 50 years, it has been only since about 1960 that an extensive examination of the characteristics of the response and the problems of control has been made. The result has been a substantial change in both method and measurement in conditioned EDR research, sufficiently so that an extended discussion of the basis for this change is necessary before the problems encountered in the literature survey can be understood.

A. Response Measurement

The most common units in which the conditioned EDR are reported are micromhos SCR and kilohms SRR. More often than not, the units are transformed with either square root or log transformations with the objectives, not necessarily achieved, of normalizing the distributions or producing a lower correlation between response amplitude and tonic level (i.e., skin conductance level, SCL, or skin resistance level, SRL). There have been some attempts at determining which transformations produce the best results for statistical purposes but the amount of information available is insufficient to argue strenuously on this basis for one transformation over the other. Since the square root and log transformations are likely to produce distributions which more closely approximate the assumptions made in the application of statistical tests, they do have that practical advantage.

Two recent recommendations for units merit consideration. Lykken,

Rose, Luther, and Maley (1966) have introduced a range-corrected score (RCS)

$$RCS = \frac{\Delta SCL}{SCL_{max} - SCL_{min}}$$

in which the left-hand side of the equation represents the response as a proportion of the total range of response that is possible. SCL_{max} is the maximum conductance level obtainable for a particular subject, with one method for estimating this maximum being the SCL obtained while the subject is blowing up a balloon to bursting. SCL_{min} is obtained during a period of relaxation. Lykken *et al.* argue that this measure will reduce the noisy influence in the range of output variable (i.e., in this case conductance). It is to be noted that Lykken *et al.* also propose a range-corrected score (RCL) for tonic levels. For example,

$$RCL = \frac{SCL - SCL_{min}}{SCL_{max} - SCL_{min}},$$

where RCL represents the measured conductance. They provide evidence that this measure does eliminate a substantial share of the individual differences which contribute to a large error term in statistical analyses.

A second recent suggestion is that of Lykken and Venables (1971). This involves measuring each response as a proportion of the subject's response to an intensely eliciting stimulus. The distinction between the two measures merits note. With the range-corrected measure, the possible ratio of change ordinarily will be less than 1.0 since the tonic level obtained during conditioning is likely to be greater than the minimum obtained during relaxation. Moreover, the ratio cannot exceed 1.0 since, presumably, the upper limit of responding is defined by the maximum tonic level employed in the equation. The proportion measure can vary from .0 to greater than 1.0. Thus, given constant tonic levels, the practical range allowable is greater with the proportion than with the range-corrected score. The former, too, would appear to be less influenced by individual differences in the tonic level obtained during conditioning.

Both measures can provide some difficulty if tonic levels do not remain constant across the conditioning session, although this difficulty exists, as well, with the measures typically employed. Since resistance and conductance changes are not independent of tonic level, it is possible (see below) for changes in magnitude across trials to be a function of shifts in tonic levels. This is particularly a problem in view of the fact that the noxiousness of the UCS can determine whether tonic levels increase or decrease throughout a conditioning session.

Most frequently SCR and SRR have been reported in magnitude units, which is to say that a zero is entered for those trials during which a response does not occur. Thus, amplitudes from response trials are averaged with zero entries from nonresponse trials. The ostensible value of this averaging is that it assumes that some size of response always occurs (Kimmel, 1968), but that an arbitrary entry is made when whatever does occur fails to meet a predetermined criterion. Clearly it has pragmatic value since, depending upon response criterion and the duration of the criterion interval, the likelihood of a response may be very high or very low. In those circumstances, if there is some interest in the size of the response, it would be a practical impossibility to plot data in small blocks of trials across all subjects unless magnitude were employed. The magnitude measure thus incorporates information about size but is substantially determined by the frequency with which subjects meet the minimal response criterion.

The magnitude measure is a complicated one and, we are inclined to believe, not a particularly useful one (Prokasy, 1969). There are several reasons for this view. First, the measure does confound frequency and amplitude. While there may be some value to the assumption, even though necessarily incorrect, that a response always occurs independent of minimal response criterion and duration of criterion interval, it is clear in several studies (Jenson, 1972; Kumpfer, 1972; Prokasy & Ebel, 1967; Prokasy, Williams, Kumpfer, Lee, & Jenson, 1973) that response frequency and response amplitude do not always covary. That is, there are instances of frequency, but not amplitude, varying with an independent variable manipulation. Under these circumstances mixing frequency and amplitude would appear to be unwise as it creates the impression that response size is changing when, in fact, it may not be.

Second, the choice of the value to use in a magnitude measure when a criterion response is not made is arbitrary and itself may determine the outcome. If the arbitrary value is far from the obtained distribution of amplitudes, then the major variance in the system will be, for all practical purposes, a frequency effect. The closer the criterion value to the bulk of the distribution of obtained frequencies, the more response size will play a role in the outcome, although the distribution itself is a problem: with many nonresponse trials the distribution is bimodal. If one is specifically interested in shifts in response amplitude, the use of an arbitrary entry for a nonresponse will reduce the likelihood of obtaining an effect if only because the within-cell variances are thereby increased.

Third, it is possible for magnitude measures to be rendered virtually meaningless with changes in tonic level across a conditioning session. In her dissertation, Kumpfer (1972) observed, with a .2-sec burst of 115-dB white noise as the UCS, a gradual increase in SCL across trials. With square root of micromhos SCR as the measure, she observed high, positive correlations between SCL and SCR. She also observed that there was an increase in SCR amplitude across blocks of trials. Given the transformation, it is apparent that the phasic and tonic levels are not independent. Under these circumstances magnitude measures could be highly misleading since response frequency decreased across trials. A further problem is that in studies employing a shock UCS, the intensity is determined by the subject, and it is clear that at least in some instances such a procedure results in a decrease in SCL across trials (e.g., Prokasy & Ebel, 1964). Any correlation between SCL and SCR could yield results not in accord with studies in which SCL either remained constant or increased.

In view of the complications with the magnitude measure, it is strongly advised that in conditioning research a separate assessment of frequency and amplitude be undertaken. Not only does this have the advantage of respecting the empirical fact that the two indices do not always co-vary, it has one major practical advantage: Most of the variance in EDR conditioning is absorbed by presence versus absence of a response, and the latter is easily measured. Employing a frequency measure avoids, for the most part, the major problems associated with tonic and phasic levels and transformations. Separate treatment of amplitude permits, moreover, a more careful assessment of the relationship between tonic and phasic values.

A note of caution is in order concerning the presence versus absence of a response. In most conditioning studies the response is defined as a minimal SRR (say, 400 Ω) even though subsequent transformations to SCR might be made. At an SRL of 40,000 Ω, the SCR would be .25 μmho, but at an SRL of 80,000 Ω, the SCR would be approximately .06 μmho. In short, if the minimum response criterion is expressed in ohms, then the minimum response in mhos will vary as a function of tonic level and vice versa. Until more is known about the distribution of amplitudes as a function of tonic levels, the definition of a response will remain quite arbitrary. One possibility to be explored is that a minimum proportion of maximum response be adopted as a criterion, given that tonic levels remain roughly constant across conditioning sessions. Conceivably a proportion criterion will separate signal from noise in a way that produces both good frequency and relative amplitude measures. See Chapter 1 of this volume for an extensive, general discussion of measurement.

B. Response Form

It has been known for some time (Bitterman, Reed, & Krauskopf, 1952; Rodnick, 1937; Switzer, 1934) that with ISIs longer than 4 or 5 sec multiple humps occur as components of the EDR. Stimulated largely by the research of Stewart, Stern, Winokur, and Fredman (1961) and of Grings, Lockhart, and Dameron (1962), it has only been in the past decade that extensive inquiry into the nature of the multiple response has been made. The first response component occurs within 3–4 sec of CS onset, the second shortly prior to the point in time at which the UCS ordinarily would occur, and the third at the point in time at which the UCR ordinarily would occur. Extensive examples from individual Ss are provided by Kimmel (1965, pp. 157–162), and some idealized forms can be found in Grings et al. (1962).

Multiple response forms pose a variety of issues: definition and nomenclature, justification for separation into multiple responses, and whether or not each is conditionable. Multiple responses are defined by latency intervals. Usually the first interval is defined as extending from about 1 to 4 or 5 sec after CS onset. The second interval is not quite so uniformly defined, and how it is employed depends upon the interstimulus interval (ISI). For example, Grings et al. (1962) defined the interval as one which is post-UCS in studies with an ISI of 5 sec. Employing slightly longer ISIs (6–8 sec), the second interval is often defined to include the span of time after a CS-elicited response ordinarily would occur but before a UCS-elicited response occurs. A typical definition with an 8-sec ISI would be: first interval from 1.0 to 4.0 sec after CS onset, second from 4.0 to 9.0, and third from 9.0 to 13.0. Just how the intervals have been defined has varied directly with ISI. With ISIs of, say, 4 sec and less, defining two pre-UCR intervals is not feasible, while with ISIs of 6 sec and longer it is possible to define not only two pre-UCR intervals but a third interval which coincides with the time span during which the UCR ordinarily would occur.

Several suggestions have been made for labeling the different responses. Stewart, Winokur, Stern, Guze, Pfeiffer, and Hornung (1959) identified four responses: an orienting response (OR), an anticipatory response (AR), a response occurring at the time a UCR ordinarily would occur and in the absence of the UCS (UCS-omission response), and the unconditioned response (UCR). The first two correspond to the first and second temporal intervals described above, while the latter two fall in a common post-UCS interval. Lockhart (1966) identified the same responses as: CS response, pre-UCS response, UCS-omission response, and UCR. Grings and Sukoneck (1971) adopted OR, AR, UCS-omission, and UCR. In earlier work, Grings et al. (1962) identified the first two by intervals: first-interval response and second-interval response, with the latter being a post-UCS response. Martin (1963b) identified, in addition, a third-interval response which, in her case, was a pre-UCR response. Prokasy and Ebel (1967) identified three response intervals as first-interval response (FIR), second-interval response, (SIR) and third-interval response (TIR). The FIR is comparable to the OR, the SIR to the AR, and the TIR to either the UCR or the UCS-omission response, depending upon the presence or absence of the UCS.

The use of OR, AR, UCS-omission, and UCR has the advantage of identifying a response with respect to either CS or UCS onset, given a long interstimulus interval. It has the disadvantages of surplus theoretical meaning and of ambiguity with respect to middle-range ISIs. The FIR, SIR, and TIR designations have the advantages of no surplus meaning and of a relative location in time following CS onset. They have the disadvantage of being ambiguous with respect to the location of the response with respect to the UCS. For the purpose of this chapter, the mnemonics provided in Table 1 will be employed. These provide for nine different labels which can identify a response location relative to both CS onset and UCS onset. These do not solve all identification problems, but they will provide a convenient shorthand.

TABLE 1

Designations for Responses Which Are Located in Time with Respect to CS Onset and UCS Onset

Post-CS interval[a]	Pre-UCS	Post-UCS UCS present	Post-UCS UCS omitted
First	FAR	FUR	FOR
Second	SAR	SUR	SOR
Third	TAR	TUR	TOR

[a] Consecutive temporal intervals following CS onset.

As a rule, the first SCR or SRR to occur in each of the intervals is defined as the response, though some investigators choose the larger of two responses in an interval (e.g., Dawson, 1970). Maximum displacement is sometimes defined as the maximum reached within an interval and sometimes as the maximum reached regardless of location given that the interval in which the response began is known. The usual procedure for determining amplitude is to define as SCL or SRL the value which exists at the point at which the response began and then to measure total displacement between that value and the peak resistance or conductance achieved.

With the advent of the Stewart *et al.* paper (1961), there was some disagreement as to whether or not first anticipatory responses (FARs) and second anticipatory responses were both conditionable and whether or not they should be treated as separate responses (e.g., Kimmel, 1964; Leonard & Winokur, 1963; Lockhart & Grings, 1963; Martin, 1963a, b; McDonald & Johnson, 1965). As is made clear in a recent review (Dengerink & Taylor, 1971), neither of these issues appears to be in doubt at the present time. Within the limits of control group procedures, there is ample evidence that FARs and second omission responses (SORs) are conditionable (e.g., Leonard & Winokur, 1963; McDonald & Johnson, 1965; Prokasy & Ebel, 1967).

That multiple responses are conditionable does not, in itself, constitute a basis for their separation. They may be, as Kimmel (1964, 1965) has argued, all part of a single, dynamic wave, the form of which changes across conditioning trials. Under these circumstances the components of a single response individually might reflect conditioning even though the separation is not entirely justified. There are two empirical ways to address this problem. The first is to determine whether or not manipulated independent variables have comparable effects on the components. The second is to search for any conditional relationships which may exist among the multiple components. If the components routinely vary in the same way with independent variable manipulation and if the correlation among the components is also high (whether negative or positive), then it would be difficult to maintain the position that the components of the EDR are separately analyzable.

At the simplest level, the FARs and SARs are distinct if only because there are studies on record in which one, but not the other, yielded evidence of conditioning. For example, Leonard and Winokur (1963) and McDonald and Johnson (1965) both obtained evidence of SAR conditioning (SAR was pre-UCR in both cases) but not of FAR conditioning. Martin (1963a, b), employing extended ISIs of 12 sec, obtained evidence of FAR, but not SAR, conditioning. A more substantial demonstration, however, is the fact that independent variable manipulation does not always result in the same outcome for FARs and SARs. For example, FAR frequency and amplitude vary with CS intensity while SAR frequency and amplitude do not (Prokasy & Ebel, 1967). In addition, FAR amplitude is greater with conditioning rather than sequential control operations, but SAR amplitude is unaffected by this treatment difference in simple conditioning. This difference occurred in spite of the fact that both FAR and SAR frequencies were greater with conditioning, rather than control, operations.

To date, the search for statistical independence of multiple responses has been limited to two published studies (Prokasy & Ebel, 1967; Prokasy et al., 1973) and two unpublished theses (Jenson, 1972; Kumpfer, 1972), and the results are generally consistent across studies. Prokasy and Ebel (1967) found that the likelihood of an SAR was not conditional upon the presence or absence of an FAR. Jenson (1972) and Kumpfer (1972) found that not only are the FARs and SARs conditionally independent, but also that their amplitudes are correlated only to a limited extent. That is, given that both FAR and SAR occurred on a given trial, no evidence of a systematic positive or negative correlation was found across trials on an S-by-S basis. One conditional relationship observed was that SAR amplitude is smaller in the presence of an FAR than in its absence. This finding, in the context of the largely negative results on other conditional relationships, suggests a peripheral response interference, possibly a kind of refractory phase, or else a measurement complication related to correlations between tonic and phasic levels.

The relative independence of FARs and SARs constitutes a strong rationale for designing conditioning experiments in such a way as to permit their separate assessment. Unless short ISIs are necessary, this would imply running conditioning experiments in which the ISI is at least 5 sec.

Although there is some variation across experiments in defining FARs, a practical upper bound is probably approximately 3.5 sec after CS onset. Response latencies to a signal onset typically are at least 1.2 sec, and only occasionally would exceed a range of from 3.2 to 3.5 sec after signal onset. Latencies in the interval from 3.5 sec after CS onset until approximately 1.2 sec after UCS onset would define responses as SARs. Obviously, the length of such an interval would be determined by the ISI. Responses recorded in the interval which ordinarily would define the location of the UCS have latencies from approximately 1.2 to 3.5 sec after UCS onset. This range would be suitable for FORs, SORs, and TORs.

C. Controls

As is the case with many autonomically mediated responses, the determination of what EDR modifications are attributable uniquely to the operations of CS–UCS pairing (or, more generally, CS–UCS contingency) is no simple task. There are many nonassociative[2] effects which exist, and to control for them requires that one consider the complications which have arisen from past research on the one hand and, on the other, incorporate into an experimental design those operations which reflect the theoretical assumptions about the behavior itself. The purpose of this section is to identify those factors which have been determined to be empirical obstacles to identifying associative effects as well as to note the (usually implicit) assumptions made when trying to control for them.

To understand the problems of control, it is necessary to examine some of the common characteristics of the EDR. Though there has been a substantial shift in the past decade, the most common form of measurement had been to record the maximum change in resistance (SRR) or conductance (SCR) which occurs between approximately 1 and 5 sec after CS onset. It is doubtful that a more delicate, or complicated, choice of CR could have been made, since signal-elicited responses have such a high initial frequency.

The frequency and amplitude of an elicited response are readily modified, and a detailed discussion is provided in Chapter 2. It is sufficient here merely to summarize some of the major changes which can occur but which are not attributable to associative effects. One of the most potent variables is signal intensity. In general, response magnitude and frequency decrease as a function of simple repetition (see, e.g., Prokasy & Ebel, 1964, 1967; Raskin, Kotses, & Bever, 1969). However, as intensity becomes quite high, it is entirely possible for magnitude to increase with repetition, For example, Raskin et al. (1969) found slight increases in SCRs and SCLs when bursts of white noise reached an intensity of 120 dB(A). Habituation to a mild or relatively nonaversive stimulus is delayed if unpaired stimuli of high intensity or aversiveness occur at unpredictable times during a session in which repetitive presentations of the relatively nonaversive signal are made (see, e.g., Prokasy, Hall, & Fawcett, 1962b). Similarly, habituation is more rapid when the average time between stimulations is reduced (Raskin et al., 1969).

---

[2] By "nonassociative" we mean effects which are attributable exclusively to the CS–UCS contingency. In a more general sense there are associative effects which are manifest in the conditioning situation but which are not the exclusive consequence of the experimenter-imposed CS–UCS relationship.

Two other EDR characteristics merit comment before turning to control operations. First, there is the offset response, as noted above. Until the past 5–10 years, most EDR conditioning was conducted with interstimulus intervals of 2 sec or less, this selection of intervals consistent with what once was thought to be an optimum interval range for conditioning (see Kimble, 1961, p. 156). With, say, a .5-sec ISI and a recording interval on test trials (i.e., trials on which the UCS is omitted) ranging out to 5 sec after CS onset, it is evident that a response to CS offset can affect the measurement. An FAR begins with a latency of 1.2–3.5 sec and will reach its peak amplitude from 1 to 3 sec later. Thus, a response to CS onset may reach its peak amplitude 4 sec after onset, but if there is an offset response to the .5-sec CS, its onset and peak could be reached, as well, within the 5-sec measuring period. It is conceivable, then, that with short ISIs the measured response is determined by both onset and offset characteristics. A further discussion of this phenomenon can be found in Badia and Defran (1970).

The second characteristic is what Grings (1960) has aptly called the "perceptual disparity response." When a signal occurs at an unexpected time, or when it is omitted at a point in time when it is expected, an EDR may occur. While such a response reflects a set of situational associations, it is to be noted that CS–UCS pairing in the usual sense is not a necessary condition for its occurrence. Given a simple conditioning situation in which a .5-sec ISI is employed with 100% CS–UCS pairing, the omission of the UCS on a test trial may result not only in a CS offset response but also in a perceptual disparity response, either or both possibly affecting the response which would ordinarily occur following CS onset.

For the most part, what experimental controls are employed are designed to control for pseudoconditioning and for sensitization. Although the two words have not been employed consistently in the literature, for present purposes the definitions provided by Kimble (1961) will suffice. Pseudoconditioning refers to the strengthening of a response to a neutral stimulus which results from the repeated elicitation of the response to another stimulus even though the two stimuli have not been paired. Sensitization refers to the strengthening of an original response to the conditioned stimulus through its pairing with an unconditioned stimulus. The emphasis in this case is on the fact that the response which is sensitized is an original response to the conditioned stimulus, and not necessarily to the unconditioned stimulus. Since the original response to both the CS and the UCS is the same in EDR conditioning, the definitions of conditioned response and sensitized response are such as to not permit a distinction between them. Since the definitions are arbitrary (i.e., not theoretically based), and since both sensitized and conditioned responses imply a pairing of stimuli, what some writers might refer to as sensitized orienting responses to the CS will be considered as CRs in this chapter.

The sequential control group is most often employed as a comparison base in simple conditioning situations. This involves the presentation, in a random, unpaired order, of CSs and UCSs with the constraint that the numbers of CSs and UCSs be the same as those encountered in the conditioning group. We call it "sequential control" to contrast the operations with an alternative set of control operations to be introduced later. An example of a sequential control can be drawn from a simple conditioning situation. If Ss in a conditioning group receive paired CS-UCS trials at an average intertrial interval of 50 sec, then the sequential control group will receive the same total number of CSs and UCSs in an unpaired order. If the time between trials in the conditioning group varies from 40 to 60 sec, then the time between successive stimulus presentation in the sequential control group would very likely vary from 20 to 30 sec.

In addition to sensitization and pseudoconditioning, the sequential control group is designed to control for the following: total number of UCS occurrences; total number of CS occurrences; average time between UCSs; average time between CSs; stimulus-specific properties; offset effects with short ISIs; and general aversiveness of the situation. Whether or not this is an adequate control for the items mentioned is moot, and is certainly not answerable in the absence of a theory of electrodermal responding. What we do know is that there are frequently (though not always) differences in FAR magnitude to the CS when it is paired with the UCS as opposed to when it is not, and the conclusion is usually drawn that the difference is a result of S associating CS and UCS (or CS and UCR in a strict S–R formulation).

There are potential problems with the sequential control group. For example, with short ISIs it is not the case that the sequential control provides an adequate baseline for comparison when perceptual disparity responses are possible. Also, it is merely a convenient assumption that the combined stimulus event rate per unit time in the sequential control group, being greater than the rate per unit time of CS–UCS pairings, is of no consequence in the comparison. The only relevant study to date (Prokasy et al., 1962b) suggests that these differential rates are not critical, but the study also provided no evidence of conditioning. Clearly with an average intertrial interval of, say, 20 sec for a conditioning group receiving 100% reinforcement, the resulting average of 10 sec between stimulus events for a sequential control group could result in complications if only because in the latter a full return to baseline might not be effected prior to the onset of the next trial. A final problem is the aversiveness of the situation. The assumption is that, with the same stimuli employed, the sequential control group is in no less aversive a situation than one in which there is a signaled aversive event. Grings (1969) did show that the unpaired UCS is judged to be more aversive than the paired UCS, but more recent research has not sustained this observation (e.g., Furedy, 1970; Furedy & Doob, 1971). Since, in addition, tonic SCLs do not differ between conditioning and sequential control groups (Prokasy & Ebel, 1964), the assumption may be acceptable.

For multiple cue, or differential, conditioning, the control operation is implicit in the procedure itself: differential responding to CS⁻ and CS⁺ is assumed to be the index of conditioning, with Ss, in effect, serving as their own controls. While the method rather economically can demonstrate differences between CS⁺ and CS⁻ responding, it does suffer from the lack of comparison with an independent baseline. One form of baseline is to run, as with the single-cue case, sequential control groups. This was done, for example, in a study by Carey, Schell, & Grings (1971). The general outcome was that CS⁻ responding tended to approximate that of the responding to the signals employed in the sequential control groups.

In his critique of pseudoconditioning control procedures Burstein (1973) suggests that a sequential control for differential conditioning be designed to approximate the differential conditioning procedure more closely. Thus, of the two neutral cues, only one would have the UCS follow it at unpaired times prior to the occurrence of the other cue. The net effect would be that one cue, a pseudo CS⁺, would be followed at least some of the time by an unpaired UCS prior to the occurrence of the pseudo CS⁻. The pseudo CS⁻ would be followed only by either the pseudo CS⁺ or another pseudo CS⁻. Though no research has been done on the problem, Burstein's position is based upon the assumption that a sequential control procedure can be interpreted as a conditioning procedure with a highly variable ISI.

An additional baseline worth mentioning is time-sampling in the absence of a signal. Time-sampling provides an index of the frequency and amplitude of nonspecific responses (Edelberg, 1967) which occur in the situation but which are not directly linked to an experimenter-controlled stimulus presentation. In one study (Prokasy et al., 1973) it was shown that with extensive differential conditioning training, not only did CS⁺ and CS⁻ performance differences disappear, but FAR frequency to both stimuli approximated nonspecific response frequency by the end of the session. Williams (1973) has shown that sequential control response rate is about the same as nonspecific response rate, and that these, in turn, approximate the levels eventually reached to a CS⁺ with extensive training.

So far the discussion of controls has been oriented primarily to what has been done to control for empirically observed effects. In the absence of a well-articulated theory of conditioning, however, it is not clear what constitutes a proper set of controls. Consider the specific contingency of pairing from a more general perspective, with the CS as event 1 and the UCS as event 2 (see, also, Prokasy, 1965). With two events there are myriad possible relationships between them. It is possible to provide a likelihood of occurrence per unit time for each of the two events and then use a random number generating system to select the time units in which each falls. Thus, event 1 may occur with a likelihood of .1 and event 2 with a likelihood of .05 per unit time, assuming in this case that each event has a duration equal to the time unit. In 1000 time units the chance expectation is that they would occur together five times if the two events were generated independently across the units. It is possible to alter the contingencies by changing the likelihood of event 2 contingent on the presence or absence of event 1. Similarly, it would be possible to alter the likelihood of either or both events as a function of the amount of time having elapsed from the last event. From this point of view, the pairing of event 1 and event 2 represents a very special contingency, the more so since, as a typical CS–UCS pairing, the precise temporal relationship between them is fixed. Similarly, the sequential control provides a special set of contingencies for S: neither event appears during a time unit in which the other exists, and it is usual for the likelihood of event 1 and event 2 to be zero for some span of time preceding and following the occurrence of either one of them.

It is easily seen that very many contingencies between events and between events as a function of time are possible, but that the typical single-cue conditioning situation has been investigated largely with only two sets of contingencies: pairing and sequential control. What has not been investigated is the extent to which modifications of EDRs occur as a function of systematic shifts in the conditional relationships between stimuli and across time in a session. The point to this is twofold. First, that a performance difference exists between a conditioning and a sequential control group in itself does not rule out effects other than the associative ones sought. Second, a wide variety of CS–UCS contingencies may result in the same class of EDR changes, which is to say that at the empirical level there may be no clear way to distinguish associative from other effects given a class of EDR performance. There is no *a priori* reason to expect that explicit, fixed ISI, pairings of CS and

UCS will result in changes in skin resistance (or conductance) or skin potential which are unique to that contingency class. What is unknown is the class of contingencies which can produce the same effects as CS–UCS pairing.

Rescorla (1967) has a position which defines a proper control for classical conditioning. From the general framework that a CS⁺ may acquire excitatory properties and CS⁻ may acquire inhibitory properties, Rescorla assumes that the proper control is a truly random control in which CS and UCS are presented randomly with respect to each other in a manner described for events 1 and 2 above. It follows from his position that the typical sequential control group for single-cue conditioning receives the nominal CS in a fashion which corresponds to a CS⁻ in a differential conditioning paradigm. Thus, if the situation is one in which inhibitory properties can be acquired by a CS⁻, then the sequential control group is not a proper control since responding to the signal would yield performance levels below that of the Ss receiving the truly random control procedure. Any excitatory properties similarly may be observed by the extent to which performance to a CS exceeds what is obtained with the truly random control group.

Not much is known about the truly random control group, and it is clear that what constitutes a random sequence of events to S is unknown. A wide variety of possible sequences can be generated from the same parameter values, and it would be surprising if each possible random sequence yielded the same outcome as all other random sequences. Nonetheless, there have been four relevant studies employing the EDR. Furedy (1971), Furedy and Schiffman (1971), and Schiffman and Furedy (1972) reported evidence only of excitatory effects. That is, there were no differences obtained between differential conditioning with a CS⁺ and CS⁻ and differential conditioning with a CS⁺ and a "truly random" signal. In both of these studies the critical comparison was a between-groups comparison. It is to be noted, as well, that the random sequence of UCSs was such as to produce no overlap between the random signal and the UCS. In this respect it was more like a CS⁻. In a more recent experiment Prokasy et al. (1973) found evidence of both excitatory and inhibitory effects, but these were not uniform across FARs and SARs. The design was such that all Ss received CS⁺, CS⁻, and RS (random signal), and of particular interest was the fact that SAR amplitude was greatest to CS⁺ and least to CS⁻. SAR probability was greatest to CS⁺, but did not differ between CS⁻ and RS. FAR probability was equivalent for CS⁺ and RS, but was reliably lower for CS⁻. The failure to obtain internal consistency raised some questions about conditioned stimuli acquiring a kind of generalized excitatory or inhibitory property.

Regardless of a final interpretation, the major point is that the control operations typically employed are not the only possible controls and that, therefore, interpretation of EDR data in terms of associative versus nonassociative effects are more precise than the experimental procedures permit.

D. Habituation and Conditioning

As noted earlier, responses are elicited with the onset (and offset) of a wide variety of stimuli from subjectively mild and neutral to subjectively intense and either highly noxious or highly pleasurable. With repeated stimulus presentation there are decreases in response frequency and amplitude. It is no surprise, then, that demonstrating conditioning with FARs or FORs is not always easy. For example, if Ss are presented with a series of neutral signals, such as tones, a decrease in response frequency will be observed. If an aversive stimulus is then paired with the tone, there results an immediate, and substantial, increase in elicited response probability with the next tone occurrence. A sequential control group given first the series of tones and then just one between-trials aversive stimulus presentation will show nearly the same increase in frequency with the next tone presentation (see, e.g., Prokasy & Ebel, 1967). Thereafter both conditioning and sequential control groups will exhibit, typically, a continued decrease in FAR probability with the sequential control yielding the more rapid decrease. Conditioning is inferred from the differential rate of FAR decrease, not from any sustained increase in responding, inasmuch as continued training seems to result in a gradual elimination of differences between sequential control group and conditioning group. Not only does this effect show up with single-cue training (e.g., Kimmel, 1959; Prokasy & Ebel, 1967), differential EDR performance disappears with extensive training (e.g., Prokasy et al., 1973; Williams, 1973). It appears likely that conditioning effects will be maintained for a longer span of training with more intense UCSs, though whether or not they would remain indefinitely provided that the UCS were intense enough to sustain a continued, reliable UCR is unknown.

Effects such as those described have led some workers (e.g., Stewart et al., 1961) to suggest that FARs or FORs are sensitized orienting responses and are not, therefore, properly classified as conditioned responses. Such a position begs the issue, of course, since one is left wondering how it is that orienting responses are differentially sensitized depending upon whether or not there is a contingency between CS and UCS. Additional interpretations are that conditioned FARs can be accounted for by the constructs of habituation and dishabituation (Raskin, 1966), or that habituation can be accounted for in terms of conditioning constructs (Stein, 1966).

As attractive interpretation of the relationship between habituation and conditioning phenomena is suggested in Razran's recent book (Razran, 1971, pp. 29–57). From an evolutionary point of view Razran sees the phenomenon of habituation as the first vestigial evidence of learning, or, more broadly, behavior modifications. Habituation reflects what Razran calls "memorial associations" which, loosely, means that in some way the organism has stored and used information from past experience with the same stimuli. That dishabituation occurs so readily with changes in modality, intensity, or temporal location constitutes *prima facie* evidence for memorial associations.

To extend Razran's ideas further, it is likely that the decreases in response frequency and amplitude which we call habituation are a direct function of contingencies between a particular signal, the static background stimulation, and the temporal characteristics (i.e., rise time. duration, between-trials average time, and variability of time between trials) of the repeated signal. Moreover, the extent to which a signal can serve as an adequate UCS is very likely a function of the same interactions. This, together with the subjective intensity or emotional tone of a signal, might very well determine the extent to which a signal can serve as an adequate UCS in providing evidence of a contingency between it and a specifically selected signal. Until further information is available, however, the relationship between habituation and conditioning phenomena is, at best, conjectural.

III. Independent Variable Manipulations

In the course of research in the area of classical conditioning, a variety of independent variables has been manipulated in an effort to understand both simple (or single-cue) and differential (two or more cues) conditioning. Included are such variables as CS intensity and modality, UCS intensity and modality, interstimulus interval, reinforcement schedules, etc. In the subsections which follow, a summary of what has been learned about the effects of these variables is provided. No attempt has been made to include all possibly relevant studies on any one topic; rather, the effort has been confined to assessing what we know in light of the sizable change in methodology in the past 10–15 years. The major emphases will be on empirical outcomes with relatively neutral, and elementary, signals as CSs.

A. Acquisition

In the methodology section a number of references was made to the characteristics of performance during acquisition training. Figure 1 provides an example of FAR, SAR, and TOR performance in simple conditioning with both magnitude and probability as dependent variables. The data come from a study by Prokasy and Ebel (1967) in which the two independent variables were CS intensity (two levels) and pairing versus sequential control. The ISI was 8 sec, which permitted identification of two pre-UCS responses. For present purposes the important outcome is that both FAR and TOR decrease in response level over training. While the SAR does not decline, more recent work (Williams, 1973) suggests that it, too, declines in strength with extended training. The FAR and TOR performance is consistent with data from other studies (e.g., Kimmel, 1959; Williams, 1973). It may be noted,

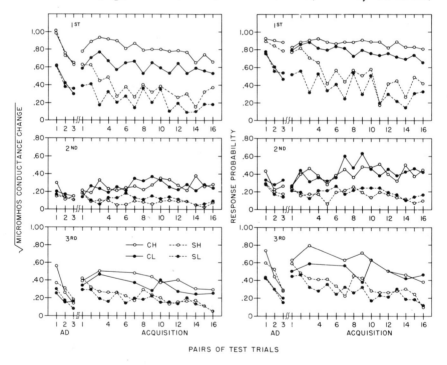

Fig. 1. Response magnitude and probability of FAR (first), SAR (second), and TOR (third) as a function of blocks of trials. Solid lines represent conditioning groups and dashed lines represent sequential control groups. Open circles represent high CS intensity and closed circles low CS intensity. (From Prokasy & Ebel, 1967, Fig. 1.)

incidentally, that the magnitude and probability functions do parallel each other in great detail, thus lending credence to the position that relative frequency is the primary determiner of what goes on with the magnitude measure.

Similar acquisition trends have been observed with the differential conditioning paradigms. Kumpfer (1972), Williams (1973), and Prokasy et al. (1973) have found that the extent of differential FAR and SAR performance first rises to a maximum and then decreases with continued training. In the former two studies this result was obtained in groups of Ss which had been informed of the conditioning contingencies as well as in those which had not been informed. In all three studies relative SAR frequency to CS⁻ approximated that obtained in the absence of any signal (i.e., approximated the nonspecific response rate) throughout a significant portion of acquisition training. For groups instructed as to the CS⁺, CS⁻ contingencies, SAR performance to CS⁻ approximated nonspecific response performance within one to five CS⁻ presentations.

The studies reported above all were done with human Ss. Employing cats as Ss, Wickens, Meyer, and Sullivan (1961) obtained comparable results with FOR magnitude at three different interstimulus intervals (simple conditioning paradigm). Their differential conditioning data exhibited (after an initial increase) an overall decline in responsivity, although differential performance itself was maintained over the 30 days of training.

Two studies constitute exceptions to the general rule that performance decreases in humans with extensive training. Gale and Ax (1968) obtained reliable differential conditioning of both FARs and SARs over 5 sessions of 60 trials each. No evidence of a permanent reduction in differential performance was obtained over the sessions. Morrow, Seiffert, and Kramer (1970) gave Ss 16 simple conditioning trials on each of 5 days and found that FOR magnitude began at a relatively high level and then decreased on each of the sessions. It appears that the rise and subsequent decay of performance is largely an intrasession phenomenon. Since the Wickens et al. (1961) data were gathered over multiple sessions, the results from cats and humans are relatively consistent.

The main summary point is that acquisition performance in EDR conditioning does not conform to the prototype learning curve: a gradual, monotonic increase in response frequency (or magnitude) to a stable limit well above control baseline. It may well be that this results from the use of mildly aversive, rather than severely punishing, UCSs, but this remains to be seen. One consequence of the nonmonotonic function is that comparing groups given different treatments is made more difficult. An independent variable may affect the rate of change upward and/or downward as well as the maximum level achieved. Since typical comparisons involve such measures as mean performance either over an entire session or on selected test (e.g., UCS omission) trials, it is likely that in many studies the full impact of the independent variable has been obscured. There is no solution to this problem short of making a careful report of changes on as small a trial-block basis as practical.

B. Interstimulus Interval

One of the most explored variables in the EDR conditioning literature is the ISI (interstimulus interval). Historically, concern with the ISI variable was rooted in the concept of the stimulus trace (Hull, 1943, pp. 41–47; Pavlov, 1927, p. 39). Hull (1943, p. 47) postulated that with the onset of a signal an afferent impulse first rose quickly to a maximum of intensity and then dropped gradually to a low level while the signal continued. With signal offset, the afferent impulse gradually diminishes to zero. The assumption was that the stimulus trace of the signal must be simultaneous with the UCR for conditioning to take place. It follows from this that an optimum ISI, i.e., one for which performance would be most pronounced, is one which ensures that the maximum afferent intensity was simultaneous with the UCS, a value, according to Hull, of approximately 450 msec. Hilgard and Marquis (1940, p. 162) suggested that the optimal delay interval (i.e., ISI) between CS and UCS onsets would be longer than the latency of the conditioned response, implying that the optimum ISI would vary as a function of response latency. Gormezano and Moore (1969, pp. 134–145) have provided a succinct summary of the basic research and theory concerned with the ISI variable, the survey including many investigated response systems and species.

1. SINGLE-CUE CONDITIONING

Beginning with the research of White and Scholsberg (1952), a series of studies (Jones, 1961; Moeller, 1954; Prokasy, Fawcett, & Hall, 1962a; Vattano & Wickens, 1963; Wickens & Cochran, 1960) have shown that, with ISIs varying from 0 to 5000 msec, FOR and FAR magnitude is maximal with an ISI of approximately 500 msec. This seems to be characteristic, as well, of performance when cats are employed as Ss, though only three ISIs have been examined (Wickens *et al.*, 1961). One example of the functional relationships is provided in Fig. 2. Of particular interest is that most of the variance in the functions is absorbed by response frequency. Magnitude of SCR parallels response frequency as a function of ISI, while SCR amplitude is relatively constant. In brief, on a test

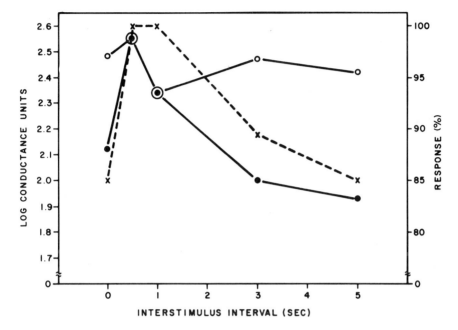

Fig. 2. First orienting response magnitude, probability, and amplitude as a function of interstimulus interval: (○) amplitude; (●) magnitude; (×) frequency. (From Prokasy, Fawcett, & Hall, 1962a, Fig. 1.)

trial following a series of paired trials, more human Ss respond at ISIs of 500–1000 msec than at other ISIs.

Morrow and Keough (1968) have conducted a systematic investigation of ISIs in steps of 4 sec from 4 to 16 sec. They divided the ISI into four 4-sec latency categories defined from CS onset: 1.5–5.5, 5.5–9.5, 9.5–13.5, and 13.5–17.5 sec. First orienting response frequency and amplitude decreased as a function of ISI. Similar ISI functions were obtained when Morrow and Keough plotted frequency and amplitude of response taken from the last scoring interval preceding UCS onset.

From these studies it appears that both FOR magnitude and frequency increase between ISIs of .0 and .5 sec and then systematically decrease as a function of ISI. First orienting response and FAR amplitudes, judging from the Morrow and Keough study (1968) and the Prokasy *et al.* study (1962a), remain at a relatively high level from an ISI of 0 to 4 or 5 sec and then decrease as a function of ISI.

The outcome of these studies is generally consistent with expectations from the Hullian formulation of the stimulus trace, but it is doubtful that the functions obtained are solely attributable to a stimulus trace. There are several reasons for this. First, in most studies cited the measured response was an FOR with the measurement range being no greater than 5 sec following CS onset. As noted earlier in this chapter, the omission of a UCS a short (e.g., 4 sec or less) ISIs itself may induce responding which affects what is measured within 5 sec of CS onset. As ISIs become longer, the effect of UCS omission will become delayed until it is beyond the scoring range. This alone on test trials could yield greater responding at the shorter intervals, although it does not account for the relatively low levels at ISIs less than .5 sec.

Second, as ISIs become longer it becomes more difficult to find a definition of response intervals. While first and second interval responses are statistically independent with ISIs of 5 to 7 or 8 sec, whether subdivisions into equal scoring intervals with even longer ISIs will yield independence is unknown. Morrow and Keough (1968) found evidence of conditioning in all of the latency intervals than employed and also found a decrease in dependent variable with longer ISIs. It may be that the decrease reflects an ISI function, but it may also be that there is a within-subject negative correlation between response levels in two adjacent scoring intervals at very long ISIs. If the latter, the decrease in level may reflect scoring categories, not strength of performance as a function of ISI.

Third, as discussed earlier, response levels in simple conditioning first increase and then decrease. Under these conditions it is entirely possible that the ISI functions obtained so far reflect different points on a non-monotonic "acquisition" function and that, therefore, the functions may not be representative either of rate of change or of performance limit.

Finally, what we label a FOR at short ISIs may actually be a combination of the effects which would be categorized as FARs and SARs at longer ISIs. If the SAR reflects in part the information value of a signal, this effect could show up at short ISIs with an increase in frequency and/or amplitude. With extremely short ISIs (e.g., less than .25 sec), the CS may not provide enough predictive information to have an effect other than that of inducing an orienting response. Regardless, the existence of a complex topography may not, as Grings, Lockhart, and Dameron (1962) have suggested, permit meaningful ISI functions to be obtained.

2. MULTIPLE-CUE CONDITIONING

The first EDR conditioning study employing a CS+ and CS- in which the ISI was also manipulated was conducted by Grings et al. (1962). They employed two independent variables: ISI (.5 vs. 5.0 sec) and average IQ of subjects (33 vs. 62). The FOR and FAR were defined as the largest decrease in resistance occurring from 1.0 to 5.0 sec after CS onset, while the SOR was defined as the largest decrease in resistance occurring from 5.0 to 10.0 sec after CS onset. Analyses were conducted only on responses occurring on UCS-omission trials. It is to be noted that the amplitudes of all responses were measured as departures from the tonic level existing at CS onset. This measure does result in correlations between FARs and SORs as well as in SORs which are, by definition, larger than FARs; consequently, some caution must be exercised in interpreting the results.

Grings et al. (1962) found clear evidence for differential conditioning of both FARs (or FORs) and for the SORs of the long ISI groups. Considerable attention was paid to the fact that the response was multiple-humped even within the 5-sec ISI and that as many as three peaks could be identified. Differential SOR performance with a 5.0-sec ISI was greater than differential FOR (FAR) performance with either the .5- or the 5.0-sec ISI, although this might well have resulted from the amplitude criterion employed. The complications implied by multiple responses led the authors to conclude that proper comparisons might not be made between responses obtained at different ISIs because different conditioning processes may be operating.

Lockhart and Grings (1964) conducted a study very similar to that of Grings et al. (1962), but with the following modifications: (1) the only independent variable was the ISI (.5 vs. 5.0); (2) a third group with a .5-sec ISI and a 5-sec duration CS was run; (3) a relative magnitude measure was employed in which magnitude during the CS was subtracted from a corresponding magnitude obtained during habituation trials; and (4) college students rather than mentally deficient children were employed as subjects. In general, the results paralleled those of the earlier study. Significant differential FOR and FAR conditioning was reported for all three ISI groups, although the largest differences were obtained with the .5-sec ISI groups. Differential conditioning of the SOR was reported for the .50-sec ISI group only when the post-UCS responses were very large. There was no differential SOR performance for the .5-sec ISI group having the 5-sec CS duration, which suggests that the contribution of CS offset is minimal.

Hartman and Grant (1962) reported that differential human eyelid conditioning performance increased as a function of ISI largely because of decreases in responding to CS⁻. In an effort to check this with the EDR, Kimmel and Pennypacker (1963) conducted a study employing ISIs of .25, .5, 1.0, and 2.0 sec. The FOR was recorded as a log transformation of the SCR. The maximum SCL achieved from 0 to 4.0 sec after CS onset was defined as the response. Those investigators found that differential responding did increase as a function of ISI and that the increase was due mainly to a drop in CS⁻ responding at a 2.0 sec ISI.

Recently Jenson (1972) examined the ISI variable in differential conditioning. The three ISI levels were .5, 3.5, and 6.7 sec. First anticipatory responses were defined as responses falling in the range from 1.2 to 4.5 sec after CS onset and SARs were defined as responses falling in the range of 4.5 to 7.8 sec after CS onset. Response frequency and amplitude were distinguished, with the amplitude measure being the square root of SCR. Differential FOR (FAR) frequency increased from an ISI of .5 to one of 3.5, and then decreased to the 6.7 ISI. In contrast, differential SAR frequency was low for ISIs of .5 and 3.5 sec but increased dramatically at an ISI of 6.7 'sec. Since previous research (Prokasy *et al.*, 1967) as well as this study showed that FAR and SAR frequencies are independent, it is clear that at least two differential ISI functions can be defined in differential conditioning: a first interval function with a peak in a shorter ISI range, and a second interval function with a peak in a longer ISI range. This is consistent with other research which shows little in the way of SOR conditioning with short (e.g., less than 5.0 sec) ISIs as well as a decrease in FAR levels with long ISIs.

Of interest in the Jenson study is the fact that SAR rate to CS⁻ was at, or slightly below, nonspecific response rates, and that this level was the same across ISIs. Thus, differential SAR performance improved at the 6.7-sec ISI as a result of an increase in CS⁺ response rate. Similarly, the increase in differential FAR performance was attributable to a greater response level to CS⁺. This need not be construed as conflicting with the Kimmel-Pennypacker results inasmuch as in that study the longest ISI employed was 2.0 sec. At the least it is clear that not all of the increase in differential FAR performance is attributable to decreases in CS⁻ performance. Whether the comparisons of first interval response performance across ISIs is independent of whether the response is pre- or post-UCS remains, however, to be seen. Until the contributions of UCS omission and CS offset to differential performance at short ISIs are understood better, the functions obtained to date are suspect. It does appear, though, that the decrease in differential performance beyond the 3.5-sec ISI is a function of decreased responding to the CS⁺ inasmuch as neither CS⁺ offset nor UCS omission directly affect FAR measurement with ISIs longer than 3.5 sec.

Some limit to the generality of the above findings is suggested by a study in which trace conditioning procedures were used (Furedy, 1970). With a 7.5-sec ISI, differential conditioning was superior with the FAR rather than the SAR. The studies cited above were uniformly conducted with delay, rather than trace, procedures, and it is entirely possible (see Section III.G) that wholly different relationships between the various interval responses and ISI exist with the trace procedure.

C. Reinforcement Schedules

Gormezano and Moore (1969) have provided a brief summary of the research in classical conditioning with reinforcement schedules (i.e., the percentage, or ratio, of reinforcement). In humans, asymptotic performance in eyelid reflex conditioning is correlated with reinforcement ratio. Across a variety of other species and measures such a uniform result has not been found. In comparing 50% and 100% schedules sometimes there is a decrement associated with the 50% schedule, sometimes not. The reverse ordering has never been observed reliably with a classical conditioning preparation. Resistance to extinction is enhanced with a 50% reinforcement schedule in human conditioning and in most instances in other species and across measures (see Gormezano & Moore, 1969, p. 166).

From a general theoretical perspective that performance increments follow reinforced trials and performance decrements follow nonreinforced trials, the effects of intermittent reinforcement schedules have been of some interest. Such a position does imply (ordinarily) that performance in acquisition should be increasingly inferior as the reinforcement ratio decreases. It does not follow theoretically, however, that resistance to extinction should be least with a 100% reinforcement schedule, and this empirical fact has led to much theorizing and speculation (see Gormezano & Moore, 1969, p. 165 ff.) about inhibitory sets, discrimination of schedule change, and cognitive factors in conditioning.

Considering the historical concern with reinforcement schedules in conditioning, it is somewhat surprising that relatively few EDR studies have been conducted in which reinforcement ratio has been an independent variable. What studies have been conducted are, at best, only somewhat consistent with the generalized outcomes described above. Concerning resistance to extinction, the evidence to date (Bridger & Mandel, 1965; Humphreys, 1940) is that FORs are more resistant to extinction following an intermittent, rather than a 100%, reinforcement schedule. The exceptions to this are two groups of Ss in the Bridger and Mandel (1965) study who were informed, after acquisition had been completed, that there would be no more UCSs. Given that instruction both (i.e., 100% and intermittent schedule) groups immediately decreased their FOR magnitude levels to a low level which did not change across extinction trials. In view of the role awareness and expectancy play in this situation (e.g., Chapter 4, this volume), it seems likely that the partial reinforcement effect in EDR conditioning is a function of the subject's expectancy about a UCS following a CS.

For simple conditioning, acquisition performance is a function of reinforcement ratio. Williams (1973) ran a study in which the independent variable was reinforcement ratio (.25, .50, .75, and 1.0). Subjects were given 72 training trials at an ISI of 6 sec, and each reinforcement ratio group had a corresponding sequential control group. The effect of the reinforcement schedule was manifest as an interaction between the percentage of reinforcement and trials: both FAR and SAR probability were a direct function of the reinforcement ratio, but over trials the effect dissipated so that by the end of training all (sequential control as well as experimental) groups reached approximately the same performance level. This contrasts, of course, with the effects usually obtained from other response systems in which the reinforcement schedule variable results in an increased divergence between groups out to an asymptotic limit (e.g., Grant, Schipper, & Ross, 1952).

Consistent with the data of Grings and Sukoneck (1971), TURs decreased in frequency as a function of increasing reinforcement ratio (Williams, 1973) in simple conditioning. Evidence was obtained for TOR conditioning in this study, and this resulted in spite of the fact that a 9-sec CS duration was employed with the 6-sec ISI. The TORs could not, therefore, be cued by CS offset.

Acquisition performance in a multiple-cue differential conditioning situation is not so obviously related to reinforcement ratio. In one study (Grings & Sukoneck, 1971) each S received four signals in a random order. The signals had associated with them (at a 10-sec ISI) the UCS on either 0, 25, 75, or 100% of the trials. The subjects were instructed that their task was to learn on what percentage of the trials the UCS followed each of the signals. Grings and Sukoneck found that FARs, SARs, and TORs all exhibited increases in magnitude as a function of the reinforcement percentage. Third unconditioned response magnitude decreased as a function of reinforcement percentage.

Öhman, Bjorkstrand, and Ellstrom (1973) conducted a study in which the CSs (8-sec duration) were statements about the likelihood and strength of a subsequent UCS. For example, the CS "25% STRONG" indicated that at CS offset there was a 25% chance of S receiving a UCS, and that, if it did occur, it would be the stronger of two intensities. Their results for FARs and SARs paralleled those of Grings and Sukoneck (1971): response magnitude increased as a function of reinforcement percentage. In contrast, however, Öhman *et al.* found that TOR magnitude was an inverted-U function of reinforcement percentage and that TUR magnitude was a U function of reinforcement percentage. The authors noted that the discrepancy between the two studies, in reflecting procedural differences, limits the generality of the TOR and TUR findings of both.

In a study in which only two stimuli (CS+ and CS−) were employed, Williams (1973) ran four groups in which the CS+ was reinforced (ISI = 6.0 sec), respectively, on 25, 50, 75, and 100% of the trials. Half of the Ss in each group were informed about the percentage of reinforcement, and half were not informed. For the uninformed Ss, FAR probability to CS+ did not vary as a function of reinforcement ratio, but it did decrease to CS− as a function of ratio to CS+. A slight, though not reliable, trend for FAR differential performance to increase as a function of ratio was observed, as well, in the informed group. In contrast, differential SAR performance increased reliably in both informed and noninformed Ss as a function of reinforcement ratio. Overall TUR frequency decreased as reinforcement ratio increased, while TOR differential performance was unrelated to reinforcement ratio. In all instances differential performance decreased across blocks of trials to a low level.

In spite of wide methodological differences, the three studies on reinforcement ratio yielded a number of common findings. First, differential FAR performance does increase with increases in reinforcement ratio. It appears that the increase is attributable to increases in CS+ responding, rather than to changes in CS− responding, when Ss have been informed about the relationships which may exist between CS and UCS. In the absence of such information, the increase in differential performance is attributable to decreases in CS− performance. All studies obtained a positive relationship between level of differential performance and reinforcement ratio, and in the Williams study this held for both informed and uninformed Ss. Why the three studies yielded different results for TURs and TORs is not clear.

A different kind of reinforcement schedule comparison was made by Longenecker, Krauskopf, and Bitterman (1952). Employing a 5-sec ISI, these investigators ran one group of subjects on a single-alteranation schedule and another group on a 50% random reinforcement schedule. During acquisition, FOR magnitude reflected the alternating pattern, with low magnitude on nonreinforced trials and high magnitude on reinforced trials. With the introduction of extinction, Ss who had been on the single alternation schedule extinguished more rapidly. It is to be noted that the alternation pattern acquired in acquisition was learned rapidly and much more clearly in the Longenecker *et al.* (1952) study than it was in a study in which the measure was the conditioned eyelid reflex (Grant, Riopelle, & Hake, 1950).

D. Backward Conditioning

The label "backward conditioning" applies to a UCS–CS pairing arrangement as opposed to the typical CS–UCS arrangement. For example, if a .2-sec shock regularly precedes a .5-sec tone by 1.0 sec, then the treatment is a backward conditioning treatment with a 1.0-sec UCS–CS interstimulus interval. The dependent variable in this example would be the response to the tone. Interest in whether or not evidence of conditioning to the tone can be obtained derives from a consideration of the temporal properties of the situation. If an association is formed between a CS and the UCR, then, from a strict contiguity viewpoint, the more temporally contiguous the CS onset and the UCR the better the conditioning. With a long-latency response system such as the EDR, it follows that if the onset of the CS were from 1.5 to 2.5 sec after the occurrence of the UCS., better contiguity between CS and UCR would be obtained, and this would imply that backward conditioning is possible.

An alternative view is that acquisition of the CR is governed by reinforcement of the CR. For example, the contiguous association of the CR with UCS offset should reinforce the CR, hence leading to further CR development. This would imply that acquisition is optimal with a forward conditioning arrangement and probably is not possible with a backward conditioning arrangement. If both CS–UCR contiguity and CR–UCS-offset contiguity are effective in determining performance, then some interactions between performance levels at selected points in training and ISI should be evident (Jones, 1962). Whether or not backward conditioning is possible has been a subject of some disagreement (Cautela, 1965; Gormezano & Moore, 1969; Razran, 1956). What is clear is that evidence for backward conditioning with measures other than the EDR is lacking: It is the EDR literature that provides positive results.

Champion and Jones (1961) ran three groups of Ss. Group TS received tone–shock pairings at a 500-msec ISI, Group ST received shock–tone pairings at 750-msec ISI, and Group T&S was a sequential control group. The two conditioning groups received shock-alone and tone-alone trials interspersed among the conditioning trials. The results were that FOR magnitude in Group TS exceeded that of Group ST, which in turn exceeded that of Group T&S. That some increase in FOR magnitude occurred in Group TS suggests that backward conditioning was obtained. Subsequent experiments by Champion (1962), Trapold, Homzie, and Rutledge (1964), and Zeiner and Grings (1968) also provide support for backward conditioning of the EDR. Zimny, Stern, and Fjeld (1966) failed to find supporting evidence.

The Zeiner–Grings study is of particular interest. These investigators ran a backward conditioning group with a 750-msec UCS–CS interval and a control group which received the CS and UCS in a random order. The result was that the backward conditioning group yielded higher performance than the unpaired control group. On the basis of S reports given between trials and of postexperimental questionnaires, Zeiner and Grings divided the backward conditioning groups into two categories: those who assigned significance to the CS to the effect that the CS should have cued the UCS, and those who assigned no significance to the CS. The latter Ss did not exhibit any conditioning relative to the sequential control group, but the former did. According to Zeiner and Grings (1968, p. 235): "If cognitive restructurings of expectations determine conditioning, then it would be predicted that Ss who anticipate shock to the CS or Ss who 'expect' a shock when a test CS is presented, or Ss who think that they were 'conditioned' to give a response to the CS similar to that elicited by the UCS, would show a higher level of responding than Ss who either ignored the CS or could see no reason for it. This is in fact what was found." The point to this is that the experimenter may structure a sequence of events, but the S may perceive a different structure and respond accordingly. In view of the ease with which conditioned EDR performance is modified with specific instructions given by the experimenter, it is not unreasonable to conclude that the S's self-instructions about the stimulus arrangements is the primary determiner of conditioning performance, independent of whether it is "forward" or "backward" pairing.

Aside from the problem of self-instructions, there is a control problem of another kind with the backward conditioning situation. Given the usual conditioning arrangement, UCR frequency and amplitude decrease across trials. However, when an unpaired UCS is presented during training, the UCR occurs at full strength. It is entirely possible that a similar phenomenon occurs when the UCS precedes the CS: responding to the CS decreases, but with the introduction of a CS-only trial after a series of pairing trials the orienting response (FOR) may return in full. Under these conditions it is doubtful that the ordinary sequential control group is adequate. This potential control problem, together with the results obtained by Zeiner and Grings (1968), raised serious questions about the interpretation of past data as support for backward conditioning within the traditional CS–UCR contiguity framework.

E. Distributional Phenomena

From at least two theoretical points of view, time between trials should affect performance. According to Hull (1943), a response should generate inhibition, thus reducing the likelihood of the same response occurring again in a short time interval. Over time between trials the inhibition dissipates and the response can be expected to occur with little in the way of inhibiting influences. For Estes (1959, pp. 424–429) the extent to which the stimulus complex on trial N is similar to the one on trial $N + 1$ is determined at least in part by the amount of time elapsing between trials: the more time between trials the less similar the stimulus complex at CS onset. From both of these positions it follows that as intertrial interval increases, average performance level should increase. In general, this is what happens with the conditioned eyelid reflex in humans (Gormezano & Moore, 1969, p. 146 ff.).

There has been but one study in the EDR literature in which the intertrial interval has been manipulated. Prokasy and Ebel (1964), employing a 500-msec ISI, compared the effects of 20- and 40-sec intertrial intervals. FOR magnitude was greater with the 40-sec intertrial interval. In addition, FOR recruitment (the amount of time elapsing between CR onset and CR peak) was greater with the longer intertrial interval. Based on performance across ten extinction trials, spaced practice yielded higher performance levels than did massed practice. Until additional information is available from studies in which SARs and FARs are measured, it cannot be known how general this result is or, for that matter, how the orienting response, which is time dependent in frequency and amplitude, interacts with the influence of time between trials on conditioning performance.

F. Conditioned Stimulus

1. Conditioned Stimulus Modality and Quality

Traditionally the CSs employed in classical EDR conditioning have been tones or lights. This follows from an S–R tradition which assumes that all detectable cues are equivalent. Although this tradition is clearly suspect in animal research (Garcia, McGowan, & Green, 1972), the evidence being that CSs must have some ecological validity for the organism, the laboratory research with humans does show that a considerable variety of stimuli can serve as effective CSs.

Usually CS onset and duration have served as the cue, but Champion (1962, 1967) has shown that tone offset is an adequate CS for FAR conditioning. Similarly, compound stimuli (Grings, 1972; Wickens, 1965), and words, synonyms, antonyms, and homonyms (e.g., Peastrel, 1961; Riess, 1940) have been employed as CSs (Diven, 1937; Lang, Geer, & Hnatiow, 1963), as are nonmeaningful verbal stimuli which were given meaning experimentally by association with scaled material (Lipton & Blanton, 1957; Phillips, 1958). As these studies suggest, the meaning of stimuli, beyond their role as predictors of the UCS, can serve as an effective CS. Proctor and Malloy (1971) and Malloy and Proctor (1973) obtained differential FAR and SAR conditioning to a rule CS, namely, the biconditional rule that shock would follow geometric figures which were "both red and square or neither red nor square." Worrall (1970) differentially conditioned Ss to their own decisions to tell a lie.

In an attempt to reduce orienting responses, Burstein and Epstein (1968) developed a circle which had rectangles of uniform size arranged along the perimeter. Whenever a moving pointer reached a rectangle, the CS occurred, and it lasted for the duration that the pointer remained on the rectangle. This procedure has been employed by Epstein and Bahm (1971) to investigate subjects' expectancies of shock, and by Swenson and Hill (1971) in a study of stimulus prediction in which the rectangles were coded to denote whether or not the CS would be followed by shock.

Thus far the stimuli described have been presented through exteroceptors. Uno (1970) has demonstrated differential interoceptive conditioning with a CS consisting of either 0 or 50-degree (C) water in an intubated balloon located between the bronchial and diaphragmatic constrictions of the esophagus. He obtained reliable conditioning of a pre-UCS response (measured from 1.5 to 10 sec after CS onset) and a post-UCS response (measured from 10 to 15 sec after CS onset).

It appears that almost any kind of signal which human beings can process can be employed as a CS. These studies demonstrate, however, only that it is possible to create circumstances in which the cues can be effective. Whether or not these laboratory observations which suggest equipotentiality generalize beyond the laboratory is unknown. While Garcia et al. (1972) have shown that which cues can serve as effective CSs is dependent upon the nature of the UCS and the UCR, the counterpart with humans has yet to be demonstrated. It is plausible, nonetheless, that there are substantial differences in which cues can serve most effectively as CSs for various UCSs and UCRs in humans outside of the laboratory setting, and that some care should be exercised in generalizing the equipotentiality principle beyond it.

2. Conditioned Stimulus Intensity

Two theoretical positions have provided the bases for research on CS intensity. Hull (1949) postulated an intensity dynamism effect, the consequence of which is that as CS intensity increases, the level of performance should increase. Perkins (1953) and Logan (1954) have proposed a modification to the dynamism effect which specifies that it is the difference between background stimulation intensity and CS intensity which is correlated with level of performance. For present purposes it is sufficient to recognize that, given that background stimulation is low intensity, either variant requires that CS performance increase with CS intensity.

Razran (1957) presented a dominance-contiguity theory of conditioning in which the attention value and the intensity of the CS relative to that of the UCS was of importance in determining the level of conditioning. It follows from his position that strength of conditioning should first increase, then decrease, as CS intensity increases.

At present the evidence points in the direction of increasing performance with increasing CS intensity, but the issue must still be declared open until a satisfactory high range of CS intensities has been employed. Kimmel (1959) reported that the level of FAR conditioning decreased with increases in CS intensity; specifically, reliable conditioning was obtained only in a low intensity group, but not in the medium or high intensity groups. Lockhart (1965), with a differential conditioning paradigm, found that differential FOR and FAR performance decreased as CS intensity increased. The unique aspect of this study was that the CS and UCS were both electric shock and in the high intensity group both CS+ and CS- (spatially separated) were of the same intensity as the UCS. More recently Prokasy and Ebel (1967) and Orlebeke and Van Olst (1968) found that FAR frequency and magnitude increased with CS intensity and that SAR frequency and magnitude were not affected by CS intensity. In the latter study it was also shown that the method of measuring CR magnitude by Kimmel (1959) very likely determined the inverse relationship he obtained between CS intensity and level of conditioning.

Two attempts to assess the Perkins–Logan hypothesis have been made in the EDR literature. Champion (1962, 1967) has shown that a shift to a low intensity from a high intensity background is correlated with FOR performance. That is, the greater the degree of shift downward, the greater the level of simple conditioning performance. While there is some evidence that the overall level of stimulation does contribute to the outcome (Champion, 1967), it seems clear that, at least for responses which occur with CS onset, the degree of change from background to CS intensity is the most critical variable.

In summary, the level of FAR and FOR performance in simple conditioning is correlated with the amount of intensity change between background and CS intensity. SAR performance is unaffected by increases in CS intensity, but what happens when the CS is a decrease in intensity is unknown. It is to be emphasized that in the studies on simple conditioning, the shift from background to CS intensity has not been of sufficient intensity, in and of itself, to support conditioning. In differential conditioning, the only evidence is that a decrease in differential FAR and FOR performance is associated with increases in CS intensity. In neither simple nor differential conditioning have attempts been made to assess conditioning in instances where the intensity shift associated with the CS is greater than that associated with the UCS. In the only studies where that might have been done (backward conditioning studies cited earlier), the measurement was taken to the second (or to the "backward") of two stimuli.

G. Trace versus Delay

Though not exclusively, duration of CS has been investigated most often in research oriented toward determining whether or not there are differences between trace and delay conditioning. In the trace conditioning paradigm, the CS is usually of brief duration (e.g., .1–.5 sec) and precedes the UCS with ISIs varying from, say, 1.0 to 10.0 sec. This contrasts with the delay procedure in which the CS terminates either with UCS onset or UCS offset, regardless of ISI. Based on the research of Pavlov (1927), it is expected that the delay procedure will result in better performance than will the trace procedure.

It is clear that trace EDR conditioning can be obtained with rather extended ISIs. First anticipatory response performance was significantly above a control baseline in single-cue studies conducted by Kimmel (1967) and by Grings and Schell (1971). The ISIs in these studies were, respectively, 5 and 6.5 sec. In our own laboratory[3] we have found reliable trace conditioning with ISIs as long as 7.0 but not 11.0 sec. Similarly, differential trace conditioning of the FAR has been obtained

[3] This unpublished research was done at the University of Utah in collaboration with William C. Williams, William Yu-Ming Lee, and William R. Jenson.

with ISIs of up to 8 sec (Baer & Fuhrer, 1968; Zeiner, 1968). Trace conditioning of the SAR seems to be a bit more equivocal. In a simple conditioning paradigm Grings and Schell (1971) report reliable SAR trace conditioning with an ISI of 5.5 sec, although we were unable to obtain a similar effect with ISIs of either 7 or 11 sec.[2] In addition, we obtained no evidence of a reliable SOR at an ISI of 3.0 sec. With a differential conditioning paradigm, evidence of reliable SAR conditioning has been found by Zeiner (1968), who employed an ISI of 5 sec.

Whether for single-cue or multiple-cue paradigms, the evidence supports the position that a trace procedure yields inferior performance to a delay procedure. While there appears to be little performance difference between the delay and trace procedures in some studies (e.g., Grings & Schell, 1971; Zeiner, 1968), Baer and Fuhrer (1968) found reliable delay SAR but not trace SAR conditioning with an 8-sec ISI. In our own unpublished research, reliable delay but not trace SAR conditioning was obtained with an ISI of 7 sec.

A cue as to why the two procedures yield different results in spite of common ISIs and intertrial intervals comes from the Baer–Fuhrer research. These investigators identified subjects as verbalizers (i.e., those who recognized the stimulus contingencies) and nonverbalizers, and found that there were more verbalizers in the delay conditioning group. It is a moot point whether the ability to verbalize a CS–UCS contingency is itself a requisite to reliable conditioning performance, but this study does show once again that superior performance is associated with the experimental treatment which results in a greater number of Ss being able to identify the CS–UCS relationships. It is entirely possible that whether or not trace conditioning will be manifest, or whether or not it will be as clearly evident as delay conditioning, depends upon the extent to which the experimental context is such that a CS–UCS contingency can be reported by S.

H. Stimulus Generalization

Stimulus generalization was first observed by Pavlov (1927). It is defined as responding by an organism to stimuli similar to, but different from, a CS originally used in conditioning. Given training on one stimulus and testing on another, any responding to the second which can be traced to the fact that CS–UCS pairings had been administered with the former as a CS would be generalized responding. Presumably, the more similar the training and test stimuli, the greater the generalized response.

In several early studies (Bass & Hull, 1934; Grant & Dittmer, 1940;

Hovland, 1937a, b, c, d; Littman, 1949) it was concluded that generalization of the FOR does occur, and the Hovland studies, in particular,
have been cited as classical examples of generalization. The evidence
also suggests that semantic generalization (see Chapter 4) exists.

In the past 20 years, the evidence for a generalization gradient as
a function of increasing distance between CS and test stimuli has been
called into question. Grant and Schiller (1953), Grant and Schneider
(1949), Hall and Prokasy (1961), and Wickens, Schroder, and Snide
(1954) all found little evidence of generalization. Grant and Schiller
(1953), for example, found larger responses to some higher intensity
generalization stimuli than to original CSs, a phenomenon mentioned
also by Hovland (1937b). Hall and Prokasy (1961), with tone intensity
as the variable, concluded that when stimulus intensity and habituation
effects were partialed out, a flat gradient existed. It is as though Ss
were responding to tones *per se*, and not to specific tonal frequency
or intensity.

Recognizing that the influences of orienting responses, conditioned
responses and perceptual disparity responses are confounded with FOR
or FAR tests of generalization, two pairs of investigators independently
tried to separate them. Van Olst and Orlebeke (1965) and Epstein and
Burstein (1966) pointed out that if the range of test stimuli is sufficiently
wide the gradient should be U shaped. The logic was that stimuli close
to the CS will show a generalization decrement, while stimuli further
from the CS will yield enhanced responding due to stimulus novelty.
The U-shaped function was obtained, although in neither study were
control groups employed.

The real doubt about the genuineness of generalization gradients
comes from two studies separated by nearly a decade. Williams (1963)
found that by presenting CS-only tones (i.e., with no pairing) and
testing for generalization on different tones, a marked increase in FAR
level was obtained as a function of the degree of discrepancy between
the habituated stimulus and the test stimuli. As she points out, the
existence of stimulus generalization can be established only if some
method can be devised for separating the contribution of novelty effects
from the contribution of a "true" generalization effect.

Öhman (1971) employed at 10-sec ISI and distinguished FARs, SARs,
and TORs. Following 24 paired trials with 67% reinforcement of a
3000-Hz tone as the CS, one presentation each of four generalization
stimuli (200, 500, 1200, and 300 Hz) were made to each S. There was
a sequential control group which received unpaired CSs and UCSs in
place of the paired trials. Test data showed that there was an increase
in SCRs as test and training stimuli differed in both conditioning and

control groups. No evidence of decremental effects was found for any of the three response measures. This study, along with the Williams study, suggests that it is doubtful that generalization decrements have been obtained to test stimuli with the conditioned EDR; that, rather, the positive evidence we have to date is as much a property of unpaired stimuli as paired stimuli.

While there appears to be little doubt that semantic generalization exists, the classical idea of a generalization gradient does not receive support in EDR conditioning when the stimuli are simple. Ordinarily what is observed is either a kind of novelty or change effect (i.e., a perceptual disparity response) or a uniform response level to the test stimuli. The former is a reasonable expectation based upon Grings' research (Grings, 1960), provided that CS-onset responses are measured and the difference between CS and test stimuli is sizable. The latter can be expected in those situations in which the controlling stimulus dimension has not been isolated and disparity responses are not in evidence.

I. Unconditioned Stimulus

1. Unconditioned Stimulus Modality

Since the EDR is one manifestation of autonomic nervous system activity, it follows that virtually any stimulus which can activate the autonomic nervous system can serve as an effective UCS. Ordinarily the signal should have at least one additional characteristic. The UCS should be capable of eliciting a UCR reliably with repeated stimulation (i.e., it should habituate slowly, if at all).

In most studies, shock has been the UCS. When Ss are permitted to set their own shock levels, habituation is likely to be more rapid (Badia & Harley, 1970; Kimmel & Schultz, 1964). This can be overcome in part by employing a fixed, relatively high, intensity. Alternatively, if Ss do not set their own shock levels, the rate of habituation can be slowed somewhat if the shock level is raised occasionally during the session.

White noise is employed quite frequently as a UCS. Since the idea of receiving a burst of white noise is not as distressing as the anticipation of shock, there is little difficulty in employing fixed, high intensity levels. As Raskin *et al.* (1969) show, there is relatively little habituation to unsignaled white noise over 30 presentations as long as the intensity is kept within the range of 100–120 dB(A).

Other stimuli which have been employed successfully as UCSs include, for example, a reaction time task cue (Baer & Fuhrer, 1969; Meyers & Joseph, 1968), a cool puff of air (Furedy, 1967; Kleist & Furedy, 1969), a parachute jump (Fenz & Epstein, 1967), and sexually arousing slides (Dean, Martin, & Streiner, 1968; Sines, 1957).

2. INTENSITY

Interest in UCS intensity and its effect on CR magnitude stems primarily from the theoretical constructs of Hull (1943) and Spence (1960). Both theories predict that the stronger the UCS intensity, the greater the level of performance. This has received support from research in human eyelid conditioning, but similar evidence with the EDR is less clear.

In two early studies, no evidence of UCS intensity effects was found. Wickens, Allen, and Hill (1963) measured FORs in extinction after acquisition with a .5-sec ISI, and Grings and Lockhart (1963) measured FARs during acquisition with a 5-sec ISI. While UCR magnitude reliably increased with UCS intensity, in neither case was CR performance a function of intensity.

More recently, Boring and Morrow (1968) reported a positive relationship between FOR magnitude in acquisition and extinction and UCS intensity with an ISI of .5 sec. Zeiner (1968), in a differential conditioning study with a 10-sec ISI, obtained reliable FAR and SOR conditioning and extinction performance as a function of UCS intensity. In this latter study, higher levels of performance to both CS⁺ and CS⁻, as well as greater differential responding to the two stimuli were obtained with the higher intensity.

Although Epstein and Clarke (1970) did not manipulate UCS intensity *per se,* they did manipulate, via instructions, the perceived intensity. Ss were instructed that they would receive a series of 20 tones, each separated by 15 sec, and that the last one would be the loudest. The three groups received different instructions, suggesting that the loudest tone would be not very loud, would be medium loud, and would be very loud, respectively. Measuring FORs to the tones which preceded the last one, Epstein and Clark found that magnitude was directly related to the instructed intensity level.

A within-Ss comparison was used by Öhman *et al.* (1973). All Ss received both high and low intensity shock UCSs, but were informed with CS onset as to whether or not the shock would be high or low intensity. Under these conditions, FAR, SAR, and TUR magnitude were greater for the higher intensity. No effect of intensity on the TOR was observed.

In general, then, FAR, FOR, SAR, SOR, and TUR performance increases as a function of UCS intensity. Whether or not the SARs and

TURs reflect the operation of intensity as a within-Ss contrast effect cannot, of course, be known until an independent-groups study is conducted.

3. DURATION

Little research has been done on the duration of the UCS. While Sullivan (1950) did report better conditioning with a 750-msec UCS as opposed to a 4000-msec UCS, this result is equivocal since the 750-msec group had an initially higher response level. Two subsequent studies (Bitterman *et al.*, 1952; Coppock & Chambers, 1959) have reported no performance differences in either acquisition or extinction as a function of UCS duration.

IV. Concluding Comments

From this review it is evident that the conditioned electrodermal response modifies substantially with independent variable manipulation. The functional relationships which do exist, though, cannot be construed as being between a stimulus input and an exclusive response output. While the experimenter selects the stimulus contingencies and the specific response to be measured, he does not "select" the skeletal and autonomic changes that are made. This follows from the simple fact that the experimenter's choice of a dependent variable does not, as a rule, differentially shape one response as opposed to any other specific response. Thus, we do not classically condition a response so much as we arrange stimulus contingencies, the consequence of which may be a variety of psychophysiological modifications. When an aversive signal is paired with a relatively neutral signal, heart rate, skin resistance, blood volume, and pupil size may be modified, to say nothing of skeletal adjustments made to the conditioning situation. That the experimenter selects but a single response as an indicator should not be interpreted to mean that changes in that response are the only consequences of the stimulus pairing.

The conditioned electrodermal response, moreover, is not simply just another conditioned response. Confining the discussion to human subjects, it is possible to consider, for example, the conditioned eyelid reflex to be a response conditioned, and shaped, as a relatively isolated response system. A human can be instructed to blink his eyes, and he does so. He may be instructed about the stimulus contingencies, and he will acquire the reflex rapidly though not necessarily immediately. In addition, to condition the eyelid reflex requires a selection from an extremely narrow set of unconditioned stimuli (specifically, those which pose a threat to the orbital area or those to which the subject has been instructed to respond rapidly).

The electrodermal response is influenced in sharply different ways. Immediate changes in response level are observed simply as a consequence of a warning that an aversive signal will follow a relatively neutral signal. However, humans cannot, as a rule, modify sweat gland activity voluntarily, and the range of stimuli which can serve as adequate unconditioned stimuli is quite wide. They include as a subset those which are adequate to support the acquisition of the conditioned eyelid reflex. In spite of the fact that one cannot employ verbally induced sets with animals, there is good reason to believe that the distinction between the autonomic and skeletal reflexes characterizes animals well. For example, it is clear that differential heart rate responding in rabbits is acquired very rapidly in situations in which a large number of trials is required before a conditioned eyelid reflex will occur (see Prokasy, 1965).

These facts suggest that some indicators, the electrodermal response among them, reflect rather directly the perceived contingencies, and that no stage of response selection (see Prokasy, in press) is necessary. Nowhere is this so evident as in the literature on instructional sets and awareness, much of which is reviewed in the following chapter. In spite of any specific training regimen, what the subject knows about present and future contingencies, or what he expects to receive in the way of stimulation is the single greatest determiner of electrodermal response levels.

It is beyond the scope of this chapter to go into these matters in any detail, but what can be said is that independent variable manipulations very likely alter the subjects' perception of the experimental circumstances, and that this, in turn, is reflected in electrodermal activity. It is doubtful that the chain of events is as direct with a discrete, skeletal conditioned response. Thus, a plausible interpretation is that changes in awareness of stimulus contingencies, or in expectations of future events, constitute one class of conditions sufficient to result in changes in electrodermal activity. Acquisition of a skeletal conditioned response may require as a necessary condition similar perceptions of the situation but, very likely, also requires response selection which is relatively UCS specific. In short, the necessary and sufficient circumstances for conditioned changes in behavior very likely differ sharply depending upon whether the measured behavior is autonomically or skeletally mediated. This means that the conditioned electrodermal response is, at best, a prototype of a *class* of conditioned responses, but is not a prototype *the* conditioned response.

Acknowledgments

This paper, and some of the research reported herein, were supported in part by NIMH Grant MH15353.

References

Badia, P., & Defran, R. H. Orienting responses and GSR conditioning: A dilemma. *Psychological Review*, 1970, **77**, 171–181.

Badia, P., & Harley, J. P. Habituation and temporal conditioning as related to shock intensity and its judgement. *Journal of Experimental Psychology*, 1970, **84**, 534–536.

Baer, P. E., & Fuhrer, M. J. Cognitive processes during differential trace and delayed conditioning of the GSR. *Journal of Experimental Psychology*, 1968, **78**, 81–88.

Baer, P. E., & Fuhrer, M. J. Cognitive factors in differential conditioning of the GSR: Use of a reaction time task as the UCS with normals and schizophrenics. *Journal of Abnormal Psychology*, 1969, **74**, 544–552.

Bass, M. J., & Hull, C. L. The irradiation of a tactile conditioned reflex in man. *Journal of Comparative Psychology*, 1934, **17**, 47–65.

Bitterman, M. E., Reed, P., & Krauskopf, J. The effect of the duration of the unconditioned stimulus upon conditioning and extinction. *American Journal of Psychology*, 1952, **65**, 256–262.

Boring, F. W., & Morrow, M. C. Effects of UCS intensity upon conditioning and extinction of the GSR. *Journal of Experimental Psychology*, 1968, **77**, 567–571.

Bridger, W. H., & Mandel, I. J. Abolition of the PRE by instructions in GSR conditioning. *Journal of Experimental Psychology*, 1965, **69**, 476–482.

Burstein, K. R. On the distinction between conditioning and pseudoconditioning. *Psychophysiology*, 1973, **10**, 61–66.

Burstein, K. R., & Epstein, S. Procedure for reducing orienting reactions in GSR conditioning. *Journal of Experimental Psychology*, 1968, **78**, 369–374.

Carey, C. A., Schell, A. M., & Grings, W. W. Effects of ISI and reversal manipulations on cognitive control of the conditioned GSR. Paper presented at the 11th annual convention of the Society for Psychophysiological Research, October 1971.

Cautela, J. R. The problem of backward conditioning. *Journal of Psychology*, 1965, **60**, 135–144.

Champion, R. A. Stimulus–response contiguity in classical aversive conditioning. *Journal of Experimental Psychology*, 1962, **64**, 35–39.

Champion, R. A. Reduced stimulus intensity as a CS in GSR conditioning. *Journal of Experimental Psychology*, 1967, **73**, 631–632.

Champion, R. A., & Jones, J. E. Forward, backward, and pseudo-conditioning of the GSR. *Journal of Experimental Psychology*, 1961, **62**, 58–61.

Coppock, H. W., & Chambers, R. M. GSR conditioning: An illustration of useless distinctions between "type" of conditioning. *Psychological Reports*, 1959, **5**, 171–177.

Dawson, M. E. Cognition and conditioning: Effects of masking the CS–UCS contingency on human GSR classical conditioning. *Journal of Experimental Psychology*, 1970, **85**, 389–396.

Dean, S. J., Martin, R. B., & Streiner, D. L. The use of sexually arousing slides as unconditioned stimuli for the GSR in a discrimination paradigm. *Psychonomic Science*, 1968, **13**, 99–100.

Dengerink, H. A., & Taylor, S. P. Multiple responses with differential properties in delayed galvanic skin response conditioning: A review. *Psychophysiology*, 1971, **8**, 348–360.

Diven, K. Certain determinants in the conditioning of anxiety reactions. *Journal of Psychology*, 1937, **3**, 291–308.

Edelberg, R. Electrical properties of the skin. In C. C. Brown (Ed.), *Methods in psychophysiology*. Baltimore, Maryland: Williams & Wilkins, 1967. Pp. 1–53.

Epstein, S., & Bahm, R. Verbal hypothesis formulation during classical conditioning of the GSR. *Journal of Experimental Psychology*, 1971, **87**, 187–197.

Epstein, S., & Burstein, K. R. A replication of Hovland's study of generalization to frequencies of tone. *Journal of Experimental Psychology*, 1966, **72**, 782–784.

Epstein, S., & Clarke, S. Heart rate and skin conductance during experimentally induced anxiety; effects of anticipated intensity of noxious stimulation and experience. *Journal of Experimental Psychology*, 1970, **84**, 105–112.

Estes, W. K. The statistical approach to learning theory. In S. Koch (Ed.), *Psychology: A study of a science*. Vol. III. New York: McGraw-Hill, 1959. Pp. 424–429.

Fenz, W. D., & Epstein, S. Gradients of physiological arousal of experienced and novice parachutists as a function of an approaching jump. *Psychosomatic Medicine*, 1967, **29**, 33–51.

Furedy, J. J. Classical appetitive conditioning of the GSR with cool air as UCS, and the roles of UCS onset and offset as reinforcers of the CR. *Journal of Experimental Psychology*, 1967, **75**, 73–80.

Furedy, J. J. Test of the preparatory adaptive response interpretation of aversive classical autonomic conditioning. *Journal of Experimental Psychology*, 1970, **84**, 301–307.

Furedy, J. J. Explicitly-unpaired and truly-random CS-controls in human classical differential autonomic conditioning. *Psychophysiology*, 1971, **8**, 497–503.

Furedy, J. J., & Doob, A. N. Autonomic responses and verbal reports in further tests of preparatory response interpretation of reinforcement. *Journal of Experimental Psychology*, 1971, **89**, 258–264.

Furedy, J. J., & Schiffman, K. Test of the propriety of the traditional discriminative control procedure in Pavlovian electrodermal and plethysmographic conditioning. *Journal of Experimental Psychology*, 1971, **91**, 161–164.

Gale, E. N., & Ax, A. F. Long-term conditioning of orienting responses. *Psychophysiology*, 1968, **5**, 307–315.

Garcia, J., McGowan, B. K., & Green, K. F. Biological constraints on conditioning. In A. H. Black & W. F. Prokasy (Eds.), *Classical conditioning II: Current theory and research*. New York: Appleton, 1972. Pp. 3–27.

Gormezano, I., & Moore, J. W. Classical conditioning. In M. T. Marx (Ed.), *Learning processes*. London: Macmillan, 1969. Pp. 121–203.

Grant, D. A., & Dittmer, D. G. An experimental investigation of Pavlov's cortical irradiation hypothesis: *Journal of Experimental Psychology*, 1940, **26**, 299–310.

Grant, D. A., & Schiller, J. J. Generalization of the conditioned galvanic skin response to visual stimuli. *Journal of Experimental Psychology*, 1953, **46**, 309–313.

Grant, D. A., & Schneider, D. E. Intensity of the conditioned stimulus and strength of conditioning: II. The conditioned galvanic skin response to an auditory stimulus. *Journal of Experimental Psychology*, 1949, 39, 35–40.

Grant, D. A., Riopelle, A. J., & Hake, H. W. Resistance to extinction and the pattern of reinforcement: I. Alternation of reinforcement and the conditioned eyelid response. *Journal of Experimental Psychology*, 1950, 40, 53–60.

Grant, D. A., Schipper, L. M., & Ross, B. M. Effects of intertrial interval during acquisition on extinction of the conditioned eyelid response following partial reinforcement. *Journal of Experimental Psychology*, 1952, 44, 203–210.

Grings, W. W. Preparatory set variables related to classical conditioning of autonomic responses. *Psychological Review*, 1960, 67(4), 243–252.

Grings, W. W. Anticipatory and preparatory electrodermal behavior in paired stimulation situations. *Psychophysiology*, 1969, 5, 597–611.

Grings, W. W. Compound stimulus transfer in human classical conditioning. In A. H. Black & W. F. Prokasy (Eds.), *Classical conditioning II: Current theory and research.* New York: Appleton, 1972. Pp. 248–266.

Grings, W. W., & Lockhart, R. A. Effects of "anxiety-lessening" instructions and differential set development on the extinction of GSR. *Journal of Experimental Psychology*, 1963, 66, 292–299.

Grings, W. W., & Schell, A. M. Effects of trace versus delay conditioning, ISI variability, and instructions on UCR diminution. *Journal of Experimental Psychology*, 1971, 90, 136–140.

Grings, W. W., & Sukoneck, H. I. Prediction probability as a determiner of anticipatory and preparatory electrodermal behavior. *Journal of Experimental Psychology*, 1971, 91, 310–317.

Grings, W. W., Lockhart, R. A., & Dameron, L. E. Conditioning autonomic responses of mentally subnormal individuals. *Psychological Monographs*, 1962, 76, No. 39 (Whole No. 58).

Hall, J. F., & Prokasy, W. F. Stimulus generalization to absolutely discriminable tones. *Perceptual and Motor Skills*, 1961, 12, 175–178.

Hartman, T. F., & Grant, D. A. Differential eyelid conditioning as a function of the CS-UCS interval. *Journal of Experimental Psychology*, 1962, 64, 131–136.

Hilgard, E. R., & Marquis, D. G. *Conditioning and learning.* New York: Appleton, 1940.

Hovland, C. I. The generalization of conditioned responses: I. The sensory generalization of conditioned responses with varying frequencies of tone. *Journal of General Psychology*, 1937, 17, 125–148. (a)

Hovland, C. I. The generalization of conditioned responses: II. The sensory generalization of conditioned responses with varying intensities of tone. *Journal of Genetic Psychology*, 1937, 51, 279–291. (b)

Hovland, C. I. The generalization of conditioned responses: III. Extinction, spontaneous recovery, and disinhibition of conditioned and generalized responses. *Journal of Experimental Psychology*, 1937, 21, 47–62. (c)

Hovland, C. I. The generalization of conditioned responses: IV. The effects of varying amounts of reinforcement upon the degree of generalizations of conditioned responses. *Journal of Experimental Psychology*, 1937, 21, 261–276. (d)

Hovland, C. I., & Riesen, A. H. Magnitude of galvanic and vasomotor response as a function of stimulus intensity. *Journal of General Psychology*, 1940, 23, 103–121.

Hull, C. L. *Principles of behavior.* New York: Appleton, 1943.

Hull, C. L. Stimulus intensity dynamisms (V) and stimulus generalization. *Psychological Review*, 1949, **56**, 67–76.

Humphreys, L. G. Extinction of conditioned psycho-galvanic responses following two conditions of reinforcement. *Journal of Experimental Psychology*, 1940, **27**, 71–75.

Jenson, W. R. Multiple EDR responding in differential classical conditioning. Unpublished M.S. thesis, University of Utah, 1972.

Jones, J. E. The CS–UCS interval in conditioning short and long latency responses. *Journal of Experimental Psychology*, 1961, **62**, 612–617.

Jones, J. E. Contiguity and reinforcement in relation to CS-UCS intervals in classical aversive conditioning. *Psychological Review*, 1962, **69**, 176–186.

Kimble, G. A. *Hilgard and Marquis' conditioning and learning*. New York: Appleton, 1961.

Kimmel, E. Judgements of UCS intensity and diminution of the UCR in classical GSR conditioning. *Journal of Experimental Psychology*, 1967, **73**, 532–543.

Kimmel, H. D. Amount of conditioning and intensity of conditioned stimulus. *Journal of Experimental Psychology*, 1959, **58**, 283–287.

Kimmel, H. D. Further analysis of GSR conditioning: A reply to Stewart, Stern, Winokur, and Fredman. *Psychological Review*, 1964, **71**, 160–166.

Kimmel, H. D. Instrumental inhibitory factors in classical conditioning. In W. F. Prokasy (Ed.), *Classical conditioning: A symposium*. New York: Appleton 1965. Pp. 148–171.

Kimmel, H. D. GSR amplitude instead of GSR magnitude: Caveat emptor! *Behavior Research Methods and Instrumentation*, 1968, **1**, 54–56.

Kimmel, H. D., & Pennypacker, H. S. Differential GSR conditioning as a function of the CS-UCS interval. *Journal of Experimental Psychology*, 1963, **65**, 559–563.

Kimmel, H. D., & Schultz, C. A., Jr. GSR magnitude and judgements of shock intensity as a function of physical intensity of shock. *Psychonomic Science*, 1964, **1**, 17–18.

Kleist, K. C., & Furedy, J. J. Appetitive classical autonomic conditioning with subject-related cool-puff UCS. *Journal of Experimental Psychology*, 1969, **81**, 598–600.

Kumpfer, K. L. Effects of instructions upon differential conditioning of the electrodermal response during acquisition, transfer, and extinction. Unpublished doctoral dissertation, University of Utah, 1972.

Lang, P. J., Geer, J., & Hnatiow, M. Semantic generalization of conditioned autonomic responses. *Journal of Experimental Psychology*, 1963, **65**, 552–558.

Leonard, C., & Winokur, G. Conditioning versus sensitization in the galvanic skin response. *Journal of Comparative and Physiological Psychology*, 1963, **56**, 169–170.

Lipton, L., & Blanton, R. L. The semantic differential and mediated generalization as measures of meaning. *Journal of Experimental Psychology*, 1957, **54**, 431–437.

Littman, R. A. Conditioned generalization of the galavanic skin reaction to tones. *Journal of Experimental Psychology*, 1949, **39**, 868–882.

Lockhart, R. A. Dominance and contiguity as interactive determinants of autonomic conditioning. Unpublished doctoral dissertation, University of Southern California, 1965.

Lockhart, R. A. Comments regarding multiple response phenomena in long interstimulus interval conditioning. *Psychophysiology*, 1966, **3**, 108–114.

Lockhart, R. A., & Grings, W. W. Comments on "An analysis of GSR conditioning." *Psychological Review*, 1963, **70**, 562–564.

Lockhart, R. A., & Grings, W. W. Interstimulus interval effects in GSR discrimination conditioning. *Journal of Experimental Psychology*, 1964, **67**, 209–214.

Logan, F. A. A note on stimulus intensity dynamism (V). *Psychological Review*, 1954, **61**, 77–80.

Longenecker, E. D., Krauskopf, J., & Bitterman, M. E. Extinction following alternating and random reinforcement. *American Journal of Psychology*, 1952, **65**, 580–587.

Lykken, D. T., & Venables, P. H. Direct measurement of skin conductance: a proposal for standardization. *Psychophysiology*, 1971, **8**, 656–672.

Lykken, D. T., Rose, R., Luther, B., & Maley, M. Correcting psychophysiological measures for individual differences in range. *Psychological Bulletin*, 1966, **66**, 481–484.

Malloy, T. E., & Proctor, S. Concept and rule utilization in the acquisition of an electrodermal response. *Journal of Experimental Psychology*, 1973, **97**, 370–377.

Martin, I. Delayed GSR conditioning and the effect of electrode placement on measurements of skin resistance. *Journal of Psychosomatic Research*, 1963, **7**, 15–22. (a)

Martin, I. A further attempt at delayed GSR conditioning. *British Journal of Psychology*, 1963, **54**, 359–568. (b)

McDonald, D. G., & Johnson, L. C. A reanalysis of GSR conditioning. *Psychophysiology*, 1965, **1**, 291–295.

Meyers, W. J., & Joseph, L. J. Response speed as related to CS prefamiliarization and GSR responsivity. *Journal of Experimental Psychology*, 1968, **78**, 375–381.

Moeller, G. The CS-UCS interval in GSR conditioning. *Journal of Experimental Psychology*, 1954, **48**, 162–166.

Morrow, M. C., & Keough, T. E. GSR conditioning with long interstimulus intervals. *Journal of Experimental Psychology*, 1968, **77**, 460–467.

Morrow, M. C., Seiffert, P. D., & Kramer, L. L. GSR conditioning and pseudoconditioning with prolonged practice. *Psychological Reports*, 1970, **27**, 39–44.

Öhman, A. Differentiation of conditioned and orienting response components in electrodermal conditioning. *Psychophysiology*, 1971, **8**, 7–21.

Öhman, A., Bjorkstrand, P., & Ellstrom, P. Effect of explicit trial-by-trial information about shock probability in long interstimulus interval conditioning. *Journal of Experimental Psychology*, 1973, **98**, 145–151.

Orlebeke, J. F., & Van Olst, E. H. Learning and performance as a function of CS intensity in a delayed GSR conditioning situation. *Journal of Experimental Psychology*, 1968, **77**, 483–487.

Pavlov, I. P. *Conditioned reflexes*. London and New York: Oxford Univ. Press, 1927. (Translated by G. V. Anrep)

Peastrel, A. Studies of efficiency: Semantic generalization in schizophrenia. Unpublished doctoral dissertation, University of Pennsylvania, 1961.

Perkins, C. C., Jr. The relation between conditioned stimulus intensity and response strength. *Journal of Experimental Psychology*, 1953, **46**, 225–231.

Phillips, L. W. Mediated verbal similarity as a determinant of the generalization of a conditioned GSR. *Journal of Experimental Psychology*, 1958, **55**, 56–61.

Proctor, S., & Malloy, T. E. Cognitive control of conditioned emotional responses: An extension of behavior therapy to include the experimental psychology of cognition. *Behavior Therapy*, 1971, **2**, 294–306.

Prokasy, W. F. Classical eyelid conditioning: Experimental operations, task demands, and response shaping. In W. F. Prokasy (Ed.), *Classical conditioning: A symposium.* New York: Appleton, 1965. Pp. 208–225.

Prokasy, W. F. Toward a complete analysis of GSR data. *Behavior Research Methods and Instrumentation,* 1969, **1,** 99–101.

Prokasy, W. F. A two-operator model account of aversive classical conditioning performance in humans and rabbits. *Learning and Motivation.* In press.

Prokasy, W. F., & Ebel, H. C. GSR conditioning and sensitization as a function of intertrial interval. *Journal of Experimental Psychology,* 1964, **67,** 113–119.

Prokasy, W. F., & Ebel, H. C. Three components of the classically conditioned GSR in human subjects. *Journal of Experimental Psychology,* 1967, **73,** 247–256.

Prokasy, W. F., Fawcett, J. T., & Hall, J. F. Recruitment, latency, magnitude, and amplitude of the GSR as a function of interstimulus interval. *Journal of Experimental Psychology,* 1962, **64,** 513–518. (a)

Prokasy, W. F., Hall, J. F., & Fawcett, J. T. Adaptation, sensitization, forward and backward conditioning, and pseudoconditioning of the GSR. *Psychological Reports,* 1962, **10,** 103–106. (b)

Prokasy, W. F., Williams, W. C., Kumpfer, K. L., Lee, W. Y., & Jenson, W. R. Differential EDR conditioning with two control baselines: Random signal and signal absent. *Psychophysiology,* 1973, **10,** 145–153.

Raskin, D. C. Habituation and the orienting reflex. Paper presented as part of a symposium entitled "Habituation: Research and Theory." Midwestern Psychological Association, Chicago, May 1966.

Raskin, D. C., Kotses, H., & Bever, J. Autonomic indicators of orienting and defensive reflexes. *Journal of Experimental Psychology,* 1969, **80,** 423–433.

Razran, G. Backward conditioning. *Psychological Bulletin,* 1956, **53,** 55–69.

Razran, G. The dominance-contiguity theory of the acquisition of classical conditioning. *Psychological Bulletin,* 1957, **5,** 1–46.

Razran, G. *Mind in evolution.* Boston, Massachusetts: Houghton, 1971.

Rescorla, R. A. Pavlovian conditioning and its proper control procedures. *Psychological Review,* 1967, **59,** 406–412.

Riess, B. F. Semantic conditioning involving the galvanic skin reflex. *Journal of Experimental Psychology,* 1940, **26,** 238–240.

Rodnick, E. H. Characteristics of delayed and trace conditioned responses. *Journal of Experimental Psychology,* 1937, **20,** 409–425.

Schiffman, K., & Furedy, J. J. Failures of contingency and cognitive factors to affect long-interval differential Pavlovian autonomic conditioning. *Journal of Experimental Psychology,* 1972, **96,** 215–218.

Sines, J. O. Conflict-related stimuli as elicitors of selected physiological responses. *Journal of Projective Techniques,* 1957, **21,** 194–198.

Spence, K. W. *Behavior theory and learning: Selected papers.* Englewood Cliffs, New Jersey: Prentice-Hall, 1960.

Stein, L. Habituation and stimulus novelty: a model based on classical conditioning. *Psychological Review,* 1966, **73,** 352–356.

Stewart, M. A., Stern, J. A., Winokur, G., & Fredman, S. An analysis of GSR conditioning. *Psychological Review,* 1961, **68,** 60–67.

Stewart, M. A., Winokur, G., Stern, J. A., Guze, S., Pfeiffer, E., & Hornung, F. Adaptation and conditioning of the GSR in psychiatric patients. *Journal of Mental Science,* 1959, **105,** 1102–1111.

Sullivan, J. J. Some factors affecting the conditioning of the galvanic skin response. Unpublished doctoral dissertation, State University of Iowa, 1950.

Swenson, R. P., & Hill, F. A. Effects of stimulus prediction in classical GSR conditioning. Paper presented at R.M.P.A., Denver, May 1971.

Switzer, St. C. A. Anticipatory and inhibitory characteristics of delayed conditioned reactions. *Journal of Experimental Psychology*, 1934, **17**, 603–620.

Trapold, M. A., Homzie, M., & Rutledge, E. Backward conditioning and UCR latency. *Journal of Experimental Psychology*, 1964, **67**, 387–391.

Uno, T. The effects of awareness and successive inhibition on introceptive and exteroceptive conditioning of the galvanic skin response. *Psychophysiology*, 1970, **7**, 27–43.

Van Olst, E. H., & Orlebeke, J. F. The role of the orientation reflex in the generalization of a conditioned GSR. *Canadian Journal of Psychology*, 1965, **19**, 56–60.

Vattano, F. J., & Wickens, D. D., Efficiency of GSR conditioning as a function of CS–UCS interval. Paper presented at the Midwestern Psychological Association, May 1963.

White, C. T., & Schlosberg, H. Degree of conditioning of the GSR as a function of the period of delay. *Journal of Experimental Psychology*, 1952, **43**, 357–362.

Wickens, D. D. Compound conditioning in humans and cats. In W. F. Prokasy (Ed.), *Classical conditioning: A symposium*. New York: Appleton, 1965. Pp. 323–339.

Wickens, D. D., & Cochran, S. W. Conditioned stimulus flash rate and efficiency of conditioning. *Journal of Comparative and Physiological Psychology*, 1960, **53**, 341–345.

Wickens, D. D., Allen, C. K., & Hill, F. A. Effect of instructions and UCS strength on extinction of the conditioned GSR. *Journal of Experimental Psychology*, 1963, **66**, 235–240.

Wickens, D. D., Meyer, P. M., & Sullivan, S. N. Classical GSR conditioning, conditioned discrimination, and interstimulus intervals in cats. *Journal of Comparative and Physiological Psychology*, 1961, **54**, 572–576.

Wickens, D. D., Schroder, H. M., & Snide, J. D. Primary stimulus generalization of the GSR under two conditions. *Journal of Experimental Psychology*, 1954, **47**, 52–56.

Williams, J. A. Novelty, GSR, and stimulus generalization. *Canadian Journal of Psychology*, 1963, **17**, 52–61.

Williams, W. C. Classical skin conductance conditioning: intermittent reinforcement. Unpublished doctoral dissertation, University of Utah, 1973.

Worrall, N. Differential GSR conditioning of true and false decisions. *Journal of Experimental Psychology*, 1970, **86**, 13–17.

Zeiner, A. R. Second interval discrimination conditioning of the GSR as a function of UCS intensity and trace and delay conditioning paradigms. *Journal of Experimental Psychology*, 1968, **78**, 276–280.

Zeiner, A. R., & Grings, W. W. Backward conditioning: a replication with emphasis on conceptualization by the subject. *Journal of Experimental Psychology*, 1968, **76**, 232–235.

Zimny, G. H., Stern, J. A., & Fjeld, S. P. Effects of CS and UCS relationships on electrodermal response and heart rate. *Journal of Experimental Psychology*, 1966, **72**, 177–181.

CHAPTER 4

Complex Variables in Conditioning

W. W. GRINGS

Department of Psychology
University of Southern California
Los Angeles, California

M. E. DAWSON

Gateways Hospital
Los Angeles, California

I. Introduction 204
II. Compound Signal Conditioning 204
    A. Compound-to-Component Transfer 205
    B. Component-to-Compound Transfer 211
III. Semantic Conditioning and Generalization 213
    A. Types of Paradigms 214
    B. Types of Methodological Issues 216
    C. Types of Theoretical Interpretations 218
    D. Variables That Affect Semantic Generalization 219
IV. Electrodermal Conditioning and the Unconditioned Response 221
    A. The Unconditioned Response as an Index of Conditioning ... 221
    B. Empirical Background: Unconditioned Response Diminution .. 223
    C. Related Concepts: Disparity 227
V. Effects of Instructional Variables on Electrodermal Conditioning .. 228
    A. Instructions That Maximize Learning Stimulus Relations 228
    B. Instructions That Minimize Learning Stimulus Relations 233
    C. Instructions That Induce Response Sets 239
VI. Individual Difference Factors 241
    A. The Drive Concept 241
    B. Introversion–Extroversion 243
    C. Other Criteria 244
    References 245

I. Introduction

This chapter is a review of five areas of electrodermal classical conditioning which are generally considered to be complex. The areas are complex in the sense that they employ stimulus manipulations or response measurements which are not simple extensions of the conditioning parameters (e.g., stimulus intensities and durations). Thus, the first two areas deal with complex conditioned stimuli, the first being compound stimuli and the second being semantic stimuli. The third area deals with unconditioned response (UCR), rather than conditioned response (CR), changes which occur during classical conditioning. The fourth area has to do with the effects of various types of verbal instructions on electrodermal conditioning and the fifth with individual differences in conditioning. The discussions of these five areas are relatively separate units and may be considered by the reader in the order and combination of his preference.

II. Compound Signal Conditioning

The concept of *the* conditioned stimulus is a convenient fiction. There is seldom, if ever, a single and unitary stimulus paired with the UCS. In addition to the nominal CS, a multitude of visual, olfactory, tactile, and proprioceptive stimuli are paired with the UCS in the classical conditioning paradigm.

The fact that the CS, even in the most controlled of laboratory situations, may consist of several components, calls for a careful examination of the controlling stimuli in classical conditioning. For example, with Pavlov's dogs, was the salivary CR controlled by (1) the ringing of the bell, solely, (2) the ringing of the bell as well as other sights, sounds, smells, and feelings, or (3) the compound of the ringing bell within the context of other sights, sounds, smells, and feelings? Stated more abstractly, is the stimulus that elicits the CR (1) the single component manipulated by the experimenter, (2) all of the components which are paired with the UCS, or (3) the entire compound and not the individual components?

One method used to answer these questions is to employ the combination of two or more stimulus components as a CS during acquisition and then subsequently to test for CR strength with each individual component as well as the entire compound. For example, one may pair the combination of light and bell with the UCS during acquisition and then subsequently test for CR strength to each individual component (light and bell) and to the entire compound (light + bell). This technique may be used to determine the amount of transfer of the CR from a compound CS to its constituent components. The following is a brief review of EDR studies which have used this experimental technique. Results based on simultaneous presentation of the components are discussed separately from those based on successive or serial presentation of the components.

A. Compound-to-Component Transfer

1. SIMULTANEOUS COMPONENTS

A simultaneous-components CS is one that has components with identical onset and offset times. As with most classical conditioning phenomena, data relevant to simultaneous components CS can be found in the pioneering research of Pavlov (1927, p. 141). Subsequent Russian and American research has been reviewed by Baker (1968) and Razran (1939b, 1965, 1971).

If a compound were used throughout acquisition, to what degree would the individual components be capable of eliciting CRs? There are several possible answers to this question, three of which have been experimentally verified, depending on the experimental parameters. First, it may be that one of the components elicits a CR equal in strength to that elicited by the entire compound while the other component elicits little or no CR (called *component overshadowing*). The results which define the phenomenon of component overshadowing are shown in Fig. 1a. The experimental conditions which are optimal for component

a. *Component overshadowing*
   compound   --→ large CR
   component$_1$ --→ large CR
   component$_2$ --→ little or no CR

b. *Component configuration*
   compound   --→ large CR
   component$_1$ --→ little or no CR
   component$_2$ --→ little or no CR

c. *Component summation*
   compound   --→ large CR
   component$_1$ --→ moderate CR
   component$_2$ --→ moderate CR

Fig. 1. Patterns of results that define the phenomena of component overshadowing, component configuration, and component summation.

overshadowing are that the components be of different sensory modalities or of unequal intensities. The second possible result is that each component elicits little or no CR while the entire compound elicits a strong CR (called *component configuration*). Hypothetical results depicting component configuration are shown in Fig. 1b. The conditions conducive to component configuration include differential reinforcement of the compound and the components and/or overtraining with the compound. The third type of finding is that each component elicits CRs equal in strength to each other but less than that elicited by the entire compound (called *component summation*). Results indicative of component summation are shown in Fig. 1c. Conditions which are favorable for component summation are that the components be of the same sensory modality and that they be of equal intensities.

There are only a small number of electrodermal conditioning experiments which have investigated the simultaneous components CS. In spite of the relatively small sample of studies, examples of component overshadowing, component configuration, and component summation may be found.

One of the earliest American studies to measure electrodermal responses while employing a compound CS was reported by Hull (1940, 1943). The subjects were college students; the components consisted of a weak light and a mild cutaneous vibrator, and the UCS was an electric shock. Hull reported that in one such experiment "the mean amplitude of reaction evoked by the compound—was exactly the same as that evoked by the stronger of the stimulus components, the cutaneous vibrator; the addition of the light to the combination seems to have added nothing to the mean amplitude of reaction [1943, p. 212]." The findings are consistent with the phenomenon of component overshadowing; however, they must be considered tentative owing to the relatively small sample size ($N = 8$) and the lack of controls for pseudoconditioning and ORs to stimulus change.

More recent electrodermal conditioning experiments have employed larger sample sizes and have included more extensive controls. In one such experiment (Grings, 1969b), the subjects were college students, the components were colored lights, and the UCS was an electric shock. During the compound acquisition phase, one pair of colored lights was associated with shock and another pair of colored lights was not associated with shock. Thus, a discrimination conditioning paradigm was employed. During the subsequent test phase, skin conductance response (SCR) magnitude was measured to each compound, to one component of the shocked compound, and to one component of the nonshocked compound. Analysis of the data indicated that, although differential conditioning to the compounds was established, there was no differential transfer to the components. The mean SCR magnitude ($\sqrt{\Delta c}$) was largest to the entire reinforced compound, smallest to the entire nonreinforced compound, and was intermediate to the individual components. These results, with minor procedural modifications, have been replicated by Grings and Zeiner (1969a). The absence of transfer from a compound to one of its components is consistent with the phenomenon of component configuration.

Another electrodermal conditioning study, using a different experimental procedure, has adduced some evidence of successful compound-to-component transfer (Grings & Shmelev, 1959). There were three sequential stages to this experiment: component training, compound training, and component testing. In the first stage, three components (colored lights) were each individually paired with an electric shock UCS. In the second stage, two of these components were presented simultaneously in order to form the compound CS. For one group, the newly formed compound was paired with the shock while for another group the compound was presented without shock. In the third stage, each component was presented individually without shock to all subjects. The major dependent variables were the SCR magnitudes elicited during the third stage by one of the components that was included in the compound and by one of the components that was not included in the compound. The results revealed that the group which had the compound reinforced responded more to the included component than to the nonincluded component, while the group which had the compound nonreinforced responded in the opposite direction. Thus, there is evidence that reinforcement of a compound can facilitate responding to one of its components. These results are consistent with the phenomenon of component summation.

In summary, there are electrodermal data which indicate the occurrence of component overshadowing (Hull, 1940, 1943), component configuration (Grings, 1969b; Grings & Zeiner, 1969a), and component summation (Grings & Shmelev, 1959). Obviously, more research is needed to determine under what conditions each will occur.

Since the effects of simultaneous components CSs tend to be quite variable (producing either component summation, component overshadowing, or component configuration), the theoretical accounts of such effects also tend to be diverse. For example, one finds statements regarding "summation of individual response strengths" to account for component summation, or "stimulus selection" to account for component overshadowing, or "discrimination between compound and component" to account for component configuration.

Probably the most unified and integrated theoretical analysis of compound-to-component transfer can be found in Hull (1943). Hull was aware of the diverse results and attempted to unify them within his learning theory.

According to the law of primary reinforcement (Hull, 1943, p. 80), each and every afferent impulse will acquire habit strength so long as it is active at the time that the to-be-conditioned response occurs and is closely followed by need reduction. Thus, each component will independently acquire habit strength and these habits may summate to produce a resultant response (p. 213). Therefore, component summation (moderate CRs to the individual components and large CRs to the entire compound) is a simple deduction from Hull's theoretical system.

However, Hull realized that not all afferent impulses acquire the same amount of habit strength. In fact, he (pp. 207–208) listed several specific stimulus properties which affect stimulus conditionability (e.g., intensity, modality, prior reinforcement history). Thus, the phenomenon of component overshadowing is not foreign to Hull's theory.

A combination of the principles of afferent neural interaction and stimulus generalization was employed by Hull (1943, pp. 216–221) to account for component configuration. According to his analysis, the concurrent afferent impulses arising from different components may appreciably modify each other so that the effective CS is quite different from the impulses due to either component presented separately. In accordance with primary stimulus generalization, the CR will be elicited by the individual components only to the degree that their afferent impulses resemble the effective CS impulse. Furthermore, since the gradient of stimulus generalization may become steeper as a function of the number of reinforcements, it would be predicted that component configuration would also be a function of the number of reinforcements. Razran (1965) has interpreted the Russian data as supporting the conclusion that component configuration is a function of the number of compound reinforcements, although recent American research suggests that this is an unsettled issue (Baker, 1968, 1969; Booth & Hammond, 1971; Thomas, Berman, & Serednesky, 1968; Wickens, Nield, Tuber, & Wickens, 1970).

2. SUCCESSIVE COMPONENTS

A successive-components CS is one whose individual component onsets appear in serial order. The components may or may not overlap within this design. Some of the possible temporal arrangements of the individual components are shown in Fig. 2. For example, the components may

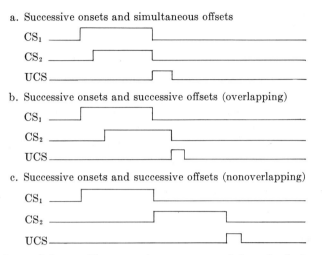

Fig. 2. Some of the possible temporal arrangements of the individual components with the successive components paradigm.

have successive onsets with either: (1) simultaneous offsets (Fig. 2a), (2) successive offsets in an overlapping arrangement (Fig. 2b), or (3) successive offsets in a nonoverlapping arrangement (Fig. 2c).

For lack of space, only an examination of experiments which studied the effects of time between component onsets (intercomponent interval) will be offered here. For almost two decades, Wickens and his co-workers have systematically investigated the effects of the intercomponent interval with successive-component CSs. A typical experimental arrangement can be found in the report of Wickens, Gelman, and Sullivan (1959). The individual components were lights and tones, the UCS was an electric shock, the Ss were college student volunteers, the independent variable was the intercomponent interval, and the dependent variable was SCR magnitude elicited by the individual components on extinction trials. In this study, all Ss were administered one of the components (called CS_2 because it always appeared second in the sequence of components) 500 msec preceding shock. The other component, CS_1, preceded the shock by 600, 700, 800, 920, 1040, 1550, 2500, and 4600 msec for different groups. Thus, the intercomponent intervals (CS_1–CS_2 interval) were 100, 200, 300, 420, 540, 1050, 2000, and 4100 msec. All components had simultaneous offsets. Analysis of SCR magnitude elicited by the individual components on the first extinction trial revealed that CR strength to CS_1 increased as the intercomponent interval increased from 100 to 420 msec, decreased for the 540-msec, and increased again for the 2000-msec interval. The CR strength to CS_2 showed the opposite trend. Thus, CS_1 was most dominant (i.e., elicited larger CRs than CS_2) when the intercomponent interval was 420 msec. A separate experiment reported by Allen, Hill, and Wickens (1963) showed that the effects of the intercomponent interval were not merely ORs to novelty produced by individual component test trials.

In another successive-components CS study, electrodermal responses were measured from the paws of cats (Wickens, Born, & Wickens, 1963). Again, the individual components were lights and tones, the UCS an electric shock, and the manipulated variable was the intercomponent interval. In essential agreement with the college student data, the CR strength to CS_1 was greatest when the intercomponent interval was 500 msec. At this "optimal" interval, SCR magnitude to CS_1 was as large as that elicited by the entire compound and significantly larger than that elicited by CS_2.

In sum, there is evidence, much of which is based on electrodermal conditioning, to suggest that the intercomponent interval is an important determiner of cue dominance with a successive-components CS paradigm. A component that precedes another component by approximately 500 msec is the dominant cue in controlling conditioned behavior. Yet, if this component precedes the other component by longer or shorter intervals, then it is not the dominant cue. The latter finding indicates that merely occurring first in the sequence of components is not the critical factor; rather, it is the intercomponent interval that is critical.

The research of Wickens (1959, 1965) and his associates regarding the effects of the intercomponent interval has been guided by a sensory conditioning hypothesis. This hypothesis assumes that when a successive compound CS is paired with a UCS, two forms of conditioning may occur. The first type is between each of the individual components and the UCR elicited by the UCS (S–R learning). The second type is between the individual components themselves (S–S learning). It is further assumed that both of these conditioning processes obey a curvilinear function between the effectiveness of conditioning and the interstimulus interval. The optimal interval, at least within the range from 0 to 2 sec, is considered to be approximately 500 msec.

Granting these assumptions, the sensory conditioning hypothesis can adequately explain most of the reported effects of the intercomponent interval. For example, consider the case where CS_2 is 500 msec in duration, CS_1 is 1200 msec in duration, and the UCS occurs at the simultaneous offset of each. In this example, the CS_1–CS_2 interval (700 msec) and the CS_1–UCS interval (1200 msec) are not optimal for conditioning but the CS_2–UCS interval (500 msec) is optimal. Therefore, CS_2 should be the dominant component (i.e., elicit larger CRs than that elicited by CS_1), and this is generally what has been found. However, if CS_1 were of 1000-msec duration, the CS_1–CS_2 interval (500 msec) would be optimal for sensory conditioning. Due to sensory conditioning, CS_1 is assumed to elicit the sensory representation of CS_2 and therefore to elicit a conditionable form of the entire compound. In this situation, CS_1 would be expected to be the dominant component and this is what has been found.

Egger and Miller (1962, 1963) have presented an interesting alternative hypothesis to account for component dominance. Stated in its strongest form, the information hypothesis asserts that a necessary condition for the classical conditioning of a component is that it provide information about the UCS occurrence. To test this hypothesis, Egger and Miller (1962) studied secondary reinforcement with successive-components CSs with two groups of rats. They found that the more informative stimulus, whether CS_1 or CS_2, was the dominant cue. Research is needed which tests the differential predictions of the sensory conditioning hypothesis and information hypothesis.

B. Component-to-Compound Transfer

Thus far, we have discussed how learning which originally occurs in the presence of a compound may transfer to the individual components. In the following discussion we will examine the converse: i.e., how learning which originally occurs in the presence of individual components may transfer to a compound. Several possible transfer outcomes may occur. First, the identity of the original components may be obscured or lost within the compound and result in no transfer (component configuration). Such an outcome would be expected when the newly formed compound possesses strong configural properties and with human Ss, at least, is perceived as a unitary stimulus object rather than an aggregate or conglomerate. Another possible outcome is that the CRs elicited by the newly formed compound are controlled completely by one of the components (component overshadowing). The latter outcome might occur when one component may mask or override the perceptual reaction of the other component. As for electrodermal component-to-compound transfer, very little work has been done with either component configuration or component overshadowing.

A third possible outcome is that when the components are presented as a compound stimulus, there is an additive function of the various response tendencies (component summation). The phenomenon of component summation has been the most extensively studied of the component-to-compound phenomena, although only the gross effects have been investigated thus far. A recent review of the relevant literature may be found in Grings (1972).

Depending upon the conditioning history of the components, one of two variations of the component summation phenomenon may be observed. If the components have been conditioned to elicit the same or similar responses, then one may observe positive component summation. That is, the newly formed compound will elicit a larger CR than either of the components when presented singly. A second variation is negative component summation, and it is in some ways of more theoretical interest. An experimental arrangement used to demonstrate negative component summation involves conditioning an excitatory tendency (e.g., EDR) to one of the components. This component is then tested in combination with another component which has negative or inhibitory tendencies. The result which defines the phenomenon of negative component summation is that the response to the combination is less than that to the excitator component alone.

Evaluations of negative component summation have been made with combinations of simple stimuli, where excitatory tendencies were developed by pairing the stimulus with a UCS and inhibitory tendencies were developed by presenting stimuli as unreinforced stimuli (CS-) in a discrimination conditioning situation (Grings & Kimmel, 1959; Grings & O'Donnell, 1956).

Rescorla (1969) has reviewed a number of stimulational arrangements which have been used to condition inhibitory forms of response tendencies appropirate for such compound stimulus transfer observations. These include the aforementioned discriminative CS-; the nonreinforcement of a previously reinforced CS; stimuli negatively correlated with the UCS; stimuli signalling UCS termination, and stimulation conducive to development of inhibition of delay. Studies endeavoring to employ the above operations in tests of compound stimulus transfer have not been as numerous with electrodermal behavior as they have with other responses.

In an attempt to evaluate conditioned inhibitory tendencies which may develop as a function of pairing a component with UCS termination, Grings and Zeiner (1969b) combined stimuli from forward and backward conditioning paradigms. Differences among major classes of stimulus compounds were obtained. That is, SCR responses to a compound of two forward conditioned components exceeded response to a compound of forward conditioned and nonconditioned stimuli (what Rescorla, 1967, calls explicitly unpaired stimuli). However, it was not possible to tell whether the component treated by the backward paradigm achieved negative (inhibitory) properties. In fact, there was strong suggestion that, for the particular circumstances of the experiment, it did not.

Still another attempt to demonstrate negative component summation was couched in the terminology of counterconditioning and employed relaxation procedures modified from those of Jacobson (1938) for developing the negative or antagonistic response (Grings & Uno, 1968). Learning was carried out over three days with compound stimulus test trials interspersed throughout the second and third days. The magnitude of SCR to the compound composed of the "fear" stimulus and the "relaxation" stimulus was less than the response to the "fear" stimulus alone.

A unique and little-studied form of stimulus compound is one which combines as components interoceptive stimuli and exteroceptive stimuli. In discussing this form of stimulus compounding, Razran (1961) predicted that combinations of this type may lead to conflict and decrementation of conditioning, rather than producing positive component summation. In a test of this situation with successive compounds of exteroceptive CSs (tones) and interoceptive CSs (temperature changes to the interior wall of the esophagus), Uno (1970) found a reduction of response to the second stimulus presented in the compound, with the amount of reduction being determined in part by the nature of the second stimulus (whether it was exteroceptive or interoceptive).

Several major methodological difficulties stand in the way of decisive tests of stimulus transfer questions with electrodermal responses of human subjects. The problems result from the extreme sensitivity of that response to any form of stimulus change. It is necessary to provide controls for evaluating the increased orienting responses which may occur to any new combination or form of stimulus presentation. With human Ss there is the further problem of controlling for verbal response sets or attitudes about the experiment which may determine the subject's response.

III. Semantic Conditioning and Generalization

A typical adult human possesses a highly developed linguistic system composed of thousands of symbols and their interrelationships. But more important than its quantity, language can be used as a powerful technique to modify or maintain various forms of human behavior. In point of fact, practically all forms of education and psychotherapy rely upon the effectiveness of language to influence human behvior. Even physiological functions can be dramatically altered through the use of verbal symbols. For example, Lacey (1959) stated that "the differential magnitude of galvanometric deflections (EDR changes) to words is one of the most reliable phenomena in psychology today! [p. 163]."

A later section of this chapter will review the effects of verbal instructions on electrodermal classical conditioning. The present section deals with how verbal symbols may become classically conditioned and how the conditioning may generalize to other such symbols. This section is divided into four parts: (1) types of semantic conditioning and generalization paradigms; (2) types of methodological problems; (3) types of theoretical interpretations of semantic generalization; and (4) variables which affect semantic generalization.

A. Types of Paradigms

Cofer and Foley (1942) distinguished three types of paradigms employed to investigate semantic generalization of classically conditioned responses. The first paradigm involves initial conditioning with a non-semantic CS (e.g., blue-colored light) and later testing for generalization with a verbal symbol which represents the CS (e.g., the word *blue*). This paradigm is called object to word generalization. The second paradigm involves initial conditioning with a verbal CS (e.g., the word *blue*) and later testing for generalization with an object represented by the symbolic CS (e.g., a blue-colored light). The second paradigm is called word to object generalization. Both of these paradigms were developed in the late 1920s and early 1930s in the Russian laboratories of Krasnogorsky and Ivanov-Smolensky. Subsequent research, mostly of Russian origin, which has extended the object to word and word to object generalization paradigm, has been reviewed by Hartman (1965).

The third paradigm originated in the United States and involves initial conditioning with a verbal CS and later testing for generalization with other verbal stimuli. The third paradigm is called word to word generalization and it was in this context that Razran (1939a) introduced the term "semantic conditioning." Of the three paradigms, the word to word generalization procedure has been the most extensively investigated in this country and therefore is the object of discussion in the following review.[1]

In his pioneering research, Razran (1939a) classically conditioned the salivary response of three college students to four visually presented words: *style, urn, freeze,* and *surf.* On later tests for CR generalization it was found that the words *fashion, vase, chill,* and *wave* elicited

---

[1] A related paradigm involves EDR conditioning to physically different but conceptually similar stimuli and later testing for generalization with a novel instance of the concept class (Proctor & Malloy, 1971; Worrall, 1970). Space does not permit a review of the interesting findings obtained with this paradigm.

greater response strength than did the words *stile, earn, frieze,* and *serf.* Thus, stimuli similar in meaning (synonyms) exhibited greater generalization than did stimuli similar in sound (homophones). Razran concluded that Ss were more conditioned to the meaning of the word than to its visual-auditory form. Subsequent Russian data which suggest a similar conclusion have been reviewed by Razran (1961).

As for electrodermal semantic conditioning and generalization, Riess (1940) paired the verbal stimuli reported earlier by Razran (*style, urn, freeze,* and *surf*) with a loud buzzer UCS. After a criterion of electrodermal classical conditioning had been attained, generalization was tested with synonyms and homophones of the CSs. Consistent with the salivary CR results reported earlier by Razran, greater electrodermal generalization was obtained to synonyms than to homophones. In a subsequent experiment, Riess (1946) employed a similar procedure with four groups differing in chronological age. The mean chronological ages of the four groups were: 7:9, 10:8, 14:0, and 18:6. To equate familiarity across the four groups, the verbal CSs were selected from the reading material in use at the educational level of each group. After conditioning, all Ss were presented homophones, antonyms, and synonyms of the original CS words. The youngest group exhibited the largest CR generalization to homophones, the next youngest group to antonyms, and the two oldest groups to synonyms.

The research discussed thus far has dealt with generalization across discrete categories of stimuli where the categories are based on extra-experimental experience (e.g., synonyms, antonyms, and homophones). Another approach is to study gradients of generalization within a single dimension, where that dimension is manipulated by preconditioning experimental training. In one of the earliest published reports using this method, Lipton and Blanton (1957) required Ss to associate eight nonsense syllables with each of eight different "concepts." There were four concepts of circularity and four of angularity presented visually in abstract designs. The designs for circularity concept were: full circle, broken circle, semicircle, and arch. The designs used to represent the triangularity concept were: full triangle, incomplete triangle, truncated triangle, and simple angle. After Ss learned to associate different nonsense syllables with each concept, electrodermal conditioning and test for generalization commenced. During conditioning, one of the nonsense syllables served as the CS and an electric shock served as the UCS. For half the Ss, the syllable previously associated with the full circle served as the CS and for the other half the syllable associated with the full triangle served as the CS. During the generalization test, electrodermal responses were found to be largest to the original CS syllable and to decrease in amplitude to syllables associated with concepts farther from the CS. For example, the group conditioned to the circularity concept gave the largest responses to the syllable associated with the full circle and then, in decreasing order, to syllables associated with the broken circle, semicircle, and arch.

Phillips (1958) used a similar approach by initially pairing five Turkish words with five discrete points along a brightness dimension (N1/, N3/, N5/, N7/, and N9/ of the Munsell colors). After these associations were firmly established, the word previously paired with the darkest stimulus (N1/) was employed as the CS in an electrodermal classical conditioning paradigm. Following conditioning, CR generalization was tested with the four remaining words. A gradient of decreasing response amplitude to words associated with the N3/, N5/, and N7/ stimuli, respectively, was found. However, the word previously associated with the brightest stimulus (N9/) elicited the largest of the generalization responses. Phillips concluded (1958, p. 61) that "the generalization gradient over the major part of this (experimentally manipulated) dimension was a decreasing function of the distance of the test stimulus from the CS."

B. Types of Methodological Issues

Feather (1965) has presented a methodological review of 25 semantic generalization experiments. The primary methodological issues discussed were: (1) controls for pseudoconditioning and sensitization, (2) controls for order effects, and (3) controls for simultaneous conditioning. Each of these methodological issues is briefly reviewed below.

1. PSEUDOCONDITIONING AND SENSITIZATION

The topics of pseudoconditioning, sensitization, and their proper control procedures are discussed in detail elsewhere in this book. The point emphasized here is that almost half of the experiments reviewed by Feather failed to include any controls for pseudoconditioning or sensitization. An encouraging trend, however, can be seen in that most of the recent studies reviewed by Feather and experiments published since his review (e.g., Brotsky & Keller, 1971; Maltzman, Langdon, & Feeny, 1970; Peastrel, Wishner, & Kaplan, 1968; Raskin, 1969) have included control stimuli. A control stimulus is one that has not been paired with the UCS and has no logical or associative relation to the CS. Differential responding between control stimulus and CS is used to infer conditioning while differential responding between control stimulus and generalization test stimulus is used to infer generalization.

2. ORDER EFFECTS

Most semantic generalization experiments test for generalization during a series of nonreinforced trials. This means that extinction will occur during the generalization test. Thus, care must be taken to avoid confounding the extinction effects with the generalization effects. Maltzman and Langdon (1969) have demonstrated that erroneous conclusions may result if such care is not taken. Counterbalancing the sequence of stimuli during the generalization or, alternatively, analyzing only the first test trial are possible methods of controlling for order effects.

3. SIMULTANEOUS CONDITIONING

If the generalization test word is a verbal associate of the CS word then the administration of CS–UCS pairings may involve conditioning simultaneously to the overt CS word and the covert generalization word. For example, consider a hypothetical case where the CS word is *needle* and the generalization test word is *scissors* (Fig. 3a). If *scissors* were

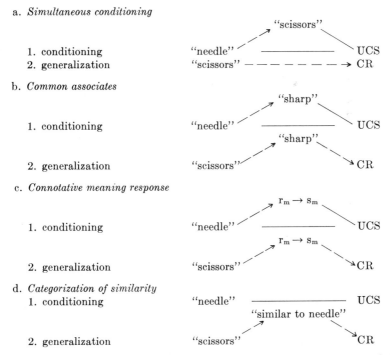

Fig. 3. Diagrammatic representation of four theoretical interpretations of the phenomenon of semantic generalization. (Dashed lines indicate learned associations; solid lines refer to experimental pairings.)

a covert verbal associate elicited by the word *needle,* then conditioning would occur simultaneously to both words. According to Feather, a CR elicited by the word *scissors* in this case would reflect the process of simultaneous conditioning and not true semantic generalization. In order to control for simultaneous conditioning, Feather suggests employing generalization test words which are semantically but not associatively linked to the CS word (Feather, 1965, p. 438).

C. Types of Theoretical Interpretations

Many investigators (e.g., Mednick, 1957; Mink, 1963; Olson, 1965) believe that simultaneous conditioning is a legitimate mediating mechanism of semantic generalization and therefore should not be conceptualized as a confounding variable. Therefore, simultaneous conditioning is presented in Fig. 3a as one possible theoretical interpretation of semantic generalization. There are three additional interpretations shown in Fig. 3 and each is discussed briefly below. A critical analysis of the various theoretical interpretations has been presented by Maltzman (1968).

Cofer and Foley (1942) suggested that the phenomenon of semantic generalization is mediated by covert responses shared in common by the CS word and the generalization test word (Fig. 3b). According to the common associates interpretation: (1) the CS word (needle) elicits covert verbal responses (e.g., sharp); (2) repetitive CS–UCS pairings result in classical conditioning of the CS word and its covert responses; (3) the generalization test word (e.g., scissors) also elicits covert responses; and (4) semantic generalization occurs to the extent that covert responses elicited by the generalization test word are the same as those elicited by the CS word (Bousfield, 1961). Data consistent with the interpretation that semantic generalization is mediated by verbal associates which the CS word and generalization test word share in common have been found by Lacey (cited by Lang, Greer, & Hnatiow, 1963, pp. 557–558).

Osgood (1961) has argued that neither simultaneous conditioning nor common associates are sufficient mechanisms to account for all occurrences of semantic generalization. Therefore, Osgood proposed that another mediating mechanism is the connotative meaning response. According to this interpretation, semantic generalization occurs as a function of the degree of similarity of the meaning of the CS word and the generalization test word (Fig. 3c). In this context, meaning ($r_m \rightarrow s_m$) is defined and measured by the multivariate profiles obtained with appropriate semantic differentials.

Still another interpretation is that Ss categorize each generalization test word in some crude fashion as being similar or dissimilar to that of the previously presented CS word. According to this interpretation (Fig. 3d), the categorization of similarity is sufficient to "control or even initiate the generalization responses [Razran, 1949, p. 362]." This interpretation differs from those discussed previously in three important ways: (1) it proposes that generalization is a discrete stepwise function rather than a continuous gradient; (2) it proposes that the mediating mechanism is operative during the generalization test and not during the initial conditioning phase; and (3) it proposes that cognitive processes play an essential role in semantic generalization. Maltzman (1968, 1971) has proposed an S–R variation of the latter interpretation. He concurs that categorization of similarity is a critical factor in semantic generalization but adds that its basis is the orienting response to the generalization test words.

D. Variables That Affect Semantic Generalization

The purpose of the following section is to review the effects of certain variables on semantic generalization and to discuss some theoretical and practical implications of these effects. The variables may be divided into three types: organismic, chemical, and instructional.

First, as was mentioned previously, Riess (1946) found that chronological age is an important determiner of semantic generalization. It was found that older subjects (14 years and above) exhibit greater generalization to synonyms than homophones while younger subjects show the reverse response pattern. Luria and Vinogradova (1959) have studied a related organismic variable. These authors investigated semantic generalization of vasomotor conditioned responses with normal and mentally retarded children (chronological ages ranged from 11 to 17). It was found that normal children generalized more to synonyms than homophones, mildly retarded children generalized equally to synonyms and homophones and severely retarded children generalized more to homophones than synonyms. In addition, Luria and Vinogradova noted that the general state of the subject (e.g., physical illness and fatigue) is an important determiner of whether semantic or phonetic generalization is dominant.

A second class of relevant variables is chemical intervention. Shvarts (cited in Razran, 1961, pp. 103–104) found that the administration of chlorohydrate caused a shift from semantic to phonetic generalization in a group of normal adult human subjects. Also, Levy and Murphy (1966) found differences in semantic and phonetic generalization as a function of alcohol ingestion. They reported that a conditioned motor response generalized more to synonyms than homophones for subjects administered a placebo while generalization was greater to homophones than synonyms for subjects administered alcohol.

Finally, a third class of relevant variables is verbal instructions. Bridger (1970) established classically conditioned electrodermal responses to the word *ship* with groups of college students. Generalization was later tested with a semantically related word (*boat*), a phonetically related word (*skip*), and an unrelated neutral word (*door*). The generalization results of two of the groups are relevant to the present discussion. One group was instructed before conditioning that the shock UCS would be associated with the word *ship* and that in a later part of the experiment no more shocks would be administered. The second group was treated identically except that they were not given these instructions. The generalization results revealed that the instructed group exhibited only phonetic generalization while the noninstructed group exhibited both phonetic and semantic generalization. A postexperimental inquiry demonstrated that the instructed group did not consciously expect the shock UCS with either *skip* or *boat* whereas the noninstructed did expect shock with the word *boat*. Thus, it was concluded that cognitive expectancy is necessary for semantic generalization whereas it is not necessary for phonetic generalization.

In summary, phonetic generalization seems to be mediated by simple and primitive mechanisms (it is dominent in young children, mental retardates, certain drug states, and in the absence of cognitive expectancy). Semantic generalization, on the other hand, appears to be mediated by higher and more complex cognitive processes (it is dominant in older children, normal intelligence levels, nondrug states, and in the presence of cognitive expectancy).

These findings may have practical and theoretical implications regarding the study of levels of cognitive functioning. A practical implication is in diagnosis of levels of cognitive functioning. Although this area has not been adequately explored, the available data are encouraging. For example, Astrup, Sersen, and Wortis (1967) have suggested that semantic generalization results are relevant to the diagnosis and prognosis of mental retardation. Also, Peastrel (1964) found greater electrodermal phonetic generalization than semantic generalization for schizophrenic patients whereas normals showed the opposite response generalization. As for theoretical implications, phonetic and semantic generalization procedures offer new avenues to investigate the conscious–unconscious or, if you prefer, first signal system–second signal interaction.

IV. Electrodermal Conditioning and the Unconditioned Response

A. The Unconditioned Response as an Index of Conditioning

In the quite extensive literature on GSR conditioning the behavior changes used as a basis for inferring learning have been of three or four main types. Postacquisition (or extinction) trials have been used most widely, with learning defined as a response to the CS after acquisition which is greater than the response before acquisition (all with reference to a control situation in which the CS is not associated with the UCS, and where considerations are given to rule out sensitization and pseudoconditioning effects). Acquisition test trials have sometimes been interspersed among reinforced trials to serve a purpose similar to postacquisition trials. Third, when the interstimulus interval is greater than response latency, electrodermal changes which follow CS onset but which antedate the UCS onset may be measured on each acquisition trial. One further measure is the UCS-omission CR derived from a response on test or extinction trials which occurs at the point where the UCS would ordinarily come on.

It is not the present purpose to evaluate the above methods for indicating learning, although it may be appropriate to mention in passing that all of the methods mentioned present difficulties. Extinction measures with the EDR are very transient, especially with human subjects where extinction may occur in one or two trials. Interspersed test trials run a risk, with electrodermal behavior, of eliciting orienting responses due to stimulus change. Anticipatory conditioned responses tend to be confused with orienting behavior (e.g., Stewart, Stern, Winokur, & Fredman, 1961); they tend to exhibit a trend over trials which peaks, then decreases (e.g., Kimmel, 1959; Silver & Kimmel, 1969); and anticipatory responses may be complex to interpret (Grings, Lockhart, & Dameron, 1962; Prokasy & Ebel, 1967; Grings, 1969a). Finally, the UCS-omission CR remains somewhat of an enigma. While it has been observed for over a decade (e.g., Stewart, Winokur, Stern, Guze, Pfeiffer, & Hornung, 1959; Grings et al., 1962) it has not been thoroughly studied and is apparently assumed by some to be a response to stimulus change (e.g., Badia & Defran, 1970).

The present interest is in examining measures of learning derived from changes in the unconditioned response which occur during conditioning trials. Three such measures will be considered. Before turning to them in some detail, note should be taken of the fact that various indirect measures of classical conditioning performance, based on changes in unconditioned behavior in contexts other than the EDR have been used for evaluating parameters of the conditioning process. One notable example is the suppression ratio based upon the degree of interference of an assumed conditioned response with performance on an operant task, such as bar pressing. As an example of such a measure in evaluations of classical conditioning parameters, one might note Kamin (1965). Other measures which have been less widely used define learning in terms of changes in an unconditioned response not presented during training itself, such as the use of the startle response as an index of conditioned fear (Brown, Kalish, & Farber, 1951). This was the forerunner of a general class of response based upon the use of probe stimuli, as in the study by Ross (1961).

Closely related to the above are some definitions, used in electrodermal conditioning, which rest on the assumption that through the conditioning process the CS comes to influence properties of the UCR (particularly its amplitude). Three of these will be discussed by name. They are stimulus (perceptual) disparity, temporal disparity, and UCR diminution. Operational definitions of these three measures are obtained as follows:

1. Stimulus disparity is based on the assumption that once a CS–UCS regularity has been established, the presentation of the UCS following a CS with which it had not been paired will cause a change in the response to UCS. Diagrammatically this may be shown as

$$CS \rightarrow UCS \rightarrow UCR,$$
$$CS' \rightarrow UCS \rightarrow UCR'.$$

In empirical situations (e.g., Grings, 1960) the response to the altered cue stimulus is one of enhancement—that is, UCR′ is greater in amplitude than UCR. The context in which the above paradigm was presented was aversive conditioning where the CS was assumed to "set" the subject for receipt of UCS. The change in CS was assumed to alter this set and dishabituate the UCR.

2. A second, related, paradigm emphasizes time relationships between signals and signaled events (CSs and UCSs). When a CS–UCS regularity has been established with a constant interstimulus interval (ISI), a temporal disparity will be created by introducing the usual UCS at some time other than that used in original conditioning (Grings, 1965, 1969a). The operational difference (usually one of response enhancement) may be diagrammed

$$CS \xrightarrow{t} UCS \rightarrow UCR,$$
$$CS \xrightarrow{t'} UCS \rightarrow UCR'.$$

3. The third concept is most commonly known as UCR diminution (e.g., Kimmel, 1966). It implies that as a CS–UCS regularity is established the UCR becomes diminished beyond the amount attributable to simple habituation and that the reduction may be attributed to the presence of the CS. For definitional purposes the concept is produced by manipulating the presence and absence of CS as in the following paradigm,

$$CS \rightarrow UCS \rightarrow UCR,$$
$$(No\ CS) \rightarrow UCS \rightarrow UCR'.$$

Again UCR' is assumed to be larger in magnitude than UCR.

The uncued UCS presentations may be administered in various ways. For example, it may be given to an S following a series of CS–UCS pairings. This method constitutes a within-group comparison, often termed a recovery measure. A between-group definition contracts UCRs of two groups, one with signaled and the other with unsignaled UCS presentations.

Of the three measures defined above, the last (UCR diminution) has received the most empirical study. All three have encountered some methodological complications which have altered the effectiveness of their use. Some of these issues can be seen from a brief review of the empirical work, considering first the UCR diminution phenomenon.

B. Empirical Background: Unconditioned Response Diminution

Although references to reduced responding to the UCS during conditioning had been made previously in an incidental manner, the phenomenon did not receive prominent attention until it was introduced almost simultaneously in two contexts, eyeblink and EDR conditioning. Kimble and Ost (1961) reported observations taken from a study by Dufort and Kimble (1958) in which diminution effects were strong enough to encourage further test. To that end, eyeblink UCRs were measured under different ISI conditions and an eventual conclusion was drawn that amount of diminution varied with that conditioning parameter. Differences were interpreted as due to conditioned inhibition. At about the same time, Lykken (1959, 1962) described instances of UCR diminution in EDR conditioning. To explain his observations Lykken proposed a form of learned change in perceived intensity of the UCS through a process he termed "preception" (Lykken, 1968).

A systematic extension of Kimble and Ost's hypotheses into electrodermal conditioning was made by Kimmel and Pennypacker (1962) who showed diminution to vary with number of reinforcement trials. Groups receiving 4, 8, or 16 CS–UCS trials showed increasing reductions of UCR with more reinforcements; and when UCS-alone trials were given, the UCR to all groups recovered to approximately their original magnitudes.

This early work was followed by a series of studies by Kimmel and his associates (Kimmel, 1966; Morrow, 1966; Baxter, 1966). Morrow used both between-groups and within-group definitions of UCR diminution and administered varying numbers of (3, 6, 12) extinction trials (CS alone) before testing UCR recovery in a CS–UCS trial. He found recovery to occur but not to be a function of the number of extinction trials. He assumed that the recovery was due to extinction of conditioned inhibition and that the extinction occurred rapidly (i.e., within three trials). An alternate explanation based on disinhibition of the conditioned inhibition due to stimulus change from acquisition to extinction was also suggested.

Baxter (1966) compared both measures of diminution under circumstances of delay and trace conditioning and argued that the duration of the CS partly determined the amount of conditioned inhibition being built up. The general conclusion reached by Kimmel (1966) from these studies was that the UCR diminution phenomenon was a viable manifestation of conditioned inhibition. Grings and Schell (1969b) repeated the essential features of the Baxter (1966) study and concluded that their data argued against the superiority of delay over trace conditioning in producing diminution. In a further replication study, Grings and Schell (1971) again found diminution under both delay and trace stimulation conditions and found differences in diminution with constant and variable ISIs. In the last instance differences in instructions about the nature of stimulus conditions interacted with the ISI variation. That is, diminution under variable ISI was more rapid when Ss were instructed on stimulus conditions than when they were not.

An earlier study (Peeke & Grings, 1968) had shown that diminution is greater for a constant ISI than when a variable ISI is used. The diminution occurred on the first trial for subjects who were instructed about stimulus relations. The last result, in particular, led those researchers to favor a perceptual set interpretation of their results.

All of the above studies were confronted with a methodological problem which was recognized by Kimble and Ost in their early article. To quote those authors:

> In obtaining these differences one main complication had to be faced: almost all of the CRs blended with the UCRs making UCR amplitudes

somewhat ambiguous for trials on which CRs occurred. Because of this ambiguity, measurements of UCR amplitude were made only on trials on which no CR occurred [Kimble & Ost, 1961, p. 152].

With the EDR, this kind of difficulty is intensified by the fact that the CS is an adequate stimulus to produce EDR behavior which could interact with the UCR, and the amount of such interference will vary with certain variables (such as intensity of the CS, and the ISI employed).

To provide instances for study of response interference in diminution-like situations, Grings and Schell (1969a) conducted the following exploratory study. The main dependent variable was the magnitude of response to a standard stimulus which occurred as the second member of a successive pair. Two variables were manipulated to produce different levels of ongoing EDR at the point of onset of the second stimulus. These were physical intensity of the first stimulus and the interstimulus interval (or time for recovery of the response to the first stimulus before the onset of the second stimulus). The results demonstrated that the magnitudes of response to the second (standard) stimulus varied inversely with intensity of the first stimulus and directly with the interval between stimuli (recovery time).

In the above experiment, the differences in magnitude of the first response resulted directly from the properties of stimulation. They are not attributable to variables of conditioning or learning. Yet it is reasonable to assume that if a learned response occurs in such an interval between paired stimuli (analogous to the CS–UCS interval in conditioning) the magnitude of response at the point of onset of the second stimulus would determine the magnitude of response to the second stimulus. This, then, becomes parallel to the situation where an anticipatory CR may interact with (or diminish) the magnitude of the response to the UCS, and hence account for diminution.

Problems created by the last-mentioned circumstances can be elaborated as follows. First, it can be asserted that, to be useful as a measure of learning, changes in UCR magnitude must be attributable to variables typically considered to be basic to learning, such as effects of trials or experience. That is, the effect should not occur independently of such practice or experience. If the presence of a CS produces a UCR different from the UCR in the absence of the CS, it should not be due merely to the fact that a CS has an intrinsic capability of producing some kind of peripheral effector fatigue which does not exist when the CS is not present. This is not the same as saying that to be useful as a measure of learning the CS must not elicit a response which could produce diminution by interfering with the UCR; for if the response produced by the CS was, in fact, itself a result of learning, the UCR would aslo be reflecting the same learning process. At that point, the issue may become whether one response or another (the CSR or the UCR) is the more sensitive indicator of learning, or whether perhaps a combination of the two would be better.

Stated differently, this becomes two issues. The first is one of control and involves the need to be certain that UCR reductions attributed to learning are not due to some nonlearning process, such as effector fatigue. The second issue is a matter of defining variables and concerns the decision of how to express most effectively an index of learning which incorporates changes in the UCR. Since work has not progressed very far on either of these issues, a closer look at the kinds of problems involved may be helpful.

Consider again Kimble and Ost's procedure of measuring diminution only on trials for which no anticipatory response occurred. On empirical grounds one might argue that selecting trials where CR and UCR do not merge is a conservative procedure tending to reduce the extent of the phenomenon. In other words, if effects of a parametric variable (like Kimble and Ost's manipulation of ISI) have a demonstrable effect with such a severe restriction imposed, it must be quite a robust phenomenon.

On a logical-theoretical basis, however, such a selection of trials leads to serious complications other than simply "diluting" the data. One such complication was pointed out by Kimble and Ost in their previously cited study (1961, p. 152): 'This rule of limiting measurements of UCR amplitude to trials on which no CR occurred created problems of its own, particularly in analysis involving the interstimulus interval. This is because the response measure occurred, on the average, earlier in conditioning in the group conditioned at favorable intervals." From the standpoint of any theory that assumes a strong dependent relation between anticipatory responding and amount of UCR, such restriction of analysis to trials on which the anticipatory response is absent could be interpreted as seriously biasing the sample of observed events in the direction of low performance learning trials. Since the degree of bias cannot at present be estimated effectively, the use of such a trial-selection procedure would be highly unwise.

One alternative approach would be to deal with the dependency directly. This would involve at least two steps: (1) estimating the nature and extent of dependency between anticipatory CRs (or ARs) and the UCRs; and (2) evaluating the factors determining the dependency so that a separation can be made between components of the AR–UCR relationship which may not be due to learning and those which are due to learning. Recent investigators have computed correlations among the various properties (e.g., magnitude, latency, and frequency) of the different response components (ORs, ARs, and UCRs). An examination of dependencies among frequency relations (Prokasy & Ebel, 1967) and exploratory factor analyses (Prescott, 1964; Slubicka, 1971; Öhman, 1972) have been made. It is likely that the future will see application of other forms of multivariate analysis to the problem (e.g., stepwise multiple regression, canonical correlation, and principal component analysis).

C. Related Concepts: Disparity

The methodological problems just described in connection with the concept of UCR diminution apply similarly to situations using the operational definitions of disparity variation. As an example, consider an experiment the purpose of which was to evaluate temporal disparity as a function of the amount of change in the time of presentation of a shock from the expected or conditioned time of presentation (Grings, 1965, 1969a). Twenty-four Ss were given a series of conditioning trials with a tone CS and shock UCS paired with a 5-sec delay interval (ISI). After a learning criterion had been met, Ss were separated randomly into three subgroups for testing with a time disparity trial (i.e., presentation of the shock at a point earlier in the delay interval). Test intervals of 1.0, 2.5, and 4.0 sec were used. Systematic differences in responses to the shock were observed in a direction supporting the notion that the greater the change in time of receipt of shock from that expected, the larger the disparity response—results in agreement with principles of disparity theory.

Unfortunately, with the EDR an equally adequate alternative explanation for the results can be given. It would call attention to the fact that the orienting responses elicited by the CS would be at different phases in their recovery cycle at the time of receipt of the shock for the various groups. Response differences observed could have resulted from interaction of ORs and UCRs (rather than from perceptual disparity differences).

This type of effector-fatigue or interference effect does not apply to the tests of disparity involving UCS presentations which are signaled differently from earlier trials. By proper arrangements of circumstances it is possible to ensure equal ORs or anticipatory CRs to the signal stimuli so that any difference in the response to the UCS is not confounded by overlap among successive reactions. Further, the data (e.g., Grings, 1960; Kimmel, 1960) are clear in indicating that response magnitudes to the same adequate stimulus are larger when that stimulus is improperly cued as compared to when it is signaled by the cue it has been previously following in time.

One explanation for the disparity results is that of a dishabituation resulting from stimulus change, rather than a response enhancement due to altered preparatory set. It is probably possible to separate experimentally the different predictions based on notions of perceptual disparity and those based on dishabituation. However, such experiments have not been conducted, and a tendency persists to lump together various response increment phenomena which accompany stimulus change and to attribute them to some common cause, like reinstatement of habituated orienting behavior. Space does not permit examining these issues in more detail at this time.

V.   Effects of Instructional Variables on Electrodermal Conditioning

Early investigators enthusiastically adopted the electrodermal measure in the study of human classical conditioning because of its assumed involuntary nature. However, before long, it became apparent that the EDR was sensitive to complex cognitive changes which commonly occur in the human conditioning situation. Thus, "researchers on electrodermal conditioning found themselves in the middle of a number of theoretical-methodological issues involving cognition [Grings, 1972b, p. 200]."

A common method used to investigate the effects of cognitive variables on EDR conditioning is the manipulation of verbal instructions. The purpose of this section is to review the effects of certain types of verbal instructions on human EDR classical conditioning. Three types of verbal instructions have been selected for review: (1) those which maximize learning of stimulus relationships, (2) those which minimize learning of stimulus relationships, and (3) those which induce response sets. The effects of the first two types of instructions are discussed separately for acquisition and extinction.

A.   *Instructions That Maximize Learning Stimulus Relations*

1.   Acquisition

The critical stimulus manipulation during acquisition of electrodermal conditioned responses is the CS–UCS relation. Instructions to be reviewed in the present section are those which supply explicit information regarding the CS–UCS relation. These instructions have been investigated within the context of two different paradigms. The first paradigm involves the measurement of electrodermal responses to a CS immediately following the instructions. No physical CS–UCS pairings intervene between the instructions and the response measurement with this paradigm. The second paradigm is similar except that CS–UCS pairings are administered following the instructions. Thus, the first paradigm permits a direct assessment of the effect of these instructions while the second paradigm permits an assessment of the interaction of these instructions with physical stimulus pairings.

In a classic example of the first paradigm (instructions without immediate pairings), Cook and Harris (1937) measured SRR magnitude and frequency to a CS before and after informing Ss of a CS–UCS relation. They found that the instructions increased magnitude and frequency of SRR's to the CS and that 30 subsequent CS–UCS pairings did not produce further increases. These findings led the authors to conclude that "conditioning of the galvanic skin response in the human adult differs from the customary conditioning procedure in that, under the conditions of this experiment, (a) this response is established by means of a process of verbal conditioning and (b) it is therefore not established as a result of a series of paired inadequate–adequate stimuli combinations [Cook & Harris, 1937, p. 209]."

The procedures employed by Cook and Harris may be criticized in that the sample size was small ($N = 6$), the instrumentation and statistical techniques were inadequate by present-day standards, and there were no controls for sensitization. However, more recent research which does not suffer from these deficiencies has confirmed the essential findings of Cook and Harris (Bridger & Mandel, 1964; Dawson & Grings, 1968). Thus, results obtained with the first paradigm support the conclusion that "behavior change similar to that which occurs through classical conditioning occurs through a process of verbalization and verbal instruction . . . and . . . the physical act of pairing external stimulus events is not necessary for this type of learning to occur [Grings, 1965, p. 85]."

In an interesting variation of the first design, Maltzman et al. (1970) found that informing Ss of the CS–UCS relation can produce electrodermal semantic generalization in the absence of physical CS–UCS pairings. Two groups of college students were instructed to perform a motor response (which would elicit EDRs) when they heard the word *light* (CS). One group then received training with the CS word, while another group did not. In a subsequent test with the word *lamp*, both groups exhibited semantic generalization. Thus, there was evidence of semantic generalization independent of prior CS–UCS pairings.

Results obtained with the second paradigm (instructions followed immediately by pairings) will not be dwelled upon. Briefly stated, electrodermal classical conditioning is facilitated by prior instructions regarding the CS–UCS relation (Block, 1962; Grings & Kimmel, 1959; Lockhart, 1968). The same effect has been reported for conditioning of heart rate (Chatterjee & Eriksen, 1962; Lacey, Smith, & Green, 1955) and eye blink (Hilgard, Campbell, & Sears, 1938; McAllister & McAllister, 1958). Razran (1955a), however, has reported that informative instructions are detrimental to human salivary classical conditioning. Whether the latter discrepancy is due to differences in response systems or type of conditioning and instruction procedures remains to be determined.

In summary, there is a general consensus regarding the effects of instructions which maximize learning of the CS–UCS relation: (1) they produce conditioned-like electrodermal responses in the absence of physical CS–UCS pairings and (2) they facilitate electrodermal conditioning when used in conjunction with physical CS–UCS pairings. There is, however, a lack of consensus regarding the theoretical integration of these findings with those of classical conditioning. One point of view is that these instructions serve to establish an expectancy of and preparation for the UCS which is the same as that established in classical conditioning by means of CS–UCS pairings (Hilgard & Marquis, 1940; Tolman, 1959; Woodworth, 1958). A quite different point of view is that the instructions produce a cognitive process which is fundamentally different than that which occurs in true classical conditioning (Grings, 1965; Martin & Levy, 1969; Razran, 1955b, 1971). According to the latter interpretation, true conditioning is a learning process which occurs best when the complex cognitive processes are minimized.

2. EXTINCTION

The critical stimulus manipulation during extinction is the termination of the CS–UCS stimulus relation. Instructions to be reviewed in the present section are those which supply explicit information that there will be no further UCS presentations (in addition, many investigators remove the UCS source). Three separate questions may be asked regarding the effects of these instructions. First, do the instructions reduce the level of general responsivity? Second, do the instructions reduce the magnitude of the conditioned response (defined as differential response magnitudes to paired and unpaired conditions)? Third, do the instructions completely and immediately abolish the previously established conditioned response?

Table 1 presents a summary of representative recent electrodermal data which are relevant to these questions. Experiments which used simple conditioning designs (paired and unpaired conditions are administered to different groups) and discrimination conditioning designs (paired and unpaired conditions are administered to different stimuli within a single group) are presented separately. The response values presented in Table 1 were transformed to permit comparisons of relative

TABLE 1

SUMMARY OF EFFECTS ON "NO FURTHER UCS" VERBAL INSTRUCTIONS ON THE ELECTRODERMAL RESPONSE (TRANSFORMED VALUES OF RESPONSE MAGNITUDE ON EARLY EXTINCTION TRIALS)

Reference	Instructed group			Noninstructed group		
	Paired conditions	Unpaired conditions	D	Paired conditions	Unpaired conditions	D
Simple conditioning						
Silverman (1960)						
.5-sec ISI	.65	.38	+.27	1.00	.74	+.26
6-sec ISI	1.09	.50	+.59	1.00	.98	+.02
Wickens *et al.* (1963)						
Weak UCS	.70	.35	+.35	1.00	.70	+.30
Strong UCS	.72	.32	+.40	1.00	.64	+.36
Discrimination conditioning						
Bridger & Mandel (1965)						
CRF	.43	.10	+.33	1.00	.16	+.84
PRF	.14	.04	+.10	1.00	.10	+.90
Mandel & Bridger (1967)						
.5-sec ISI	.64	.36	+.28	1.00	.64	+.36
5-sec ISI	.28	.17	+.11	1.00	.55	+.45

response strengths between various experiments. The method of transformation was the following: (1) the mean response magnitude on early extinction trials for the paired and unpaired conditions for the instructed and noninstructed groups were obtained[2] and (2) the ratio of each obtained value to that of the paired–noninstructed condition was calculated. For example, in Silverman's (1960) .5-sec ISI group, the response magnitude (in log $\bar{X}$ conductance units) for the paired–noninstructed, unpaired–noninstructed, paired–instructed, and unpaired–instructed

[2] In some cases these values were estimated from published figures.

conditions were 2.49, 1.84, 1.63, and .94, respectively. The ratios were 1.00 (2.49/2.49), .74 (1.84/2.49), .65 (1.63/2.49), and .38 (.94/2.49). The difference (D) between the transformed values for the paired and unpaired conditions is the index of conditioning.

How do the data presented in Table 1 relate to the three experimental questions listed previously? First, regarding the level of general responsivity, the appropriate comparisons are between each instructed and noninstructed value. Of the 16 possible comparisons, 15 indicate that the level of responsivity is less for the instructed group than for the noninstructed group. Results of other experiments, not shown in Table 1, also indicate that "no more UCS" instructions reduce the level of electrodermal responsivity (Cook & Harris, 1937; Grings & Lockhart, 1963; Koenig & Castillo, 1969; Mowrer, 1938). Reduced responsivity as a function of "no more UCS" instructions has also been reported with the conditioned cardiac response (Chatterjee & Eriksen, 1962), vasomotor response (Shean, 1968a), and eye-blink response (Hartman & Grant, 1962). Thus, it may be concluded that instructions which inform S of a termination of the CS–UCS relation significantly reduce the overall level of autonomic responsivity.

As to whether these instructions reduce the magnitude of the conditioned response, the appropriate comparison is between the D values for the instructed and noninstructed groups. Examination of these data suggests different conclusions for the simple and discrimination conditioning paradigms. For the simple conditioning designs, the CR index is larger for the instructed groups than for the noninstructed groups. For the discrimination conditioning paradigms, the reverse is true. However, there is a critical procedural difference between the simple and discrimination conditioning paradigms; namely, with the simple conditioning design, Ss who failed to completely believe the "no more UCS" instructions were included in the data analysis whereas these Ss were excluded with the discrimination conditioning design. Thus, the apparent differences due to conditioning paradigms may reflect the differential treatment of Ss who failed to believe the instructions.

Finally, to determine whether the instructions completely and immediately abolished the conditioned response, one should examine the D values for each instructed group shown in Table 1. All of the D values (CR indices) for the instructed groups are positive and statistically significant; thus, the conditioned responses were not completely or immediately abolished. The fact that the conditioned electrodermal response persists despite the "no more UCS" instructions is consistent with the clinical findings that "cognitive control conspicuously fails to extinguish neurotic anxiety reactions [Rachman & Teasdale, 1969, p. 315]."

The finding that classically conditioned responses persist despite the administration of "no more UCS" instructions has been interpreted as evidence that there are two levels of learning produced by CS–UCS pairings, mediational and nonmediational (Bridger & Mandel, 1964, 1965). The essential assumption of this interpretation is that the administration of these instructions completely and immediately abolishes appropriate cognitive mediation (expectancy of the UCS) without having a similar effect on the autonomic CR. Support for the assumption rests solely upon S's report of belief of the instructions stated during a postexperimental inquiry (Bridger & Mandel, 1965; Mandel & Bridger, 1967).

However, it must be emphasized that the postexperimental inquiry requires the suspicious S to openly state to the experimenter that he considered the experimental instructions to be possibly false. Some Ss may have difficulty in reporting their suspicion for any one or combination of the following reasons: (1) S may perceive E as an authority figure, which inhibits statements of suspicion; (2) the instructions have been confirmed by means of extinction trials, thus making suspicion appear foolish and incorrect; and (3) S may perceive the report of suspicion as being a sign of being a bad subject or as ruining the experiment. Research which controls for these demand characteristics is needed in order to clarify the theoretical interpretation of the effects of "no more UCS" instructions.

Wilson (1968) has reported on an interesting variation of the "no more UCS" instructions. Following initial acquisition with a discrimination conditioning paradigm, Wilson verbally instructed Ss that the previously reinforced CS would no longer be associated with the UCS but that the previously nonreinforced CS would be paired with the UCS. Unknown to the Ss, no UCSs were administered following these instructions. Analysis of SRR magnitude data revealed an immediate reversal, i.e., more responding to the previously unreinforced CS than to the previously reinforced CS. The author concluded that "the present study finds no evidence to support the contention that some part of a conditioned autonomic response is 'simple' in the sense that it is not mediated by S's perception of stimulus contingencies [Wilson, 1968, p. 493]."

B. Instructions That Minimize Learning Stimulus Relations

1. ACQUISITION

There have been several attempts to study the acquisition of human electrodermal classical conditioning in situations designed to minimize learning of the CS–UCS relation. One common experimental method is to embed the CS–UCS pairing within a masking task and administer verbal instructions which are misleading about the purpose of the experiment. The masking task and misleading instructions are intended to direct S's attention to an irrelevant aspect of the situation and make it unlikely that he will become aware of the CS–UCS relation. The primary experimental question of these experiments has been: Can human classical conditioning occur when awareness of the CS–UCS relation is eliminated or, at least, minimized?

Table 2 presents a summary of representative experiments which have included masking tasks and misleading instructions to minimize learning of the CS–UCS relation. Table 2 includes the reference, type of response measure, type of masking task, and type of questionnaire used to verify that awareness was minimized.

There are several interesting facts which emerge from an examination of Table 2. First, the majority of experiments measured electrodermal responses. Second, the majority of experiments employed a word-association masking task originally introduced by Diven (1937). Third, the conclusions of the studies are quite discrepant. The upper six studies reported that conditioning did occur in the absence of awareness while the lower six studies reported that it did not occur.

The methods and findings of the experiments presented in Table 2 are briefly reviewed. Haggard (1943) presented a series of 42 words to which Ss were instructed to free-associate and tap their index finger. The CS word (*sword*) was presented five times during the series and was followed each time in 10–12 sec by an electric shock UCS. Upon being asked if they could predict when they were going to receive the shock, 9 of 18 Ss correctly stated that the shock followed *sword*. Analysis of SCR magnitude revealed that the responses of the unaware group were larger than those of the aware group.

Lacey and Smith (1954) pointed out that the procedures used by Haggard, as well as those of Diven, did not provide an adequate test of whether human autonomic classical conditioning occurred (much less whether it occurred in the absence of awareness). Therefore, Lacey and Smith used a similar masking task with an improved conditioning design. Following the conditioning session, each S was administered an extensive interview which included the question, "Did you know when you were going to get shocked?" Twenty-two of the 31 Ss failed to verbalize the correct word–shock relation and yet analysis of their heart rate indicated successful conditioning and semantic generalization. Wieland, Stein, and Hamilton (1963) varied the intensity of the UCS and essentially replicated the Lacey and Smith findings.

TABLE 2

SUMMARY OF HUMAN AUTONOMIC CONDITIONING EXPERIMENTS WHICH
EMBEDDED CS–UCS PAIRINGS IN A MASKING TASK

Reference	Response	Masking task	Question-naire[a]
Conditioning in absence of awareness			
Haggard (1943)	SCR	Word association and motor tapping	Short recall
Lacey and Smith (1954)	HR	Word association and motor tapping	Short recall
Golin (1961)	SCR	Word association and motor tapping	Long recognition
Wieland, Stein, and Hamilton (1963)	HR	Word association and motor tapping	Short recall
Lockhart (1966)	SCR	Musical quiz	Short recognition
Fuhrer and Baer (1969)	SCR	Probability learning	Long recall
No conditioning in absence of awareness			
Chatterjee and Eriksen (1960)	SCR	Word association	Long recognition
Chatterjee and Eriksen (1962)	HR	Word association	Long recognition
Shean (1968a)	Vasomotor	Word association	Long recognition
Dawson and Grings (1968)	SCR	Paper and pencil "mental test"	Short recognition
Dawson (1970, Experiment I)	SCR	Sound–pitch discrimination	Long recognition
Dawson (1970, Experiment II)	SCR	Sound–pitch discrimination	Short recognition

[a] Description of the various types of questionnaires:

Short recall: The subject is required to verbalize the correct CS–UCS relation in response to one or two brief open-ended questions (e.g., "Did you know when you were going to receive the UCS?").

Long recall: The subject is required to verbalize the correct CS–UCS relation in response to a lengthy series of questions which become progressively more specific.

Short recognition: The subject is required to select the correct CS–UCS relation from a series of choices on a multichoice questionnaire.

Long recognition: The subject is required, upon being presented several CSs, to state a high probability of the UCS being associated with the reinforced CS.

Eriksen (1958) criticized the questionnaire methods employed by previous investigators. The criticism is essentially that although Ss may not be able to verbalize the specific CS–UCS relation on an open-ended recall questionnaire, they might be able to correctly recognize the reinforced CS. Based on this line of reasoning, Chatterjee and Eriksen (1960) replicated the Lacey and Smith procedures except that (1) SCR, rather than heart rate, was recorded, and (2) a multiple-choice recognition questionnaire in addition to a recall questionnaire was administered. Analysis of their data led the authors to conclude that "conditioning of the autonomic response (GSR) was no more specific than S's verbalizations [p. 403]." In a subsequent study, Chatterjee and Eriksen (1962) recorded heart rate and found "clear evidence of heart rate conditioning . . . only in those cases where S could verbalize the relationship between the CS and UCS [p. 279]." Shean (1968a) used a similar masking task and a recognition questionnaire and failed to find evidence of vasomotor conditioning in the absence of awareness. Golin (1961), on the other hand, used a similar masking task and recognition questionnaire and did report successful electrodermal conditioning in the absence of awareness.

All of the experiments discussed thus far have used a similar masking task; namely, requiring S to verbally free-associate to a series of words while the UCS is administered following one particular word. However, based on their experience with this masking task, Chatterjee and Eriksen concluded that "there are so many uncontrolled and confounded sources of variance in this design so as to render virtually impossible an answer to the basic question of conditioning without awareness [1960, p. 402]." More recent studies have employed different masking tasks to minimize learning of the CS–UCS relation.

Lockhart (1966), for example, devised a "musical quiz" masking task. The Ss listened to a tape-recorded musical collage and were "busily engaged in reading a 4-page mimeographed 'musical quiz' to which they were oriented prior to the experiment [p. 441]." Lockhart employed a recognition postconditioning questionnaire and reported successful temporal conditioning of the EDR in the absence of awareness of the correct inter-UCS interval.

Dawson and Grings (1968) embedded CS–UCS pairings within a paper and pencil mental test masking task. Their postconditioning assessment of awareness included a recognition questionnaire and they failed to find SCR conditioning in the absence of awareness. However, as the authors noted, the masking task may have partially prevented perceptual discrimination of the individual CSs in addition to minimizing awareness. Therefore, Dawson (1970, Experiment I; Experiment II) devised an auditory discrimination masking task which required that Ss attend to and discriminate between the individual CSs. Awareness was measured by recognition questionnaires and no evidence of SCR conditioning in the absence of awareness was found. However, Fuhrer and Baer (1969) also noted the problem of CS perception involved in the task used by Dawson and Grings and therefore employed a probability learning masking task. Fuhrer and Baer used a long recall postconditioning questionnaire and reported successful electrodermal classical conditioning in the absence of awareness.

What can one conclude on the basis of these widely discrepant results? When the methods used to measure awareness are examined it can be seen that the results, although discrepant, are not totally inconsistent. Of the studies in Table 2 which failed to find conditioning in the absence of awareness, all six employed some form of recognition questionnaire. And, of the six studies which found evidence of conditioning in the absence of awareness, four employed some form of recall questionnaire and two used recognition questionnaires. Thus, there is a strong, although not perfect, correlation between the conclusion of an experiment and the method used to measure awareness. In addition, both of the studies which are exceptions to this correlation (Golin, 1961; Lockhart, 1966) administered the questionnaires following an extinction session. Spielberger and DeNike (1966) have indicated that presenting an extinction session before the questionnaire may invalidate the questionnaire data.

Given that recognition questionnaires yield different results than do recall questionnaires, it is reasonable to ask which questionnaire is correct. Logical considerations indicate that the recognition questionnaire is the appropriate measure (Dawson, 1973; Eriksen, 1958). However, an empirical approach to the issue of questionnaire validity is possible. One can test the construct validity of any measurement technique by employing it in situations where the construct to be measured will vary. If the measurement technique is valid, then its scores will vary as the situation varies (Cronbach & Meehl, 1955).

Dawson and Reardon (1973) tested the construct validity of various recall and recognition questionnaires. They employed the questionnaires in situations where the construct of awareness would vary. Thus, the situation in which awareness was likely to occur was one in which Ss were instructed prior to conditioning that there may be a CS–UCS relation. A situation in which the occurrence of awareness was unlikely was one in which the UCS was presented in essentially an unpredictable manner. It was found that a short recognition questionnaire was best at discriminating between the rates of awareness in these conditions. Recall questionnaires were the poorest at such discrimination. In addition, the only evidence of conditioning in the absence of awareness was found among a subsample of Ss who were rated unaware with the short recall questionnaire but aware with the short recognition questionnaire. These results suggest that previous studies which used recall questionnaires, especially the short variety, did not adequately measure awareness and therefore may not have conducted valid tests of whether human conditioning can occur in the absence of awareness.

Obviously, a great deal more research is needed to determine whether, and under what conditions, human conditioning may occur in the absence of awareness. At the present time, it appears that unaware conditioning has not been reliably demonstrated when a valid measure of awareness is employed. The validity of various postconditioning questionnaires needs to be further investigated. In fact, it may be that all postconditioning questionnaires are invalid in comparison to one which occurs repeatedly during conditioning.

The possibility that measures of awareness which occur during conditioning are more valid and useful than those which occur after conditioning is not a new concept (Grant, 1939, p. 338; Hamel, 1919, p. 26). Nevertheless, previous attempts to relate such measures with conditioning performance, although encouraging, have met with only moderate success (Epstein & Bahm, 1971; Fuhrer & Baer, 1965; Hilgard, Campbell, & Sears, 1937; Shean, 1968b).

2. EXTINCTION

To these authors' knowledge, there are no published experiments which have measured electrodermal extinction while S's awareness of the extinction procedure was minimized. In other words, there is no research to answer the question: Will electrodermal conditioned responses extinguish when S is made unaware of the termination of the CS–UCS relation? This lack of research is surprising for two reasons. First, there has been extensive study of other types of cognitive factors in electrodermal conditioning. Second, this issue of awareness during extinction has been recently an active area of research with human eyelid conditioning (Ross, 1971; Spence, 1966).

Although there is no directly relevant evidence, there is reason to believe that electrodermal extinction will not occur as long as S continues to expect UCS following the CS. For example, consider a group that was told that two strong electric shocks would be paired with a CS (Bridger & Mandel, 1964). Following these instructions, a total of 20 CS-alone trials (acquisition or extinction?) were administered. At no time was shock ever administered to this group. The SCR data indicated that this group exhibited significant conditioned-like behavior for all 20 trials. In fact, over the last 10 trials, the SCR data of this group did not differ from that of another group which was administered physical

CS–UCS pairings. Thus, there was no indication of electrodermal extinction despite 20 nonreinforced trials.

C. Instructions That Induce Response Sets

It has been known for many years that verbal instructions which induce response sets can markedly affect conditioned eyeblink performance (Gormezano & Moore, 1962; Hilgard & Humphreys, 1938; Nichols & Kimble, 1964; Norris & Grant, 1948). However, only recently have the effects of these instructions been investigated with conditioned electrodermal responses. Hill (1967) induced different response sets by instructing one group that it was "the most adaptive, sensible, and intelligent thing *to become conditioned*" (facilitory instructions) and a second group that it was "the most adaptive, sensible, and intelligent thing *not to become conditioned*" (inhibitory instructions). The results revealed that the magnitude of the SCR elicited by the CS during conditioning was significantly larger for the facilitory group than for the inhibitory group. These findings were essentially replicated by Dawson and Reardon (1969), who added a neutral instruction group and a pseudoconditioning control group. The latter study showed that, although both groups conditioned (i.e., responded more than the control group), the SCR magnitude of the facilitory group was significantly larger than that of the inhibitory group.

Hughes and Shean (1971) have reported a variation of the inhibitory instructions. Before being administered a series of CS–UCS pairings, two groups were explicitly instructed to "keep your responses at as low a level as you possibly can [p. 309]." One group was given feedback after each trial as to the success of response inhibition. The second group was not given feedback. The SCR magnitude elicited by the CS demonstrated that the feedback group responded at a significantly lower level than did a noninstructed control group. The response magnitude of the nonfeedback group did not differ from that of the control group. Thus, successful inhibition of electrodermal conditioned responses as a result of explicit instructions occurred only in the presence of feedback.

Martin and Dean (1970) reported a series of experiments which varied instructions regarding response sets within an electrodermal classical conditioning paradigm. In the first experiment, one group was instructed to respond one CS and not respond to another CS. In addition, electric shock was avoided on trials in which responses were successfully facilitated or inhibited. A second group was administered the same instructions but shock was presented on a yoked schedule. It was found that both groups responded more to the facilitory CS than to the inhibitory CS while a noninstructed control group did not respond differentially to the two CSs. Thus, the instructions modified electrodermal reactivity in the appropriate direction independently of contingent reinforcement. Other data reported by the authors demonstrated these findings to hold true only for electrodermal ARs and not ORs.

Does the effect of instructions on conditioned EDRs reflect a difference in associative strength (habit) or merely general responsivity (drive)? Hill (1967) interpreted the finding that the facilitory and inhibitory groups extinguished at similar rates as evidence that differences in response magnitude did not reflect true associative differences. Harvey and Wickens (1971) have reported additional evidence that the effects of the instructions are on general responsivity rather than learning *per se*. These authors replicated the procedures of Hill with the addition of uncued UCS presentations. They found, as did Hill (1967) and Dawson and Reardon (1969), that SCR magnitude elicited by the CS was larger for facilitory groups than for the inhibitory group. In addition, the authors found that UCR magnitude elicited by uncued UCSs was larger for the facilitory group than for the inhibitory group. The latter finding is consistent with the notion that response sets affect general responsivity and not necessarily associative strength.

Several interesting possibilities are suggested by the fact that humans can modulate, to a degree, their conditioning performance. One possibility is that the effect of certain variables on conditioning may be mediated by response sets. For example, Ss who experience extinction following continuous reinforcement may try to inhibit their responding more than those who experience extinction following partial reinforcement (Spence, 1966). Another possibility is that variability in conditioning results (whether in the laboratory or clinic) may be reduced by ensuring similar response sets prior to conditioning. Still another possibility is that there are important individual differences in ability to modulate electrodermal conditioning. Research dealing with individual differences has been rather disappointing thus far. Hill (1967) failed to find differences in ability to modulate conditioning as a function of "need for approval" (Crowne & Marlowe, 1960) and Hughes and Shean (1971) failed to find a difference as a function of neuroticism or extroversion–introversion (Eysenck, 1967). However, in controlling rate of spontaneous electrodermal response, Stern and Lewis (1968) found that method actors are better than nonmethod actors and that Ss who report sweating to be a physiological manifestation of anxiety are better than those who do not report this effect.

In summary, instructions which induce response sets do affect magnitude of electrodermal CRs. The amount of research in this area is very small so that the theoretical mechanisms, controlling variables, limiting conditions, and implications are largely unknown.

VI. Individual Difference Factors

It is reasonable to assume that conditioning of autonomic behavior, like the EDR, will be determined in part by the personal characteristics of the learner. Among obvious candidates for such variables are the subject's age, sex, and intelligence. The crucial task for research becomes the identification of the individual characteristics, description of the extent of their influence, and the explanation of why they are important. There has been at least the beginning of systematic work on this task and, although much of the work has been done with other conditioned responses (especially the eye blink), there is enough electrodermal research to be noted here.

For convenience, the research will be divided among several classes according to underlying explanations of predicted effects. One class will be derived from the concept of motivation or drive, another from personality traits of introversion and extroversion, and the third from general social–medical–psychiatric criteria.

A. The Drive Concept

Much work on individual differences in conditioning was stimulated by the arguments of Spence (1958) that emotionality operates as a drive which may influence performance or acquisition in conditioning situations. The response most frequently studied was eye blink rather than electrodermal response (EDR) (Spence, 1964) and the drive variable was most often defined by means of the Taylor Manifest Anxiety Scale (MAS). However, in at least one case (Runquist & Ross, 1959) electrodermal behavior was used in defining the drive variable. Prior to conditioning, those investigators gave their subjects 15 trials on the UCS (an air puff) during which they measured change in skin resistance and heart rate. High and low drive groups were selected on the basis of the single physiological measures or a combination of the two. Then an eye-blink conditioning series was given during which significantly better performance was observed for high drive groups on the single indices and almost significant difference on the combined index. They concluded that conditioning performance is a function of the drive level of the two groups.

There are relatively few studies defining drive in terms of inventory scores which employ electrodermal conditioning. Of these, the experiment of Becker and Matteson (1961) will serve as an example. They selected four groups of 10 subjects each from 273 introductory psychology students to represent extreme high and low anxiety and high and low extroversion subjects. Cattell's Anxiety (A) Scale was used as the drive measure and was reported to correlate .85 with the MAS. (The extroversion data will be ignored for the time being.) Unadjusted differences in mean amplitude conditioning scores favored the high drive groups but were statistically insignificant. However, differences in basal resistance level were noted and an analysis of covariance was performed to adjust for that variable. When that was done, the adjusted mean conditioning scores were significantly larger for the high than for the low anxiety groups, supporting Spence's assertion. The study has been criticized (Eysenck, 1965) for failure to ensure equal strength of UCS between groups. A later study (Davidson, Payne, & Sloane, 1968) separated Ss on the MAS and reported negative results, but this study also contained methodological problems in definition of conditioning indices.

Using a clinical index of anxiety with normal Ss, Bitterman and Holtzman (1952) found the SRR to condition more readily and to extinguish less quickly in a high as compared to a low anxiety group. Streiner and Dean (1968) used the Sarason test anxiety scale to separate high and low anxiety groups who were found not to differ in SCR conditioned acquisition performance but to differ in rate of extinction (the high anxiety group extinguished more slowly). Closely related to these studies with inventory-defined drives are those that employ patients exhibiting symptoms of manifest anxiety as the high drive group. For example, Welch and Kubis (1947a, b) compared normals and anxiety patients and found the patients required fewer trials to condition and showed greater resistance to extinction. The anxiety-drive variable has also been identified by some workers with the neuroticism scale on inventories like the Maudsley Personality Inventory, under the assumption that such scales reflect a form of neurotic arousal or drive. An example of such a study is that of Martin (1960) where no relationship was found between conditioning and neuroticism.

Although the above studies do not exhaust the research on the question, they show how complicated and diverse the observed relations have been. Many different indices of drive have been used. Much difficulty exists in separating sensitization effects from associative effects, particularly where extinction rates are compared between patient groups and normals. The base level of electrodermal behavior is significantly related to the various drive measures so that general reactivity levels of comparison groups cannot be equated (except for some adjustment procedure like that used by Becker and Matteson).

B. Introversion–Extroversion

One might hope for a simpler basis for prediction from traits which do not purport to reflect general arousal or reactivity level. Such a trait is introversion–extroversion, which Eysenck argues should be related to conditioning through the underlying processes of excitation and inhibition which that trait is assumed to tap. The relation between conditioning and introversion is based on two assumptions: that extroversion is related to relative ease of arousal or cortical excitation and inhibition, extroverts showing greater inhibition, introverts greater excitation; and, that cortical inhibition depresses conditioning and facilitates extinction. Limiting conditions affecting the manifestation of the relation are provided by circumstances assumed to be productive of inhibition, such as (1) partial as compared with complete reinforcement, (2) weak as opposed to strong CS and UCS, and (3) discrimination learning as opposed to single stimulus conditioning. Inhibition is assumed to be generated during the unreinforced trials interspersed with the reinforced trials.

In a review of data using electrodermal conditioning, relevant to the above predictions, Eysenck (1965) cites nine studies of which five concluded in favor of predicted relations and four found no relationship. In general, the negative results were attributed by Eysenck to the use of very strong UCS (studies of Becker, 1960; Becker & Matteson, 1961; and Davidson, Payne, & Sloane, 1964). The positive results included a correlation of −.25 between an index of conditioning and scores on Guilford's R scale (Franks, 1956); instances where introverts (on the Maudsley Personality Inventory) required fewer trials to reach a criterion than did extroverts (Vogel, 1960, 1961); and a study comparing sociopaths (shown to be extroverted on the MMPI) and normals, where the sociopaths showed less conditioning.

Since the time of Eysenck's review there have been few reported tests with electrodermal responses. Three, of which the authors are aware, have yielded largely negative results (Purhoit, 1966; Morgenson & Martin, 1969; Cowan, 1968) although two of these studies expressed qualifications about the conclusiveness of tests made. Variables of cognition and responsivity level were discussed as complicating factors. In general, then, introversion–extroversion joins manifest anxiety as an individual difference variable whose role in conditioning remains unclear.

C. Other Criteria

A wide range of other individual characteristics has been explored for possible determiners of EDR conditioning, including age, sex, and intelligence, as well as various medical-psychiatric criteria. At least three investigations have reported age differences in performance during EDR conditioning, two with discrimination arrangements and the other with a single CS.

Morrow, Boring, Keough, and Haesly (1969) compared children, young adults, and aged adults on differential conditioning trials. There were no differences among the groups on the amount of differential conditioning, but the groups did differ on responsivity. The younger Ss gave significantly larger SRRs to the CS+ than did the aged group, as well as marginally significantly greater response to the CS- as well. The authors concluded "that aging most probably affects the response mechanism rather than conditioning [Morrow et al., 1969, p. 299]." A similar interpretation might be given to the results of Botwinick and Kornetsky (1960) who employed simple conditioning to a tone and found that the aged groups took fewer trials to habituate to the tone prior to conditioning and gave fewer CRs during 15 conditioning trials than did a younger group. They concluded that the older group was less reactive than the younger group.

Adding the variable of sex to that of age, Shmavonian, Miller, and Cohen (1968) ran four groups, young and aged, men and women, in a discrimination conditioning study. They found the younger groups to give better discrimination than the older groups and the older females to be somewhat better than the older males. They correlated their results with differences in cognitive reactions to the study by the different groups.

Intelligence as a determiner of conditioning has been studied in a number of ways, mostly with extreme groups. Grings et al. (1962) compared two groups of mentally deficient adolescents (one with a mean IQ of 34, the other with a mean of 63) and found no significant differences between the discrimination conditioning performance of the groups, both of whom conditioned readily. In a comparison of retardates and normals, Baumeister, Beedle, and Urquhart (1964) found the retardates to condition as well as the comparison group on the mean number of EDRs to a tone CS in a simple conditioning paradigm. In contrast, Lobb (1968) found superior conditioning for normal controls over mentally retarded Ss for a limited range of interstimulus intervals in a study which varied ISI and drug administration variables as well as intelligence.

Further comparisons with special groups of children include comparisons of conditioning and extinction of two groups of brain-injured children, a group of mongloid, and a small group of normal children (Birch & Demb, 1959). It was found that the brain-injured children who were characterized as being hyperactive or distractable required a significantly larger number of paired presentations of light and shock to reach the criterion for conditioning than did the groups of brain-injured children not so classified. The mongloid Ss required even longer to reach acquisition criterion. With an emphasis on habituation of the EDR, Pilgrim, Miller, and Cobb (1969) found no significant differences in rates of habituation between groups of mildly retarded persons and normals.

At least two studies have shown conditioning differences attributable to the trait of psychopathic personality, as manifested in criminal populations. Lykken (1957) observed "primary" sociopaths (as defined by the criteria of Cleckley) to show less reactivity to a conditioned stimulus associated with shock, as compared to normals. When 24 penitentiary inmates were divided into psychopathic and nonpsychopathic samples, the former were found to condition more slowly and to show less generalization to new stimuli (Hare, 1965).

Several theories of schizophrenic behavior have predicted unique generalization behavior for such Ss. One hypothesis is that schizophrenics would generalize a conditioned EDR relatively more to the homonym of a CS and relatively less to the synonym than normals. Peastrel (1964) presented data which he concluded demonstrated this "interaction between the 'normal–schizophrenic' variable and generalization to synonyms and homonyms [p. 446]." In a study with high and low anxious and reactive and process schizophrenic Ss, Jongsma, Sullivan, and Martin (1969) found that acute, highly anxious reactive Ss conditioned and generalized more than the chronic, low anxious reactive Ss, and that the reverse was true in the process subgroups.

Acknowledgments

The authors wish to acknowledge aid from National Institute of Mental Health Grants, MH03916 (Grings) and MH18411 (Dawson).

References

Allen, C. K., Hill, F. A., & Wickens, D. D. The orienting reflex as a function of the interstimulus interval of compound stimuli. *Journal of Experimental Psychology*, 1963, 65, 309–316.

Astrup, C., Sersen, E. A., & Wortis, J. Conditioned reflex studies in mental retardation: A review. *American Journal of Mental Deficiency*, 1967, **71**, 513–530.

Badia, P., & Defran, R. H. Orienting responses and GSR conditioning: A dilemma. *Psychological Review*, 1970, **77**, 171–180.

Baker, T. W. Properties of compound conditioned stimuli and their components. *Psychological Bulletin*, 1968, **70**, 611–625.

Baker, T. W. Component strength in a compound CS as a function of number of acquisition trials. *Journal of Experimental Psychology*, 1969, **79**, 347–352.

Baumeister, A. A., Beedle, R., & Urquhart, D. GSR conditioning in normals and retardates. *American Journal of Mental Deficiency*, 1964, **69**, 114–120.

Baxter, R. Diminution and recovery of the UCR in delayed and trace classical GSR conditioning. *Journal of Experimental Psychology*, 1966, **17**, 447–451.

Becker, W. C. Cortical inhibition and extraversion–introversion. *Journal of Abnormal and Social Psychology*, 1960, **61**, 52–66.

Becker, W. C., & Matteson, H. H. GSR conditioning, anxiety, and extroversion. *Journal of Abnormal and Social Psychology*, 1961, **62**, 427–430.

Birch, H. G., & Demb, H. The formation and extinction of conditioned reflexes in "brain-damaged" and Mongoloid children. *Journal of Nervous and Mental Disease*, 1959, **129**, 162–170.

Bitterman, M. E., & Holtzman, W. H. Conditioning and extinction of the galvanic skin response as a function of anxiety. *Journal of Abnormal and Social Psychology*, 1952, **47**, 615–623.

Block, J. D. Awareness of stimulus relationships and physiological generality of response in autonomic discrimination. In J. Wortis (Ed.), *Recent advances in biological psychiatry*. New York: Plenum, 1962.

Booth, J. H., & Hammond, L. J. Configural conditioning: Greater fear in rats to compound than component through overtraining of the compound. *Journal of Experimental Psychology*, 1971, **87**, 255–262.

Botwinick, J., & Kornetsky, C. Age differences in the acquisition and extinction of the GSR. *Journal of Gerontology*, 1960, **15**, 190–192.

Bousfield, W. A. The problem of meaning in verbal learning. In C. N. Cofer (Ed.), *Verbal learning and verbal behavior*. New York: McGraw-Hill, 1961.

Bridger, W. H. The role of cognitive set and stress in generalization of conditional responses to verbal stimuli. *International Journal of Psychobiology*, 1970, **1**, 39–42.

Bridger, W. H., & Mandel, I. J. A comparison of GSR fear responses produced by threat and electric shock. *Journal of Psychiatric Research*, 1964, **2**, 31–40.

Bridger, W. H., & Mandel, I. J. Abolition of the PRE by instructions in GSR conditioning. *Journal of Experimental Psychology*, 1965, **69**, 476–482.

Brotsky, S. J., & Keller, W. H. Semantic conditioning and generalization of the galvanic skin response: Locus of mediation in classical conditioning. *Journal of Experimental Psychology*, 1971, **89**, 383–389.

Brown, J. S., Kalish, H. I., & Farber, I. E. Conditioned fear as revealed by magnitude of startle response to an auditory stimulus. *Journal of Experimental Psychology*, 1951, **41**, 317–328.

Chatterjee, B. B., & Eriksen, C. W. Conditioning and generalization of GSR as a function of awareness. *Journal of Abnormal and Social Psychology*, 1960, **60**, 396–403.

Chatterjee, B. B., & Eriksen, C. W. Cognitive factors in heart rate conditioning. *Journal of Experimental Psychology*, 1962, **64**, 272–279.

Cofer, C. N., & Foley, J. P. Mediated generalization and the interpretation of verbal behavior: I. Prolegomena. *Psychological Review*, 1942, **49**, 513–540.

Cook, S. W., & Harris, R. E. The verbal conditioning of the galvanic skin response. *Journal of Experimental Psychology*, 1937, **21**, 202–210.

Cowan, C. O. Cognitive process, anxiety, extroversion and GSR responsiveness in classical differential GSR conditioning. *Dissertation Abstracts*, 1968, **28**, 5201.

Cronbach, L. J., & Meehl, P. E. Construct validity in psychological tests. *Psychological Bulletin*, 1955, **52**, 281–302.

Crowne, D. P., & Marlowe, D. A new scale of social desirability independent of psychopathology. *Journal of Consulting Psychology*, 1960, **24**, 349–354.

Davidson, P. O., Payne, R. W., & Sloane, R. B. Introversion, neuroticism, and conditioning. *Journal of Abnormal and Social Psychology*, 1964, **68**, 136–143.

Davidson, P. O., Payne, R. W., & Sloane, R. B. Conditionability in normals and neurotics. *Journal of Experimental Research in Personality*, 1968, **3**, 107–113.

Dawson, M. E. Cognition and conditioning: Effects of masking the CS-UCS contingency on human GSR classical conditioning. *Journal of Experimental Psychology*, 1970, **85**, 389–396.

Dawson, M. E. Can classical conditioning occur without contingency learning?: A review and evaluation of the evidence. *Psychophysiology*, 1973, **10**, 82–86.

Dawson, M. E., & Grings, W. W. Comparison of classical conditioning and relational learning. *Journal of Experimental Psychology*, 1968, **76**, 227–231.

Dawson, M. E., & Reardon, P. Effects of facilitory and inhibitory sets on GSR conditioning and performance. *Journal of Experimental Psychology*, 1969, **82**, 462–466.

Dawson, M. E., & Reardon, P. Construct validity of recall and recognition postconditioning measures of awareness. *Journal of Experimental Psychology*, 1973, **98**, 308–315.

Diven, K. Certain determiners of the conditioning of anxiety reactions. *Journal of Psychology*, 1937, **3**, 291–308.

Dufort, R. H., & Kimble, G. A. Ready signals and the effect of interpolated UCS presentations in eyelid conditioning. *Journal of Experimental Psychology*, 1958, **56**, 1–7.

Egger, M. D., & Miller, N. E. Secondary reinforcement in rats as a function of information value and reliability of the stimulus. *Journal of Experimental Psychology*, 1962, **64**, 97–104.

Egger, M. D., & Miller, N. E. When is a reward reinforcing?: An experimental study of the information hypothesis. *Journal of Comparative and Physiological Psychology*, 1963, **56**, 132–137.

Epstein, S., & Bahm, R. Verbal hypothesis formulatin during classical conditioning of the GSR. *Journal of Experimental Psychology*, 1971, **87**, 187–197.

Eriksen, C. W. Unconscious processes. In M. R. Jones (Ed.), *Nebraska symposium on motivation*. Lincoln: Univ. of Nebraska Press, 1958.

Eysenck, H. J. Extraversion and the acquisition of eyeblink and GSR conditioned responses. *Psychological Bulletin*, 1965, **63**, 258–270.

Eysenck, H. J. *The biological basis of personality*. Springfield, Illinois: Thomas, 1967.

Feather, B. W. Semantic generalization of classically conditioned responses: A review. *Psychological Bulletin*, 1965, **63**, 425–441.

Franks, C. M. Conditioning and personality: A study of normal and neurotic subjects. *Journal of Abnormal and Social Psychology*, 1956, **52**, 143–149.

Fuhrer, M. J., & Baer, P. E. Differential classical conditioning: Verbalization of stimulus contingencies. *Science*, 1965, **150**, 1479–1481.

Fuhrer, M. J., & Baer, P. E. Cognitive processes in differential GSR conditioning: Effects of a masking task. *American Journal of Psychology*, 1969, **82**, 168–180.

Golin, S. Incubation effect: Role of awareness in an immediate versus delayed test of conditioned emotionality. *Journal of Abnormal and Social Psychology*, 1961, **63**, 534–539.

Gormezano, I., & Moore, J. W. Effects of instructional set and UCS intensity on the latency, percentage, and form of the eyelid response. *Journal of Experimental Psychology*, 1962, **63**, 487–494.

Grant, D. A. The influence of attitude on the conditioned eyelid response. *Journal of Experimental Psychology*, 1939, **25**, 333–346.

Grings, W. W. Preparatory set variables related to classical conditioning of autonomic responses. *Psychological Review*, 1960, **67**, 243–252.

Grings, W. W. Verbal-perceptual factors in conditioning of autonomic responses. In W. F. Prokasy (Ed.), *Classical conditioning: A symposium*. New York: Appleton, 1965.

Grings, W. W. Anticipatory and preparatory electrodermal behavior in paired stimulation situations. *Psychophysiology*, 1969, **5**, 597–611. (a)

Grings, W. W. Transfer of response from compound conditioned stimuli. *Psychonomic Science*, 1969, **15**, 187–188. (b)

Grings, W. W. Compound stimulus transfer in human classical conditioning. In A. H. Black & W. F. Prokasy (Eds.), *Classical conditioning II: Current research and theory*. New York: Appleton, 1972.

Grings, W. W. Cognitive factors in electrodermal conditioning. *Psychological Bulletin*, 1973, **79**, 200–210.

Grings, W. W., & Kimmel, H. D. Compound stimulus transfer for different sense modalities. *Psychological Reports*, 1959, **5**, 253–260.

Grings, W. W., & Lockhart, R. A. Effects of "anxiety-reducing" instructions and differential set development on the extinction of the GSR. *Journal of Experimental Psychology*, 1963, **66**, 292–299.

Grings, W. W., & O'Donnell, D. Magnitude of response to compounds of discriminated stimuli. *Journal of Experimental Psychology*, 1956, **52**, 354–359.

Grings, W. W., & Schell, A. M. Magnitude of electrodermal response to a standard stimulus as a function of intensity and proximity of a prior stimulus. *Journal of Comparative and Physiological Psychology*, 1969, **67**, 77–82. (a)

Grings, W. W., & Schell, A. M. UCR diminution in trace and delay conditioning. *Journal of Experimental Psychology*, 1969, **79**, 246–248. (b)

Grings, W. W., & Schell, A. M. Effects of trace versus delayed conditioning, interstimulus interval variability, and instructions on UCR diminution. *Journal of Experimental Psychology*, 1971, **90**, 136–140.

Grings, W. W., & Shmelev, V. N. Changes in GSR to a single stimulus as a result of training on a compound stimulus. *Journal of Experimental Psychology*, 1959, **58**, 129–133.

Grings, W. W., & Uno, T. Counterconditioning: Fear and relaxation. *Psychophysiology*, 1968, 4 479–485.

Grings, W. W., & Zeiner, A. Compound stimulus transfer. *Psychonomic Science*, 1969, **16**, 299–300. (a)

Grings, W. W., & Zeiner, A. Compound stimulus transfer among forward and backward conditioning situations. *Psychonomic Science*, 1969, **17**, 353–354. (b)

Grings, W. W., Lockhart, R., & Dameron, L. Conditioning autonomic responses of mentally subnormal individuals. *Psychological Monographs*, 1962, **76**, No. 39 (Whole No. 558).

Haggard, E. A. Experimental studies in affective processes: I. Some effects of cognitive structure and active participation on certain autonomic reactions during and following experimentally induced stress. *Journal of Experimental Psychology*, 1943, **33**, 257–284.

Hamel, I. A. A study and analysis of the conditioned reflex. *Psychological Monographs*, 1919, **27** (Whole No. 118).

Hare, R. D. Acquisition and generalization of a conditioned-fear response in psychopathic and nonpsychopathic criminals. *Journal of Psychology*, 1965, **59**, 367–370.

Hartman, T. F. Dynamic transmission, elective generalization, and semantic conditioning. In W. F. Prokasy (Ed.), *Classical conditioning: A symposium*. New York: Appleton, 1965.

Hartman, T. F., & Grant, D. A. Effects of pattern of reinforcement and verbal information on acquisition, extinction, and spontaneous recovery of the eyelid CR. *Journal of Experimental Psychology*, 1962, **63**, 217–226.

Harvey, B., & Wickens, D. D. Effect of instructions on responsiveness to the CS and to the UCS in GSR conditioning. *Journal of Experimental Psychology*, 1971, **87**, 137–140.

Hilgard, E. R., & Humphreys, L. G. The effect of supporting an antogonistic voluntary instructions on conditioned discrimination. *Journal of Experimental Psychology*, 1938, **22**, 291–304.

Hilgard, E. R., & Marquis, D. G. *Conditioning and learning*. New York: Appleton, 1940.

Hilgard, E. R., Campbell, A. A., & Sears, W. N. Conditioned discrimination: The development of discrimination with and without verbal report. *American Journal of Psychology*, 1937, **49**, 564–580.

Hilgard, E. R., Campbell, R. K., & Sears, W. N. Conditioned discrimination: The effect of knowledge of stimulus relationships. *American Journal of Psychology*, 1938, **51**, 498–506.

Hill, F. A. Effects of instructions and subjects' need for approval on the conditioned galvanic skin response. *Journal of Experimental Psychology*, 1967, **73**, 461–467.

Hughes, W. G., & Shean, G. D. Ability to control GSR amplitude. *Psychonomic Science*, 1971, **23**, 309–311.

Hull, C. L. Explorations in the patterning of stimuli conditioned to the GSR. *Journal of Experimental Psychology*, 1940, **27**, 95–110.

Hull, C. L. *Principles of behavior*. New York: Appleton, 1943.

Jacobson, E. *Progressive relaxation*. Chicago, Illinois: Univ. of Chicago Press, 1938.

Jongsma, A., Sullivan, D., & Martin, R. B. Adjustment and chronicity in simple and complex learning of schizophrenics and normals. *Journal of Clinical Psychology*, 1969, **25**, 152–155.

Kamin, L. J. Temporal and intensity characteristics of the conditioned stimulus. In W. F. Prokasy (Ed.), *Classical conditioning*. New York: Appleton, 1965.

Kimble, G. A., & Ost, J. W. P. A conditioned inhibitory process in eyelid conditioning. *Journal of Experimental Psychology*, 1961, **61**, 150–156.

Kimmel, H. D. Amount of conditioning and intensity of conditioned stimulus. *Journal of Experimental Psychology*, 1959, **58**, 283–288.

Kimmel, H. D. The relationship between direction and amount of stimulus change and amount of perceptual disparity response. *Journal of Experimental Psychology*, 1960, **59**, 68–72.

Kimmel, H. D. Inhibition of the unconditioned response in classical conditioning. *Psychological Review*, 1966, **73**, 232–240.

Kimmel, H. D., & Pennypacker, H. S. Conditioned diminution of the unconditioned response as a function of the number of reinforcements. *Journal of Experimental Psychology*, 1962, **64**, 20–23.

Koenig, K. P., & Castillo, D. D. False feedback and longevity of the conditioned GSR during extinction: Some implications for aversion therapy. *Journal of Abnormal Psychology*, 1969, **74**, 505–510.

Lacey, J. I. Psychophysiological approaches to the evaluation of psychotherapeutic process and outcome. In E. A. Rubinstein & M. B. Parloff (Eds.), *Research in psychotherapy*. Washington, D.C.: Amer. Psychol. Assoc., 1959.

Lacey, J. I., & Smith, R. L. Conditioning and generalization of unconscious anxiety. *Science*, 1954, **150**, 1045–1052.

Lacey, J. I., Smith, R. L., & Green, A. Use of conditioned autonomic responses in the study of anxiety. *Psychosomatic Medicine*, 1955, **17**, 208–217.

Lang, P. J., Geer, J., & Hnatiow, M. Semantic generalization of conditioned autonomic responses. *Journal of Experimental Psychology*, 1963, **65**, 552–558.

Levy, C. M., & Murphy, P. H. The effects of alcohol on semantic and phonetographic generalization. *Psychonomic Science*, 1966, **4**, 205–206.

Lipton, L., & Blanton, R. L. The semantic differential and mediated generalization as measures of meaning. *Journal of Experimental Psychology*, 1957, **54**, 431–437.

Lobb, H. Trace GSR conditioning with benzedrine in mentally defective and normal adults. *American Journal of Mental Deficiency*, 1968, **73**, 239–246.

Lockhart, R. A. Temporal conditioning of GSR. *Journal of Experimental Psychology*, 1966, **71**, 438–446.

Lockhart, R. A. Distinguishing component processes reflected in autonomic behavior of human subjects during classical conditioning. Paper presented at Symposium on Higher Nervous Activity of the Collegium Internationale Activitatis Nervosae Superioris, Milan, Italy, October, 1968.

Luria, A. R., & Vinogradova, O. S. An objective investigation of the dynamics of semantic systems. *British Journal of Psychology*, 1959, **50**, 89–105.

Lykken, D. T. A study of anxiety in the sociopathic personality. *Journal of Abnormal and Social Psychology*, 1957, **55**, 6–9.

Lykken, D. T. Preliminary observations concerning the "preception" phenomenon. *Psychophysiological Measurements Newsletter*, 1959, 5, 2–7.

Lykken, D. T. Preception in the rat: Autonomic response to shock as a function of length of warning interval. *Science*, 1962, **137**, 665–666.

Lykken, D. T. Neuropsychology and psychophysiology in personality research. In E. F. Borgatto & W. W. Lambert (Eds.), *Handbook of personality research*. New York: Rand McNally, 1968.

Maltzman, I. Theoretical conceptions of semantic conditioning and generalization. In T. R. Dixon & D. L. Horton (Eds.), *Verbal behavior and general behavior theory*. Englewood Cliffs, New Jersey: Prentice-Hall, 1968.

Maltzman, I. The orienting reflex and thinking as determiners of conditioning and generalization to words. In H. H. Kendler & J. T. Spence (Eds.), *Essays in neobehaviorism*. New York: Appleton, 1971.

Maltzman, I., & Langdon, B. Semantic generalization of the GSR as a function of semantic distance or the orienting reflex. *Journal of Experimental Psychology,* 1969, **80,** 289–294.

Maltzman, I., Langdon, B., & Feeney, D. Semantic generalization without prior conditioning. *Journal of Experimental Psychology,* 1970, **83,** 73–75.

Mandel, I. J., & Bridger, W. H. Interaction between instructions and ISI in conditioning and extinction of the GSR. *Journal of Experimental Psychology,* 1967, **74,** 36–43.

Martin, I. Variations in skin resistance and their relationship to GSR conditioning. *Journal of Mental Science,* 1960, **106,** 281–287.

Martin, I., & Levy, A. B. *The genesis of the classically conditioned response.* New York: Pergamon, 1969.

Martin, R. B, & Dean, S. J. Instrumental modification of the GSR. *Psychophysiology,* 1970, **7,** 178–185.

McAllister, W. R., & McAllister, D. E. Effect of knowledge of conditioning upon eyelid conditioning. *Journal of Experimental Psychology,* 1958, **55,** 579–583.

Mednick, M. T. Mediated generalization and incubation effect as a function of manifest anxiety. *Journal of Abnormal and Social Psychology,* 1957, **55,** 315–321.

Mink, W. D. Semantic generalization as related to word association. *Psychological Reports,* 1963, **12,** 59–67.

Morgenson, D. F., & Martin, I. Personality, awareness and autonomic conditioning. *Psychophysiology,* 1969, **5,** 536–547.

Morrow, M. C. Recovery of conditioned UCR diminution following extinction. *Journal of Experimental Psychology,* 1966, **71,** 883–888.

Morrow, M. C., Boring, F. W., Keough, T. E., & Haesly, R. R. Differential GSR conditioning as a function of age. *Developmental Psychology,* 1969, **1,** 299–302.

Mowrer, O. H. Preparatory set (expectancy)—A determinant in motivation and learning. *Psychological Review,* 1938, **45,** 62–91.

Nicholls, M. F., & Kimble, G. A. Effect of instructions upon eyelid conditioning. *Journal of Experimental Psychology,* 1964, **67,** 400–402.

Norris, E. B., & Grant, D. A. Eyelid conditioning as affected by verbally induced inhibitory set and counter-reinforcement. *American Journal of Psychology,* 1948, **61,** 37–49.

Öhman, A. Factor analytically derived components of orienting, defensive, and conditioned behavior in electrodermal conditioning. *Psychophysiology,* 1972, **9,** 199–209.

Olson, R. K. Generalization to similar and opposite words. *Journal of Experimental Psychology,* 1965, **70,** 328–331.

Osgood, C. E. Comments on professor Bousfield's paper. In C. N. Cofer (Ed.), *Verbal learning and verbal behavior.* New York: McGraw-Hill, 1961.

Pavlov, I. P. *Conditioned reflexes.* London and New York: Oxford Univ. Press, 1927.

Peastrel, A. L. Studies in efficiency: Semantic generalization in schizophrenia. *Journal of Abnormal and Social Psychology,* 1964, **69,** 444–449.

Peastrel, A. L., Wishner, J., & Kaplan, B. E. Set, stress, and efficiency of semantic generalization. *Journal of Experimental Psychology,* 1968, **77,** 116–124.

Peeke, S. C., & Grings, W. W. Magnitude of UCR as a function of variability in the CS-UCS relationship. *Journal of Experimental Psychology,* 1968, **77,** 64–69.

Phillips, L. W. Mediated verbal similarity as a determinant of the generalization of a conditioned GSR. *Journal of Experimental Psychology,* 1958, **55,** 56–61.

Pilgrim, D. L., Miller, F. D., & Cobb, H. V. GSR strength and habituation in normal and nonorganic mentally retarded children. *American Journal of Mental Deficiency,* 1969, **74,** 27–31.

Prescott, J. W. A factor analysis of electrodermal response measures: A study in human conditioning. Unpublished doctoral dissertation, McGill University, 1964.

Proctor, S., & Malloy, T. E. Cognitive control of conditioned emotional responses: An extension of behavior therapy to include the experimental psychology of cognition. *Behavior Therapy,* 1971, **2,** 294–306.

Prokasy, W. G., & Ebel, H. C. Three components of the classically conditioned GSR in human subjects. *Journal of Experimental Psychology,* 1967, **73,** 247–256.

Purhoit, A. P. Personality variables, sex-differences, GSR responsiveness and GSR conditioning. *Journal of Experimental Research on Personality,* 1966, **1,** 166–173.

Rachman, S., & Teasdale, J. D. Aversion therapy: An appraisal. In C. M. Franks (Ed.), *Behavior therapy: Appraisal and status.* New York: McGraw-Hill, 1969.

Raskin, D. C. Semantic conditioning and generalization of autonomic responses. *Journal of Experimental Psychology,* 1969, **79,** 69–76.

Razran, G. A quantitive study of meaning by a conditioned salivary technique (semantic conditioning). *Science,* 1939, **90,** 89–90. (a)

Razran, G. Studies in configural conditioning: 1. History and preliminary experimentation. *Journal of General Psychology,* 1939, **21,** 307–330. (b)

Razran, G. Some psychological factors in the generalization of salivary conditioning to verbal stimuli. *American Journal of Psychology,* 1949, **62,** 247–256.

Razran, G. A direct laboratory comparison of Pavlovian conditioning and traditional associative learning. *Journal of Abnormal and Social Psychology,* 1955, **51,** 649–652. (a)

Razran, G. Conditioning and perception. *Psychological Review,* 1955, **62,** 83–95. (b)

Razran, G. The observable unconscious and the inferable conscious in current Soviet psychophysiology: Interoceptive conditioning, semantic conditioning, and the orienting reflex. *Psychological Review,* 1961, **68,** 81–147.

Razran, G. Empirical codifications and specific theoretical implications of compound-stimulus conditioning: Perception. In W. F. Prokasy (Ed.), *Classical conditioning.* New York: Appleton, 1965.

Razran, G. *Mind in evolution.* Boston: Houghton, 1971.

Rescorla, R. Pavlovian conditioning and its proper control procedures. *Psychological Review,* 1967, **74,** 71–80.

Rescorla, R. Pavlovian conditioned inhibition. *Psychological Bulletin,* 1969, **72,** 77–94.

Riess, B. F. Semantic conditioning involving the galvanic skin reflex. *Journal of Experimental Psychology,* 1940, **26,** 238–240.

Riess, B. F. Genetic changes in semantic conditioning. *Journal of Experimental Psychology,* 1946, **36,** 143–152.

Ross, L. E. Conditioned fear as a function of CS-UCS and probe stimulus intervals. *Journal of Experimental Psychology,* 1961, **61,** 265–273.

Ross, L. E. Cognitive factors in conditioning: The use of masking tasks in eyelid conditioning. In H. H. Kendler & J. T. Spence (Eds.), *Essays in neobehaviorism.* New York: Appleton, 1971.

Runquist, W. N., & Ross, L. E. The relations between physiological measures of emotionality and performance in eyelid conditioning. *Journal of Experimental Psychology,* 1959, **57,** 329–332.

Shean, G. D. Vasomotor conditioning and awareness. *Psychophysiology,* 1968, **5,** 22–30. (a)

Shean, G. D. The relationship between ability to verbalize stimulus contingencies and GSR conditioning. *Journal of Psychosomatic Research,* 1968, **12**, 245–249. (b)

Shmavonian, B. M., Miller, L. H., & Cohen, S. I. Differences among age and sex groups in electro-dermal conditioning. *Psychophysiology,* 1968, **5**, 119–131.

Silver, A. I., & Kimmel, H. D. Resistance to extinction in classical GSR conditioning as a function of acquisition trials beyond peak CR size. *Psychonomic Science,* 1969, **14**, 53.

Silverman, R. E. Eliminating a conditioned GSR by the reduction of experimental anxiety. *Journal of Experimental Psychology,* 1960, **59**, 122–125.

Slubicka, B. Changes in electrodermal responses during classical conditioning and their relationship to personality and awareness. Unpublished doctoral dissertation, University of London, 1971.

Spence, K. W. A theory of emotionally based drive and its relation to performance in simple learning situations. *American Psychologist,* 1958, **13**, 131–141.

Spence, K. W. Anxiety level and performance in eyelid conditioning. *Psychological Bulletin,* 1964, **61**, 129–139.

Spence, K. W. Cognitive and drive factors in the extinction of the conditioned eyeblink in human subjects. *Psychological Review,* 1966, **73**, 445–458.

Spielberger, C. D., & DeNike, L. D. Descriptive behaviorism versus cognitive theory in verbal operant conditioning. *Psychological Review,* 1966, **73**, 306–326.

Stern, R. M., & Lewis, N. L. Ability of actors to control their GSRs and express emotions. *Psychophysiology,* 1968, **4**, 294–299.

Stewart, M. A., Stern, J. A., Winokur, G., & Fredman, S. An analysis of GSR conditioning. *Psychological Review,* 1961, **68**, 60–67.

Stewart, M. A., Winokur, G., Stern, J., Guze, S., Pfeiffer, E., & Hornung, F. Adaptation and conditioning of the galvanic skin response in psychiatric patients. *Journal of Mental Science,* 1959, **105**, 1102–1111.

Streiner, D. L., & Dean, S. J. Expectancy, anxiety and the GSR. *Psychonomic Science,* 1968, **10**, 293–294.

Thomas, D. R., Berman, D. L., Serednesky, G. E., & Lyons, J. Information value and stimulus configuring as factors in conditioned reinforcement. *Journal of Experimental Psychology,* 1968, **76**, 181–189.

Tolman, E. C. Principles of purposive behavior. In S. Koch (Ed.), *Psychology: A study of a science.* Vol. 2. New York: McGraw-Hill, 1959.

Uno, T. The effects of awareness and successive inhibition on interoceptive and exteroceptive conditioning of the galvanic skin response. *Psychophysiology,* 1970, **7**, 27–43.

Vogel, M. D. The relation of personality factors to GSR conditioning of alcoholics: An experimental study. *Canadian Journal of Psychology,* 1960, **14**, 275–280.

Vogel, M. D. GSR conditioning and personality factors in alcoholics and normals. *Journal of Abnormal and Social Psychology,* 1961, **63**, 417–421.

Welch, L., & Kubis, J. Conditioned PGR (psychogalvanic response) in states of pathological anxiety. *Journal of Nervous and Mental Disease,* 1947, **105**, 372–381. (a)

Welch, L., & Kubis, J. The effect of anxiety on the conditioning rate and stability of the PGR. *Journal of Psychology,* 1947, **23**, 83–91. (b)

Wickens, D. D. Conditioning to complex stimuli. *American Psychologist,* 1959, **7**, 180–188.

Wickens, D. D. Compound conditioning in humans and cats. In W. F. Prokasy (Ed.), *Classical conditioning.* New York: Appleton, 1965.

Wickens, D. D., Allen, C. K., & Hill, F. A. Effect of instructions and UCS strength on extinction of the conditioned GSR. *Journal of Experimental Psychology,* 1963, **66**, 235–240.

Wickens, D. D., Born, D. G., & Wickens, C. D. Response strength to a compound conditioned stimulus and its elements as a function of the ISI. *Journal of Comparative and Physiological Psychology,* 1963, **56**, 727–731.

Wickens, D. D., Gelman, R. S., & Sullivan, S. N. The effect of differential onset time on the conditioned response strength to elements of a stimulus complex. *Journal of Experimental Psychology,* 1959, **58**, 85–93.

Wickens, D. D., Nield, A. F., Tuber, D. S., & Wickens, C. D. Classically conditioned compound-element discrimination as a function of length of training, amount of testing and CS-UCS interval. *Learning and Motivation,* 1970, **1**, 95–109.

Wieland, W. F., Stein, M., & Hamilton, C. L. Intensity of the unconditioned stimulus as a factor in conditioning out of awareness. *Psychosomatic Medicine,* 1963, **25**, 124–132.

Wilson, G. D. Reversal of differential GSR conditioning by instructions. *Journal of Experimental Psychology,* 1968, **76**, 491–493.

Woodworth, R. S. *Dynamics of behavior.* New York: Holt, 1958.

Worrall, N. Differential GSR conditioning of true and false decisions. *Journal of Experimental Psychology,* 1970, **86**, 13–19.

CHAPTER 5

Instrumental Conditioning

H. D. KIMMEL

Department of Psychology
University of South Florida
Tampa, Florida

I. Background and Definitions 255
II. Literature Review 258
    A. Reward Conditioning 258
    B. Punishment Conditioning 265
    C. Avoidance Conditioning 266
    D. Discrete-Signaled Reward Conditioning 275
III. Summary and Theoretical Implications 276
    References 280

I. Background and Definitions

The distinction between classical and instrumental conditioning, first explicitly drawn by Miller and Konorski (1928) and later elaborated by Schlosberg (1937) and Skinner (1938), rests largely on what is meant by the term "reinforcement." For Pavlov, who first used the term, reinforcement referred to the presentation of the unconditioned stimulus (UCS) in close temporal contiguity following the conditioned stimulus (CS). In classical conditioning reinforcement is administered independently of the subject's (S's) behavior. It is neither a reward (in classical appetitive conditioning) nor a punishment (in classical aversive conditioning), since in neither case is its delivery in any way contingent upon the occurrence of a conditioned response (CR). In instrumental conditioning, "reinforcement" may refer to the delivery of an appetitive stimulus contingent upon the occurrence of a response (reward), the delivery of an aversive stimulus contingent upon the occurrence of a response (punishment), the delivery of an appetitive stimulus contingent upon the absence of a response (omission), the delivery of an aversive stimulus contingent upon the absence of a response (avoidance), or the termination of an aversive stimulus contingent upon the occurrence of a response (escape). The observed effectiveness of a response-reinforcement contingency in increasing or decreasing the tendency to respond determines whether instrumental reinforcement has, in fact occurred. This circular definition of reinforcement, commonly referred to as the empirical law of effect, has the apparent advantage of avoiding *a priori* commitment to theoretical conceptions regarding the reinforcement process. It has the disadvantage of implying commonality among all forms of instrumental reinforcement, however.

Instrumental conditioning may involve discrete trials which are signaled by a regular CS (as in signaled or "classical" avoidance, escape or straight-alley reward conditioning), or it may involve no regular signal at all (as in free operant or unsignaled, Sidman avoidance conditioning). In discriminative operant conditioning, a continuous signal, referred to as the positive discriminative stimulus (S^D), is present whenever responding is to be reinforced. Its absence, or the continuous presence of the negative discriminative stimulus (S^Δ), identifies a period of nonreinforcement. Although there is a tendency for the word "operant" to be used interchangeably with "instrumental," the latter will be used generically in this chapter to include all conditioning procedures in which an explicit response-reinforcement contingency is operative, while the former will be reserved for those unique instrumental conditioning procedures which have emerged from the work of Skinner (1938) and which normally begin with unelicited responses.

When Miller and Konorski (1928) first attempted to identify the differences between classical and instrumental conditioning (labeled type 1 and type 2 by them), they proposed that responses mediated by the autonomic nervous system are modifiable only by classical but not by instrumental conditioning. Their proposition was based on the belief that autonomic nervous system responses are not instrumental in nature. Although expressing some reservations based upon the observation that children seem to learn to cry "real" tears in relation to their consequences, Skinner (1938) adopted Miller and Konorski's position and even extended it to the point of questioning whether nonautonomic behavior can be modified by classical conditioning. He attempted an exploratory study of instrumental conditioning of digital vasomotor behavior and reported no evidence of success. At about the same time, Mowrer (1938) found negative results in an exploratory study of avoidance conditioning of the skin resistance response (SRR). In the context of this meager evidence, the proposition that autonomic nervous system behavior could not be conditioned instrumentally was accepted almost universally for more than 30 years following Miller and Konorski's original paper, although no systematic empirical evaluation of it was undertaken until about 1958.

It is of more than passing historical interest than this scientific cul de sac was ever seriously entered, considering the fact that Bernard (1859) had long before drawn scientific attention to the significance of the internal environment. What Miller and Konorski (1928) meant by the phase "not instrumental in nature" was that autonomic responses do not ordinarily have any effect upon the external environment, except under very unusual circumstances (e.g., when children cry "real" tears and thereby attain their goals). That these responses may be instrumental in their influence upon the internal environment hardly needs to be pointed out.

Beginning in 1958, a program of research on the instrumental modifiability of autonomically mediated responses was undertaken by the author and his students, at first using the SRR in human Ss. This research endeavor was soon joined by related programs in other laboratories using SRR and skin potential response (SPR) as well as other autonomic nervous system responses with other organisms than humans. In the decade of the 1960s some 80–100 studies of instrumental conditioning of autonomic responses were published, the great majority of which reported positive results. Almost half of these studies involved the electrodermal behavior of humans.

The weight of this empirical evidence has resulted in complete rejection of the earlier erroneous belief that autonomic responses are not instrumentally conditionable. In fact, the dogma pendulum appears to have swung too sharply to the other extreme, with some indications of an equally uncritical acceptance of autonomic responses into the elite domain of the instrumentally modifiable, without any reservations regarding obvious differences between them and skeletal responses (cf. Konorski, 1969).

In subsequent sections of this chapter, the empirical work on instrumental conditioning of electrodermal responses will be reviewed and summarized and significant methodological issues examined. The chapter will conclude with some theoretically based suggestions for future research directions, some of which are now being explored by the author and other investigators in this field.

II. Literature Review

A. *Reward Conditioning*

Ingenuous acceptance of Skinner's (1938) definition of operant behavior as comprising those responses whose occurrence is not preceded by reliable, identifiable stimulation led Kimmel and his associates to attempt to modify the frequency of unelecited (i.e., operant) SRRs by presenting potentially reinforcing events contingent upon their occurrence. An exploratory study (Kimmel & Hill, 1960) used brief pleasant or unpleasant odors as potential reinforcers. Although the results of this study were, at best, suggestive, its procedures uncovered several methodological problems whose solution resulted in improved future research. In order to provide a standard response whose amplitude could be used to establish a criterion for determining when a reinforcable response had occurred, a series of five weak electric shocks were administered before conditioning and one-half of the average amplitude of the SRRs they elicited was taken as the reinforcement criterion for each S during conditioning. The preliminary shocks had the effect of reducing significantly the rate of occurrence of unelicited SRRs (Kimmel & Hill, 1961) as well as greatly attenuating the frequency with which reinforcement could be delivered. Neither the pleasant nor the unpleasant odors had the effect during conditioning of influencing the rate of responding of Ss receiving response-contingent reinforcement as compared with the controls who received the same number of pleasant or unpleasant odors per minute, but at times of nonresponding. At the end of 20 minutes of reinforcement, an extinction session was run, consisting of complete omission of reinforcement. The effect of the response-reinforcement contingency was seen in the fact that the contingent-reinforcement Ss abruptly increased in response rate while the controls decreased. This was true for both types of odor.

Because of the response-suppressing effect of the preliminary shocks, our subsequent studies of reward conditioning did not involve electric shock. Also, since the use of odors required a delay of reinforcement of over 2 sec, and since the pleasant and unpleasant odors appeared to have similar effects, the next study in our laboratory (Fowler & Kimmel, 1962) used as reinforcement a dim white light presented to an S seated in a totally dark room. The duration of the light was precisely controllable and delay of reinforcement was reduced to a negligible amount. The light intensity deliberately was greatly attenutated so that it could be seen only in a dark room. With the preliminary shocks

eliminated, Fowler and Kimmel (1962) measured the amplitude of unelicited responses for 2 min prior to beginning reinforcement and used
one-half of their average amplitude as a reinforcement criterion. Two
response-contingent reinforcement groups were employed, one receiving
the reinforcement for 8 min prior to extinction and the other receiving
it for 16 min. As in the Kimmel and Hill study, control Ss were run
who were matched to response-contingent Ss in the number of lights
received each minute, delivered at times of nonresponding. Figure 1
presents the average relative response frequencies during the reinforcement period.

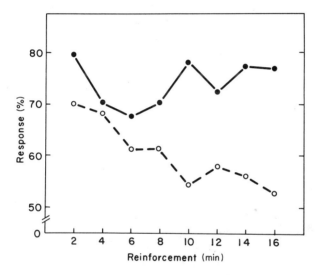

Fig. 1.   Relative frequency of SRR in contingent (●) and noncontingent (○)
groups in 2-min blocks of reinforcement. (From Fowler & Kimmel, 1962.)

Both contingent-reinforcement groups and both groups of controls
showed a reduction in frequency of response for the first 6 min of reinforcement. Thereafter, particularly noticeable in the 16-min contingent-
reinforcement group, response frequency began to increase. The 16-min
controls continued to decline in responding throughout the reinforcement
period. Analysis of the data of only the two 16-min groups indicated
that their divergence in the last several minutes of reinforcement was
significant, as was the difference between their average frequencies of
response during the last 2 min taken separately. In extinction, likewise,
the frequency of response in the contingent groups was significantly
higher than in the controls, especially following 16 min of reinforcement.
The response frequency curves of the contingent and control groups

tended to converge during extinction, with the contingent groups show-ing a reduction in response frequency and the controls showing an increase.

Because the reinforcing stimulus tends to elicit an SRR, both the Kimmel and Hill (1960) and the Fowler and Kimmel (1962) studies employed a 5-sec period of time out from reinforcement following each reinforcement. During this time-out period, responses were neither rein-forced nor counted, since they could not be considered unelicited. In a replication of the Fowler and Kimmel (1962) study (Kimmel & Kim-mel, 1963), the time-out period was shortened to 3 sec because it tends to introduce bias against the controls and because it attenuates the num-ber of possible reinforcements. In addition to reducing the time-out period, the duration of the light reinforcer was reduced from 1.0 to .1 sec and the initial period of nonreinforcement and the extinction period were both increased to 10 min. The initial period was increased because it was suggested by Fowler and Kimmel (1962) that the drop in response frequency during the early part of reinforcement might have resulted from the failure to allow the Ss enough time before conditioning to become acclimated to the experimental situation. Only one response-contingent group was run, receiving 20 min of reinforcement and a nonresponse-contingent control similar to those of the earlier studies was also included. Figure 2 shows the principal findings of this study.

Not only was the difference in relative response frequency between the response-contingent and nonresponse-contingent groups highly sig-nificant, both during acquisition and extinction, the procedure of length-ening the initial operant period to 10 min also had the desired effect of eliminating the previously observed tendency toward an initial decline in responding. The fact that acquisition response frequency is expressed relative to average response frequency during the last 2 min of initial rest accounts for the rather high level of responding shown in Fig. 2, since the Ss drop to a low level of responding by the last 2 min of the initial operant period (this is, of course, also true for the nonre-sponse-contingent controls, so that it in no way reduces the importance of the difference betwen the two groups).

Following the publication of the earliest studies done in our labora-tory, confirmation of their findings was reported by Shapiro, Crider, and Tursky (1964), using SPR rather than SRR as the reinforced re-sponse and reporting measures of heart rate and respiration as well. They reported the results of their study in complete accord with those reported by Fowler and Kimmel (1962) and Kimmel and Kimmel (1963) and, importantly, showed that the electrodermal changes were independent of basal levels of skin potential (SP) and heart rate as well as being unrelated to respiration changes. The use of simultaneously recorded heart rate and respiration by Shapiro *et al.* (1964) was the first published attempt to deal with the possibility that observed changes in electrodermal behavior resulting from response-contingent reinforcement might be an artifactual consequence of instrumental modification of some other response, especially some skeletal response. Their study was important also because it showed that autonomic responses other than those which are reinforced are not necessarily also modified by the reinforcement.

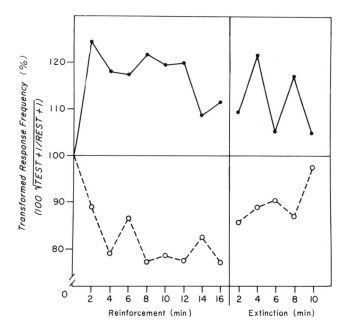

Fig. 2. Relative frequency of SRR in contingent (●) and noncontingent (○) groups, in 2-min blocks of reinforcement and extinction. (From Kimmel & Kimmel, 1963.)

The possibility that skeletal behavior may be influenced by the reinforcement and then serve as a mediator of observed changes in the autonomic response was also examined using the electromyogram (EMG), in subsequent studies by Rice (1966) and Van Twyver and Kimmel (1966). In both studies, the EMG electrodes were placed on the S's arm on the same side of the body as the hand containing the skin electrodes. This site was chosen because it is the most likely source of movement-elicited electrodermal changes in the hand in question.

In the Van Twyver and Kimmel (1966) study, respiration records were also taken during the conditioning session and both respiration rate and frequency of respiration irregularities were reported. When Van Twyver and Kimmel eliminated from consideration all SRRs which occurred in close temporal contiguity to EMG responses or respiration irregularities, the results shown in Fig. 3 were obtained.

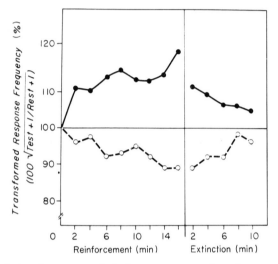

Fig. 3. Relative frequency of SRRs not associated with EMGs or respiration irregularities in contingent (●) and noncontingent (○) groups, in 2-min blocks of reinforcement and extinction. (From Van Twyver & Kimmel, 1966.)

As is indicated in the figure, evidence supporting the instrumental conditionablity of the SRR via reward training was quite pronounced, even under the highly controlled conditions described. Van Twyver and Kimmel (1966) also showed that no differences in any of the other measures were found betwen the two groups of Ss, nor did any of the other measures change systematically during the experimental session.

Also of some importance in these early studies was the gradual realization that the control procedure of delivering reinforcement at times when the S was not making unelicited SRRs was actually, itself, an instrumental conditioning procedure. The data in Figs. 2 and 3 illustrate quite clearly that the nonresponse-contingent controls showed a reduction in responding during conditioning and an increase in responding during extinction. The fact that the response rate increases in extinction, when the nonresponse–reinforcement contingency is removed, establishes that the reduction of responding during conditioning is not merely attributable to a nonassociative decremental process, such as habituation. This phenomenon was actually observable in the data of both the Fowler and Kimmel (1962) and the Kimmel and Kimmel (1963) studies, but its significance was not fully appreciated until the Van Twyver and Kimmel (1966) study was completed. A more appropriate control procedure for comparison with the response-contingent reinforcement procedure would be one in which the reinforcement is delivered totally independently of the control S's responding, although this would entail the possibility of fortuitous response-contingent reinforcement and nonresponse-contingent reinforcement.

In the Rice (1966) study, reinforcement was withheld during conditioning unless the SRR occurred in the absence of an immediately preceding EMG. In addition, Rice divided his Ss into two groups based upon their initial response rates. His high initial responders showed results similar to those found by Van Twyver and Kimmel, i.e., instrumental conditioning of SRR, but his low initial responders failed to show the conditioning effect. It is possible that the elimination of all SRRs that could have been elicited by skeletal responses, in Ss who were low frequency responders to begin with, may have reduced the number of potentially reinforceable responses to a level at which reinforcement is not effective. It is also possible that Ss who make very few unelicited SRRs are not easily conditionable, for reasons presently unknown.

A somewhat different attempt to deal with the question of skeletal mediation was described by Birk, Crider, Shapiro, and Tursky (1966). In this study, one S (Birk) volunteered to be partially curarized, so that bodily movements which could mediate electrodermal changes were greatly reduced. Obviously, for reasons of safety, the S could not be dramatically curarized[1] and artificially respirated. Nevertheless, the S's skeletal behavior was reduced to a minimum (breathing without difficulty was possible and some slight head movement, with difficulty). Instrumental conditioning of SPR was found, as in the earlier studies without curare, and no associated changes in respiration or basal potential occurred. Although only a single S was involved in this study, and complete blockage of the neuromuscular junction could not be employed, its findings surely mitigate against hasty acceptance of the belief that skeletal mediation underlies reported instances of instrumental electrodermal conditioning. Along with the Rice (1966) and Van Twyver and Kimmel

---

[1] Research on subhumans (Miller, 1969) has employed curarization sufficient to block the neuromuscular junction totally and has employed artificial respiration to maintain the animals during curarization.

(1966) studies, this study permitted experimental attention to be shifted to other questions of importance.

While some of the experiments on reward conditioning of the unelicited SRR or SPR have employed stimuli with *a priori* assumed reinforcing properties, such as pleasant odors, pictures of naked women, or lights and sounds which represented monetary rewards, several studies used nothing but a dim light presented to a person seated in a totally dark room. Implicit in the use of a dim white light as a potential reinforcer is the assumption that its delivery in some way is motivationally appropriate, so that its response-contingent delivery results in an increase in the tendency to respond. To be sure, no empirical consideration of this question has appeared until very recently, probably because the investigators in question have been content to define reinforcement completely empirically, in terms of its behavioral consequences. Coffman and Kimmel (1971) attempted to determine experimentally whether the response-contingent presentation of a dim white light to a person seated in the dark has reinforcing effects because the S has been light-deprived or for other reasons. Half of their contingent-reinforcement Ss were seated in a totally dark room and were given response-contingent presentations of a dim white light each time an SRR occurred. The other half of their contingent-reinforcement Ss sat in the experimental room with the dim white light continuously on and were given response-contingent presentations of light-off each time an SRR occurred. Two nonresponse-contingent controls were run, matched to the Ss in the first two groups in number of reinforcements per minute, but receiving them at times of nonresponding. The major finding of this study was that both response-contingent reinforcement groups showed higher response frequencies than their nonresponse-contingent controls, both during acquisition and extinction. Coffman and Kimmel (1971) speculated that the explanation of this result was that interruption of invariant ongoing stimulation occurs when reinforcement is delivered, regardless of whether it consists of light-onset or light-offset, and that this interruption is an adequate stimulus for eliciting an orienting reflex. Examination of SRRs elicited by the light-on and light-off events indicated that they were equally effective stimuli in that respect. It will be recalled that Kimmel and Hill (1960) had found that both pleasant and unpleasant response-contingent odors had similar effects as compared with their nonresponse-contingent controls, possibly for the same reason.

Although the majority of subsequent published work on reward conditioning of unelicited SRR and SPR has reported positive evidence of instrumental conditioning (Coffman & Kimmel, 1971; Crider, Shapiro, & Tursky, 1966; Gavalas, 1967; Greene, 1966; Greene & Nielsen, 1966;

Kimmel & Kimmel, 1967; May & Johnson, 1969; Milstead, 1968; Schwartz & Johnson, 1969; Shapiro & Crider, 1967), a few studies have been reported which do not fully conform to this pattern. In particular, Edelman (1970) found evidence for instrumental maintenance of elevated skin potential (using a light which signaled that one cent was earned as reinforcement) only when the Ss were reinforced for all responses, but not when responses associated with EMGs were nonreinforced. Edelman's Ss, in addition, reported that they believed that skeletal events were responsible for the reinforcement. However, electric shock was employed in this study to attain an initial increase in SP, and there was an observed tendency for deep breathing following the shock. Two other studies have been interpreted as negative (Stern, 1967; Stern, Boles, & Dionis, 1968), although the latter involved differences similar to those found by others but which were attributed to cognitive mediation on the part of the Ss. In the study by Stern (1967), no significant differences were found in support of an instrumental conditioning conclusion, but the experimenter again reported that his Ss were aware of the reinforcement contingency. Neither of the latter two studies involved the degree of situational control which has been characteristic of the positive studies.

B. Punishment Conditioning

The earliest published study using an explicit punishment reponse-reinforcement contingency and electrodermal behavior was done by Senter and Hummel (1965). These researchers used an electric shock to the fingertips to punish unelicited SRRs and reported a decrease in the frequency of this behavior as a consequence of the aversive contingency. Control Ss received the shocks randomly and showed an increase, rather than a decrease, in unelicited SRR frequency. Somewhat similarly, but with more impressive results, Johnson and Schwartz (1967) found that a response-contingent loud sound was effective in suppressing unelicited SRRs, in contrast with the effect of noncontingent sounds. Since Johnson and Schwartz (1967) also measured EMG and found no evidence to support a skeletal-mediation explanation of their SRR results, their study provides strong support for the proposition that a punishment instrumental reinforcement contingency is effective in modifying electrodermal behavior. Further support for this conclusion has been found by May and Johnson (1969), Martin, Dean, and Shean (1968), and by Crider, Schwartz, and Shapiro (1970), in the last case with the SPR as the response measure. In the Crider et al. (1970) study, punishment under continuous reinforcement was effective in

reducing the unelicited SPR by 50% and there was no recovery of responding during extinction. Partial reinforcement produced less dramatic reductions in response rate. Shean (1970) reported that a punishment
contingency resulted in reductions in SRR magnitude, but attributed
these findings to the intermediation of cognitive and skeletal behaviors.
In a study designed for different purposes, Kimmel and Kimmel (1968)
presented a red light contingent upon SRR to one group of Ss while
the Ss in another group could turn off the red light by making SRRs.
Two matched noncontingent control groups were also run in this experiment. The only group that showed an average increase in response frequently was the contingent light-off reinforcement group. In addition,
the Ss whose SRRs were followed by the presentation of the red light
showed the lowest average level of resonding and, during extinction,
did not recover to their original level of response frequency. Kimmel
and Kimmel (1968) interpreted the results of this study by assuming
that the red light was an aversive stimulus to their Ss, so that its onset
was punishing and the oportunity to turn it off by responding was positively reinforcing (i.e., by escape conditioning).

C. Avoidance Conditioning

The earliest experiment with positive results, using an aversive response–reinforcement contingency with an autonomic nervous system
response, was done by Kimmel and Baxter (1964). Two groups of Ss
were employed in this study. The first group received a tone of 1-sec
duration and an electric shock 4 sec after tone offset, unless the S made
an SRR of criterion magnitude during the 4-sec period between the
end of the tone of the shock. The Ss in the other group were run as
classical conditioning yoked controls. They were matched, one S at a
time, to the Ss in the avoidance group, so that they received exactly
the same trial-by-trial pattern of tones and shocks, except the pattern
was in no way contingent upon their behavior. Figure 4 presents the
average SRR magnitudes for the two groups during the conditioning
session.

The avoidance Ss' average SRR magnitude was significantly greater
than that of the yoked classical controls, a result which Kimmel and
Baxter (1964) interpreted to mean that the instrumental avoidance contingency was effective in modifying the magnitude of the SRR of the
avoidance Ss. It must be noted that there is no *a priori* reason to expect
such a difference, even assuming that SRR magnitude is sensitive to
the avoidance contingency. That is, it could have turned out that the
classical procedure employed with the yoked controls was just as effec-

tive as the instrumental procedure used for the avoidance group. If
that had happened, of course, Kimmel and Baxter (1964) would have
been unable to conclude that avoidance conditioning had occurred, since
the performance of the avoidance Ss would not have been differentiable
from that of the classical Ss. The observed superiority of the avoidance
group is, thus, strong support for the conclusion that the instrumental
avoidance procedure was effective.

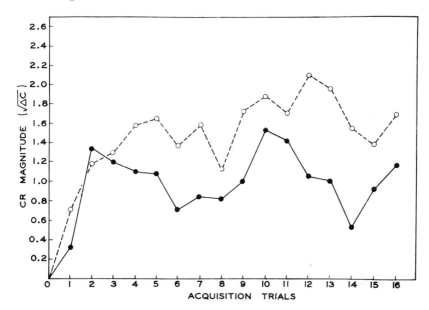

Fig. 4. Average SRR magnitudes of avoidance and yoked control groups during
16 min of conditioning: (●) control; (○) experimental. (From Kimmel & Baxter,
1964.)

As had been noted earlier by Moore and Gormezano (1961), the
superiority of an avoidance group over its yoked classical controls is
not necessarily due to the operation of the law of effect, in the usual
sense. Both groups may be conceptualized as receiving a partial reinforcement, classical conditioning procedure, with the Ss in the avoidance
group receiving the classical UCS only at times when no CR has occurred and the control Ss sometimes receiving it when a response has occurred and sometimes when a response has not occurred. If one may assume
that classically conditioned Ss need the UCS on trials when they have
not made a CR but do not need it on trials when they have made
one, it would follow that the avoidance Ss may be receiving what constitutes a more effective classical conditioning procedure than that which

the controls receive. Although Moore and Gormezano's (1961) novel assumption that the classicaly conditioned S needs the UCS only on trials on which no CR has occurred has not been evaluated in the classical conditioning literature, it is not inconsistent with recent findings that resistance to extinction in classical SRR conditioning is reduced when Ss receive more than a few paired CS–UCS trials (Kimmel, 1970).

One of the reasons why interpretive complications arise in studies such as Kimmel and Baxter's (1964) is that discrete signals, which may serve as classical CSs, mark the occasions for the performance of the avoidance response. The traditional avoidance conditioning procedure involves the same CS and UCS as are used in classical conditioning, with the only difference being the possibility of prevention of the UCS via the performance of an anticipatory CR. Thus, not only is it often possible that a classical conditioning interpretation may be indicated, but, in addition, any response that may be elicited by the signal may be capable of either preventing an instrumental effect from occurring or obscuring its occurrence. It is also possible for such responses to create the false impression that an instrumental effect has occurred, as has been pointed out by Church (1964).

Following the Kimmel & Baxter study, Thysell and Huang (1968) reported an independent replication of their findings, again using SRR. Additional replications with approximately the same results were conducted by Kimmel, Sternthal, and Strub (1966) and by Kimmel and Sternthal (1967). In the latter study, Ss were very carefully matched in initial responsiveness and classical conditionability. The strength of the effect (the relative extent of difference in average SRR magnitude between avoidance and yoked controls groups) found by Kimmel and Sternthal (1967) was substantially smaller than had previously been reported in studies with unmatched Ss in the different conditions. Furthermore, no difference in size of SRR during extinction was found, unlike the results of the Kimmel, Sternthal, and Strub (1966) study. Within-S avoidance conditioning of SRR has been reported by Martin and Dean (1970) and by Martin et al. (1968).

In addition to avoidance conditioning studies involving the magnitude of SRR, there have been some studies using other electrodermal response measures. Shnidman (1969) found that Ss receiving an avoidance conditioning procedure make significantly more SPRs during extinction than do their yoked controls. The Shnidman study appears to be the only one in the literature in which frequency of the SPR is the dependent variable. An earlier study by Grings and Carlin (1966) used frequency and magnitude of SRR and investigated both avoidance and punishment contingencies. In the Grings and Carlin study, a red triangle of 5 sec duration served as the CS; the UCS was electric shock, delivered at the instant of termination of the CS on trials on which the avoidance S failed to respond, or on trials on which the punishment S responded. The Ss were matched in initial responsiveness to the tone before being assigned to the avoidance and punishment (and yoked control) conditions. Grings and Carlin (1966) found that the avoidance Ss made significantly more SRRs than their yoked controls, but this difference was greatest on the first day of conditioning and did not increase thereafter. Peculiarly, the yoked controls' SRRs were significantly larger than those of the avoidance Ss, a finding which conflicts with Kimmel and Baxter's (1964) and Thysell and Huang's (1968) results as well as being seemingly inconsistent with their own difference in frequency between groups in the opposite direction.

Comparison of Grings and Carlin's (1966) experimental procedure with the procedures employed by Kimmel and Baxter (1964) and by Thysell and Huang (1968) reveals that they used a different CS duration than had been used by the others. Their CS remained on for 5 sec on every trial, regardless of whether an avoidance response had been made. Since the avoidance SRR normally occurs with a latency of about 2–3 sec, the optimal procedure for obtaining avoidance conditioning would be to employ response-contingent termination of the CS, on the assumption that the CS has conditioned aversive properties. Kimmel and Baxter (1964) actually employed a response-contingent CS-termination procedure in a pilot study for their published experiment, but decided that CS termination in the yoked controls provides information to the control Ss regarding whether or not shock will be delivered on each trial, introducing a highly complicating factor which probably biases the results in favor of apparent avoidance conditioning.[2] They circumnavigated this problem (as did Thysell & Huang; Kimmel, Sternthal, & Strub; and Kimmel & Sternthal) by using a CS only 1 sec in

[2] The control S may recognize that shock is delivered only on those trials on which the CS is protracted but not on those trials on which the CS is terminated after only 2 or 3 sec. This differentiation may provide a basis for differential responding (i.e., larger responses on long-CS trials than on short-CS trials, which would complicate the interpretation of any observed differences in magnitude of SRR between avoidance and yoked controls) and, possibly, tend to favor the avoidance group. To eliminate this problem, it is necessary to use a very short CS which cannot be terminated by the SRR because it terminates automatically before the SRR can occur. The only differentiation between the avoidance condition and the controls, under the latter condition, would have to be related to the response-avoidance contingency. It is recognized that the short-CS condition is not ideal, either for establishing a classically conditioned SRR or for instrumental reinforcement of an avoidance SRR.

duration, so that its automatic offset always occurred before the SRR avoidance response occurred. Although the exact mechanism is not obvious, it seems reasonable to attribute Grings & Carlin's somewhat paradoxical results to the peculiarities of their nonoptimal avoidance conditioning procedure. Since their frequency data were in accord with an avoidance conditioning interpretation, although weakly, it may be simply that frequency of SRR is more sensitive to the law of effect than is magnitude of SRR. Why the magnitude of SRR was significantly smaller in the avoidance group than in the yoked controls remains to be determined. It is apparent that a reversed difference has greater significance than no difference at all.

The frequency of SRR has also been employed as a dependent variable in unsignaled (Sidman) avoidance conditioning, in an unpublished study done in the author's laboratory.[3] Subjects were given electric shock on a shock–shock interval of 25 sec and could delay the shock for 50 sec by making an unelicited SRR. Following 24 min of this treatment, the S was either extinguished or reversed to response-contingent punishment. Figure 5 shows the data from one S who received Sidman avoidance training with a response-shock interval of 50 sec and then was shifted to punishment. As is indicated in the figure, this S showed a slight tendency toward increased rate of responding near the end of avoidance training and a reduction in response rate when punishment was introduced. These data conform to instrumental conditioning expectations. However, as is shown in Fig. 6, the identical procedure in another S produced essentially negative results, since the rate did not change appropriately during training (other than a slight decline near the end) and no effect of the reversal can be seen. Similarly, as shown in Fig. 7, another S run under the same conditions showed a slight increase in response rate at the beginning of avoidance training, but this effect vanished later in training and there was no change in extinction. It is clear from data of this type that SRR did not yield in any conventional way to unsignaled avoidance conditioning procedures.

As was noted briefly above, Church (1964) has criticized the use of yoked control designs on the grounds that data tending to support the conclusion that avoidance conditioning has occurred may result from systematic bias incorporated within the yoked design itself. His argument is that random differences in responsiveness or classical conditionability, etc., between members of a yoked pair may tend to favor the avoidance S, when he is the more responsive or the better classical conditioner, but should not tend to favor the yoked control in reciprocal fashion,

[3] H. D. Kimmel, and F. R. Terrant, unpublished study.

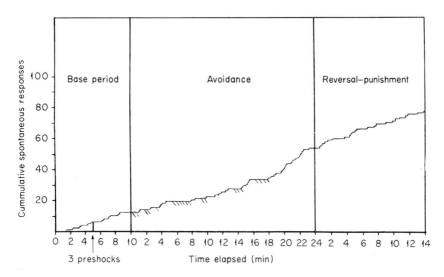

Fig. 5. Cumulative record of SRR during Sidman avoidance and punishment. (From Kimmel & Terrant, unpublished.)

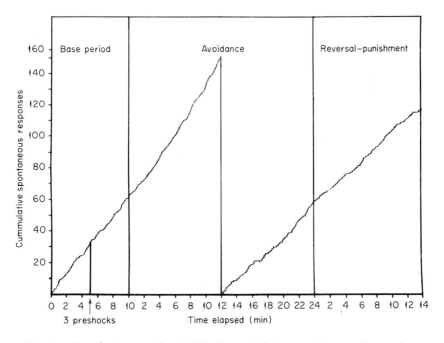

Fig. 6. Cumulative record of SRR during Sidman avoidance and punishment. (From Kimmel & Terrant, unpublished.)

271

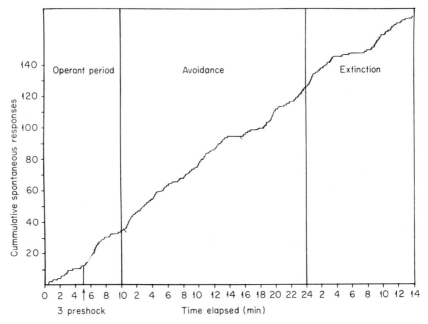

Fig. 7. Cumulative record of SRR during Sidman avoidance and extinction. (From Kimmel & Terrant, unpublished.)

when he is the more responsive or the better classical conditioner. On the basis of his analysis, Church (1964) recommends that either the yoked control design not be used or that it only be used when Ss can be well matched in responsiveness. Although some of Church's assumptions have been seriously questioned (Crider, Schwartz, & Shnidman, 1969), especially in the case of electrodermal behavior, there has been an increasing tendency for some type of matching to be used since his criticism was first published. As was mentioned above, Kimmel and Sternthal (1967) matched their avoidance and yoked control Ss in both SRR responsiveness and classical conditionability, and found that the avoidance Ss' SRRs were only slightly larger than those of the controls during conditioning and that there was no difference whatsoever during extinction.

The possibility exists, however, that preliminary classical conditioning trials, which are necessary to provide a basis for matching Ss in classical conditionability, may interfere with the later acquisition of instrumental avoidance. This was suggested by Kimmel and Sternthal (1967), in discussing their results, but no evidence supporting this conjecture existed at that time. Since then, Solomon and his associates (e.g., Maier,

Seligman, & Solomon, 1969) have described a series of experiments on shuttle-box avoidance in dogs, in which preliminary unavoidable and inescapable shocks, whether signaled or unsignaled, were shown to produce a state referred to as "learned helplessness." Following the development of this condition, the animals do not acquire the avoidance response. On the assumption that human Ss are also (or even more) prone to this type of adjustment to unavoidable and inescapable shock, it may be that effective avoidance conditioning cannot be preceded by classical conditioning trials.

One way to minimize the effect of preliminary classical conditioning trials on subsequent avoidance conditioning would be to follow the classical conditioning trials with classical extinction. Kimmel, Kimmel, and Silver (1969) used this method and conducted the classical conditioning part of their study 2 months prior to the avoidance conditioning part. Nevertheless, they found no difference in magnitude of SRR between avoidance and matched yoked control Ss, either during avoidance acquisition or extinction. Since their Ss showed significant spontaneous recovery of the classically conditioned SRR between the end of extinction in the first session and the beginning of the avoidance session 2 months later, it may be that there is no reasonable way to precede an avoidance conditioning session with preliminary classical conditioning without interfering greatly with the acquisition of avoidance responding.

Further illustration of the possible futility of attempts to attain instrumental reinforcement effects following classical conditioning of the SRR may be seen in a recent study by Kimmel and Lucas (1973). Subjects received classical conditioning trials only to the point of the peak SRR magnitude (about four or five trials) and then were shifted to instrumental secondary reinforcement of the SRR, by means of turning off the CS contingent upon the SRR. No additional UCSs were given following the shift. In addition, controls were run which were yoked in duration of the CS. Another control group received standard extinction with the full 8-sec CS duration. No reliable differences were found in resistance to extinction among the three groups in question, either in average number of trials to reach an extinction criterion or in magnitude of SRR during extinction. In other words, permitting the S to terminate the conditioned aversive stimulus by making an SRR did not result in increased maintenance of the SRR.

A rather different approach to dealing with Church's (1964) criticism of yoked control designs in electrodermal avoidance conditioning was taken by Terrant (1968). Terrant's study is probably the most elaborate investigation of aversive instrumental conditioning of autonomic behavior that has been conducted to date. He used a reciprocal yoked control design (Kimmel & Terrant, 1968) in which two CSs are presented to each S. Within a yoked pair, an avoidance (or punishment) contingency is in effect for one of the CSs for one S, with another S serving as yoked control on that CS. For the other CS, the Ss' roles are reversed. In this way, each S is both an avoidance (or punishment) S and a yoked control. Terrant did four separate experiments. In the first, the reciprocal yoked control design was used to study avoidance conditioning of SRR. In the second, the design was used to study punishment conditioning of SRR. The third study had one S in an avoidance contingency on one CS and the other S is a punishment contingency on the other CS. Each S served as a yoked control for the other S as in the first two studies. In the fourth experiment, one S had an avoidance contingency on one CS and a punishment contingency on the other CS, while the other S was yoked on both CSs.

In Terrant's first experiment, involving 20 yoked pairs of Ss, there was no evidence of an avoidance conditioning effect in the SRR data. The average magnitude of SRR under the avoidance contingency was almost identical to the average magnitude of the SRR in the yoked control condition, and neither condition showed any change in SRR magnitude over 16 conditioning trials. In his second experiment, again involving 20 yoked pairs, there was no difference whatsoever in average SRR magnitude between the punishment and yoked control conditions. However, in this experiment both conditions showed a significant systematic decline in SRR magnitude during conditioning. Only in Terrant's third experiment was there evidence of an intrumental reinforcement effect on the magnitude of the SRR. The data from these 20 pairs of Ss showed a gradual increase in SRR magnitude in the avoidance condition, coupled with a decrease in the avoidance yoked control condition, and a gradual decrease in SRR magnitude in the punishment condition, coupled with an increase in the punishment yoked control condition. However, this apparent instrumental reinforcement effect may have been due to differences in responsiveness between Ss in the two groups, since the significant interaction in question basically involved changes over trials in between-group differences. The 20 pairs of Ss in the fourth experiment, in which the avoidance-punishment comparison was within-S, showed differences which could most parsimoniously be attributed to classical SRR conditioning.

It would appear that no firm conclusion regarding the effectiveness of avoidance conditioning of electrodermal behavior may be stated. Some of the earlier studies indicated that larger and more frequent SRRs and SPRs may result from the avoidance procedure in comparison with yoked controls. However, when Ss are carefully matched in responsiveness and classical conditionability, differences between avoidance and yoked control conditions either vanish or shrink noticeably. Since most of the studies of electrodermal avoidance conditioning have involved discrete trials initiated by a CS, it may be that the response-eliciting capability of the CS introduces complications which either render avoidance conditioning impossible or which obscure whatever conditioning may actually occur. Within-S manipulations, such as those employed in Terrant's (1968) reciprocal yoked control design, may also be more complicating than clarifying. In any case, it seems certain that additional research in this area is needed.

D. Discrete-Signaled Reward Conditioning

Only a few studies have been done in this area, possibly because of the complexities involved when elicited responses are followed by positive reinforcement. The first published study (Kimmel, Pendergrass, & Kimmel, 1967) used candy and verbal reinforcement contingent upon either the occurrence or nonoccurrence of a short-latency SRR elicited by simple geometric visual stimuli. The Ss in this study were mentally retarded and normal children. The children received 30 conditioning trials, consisting of a 3-sec presentation of either a circle, square, or triangle. For half of the Ss a reward procedure was used, so that a short-latency SRR (within 3 sec) resulted in delivery of the candy and verbal reinforcement. For the other half of the S an omission procedure was used in which the reinforcement was delivered only when no SRR occurred during the 3 sec. Immediately following the conditioning session, the S was taken to another room and tested with the Seguin form board, having been tested previously on the form board 3 months earlier. The only condition which resulted in systematic increase in the magnitude of the SRR was the omission condition, when it was applied to the intellectually normal children. The reward procedure did not result in any change in the size of the SRR. Of the eight normal children who received reward conditioning, seven showed improvement in their performance on the Seguin, while one got poorer. On the other hand, of the ten normal children run under the omission contingency, six improved and four got poorer on the form board. Twelve retarded children were run under reward and eleven showed improvement on the form board, while one got poorer. Of the eleven retarded children run with the omission contingency, six showed improvement and five got poorer. Ten additional children who received no conditioning procedure but were tested twice on the form board showed no differential tendency toward improvement or impairment. Thus, even though there was little evidence to support an instrumental conditioning conclusion in the SRR data, the performance on the form board suggested that reinforcement of orienting behavior (in the form of short-latency SRR) may result in better utilization of visual shape cues in perceptual-motor performance.

Shnidman (1970) followed up on the Kimmel *et al.* (1967) study, improving on their methodology by matching Ss based upon initial habituation SPR performance. She found that rewarded orienting responses (SPR) tended to increase in frequency in comparison to SPRs made by a group of yoked controls. Shnidman, however, did not employ an omission procedure in her experiment. Another experiment in which a yoked control procedure was employed in reward training, in this case using SRR amplitude, has been reported by Helmer and Furedy (1968). The contingent reinforcement Ss in this study received five cents each time a nonzero SRR occurred in response to a yellow light. The yoked controls simply received the same reinforcement schedule as the contingent Ss, in noncontingent fashion. Relative SRR amplitude increased for the contingent reinforcement Ss, but remained constant for the yoked controls, again supporting the conclusion that instrumental conditioning occurred. Also, in the only published study using a discriminative operant reward procedure, Defran, Badia, and Lewis (1969) reported that stimulus control of SRR was present during extinction, although it had not been present during training.

III. Summary and Theoretical Implications

In a review of the empirical research on instrumental conditioning of autonomic behavior written by the present author in 1966 (Kimmel, 1967), the hope was expressed that the subsequent few years would provide the theoretical structure which appeared to be required by the growing body of positive evidence. Although, as has been shown in this chapter, a large number of additional studies using electrodermal measures (and several with other responses, not germane to this book) have been added to the positive roster (plus a few on the negative side), no generally acceptable theoretical systematization has yet appeared. As has been mentioned very briefly, a tendency toward uncritical acceptance of autonomic responses into the family of operant behavior may be evidenced by Skinner's generous translation of the original 1928 Miller and Konorski article for publication in the *Journal of Experimental Analysis of Behavior*, along with a solicited up-to-date postscript by Konorski (1969). Are these responses which were not instrumental in nature now presumably subject to the same quality and degree of control via reinforcement as the rat's bar press and the pigeon's peck? Would that the world were that simple!

On the other hand, there are those (e.g., Katkin & Murray, 1968) who cannot conceive of human behavioral change that does not depend upon cognition. For these writers, the instrumental autonomic conditioning results with curarized subhumans are persuasive, but the human studies are corrupted by cognitive mediation. Those who take this theoretical approach become most fervent regarding instrumental conditioning of human electrodermal behavior, since cognitive variables so demonstrably influence the human electrodermal response system. The fact remains, however, that humans cannot generally make electrodermal responses on instruction and, more importantly, they cannot report having made them when they have. There is nothing more informative in this regard than a brief session with skin electrodes on one's own hand and one's own live record before one's eyes.

Self-instructed skeletal behavior (obviously also involving cognitive mediation), which elicits SRRs or SPRs, however, is a ubiquitous possibility that can only be dealt with effectively by means of concomitant EMG measurement. To the extent that this has been done (e.g., Rice, 1966; Van Twyver & Kimmel, 1966), the results indicate that unsignaled reward and punishment of electrodermal responses produce instrumental conditioning effects, but that signaled avoidance and, possibly, signaled reward are not as consistently effective. The subhuman studies using curare (Miller, 1969), powerful as they are, do not completely deal with this problem, since rats and humans may be assumed to differ principally in the domain of cognitively mediated behavior. The one study involving curarization in humans (Birk et al., 1966) is reassuring but only a beginning.

Some writers (Black, 1967; Konorski, 1967) are not satisfied even that curarization (even in subhuman studies) completely eliminates the problem of skeletal mediation. While these theorists differ regarding specific details, both have suggested that mediation of autonomic responding via the central nervous system may occur, even if the peripheral neuroeffector junction is totally blocked by curarization. There is no a priori reason why such a proposition may not be true, but its acceptance would surely require more than armchair speculation. After all, elimination of overt skeletal behavior by curarization also eliminates proprioception from skeletal action. It is difficult to imagine how skeletal behavior, itself, could be modifiable instrumentally without its own proprioceptive feedback available to the central nervous system.

Konorski's (1967) position on this question bears some scrutiny, both because it exemplifies for behavioral psychologists the logical difficulties associated with mediational models and because it seems to fit some of the results summarized in this chapter. In particular, he suggests that only those responses can be instrumentalized which are mediated by what he refers to as the "central behavioral system." These are responses which "are performed by the organism itself and are not forced upon it, as is the case with passive movements or movements elicited by stimulation of efferent pathways [Konorski, 1967, p. 479]." Forty years of difficult scientific work and we are still ensnared in the web of voluntarism! What is the difference between a response which the organism performs by itself and one which is elicited by some antecedent stimulus? And, in any case, even if Konorski wishes to isolate passive movements and efferently stimulated responses, he still is left with internally elicited (not efferently) autonomic responses and internally elicited skeletal responses under a common rubric.

It becomes necessary for Konorski to segregate still another type of instrumentalizable act, that which takes its origin from a particular unconditioned reflex, such as scratching, licking the anus, or yawning. This category also includes most if not all autonomically mediated responses. These differ from responses of the central behavioral system because the stimulus that elicits them is concurrent with the drive state-reinforcement process resulting in instrumental conditioning. Accordingly, the drive state becomes associated with the eliciting stimulus and becomes capable of activating appropriate sensory units on future occasions. "Thus, it may be assumed that the animal starts to perform the (formerly elicited) motor response because he 'feels' the stimulus provoking that response although this stimulus is no longer administered [Konorski, 1967, p. 482]." Konorski leaves no doubt that he is writing about instrumental autonomic conditioning in this discussion, and that he is suggesting that the S must experience an image or hallucination of the eliciting stimulus. There is little evidence from extensive postexperimental interviews with human Ss who have served in instrumental autonomic conditioning experiments that imagined or hallucinated stimuli are responsible for eliciting their autonomic responses, although some authors have reported that movements are sometimes implicated.

As Skinner correctly noted (1938), the identification of operants as reponses which occur in the absence of identifiable eliciting stimulation should not be taken to imply that no antecedent elicitors exist. What was important about operants, to Skinner, was the fact that their rate of occurrence could be influenced by their consequences. That this influence of their consequences on their rate of occurrences might depend upon the manner of their elicitation was not a matter of importance to him, nor was the possibility even explicitly mentioned. Now that we have abundant empirical data that show that autonomic responses are amenable to instrumental reinforcement, at least under certain circumstances, it becomes important to determine exactly what those circumstances actually may be.

Electrodermal behavior (along with some of the other peripheral autonomic responses) lends itself most readily to experimental examination of the role of eliciting events in instrumental autonomic conditioning, since the SRR and SPR are, at once, highly reliable components of the orienting reaction to novel stimuli and spontaneous potential operants. As elicited components of the orienting reaction, SRR and SPR are easily habituated and transformed into classical CRs under conditions of regular CS–UCS pairing. Unelicited SRRs, on the other hand probably do not habituate as readily (Greene & Kimmel, 1966), especially when they are initially of low amplitude. The reason for this possible difference in habituability (Kimmel, 1973) may be that unelicited SRRs are actually elicited by highly variable antecedent stimuli while elicited SRRs are usually defined in the context of great regularity of antecedent stimulation. Kimble and Ray (1965) have demonstrated that the wiping reflex of the frog, elicited by tactile stimulation with a von Frey bristle, habituates under repetitive stimulation only when the bristle is applied to the same precise spot on each presentation. When the location of application of the tactile stimulus is varied from trial to trial, the reflex shows sensitization rather than habituation. If the habituability of autonomic responses, specifically electrodermal responses, varies as a function of the degree of variability of eliciting stimulation, it may also be possible that their habituability is a determiner of whether or not, and to what degree, autonomic responses are classically or instrumentally conditionable. In other words, regular elicitation of an autonomic response by a consistent antecedent stimulus, as in the classical conditioning paradigm, may provide the perfect condition for habituation of the autonomic response and its replacement by an anticipatory CR based upon the response to the UCS. On the other hand, under highly variable antecedent stimulus circumstances, as in free operant autonomic conditioning, the habituability of the autonomic response may be greatly reduced or even eliminated, in which case the reinforcement could result in instrumental rather than classical conditioning.

For instrumental conditioning of SRR and SPR, the foregoing would suggest that unsignaled reward and punishment would be more promising than signalled reward, punishment, or avoidance. In a general way, the data appear to conform to this expectation, but there are specific exceptions which cannot be overlooked (e.g., Grings & Carlin, 1966; Shnidman, 1970). Nevertheless, the most consistent positive results have been obtained under unsignaled conditions and the most frequent negative results under signaled conditions. In spite of the incompatibility of some of the data with the foregoing generalization, it is possible that further research done in its explicit context might result in clarification of the present inconsistencies.

Acknowledgments

Done under USPHS Grant MH-16839. Ms. Joan Snyder assisted the author in compiling the bibliography.

References

Bernard, C. *Leçons sur les propriétés physiologiques et les alterations pathologique des liquides de l'organisme*. Paris: Balliere, 1859.

Birk, L., Crider, A., Shapiro, D., & Tursky, B. Operant electrodermal conditioning under partial curarization. *Journal of Comparative and Physiological Psychology*, 1966, **62**, 165–166.

Black, A. H. *"Operant Conditioning of Heart Rate under Curare"* Technical report #12. McMaster University, October 1967.

Church, R. M. Systematic effect of random error in the yoked control design. *Psychological Bulletin*, 1964, **62**, 122–131.

Coffman, M., & Kimmel, H. D. Instrumental conditioning of the GSR: a comparison of light deprivation and monotony hypotheses. *Journal of Experimental Psychology*, 1971, **89**, 410–413.

Crider, A., Schwartz, G. E., & Shapiro, D. Operant suppression of electrodermal response rate as a function of punishment schedule. *Journal of Experimental Psychology*, 1970, **83**, 333–334.

Crider, A., Schwartz, G., & Shnidman, S. On the criteria for Instrumental Autonomic Conditioning: A reply to Katkin and Murray. *Psychological Bulletin*, 1969, **71**, 455–461.

Crider, A., Shapiro, D., & Tursky, B. Reinforcement of spontaneous electrodermal activity. *Journal of Comparative and Physiological Psychology*, 1966, **61**, 20–27.

Defran, R. H., Badia, P., & Lewis, P. Stimulus control over operant galvanic skin responses. *Psychophysiology*, 1969, **6**, 101–106.

Edelman, R. I. Effects of differential afferent feedback on instrumental GSR conditioning. *Journal of Psychology*, 1970, **74**, 3–14.

Fowler, R. L., & Kimmel, H. D. Operant conditioning of the GSR. *Journal of Experimental Psychology*, 1962, **63**, 563–567.

Gavalas, R. J. Operant reinforcement of an autonomic response: Two studies. *Journal of Experimental Analysis of Behavior*, 1967, **10**, 119–130.

Greene, W. A. Operant conditioning of the GSR using partial reinforcement. *Psychological Reports*, 1966, **19**, 571–578.

Greene, W. A., & Kimmel, H. D. Habituation of large and small GSRs. *Psychological Reports*, 1966, **19**, 587–591.

Greene, W. A., & Nielsen, T. C. Operant GSR conditioning of high and low autonomic perceivers. *Psychonomic Science*, 1966, **6**, 359–360.

Grings, W. W., & Carlin, T. Instrumental modification of autonomic behavior. *Psychological Record*, 1966, **16**, 153–159.

Helmer, J. E., & Furedy, J. J. Operant conditioning of GSR amplitude. *Journal of Experimental Psychology*, 1968, **78**, 463–467.

Johnson, H. J., & Schwartz, G. E. Suppression of GSR activity through operant reinforcement. *Journal of Experimental Psychology*, 1967, **75**, 307–312.

Katkin, E. S., & Murray, E. N. Instrumental conditioning of autonomically mediated behavior: Theoretical and methodological issues. *Psychological Bulletin*, 1968, **70**, 52–68.

Kimble, D. P., & Ray, R. S. Reflex habituation and potentiation in *Rana pipiens*. *Animal Behavior*, 1965, **13**, 530–533.

Kimmel, H. D. Instrumental conditioning of autonomically mediated behavior. *Psychological Bulletin*, 1967, **67**, 337–345.

Kimmel, H. D. Essential events in the acquisition of classical conditioning. *Conditional Reflex*, 1970, **5**, 156–164.

Kimmel, H. D. Habituation, habituability, and conditioning. In H. V. S. Peeke & M. J. Herz (Eds.), *Habituation*. Vol. 1, *Behavioral Studies*. New York: Academic Press, 1973.

Kimmel, H. D., & Baxter, R. Avoidance conditioning of the GSR. *Journal of Experimental Psychology*, 1964, **68**, 482–485.

Kimmel, H. D., & Hill, F. A. Operant conditioning of the GSR. *Psychological Reports*, 1960, **7**, 555–562.

Kimmel, H. D., & Hill, F. A. Two electrodermal measures of response to stress. *Journal of Comparative and Physiological Psychology*, 1961, **94**, 395–397.

Kimmel, E., & Kimmel, H. D. A replication of operant conditioning of the GSR. *Journal of Experimental Psychology*, 1963, **65**, 212–213.

Kimmel, E., & Kimmel, H. D. Instrumental conditioning of the GSR: Serendipitous escape and punishment training. *Journal of Experimental Psychology*, 1968, **77**, 48–51.

Kimmel, H. D., & Kimmel, E. Intereffector influences in instrumental autonomic conditioning. *Psychonomic Science*, 1967, **9**, 191–192.

Kimmel, H. D., & Lucas, M. E. Attempted maintenance of the classically conditioned GSR via response-contingent termination of the CS. *Journal of Experimental Psychology*, 1973, **97**, 278–280.

Kimmel, H. D., & Sternthal, H. S. Replication of GSR avoidance conditioning with concomitant EMG measurement and subjects matched in responsivity and conditionability. *Journal of Experimental Psychology*, 1967, **74**, 144–146.

Kimmel, H. D., & Terrant, F. R. Bias due to individual differences in yoked control designs. *Behavior Research Methods and Instrumentation*, 1968, **1**, 11–14.

Kimmel, H. D., Kimmel, E., & Silver, A. I. The effect of UCS intensity in classical and avoidance GSR conditioning. *Conditional Reflex*, 1969, **4**, 32–51.

Kimmel, H. D., Pendergrass, V. E., & Kimmel, E. Modifying children's orienting reactions instrumentally. *Conditional Reflex*, 1967, **2**, 227–235.

Kimmel, H. D., Sternthal, H. S., & Strub, H. Two replications of avoidance conditioning of the GSR. *Journal of Experimental Psychology*, 1966, **72**, 151–152.

Konorski, J. *Integrative activity of the brain*. Chicago, Illinois: Univ. of Chicago Press, 1967.

Konorski, J. On a particular type of conditioned reflex. *Journal of Experimental Analysis of Behavior*, 1969, **12**, 187–189.

Maier, S. F., Seligman, M. E. P., & Solomon, R. L. Pavlovian fear conditioning and learned helplessness. In B. A. Campbell, & R. M. Church (Eds.), *Punishment and aversive control.* New York: Appleton, 1969.

Martin, R. B., & Dean, S. J. Instrumental modification of the GSR. *Psychophysiology,* 1970, 7, 178–185.

Martin, R. B., Dean, S. J., & Shean, F. Selective attention and instrumental modification of the GSR. *Psychophysiology,* 1968, 4, 460–467.

May, J. R., & Johnson, H. J. Positive reinforcement and suppression of spontaneous GSR activity. *Journal of Experimental Psychology,* 1969, 80, 193–195.

Miller, N. E. Learning of visceral and glandular responses. *Science,* 1969, 163, 434–445.

Miller, S., & Konorski, J. Sur une forme particulière des réflexes conditionels. *Comptes Rendues Société Biologique Paris,* 1928, 99, 1155–1177.

Milstead, J. R. Operant GSR conditioning using a within-S design. *Psychonomic Science,* 1968, 13, 215–216.

Moore, J. W., & Gormezano, I. Yoked comparisons of instrumental and classical eyelid conditioning. *Journal of Experimental Psychology,* 1961, 62, 552–559.

Mowrer, O. H. Preparatory set (expectancy)—a determinant in motivation and learning. *Psychological Review,* 1938, 45, 61–91.

Rice, D. G. Operant conditioning and associated electromyogram responses. *Journal of Experimental Psychology,* 1966, 71, 908–912.

Schlosberg, H. The relationship between success and the laws of conditioning. *Psychological Review,* 1937, 44, 379–394.

Schwartz, G. E., & Johnson, H. J. Affective visual stimuli as operant reinforcers of the GSR. *Journal of Experimental Psychology,* 1969, 80, 28–32.

Senter, R. J., & Hummel, W. F., Jr. Suppression of an autonomic response through operant conditioning. *Psychological Record,* 1965, 15, 1–5.

Shapiro, D., & Crider, A. Operant electrodermal conditioning under multiple schedules of reinforcement. *Psychophysiology,* 1967, 4, 168–175.

Shapiro, D., Crider, A. B., & Tursky, B. Differentiation of an autonomic response through operant reinforcement. *Psychonomic Science,* 1964, 1, 147–148.

Shean, G. D. Instrumental modification of the galvanic skin response: Conditioning or control? *Journal of Psychosomatic Research,* 1970, 14, 155–160.

Shnidman, S. R. Avoidance conditioning of skin potential responses. *Psychophysiology,* 1969, 6, 38–44.

Shnidman, S. R. Instrumental conditioning of orienting responses using positive reinforcement. *Journal of Experimental Psychology,* 1970, 83, 491–494.

Skinner, B. F. *The behavior of organisms.* New York: Appleton, 1938.

Stern, R. M. Operant conditioning of spontaneous GSRs: Negative results. *Journal of Experimental Psychology,* 1967, 75, 128–130.

Stern, R. M., Boles, J., & Dionis, J. Operant conditioning of spontaneous GSRs: two unsuccessful attempts, *Technical Report No. 13.* Office of Naval Research, Indiana University, 1968.

Terrant, F. R. Effects of instrumental avoidance and punishment contingencies on the conditioned and unconditioned GSR. Unpublished Ph.D. dissertation, Ohio University, 1968.

Thysell, R. V., & Huang, C. Avoidance conditioning of the GSR. *Journal of Experimental Psychology,* 1968, 78, 534–535.

Van Twyver, H. B., & Kimmel, H. D. Operant conditioning of the GSR with concomitant measurement of two somatic variables. *Journal of Experimental Psychology,* 1966, 72, 841–846.

CHAPTER 6

Personality and Psychopathology

JOHN A. STERN

Department of Psychology
Washington University
St. Louis, Missouri

CYNTHIA L. JANES

Department of Child Psychiatry
Washington University School of Medicine
St. Louis, Missouri

I.	Introduction	284
II.	Schizophrenia	284
	A. Resting Level of Skin Conductance, Admittance, or Potential	285
	B. Nonspecific Responses	288
	C. Response to Stimulation	288
	D. Conditionability	293
III.	Depression	295
	A. Tonic Measures	295
	B. Responsivity	296
	C. Habituation	297
	D. Conditioning	298
IV.	Psychopathy	299
	A. Resting Level of Skin Conductance	299
	B. Response to Stimulation	300
V.	Mental Retardation	301
	A. Resting Levels	302
	B. Nonspecific Responses	304
	C. Responsiveness	305
	D. Habituation	313
	E. Conditioning	314
VI.	Central Nervous System Damage	316
VII.	Anxiety	322
	A. Normal Subjects	323
	B. General Psychiatric Population	328
	C. Anxiety States	330
VIII.	Introversion–Extroversion	333
	References	337

283

I. Introduction

Previous publications from our laboratory have reviewed the literature relating psychophysiological measures to personality variables (Stern & McDonald, 1965) and have more recently reveiwed the problems of clinical psychology that have been assessed with the use of psychophysiological techniques (Stern & Plapp, 1969). This chapter hopes to deal in some depth with only one physiological measure—electrodermal activity—as it relates to highly selected aspects of personality functioning and/or psychopathology. The specific areas of personality functioning or malfunctioning chosen for discussion here should be considered representative of this area, rather than constituting an exhaustive review of the field. Both time constraints as well as the interests of the authors determined the specific areas selected. We have attempted to obtain some breadth of coverage by sampling the major psychiatric "diseases," organic conditions, as well as neurotic disturbances. We further have attempted to liven up our review not only by being critical of the research reported, but by occasionally engaging in flights of fancy with respect to what we believe may be desirable lines of research that should be pursued.

II. Schizophrenia

Research involving electrodermal activity as related to schizophrenia has had a long and by no means consistent history. Part of the problem, of course, is in the definition of schizophrenia; another confounding variable is the armamentarium of drugs that have been made available for "managing" some of the symptoms of schizophrenia, and, of course, always the problem of the effect of various techniques for measuring the phenomena under investigation. This problem has been recognized for a long time, but little has been done to solve it. Though Paintal (1951) compounded the problem by lumping all psychiatric patients together, rather than grouping them by even crude diagnostic groups, the opening paragraph to his paper is still worth quoting:

> Several investigations have been made on psychiatric patients by the electrodermal method. However, entire agreement between any two workers does not exist. For instance, Peterson and Jung (1897) found normal reactions, McCowan greater, while Ödegaard (1932) and Syz and Kinder (1931) found diminished responses. Such differences in conclu-

sions are in some measure due to variations in stimulus and techniques used [p. 425].

A. Resting Level of Skin Conductance, Admittance, or Potential

Though the methodologically sophisticated reader may wince slightly at the jumbling together of the above measures and abstracting and interpreting them in terms of "arousal" or alertness, we find it both convenient and hopefully instructive to do so. Arousal, within the context of this exposition, should be read as electrodermal measure of arousal since such measures of arousal correlate far from perfectly with other measures of arousal, such as electroencephalograph (EEG), heart rate (HR), etc. As a matter of fact, it is not unusual for system A to demonstrate marked arousal, while system B demonstrates marked quiescence (Lacey, 1967)

We would further like to point out that arousal as measured from different aspects of activity in the same physiological response system may not give identical information. Thus, arousal as measured by resting level of skin conductance and arousal as measured by nonspecific electrodermal responses are not always found to be highly correlated (Zahn, Rosenthal, & Lawlor, 1968).

We will subdivide our discussion of this measure into (1) studies which are concerned only with measures of resting levels at a given point in time and (2) studies which esentially evaluate such resting levels at various points in time where this time period is one in which subjects are also stimulated in a variety of ways (habituation, conditioning, relaxation, etc.) and (3) studies utilizing nonspecific responses as the measure of arousal.

Table 1 presents a listing of studies in which resting levels of electrodermal measures are identified. As is obvious, if one looks at a representative sample of the literature, one can find higher values, lower values, or no difference in resting levels of electrodermal activity. One possible reason for these differences is well documented in the studies by Bernstein (1969). This author finds that the variables of drugs and degree of confusion (apathetic, uncommunicative, disoriented, disorganized) are important factors to be taken into consideration. Thus patients who are not confused and free of phenothiazines are more aroused than control subjects, while confused patients medicated with phenothiazines are less aroused than control subjects. Patients who are confused and not on phenothiazines and patients who are clear and on phenothiazines manifest levels of arousal comparable to that of the control group.

Goldstein and Acker (1967) come to a similar conclusion with respect to the relationship between skin resistance level (SRL) and severity of pathology (as measured by responses to a word association test). Increasing levels of thought disturbance were found to be associated with decreasing levels of arousal.

TABLE 1

Resting level Lower "arousal" (higher resistance)	Higher "arousal" (lower resistance)	Equal "arousal" (no difference)
	Ax *et al.* (1970)	Bernal and Miller, 1971 (child)
Crooks and McNulty (1966)	Burdick (1968)	Paintal (1951)
Goldstein, I. (1965)	Bernstein (clear patterns) (1969)	Bernstein (confused patterns) (1969)
Howe (1958)	Wenger (1966)	Bernstein (clear patterns on drugs) (1969)
Williams, M. (1953)	Zahn *et al.* (1969)	Goldstein and Acker (1967)—low or moderate thought disturbance
Bernstein—(confused patterns on drugs) (1969)		Taylor (1971)
Goldstein and Acker high thought disturbance (1967)		
Fenz and Velner (1970)		
Fenz and Steffy (1968)		
Pfister (1938)		
Venables (1964)		

Zahn *et al.* (1968) utilized a group of drug-free chronic schizophrenic patients; the parameter of confusion was not identified in this study. Zahn evaluated skin conductance level (SCL) on two occasions separated by 1–3 weeks. On the first occasion he saw marked differences in SCL between his control and patient group; on second testing this difference was markedly attenuated though on both occasions his schizophrenic group was significantly more aroused than his control group. This suggests that heightened arousal in schizophrenics may be situationally determined rather than being characteristic of the illness(es). It is quite possible that novel, strange, and perhaps threatening situations may have a more arousing effect on hospitalized schizophrenics for whom even slight changes in routine (if they have been hospitalized for a long period of time) may be out of the ordinary. Similarly, acutely ill schizophrenic patients may be threatened by all aspects of the hospital situations. Normal control subjects, on the other hand, who cognitively know what is going on and who have no reason not to trust the experimenters are much less aroused by the experimental situation. Fenz and Steffy (1968) related a measure of social responsiveness (minimal social behavior scale) and one of psychoticism (psychotic reaction profile) to SCL at time of initiation of an intensive behavioral treatment program for patients, sometime during treatment, and again a year after the first measurement. They found higher SCL to be positively correlated with amount of appropriate social behavior. Socially responsive subjects also were more responsive to the task demands of their experimental situation by demonstrating increases in SCL during the period of a laboratory experiment while socially nonresponsive subjects demonstrated decreases in SCL. With respect to their measures of psychoticism, significant correlations were obtained between SCL and paranoid belligerence ($\rho + .44$), withdrawal ($\rho - .52$), and thought disorder ($\rho - .64$).

With respect to changes in SCL over the 1-year period, it was found that normal subjects demonstrated a significant drop in SCL over the three sessions while the psychotic group demonstrated a significant increase in SCL from the first to the third session. This increase is attributed to the behavioral intervention program which made the patients more responsive to environmental inputs.

Venables (1963) has demonstrated that "withdrawn" schizophrenics are more highly aroused than "active" schizophrenics as measured by skin potential level (SPL). Thus behavioral withdrawal may well be associated with considerable autonomic turmoil. This discrepancy between behavior and physiology is not unique to schizophrenia. Patients suffering from psychotic depressions are behaviorally lethargic and suffer from psychomotor retardation: Yet, when one measures muscle activity (EMG), they are found to be hyperactive (Whatmore & Ellis, 1959); or if one observes their eyelids, they demonstrate significantly more eyelid tremulousness than is true of either normal subjects or patients with other diagnoses—including schizophrenia (Schwarz & Stern, 1968).

Howe (1958) reported not only that his schizophrenic group had a significantly higher SRL than either an anxious or a control group, but what may be equally important, that the within-group variability of skin resistance in his schizophrenic group was significantly larger than that of the control or an anxious group. (The latter group demonstrated significantly less variability than the control group). What is important here, of course, is an answer to the question of whether this variability is only a function of the group or whether such variability is in part accounted for by a high within-individual variability. It has been suggested that schizophrenics have greater within-subject variability on a variety of measures. Unfortunately, few data are available with respect to SRL. Fenz and Steffy correlated resting levels across three points in time, the first and third measures separated by 1 year. The correlations between sessions were as follows: 1 and 2, .50; 1 and 3, .77; and 2 and 3, .47. These correlations were all significant beyond the .01 level. They are, however, considerably lower than the correlation obtained by Corah and Stern (1963) for children in which comparisons were made of SRL on two successive days. The correlation here was .86.

B. Nonspecific Responses

The literature with respect to nonspecific responses (spontaneous fluctuations), though not as large as that on resting levels, is equally inconsistent with respect to whether schizophrenics produce more or fewer such responses. Thayer and Silber (1971) and Bernal and Miller (1971) found no significant differences in such responses betwen schizophrenics and controls. Fenz and Velner (1970) report fewer such responses in both reactive and process schizophrenics when compared to normals, and Zahn, et al. (1968) and Pugh (1968) obtained significantly more such responses in a schizophrenic population.

Bernstein (1969) utilized two variables to divide his population of schizophrenics into subgroups. The first of these was medication; the patient either was (D), or was not medicated with phenothiazines (ND). The second was based on Montrose Rating Scale evaluations (MRS). Patients were divided into two groups, those high (MRSH) and those low (MRSL) on the MRS, the lower the rating the more serious the degree of impairment. Bernstein thus ended up with four subgroups, namely, D, MRSH; ND, MRSH; D, MRSL; and ND, MRSL. For the non-drug low MRS group he reports an increase in nonspecific responses over the course of the experiment, high MRS demonstrated an inconsistent pattern over time, while control subjects demonstrated a decrease over time. The effect of phenothiazines was to decrease the slope (rate of change) of the response over time for the low MRS patient group.

C. Response to Stimulation

Table 2 presents data on studies which have compared responsiveness to relatively innocuous as well as noxious stimuli in schizophrenic as compared to control populations. Simplified tables such as the above are both instructive and confusing since they cannot take into consideration other dimensions which may be important in determining whether schizophrenics are more or less responsive than controls. The data in our table suggest, in general, that schizophrenics either are less responsive or do not differ in responsiveness from controls. Let us briefly discuss a few of these dimensions.

TABLE 2

Response to innocuous stimuli and habituation	Response to noxious stimulation
More responsive	*More responsive*
Goldstein *et al.* (1969): good premorbid versus poor premorbid	Ax *et al.* (1970)
Zahn *et al.* (1968)	Lykken and Maley (1968)
Ax *et al.* (1970)	
Mednick and Schulsinger (1968)	
Equally responsive	*Equally responsive*
Fenz and Velner (1970): reactive-inconsistent	
Fuhrer and Baer (1970)	
Howe (1958)	
Spohn *et al.* (1970)	
Taylor, J. (1971)	
Thayer and Silber (1971)	
Less responsive	*Less responsive*
Ax *et al.* (1970)	Astrup (1966)
Bernal (1971)	Howe (1958)
Dmitriev *et al.* (1968)	Paintal (1951): *threat* of shock
Fenz and Velner (1970): process schizophrenia	Pugh (1968): effect of drug
Wyatt and Grinspoon (1969)	
Bernstein (1970): dependence on stimulus intensity and confusion level (1969)	
Smith (1968)	

1. STIMULUS INTENSITY

Two sets of studies have concerned themselves with the problem of stimulus intensity. The first are those by Bernstein (1969) who utilized three intensities of auditory stimuli (90, 75, 60 dB) and demonstrated that confused schizophrenics as compared to both clear schizophrenics and controls were less responsive to low-intensity tones (60 and 75 dB) while with a 90-dB tone they responded very much like normals. The lower level of responsiveness was evaluated both by comparing the number of subjects who did or did not respond to the first trial of stimulation at each of the intensities used as well as by rapidity of habituation. With the habituation to criterion measure (number of trials to two or three consecutive no responses) he found that both of his schizophrenic groups habituated more rapidly than the control group.

Zahn *et al.* (1968) arrive at essentially diametrically opposed conclusions. They report their results as demonstrating that the weaker the stimulus intensity, the greater the autonomic responsiveness of schizophrenic patients. They further find that with the intensities of stimulation utilized (300-Hz, 72-dB tone and a 15-W light) there was significantly *slower* habituation for their schizophrenic subjects. With respect to the response for first trial of stimulation their results for tone stimulation accord with Bernstein's in that significantly fewer schizophrenics than normals responded.

2.   DEFINITION OF CONCEPT OF HABITUATION

The slower habituation for the schizophrenic subjects of Zahn *et al.* (1968) at first blush appears to be inconsistent with the above conclusion. Their measure of habituation, however, was somewhat different from Bernstein's in that they counted all ORs made to a fixed number of stimuli rather than counting number of responses to a criterion of habituation. This distinction appears to be important since Zahn *et al.* report that their schizophrenic group was characterized by an erratic pattern of responding. We suspect that if they had utilized Bernstein's criteria for the assessment of habituation, then results might not have been as discrepant as they appear. Our suspicion is that they would have found more rapid habituation for their schizophrenic group. This would be comparable to Bernstein's results. However, an additional finding of importance might have been observed, namely, that schizophrenics manifest more disinhibition of habituation when compared to control groups. Disinhibition of habituation is manifested by the number of orienting responses, usually randomly distributed with respect to time of occurrence, that are obtained once a criterion of habituation is met. Thus, defining habituation in terms of number of trials to criterion, as compared to defining it in terms of number of responses produced over a fixed number of trials, may well lead to different results. Though there are reports in the literature that these two measures of habituation are highly correlated, that generalization, based on studies of college students, is probably not applicable to schizophrenic patients.

3.   PHARMACOLOGICAL AGENT

There is no question that psychoactive agents such as tranquilizers exert effects not only on patient behavior but on psychophysiological responses as well. Thus, in evaluating the research literature, one needs to take into consideration the question of whether patients are on or off medication. If off, the question is, how long has it been since they were taken off medication. Traces of many psychoactive drugs can be found in the blood as long as a month after treatment termination. Acute withdrawal produces behavioral side effects such as feelings of nervousness or jitteriness which undoubtedly affect physiological responsiveness (Lykken & Maley, 1968). Thus studies in which patients have been drug-free for 24 hr cannot be compared to those in which patients have been drug-free for weeks or months.

What effect do phenothiazines, one of the common classes of tranquilizers prescribed for patients with schizophrenia, have on electrodermal responses? Astrup (1966) reports that chlorpromazine produces marked inhibition of unconditional responses with less inhibition of responses to conditional signals. Goldstein, Judd, Rodnick, and LaPolla (1969) report that phenothiazines reduce arousal in most schizophrenics as measured by increases in skin resistance. In response to a startling stimulus, however, these authors report no significant drug effects. Pugh (1968) reports that phenothiazines produce increases in SRL, a decrease in nonspecific SRRs, decrease in amplitude of response to unpleasant stimuli, and no change in amplitude of response to neutral stimuli. Spohn, Thetford, and Woodham (1970) report that phenothiazines increase SRL, with amount of increase proportional to drug dosage. Bernstein (1969) reports that phenothiazines do not significantly affect incidence of phasic ORs. Tonic levels are, however, markedly affected by these drugs; like others, Bernstein reports higher levels of skin resistance in drug-treated patients. Parsons and Chandler (1969) report no significant differences between controls and schizophrenics at the beginning of an experiment. The schizophrenic group, however, demonstrated a consistent trend toward lower skin conductance levels during the experiment. To recapitulate, most authors report higher resting levels of skin resistance in patients treated with tranquilizers. The effect of these drugs on response to both innocuous as well as noxious stimuli, in general, is a depression or no change of responsiveness.

4. Diagnostic Subgroups

A variety of groupings of schizophrenics are utilized in the studies reviewed. Some studies classify them on the basis of responses to rather specific instruments, such as the Montrose Rating Scale (Bernstein, 1969) which classifies patients with respect to degree of confusion, chronicity (as measured by number of years of continuous hospitalization), process or reactive (Phillips scale), and conventional clinical groupings (paranoid, hebephrenic, simple, affective, etc.). Bernstein (1969) reports that confused patients are less responsive than clear patients. A number of authors report differences in responsiveness between paranoid and non-paranoid schizophrenics, all finding the paranoid group to be more responsive than other groups (Lykken & Maley, 1968; Stern, Surphlis & Koff, 1965; Venables, 1964). Similarly, reactive schizophrenics behave more like normal subjects than is true of chronically ill schizophrenics patients.

Dmitriev, Belyakova, Bondarenko, and Nikolaev (1968) report that orienting and defensive response alteration are dependent on "stages" of the psychosis. They discriminate between "early," "critical," and "terminal" stages of schizophrenia, and report that inhibition of orienting responses begins in the early stages of the psychosis and gradually increases as a function of severity of the disturbance. Defensive reflexes were not affected in autonomic response measures.

Thus type of schizophrenic disturbances (reactive versus functional; paranoid versus nonparanoid), duration of illness, contact with reality, are all important attributes which affect electrodermal responsiveness measures.

5. Response Measure

A number of different attributes of responses to stimulation can be measured. These are (1) latency of response, i.e., time from stimulus onset to response onset, (2) amplitude of response, (3) time to peak, (4) recovery, i.e., time to return to basal level. Most studies to date have concerned themselves principally with amplitude of responses. A few have focused on other characteristics of the response. Mednick and Schulsinger (1968) have utilized information from the recovery limb portion of the electrodermal response to discriminate between children with high risk for developing schizophrenia and a control sample. The high risk group not only produced greater amplitude responses to stimulation, but also demonstrated faster recovery of the response. Mednick's recovery measure was rate of change or slope. Ax and Bamford (1970) utilized both the Mednick and Schulsinger measure of recovery as well as one more recently devised by Edelberg (1970). Edelberg measures the time it takes for the response to return to a level midway between the peak and resting amplitudes, and identifies this as recovery *time* while the Mednick measure deals with recovery *rate*. Ax and Bamford (1970) report significant differences ($p < .01$) between schizophrenics and controls on the recovery time measure both for response to warning signals (OR) and in responding to a noxious shock stimulus. They evaluated the Mednick measure and found it to be significantly correlated with response amplitude, while the relationship between response amplitude and recovery time was not found to be significant. They thus conclude that, "The rate of recovery measure as used by Mednick worked fine on his data because his high risk group also had much larger GSRs so that in effect, his rate of recovery measure combined both the amplitude and more rapid recovery effects into one index, which probably accounts for this 'rate index' being the best criterion group discriminator [p. 147]."

We suspect that future researchers will pay more attention to the recovery time measure than has been true in the past.

D. Conditionability

The literature on conditionability of electrodermal phenomena in schizophrenia is as confused and confounded as the literature on electrodermal conditioning in general. The interested reader is referred to a chapter by Stern (1972) in the *Handbook of Psychophysiology*, for his critique of the classical conditioning of electrodermal response(s) literature. We would only like to point out here that one cannot talk of "the" conditional electrodermal response even in the simplest type of classical conditioning paradigm. A number of responses are conditionable, including the orienting response to the CS, a response in anticipation of the UCS, and a response which may occur when the UCS is omitted. Unfortunately, the conditioning literature in the area of schizophrenia, and until recently in the literature on conditioning, did not discriminate between these various responses. Thus the lack of replicability of classical conditioning studies in schizophrenia is readily rationalized.

What is generally reported in the classical conditioning of electrodermal responses is that most such responses are affected by cognitive factors. If the subject can figure out, or is told the contingencies between the CS and the UCS, conditioning occurs; where he remains naive about the contingencies, conditioning does not occur. Baer and Fuhrer (1969) and Fuhrer and Baer (1970) have convincingly demonstrated this in a differential conditioning paradigm, utilizing a delay conditioning procedure (8-sec interval between CS and UCS) in which the unconditioned electrodermal response was mediated by having the subject perform a reaction time task. In the Baer and Fuhrer study, subjects were allowed to figure out for themselves the contingency between the CS+ and the UCS. Twelve out of 22 normals and 3 out of 22 schizophrenics were able, at termination of the experiment, to verbalize their awareness of which CS was followed by the UCS. In the normal group significant SCR conditioning was found, while no conditioning occurred in the patient group.

In the Fuhrer and Baer (1970) study both normals and schizophrenics were informed of the CS–UCS contingencies by the use of "exhortative instructions." Good conditioning of both the orienting (first interval) and the anticipatory (second interval) response was obtained in both normals and schizophrenics. They summarize their results as follows:

> Results of the present study do not substantiate the alternative interpretation that schizophrenics failed to condition because of deficient electrodermal reactivity or impairments in the excitatory and inhibitory mechanisms that underlie the differential conditioning process. Instead, the present results indicate clearly that schizophrenics can be differentially conditioned with a non-aversive UCS when they have knowledge of the stimulus relations [p. 484].

These authors did, however, find that their third interval response (response to the omission of the UCS on nonreinforced trials) discriminated between their normal and schizophrenic samples with the normal group demonstrating better differentiation. It could not be determined from their report whether this differentiation was based on the development of greater amplitude responses to the CS+ over conditioning trials or the inhibition of responding to the CS- stimulus.

We doubt that all conditional electrodermal responses can be accounted for on the basis of cognitive factors, though much of the evidence supports this conclusion. As reviewed in Section V, there are data by Lockhart and Grings (1964) which indicate that some conditional responses may not be subject to this restriction. Specifically these authors report the development of ED conditional responses in the absence of cognition for their MR group. Conversely, Fuhrer and Baer's study presents data that cognition can occur in the absence of conditioning; namely, the third interval response (response at latency of the UCR on nonreinforced trials) discriminates between their two groups of subjects. Thus, though cognition was controlled for by having all subjects well aware of the contingencies of stimulation, the control sample demonstrated significantly better differentiation (differential responding to CS+ and CS-) than the patient group.

A study by Pishkin and Hershiser (1963) demonstrates some other problems one needs to be concerned with in the conditioning of schizophrenics. One of these is the response to the UCS. Astrup, as well as these authors, point out that schizophrenics are less responsive to noxious stimulation, and that they demonstrate more habituation to such stimuli than is true of normal subjects. It would appear not unreasonable to assume that if the UCS is unable to elicit a response, then the likelihood of conditioning would be rather small. Sokolov (1963) has also demonstrated that if there is no response to the CS, presumably as a function of prior habituation, then conditioning also is not likely to occur.

III. Depression

Comparison of investigations of depression as related to electrodermal activity is rendered infeasible at the outset by two unfortunate facts regarding the classification of depression. First, the rather amorphous pie called depression can be divided in a number of equally appealing ways; and second, we have at our disposal an arsenal of diagnostic knives with which to slice the pie. With reference to the first point, depressions have been categorized along the following dimensions (Beck, 1967; Lader & Wing, 1969): (1) etiological (endogenous versus exogenous factors), (2) responsivity to external environment (autonomous versus reactive), (3) degree of activity (agitated versus retarded), (4) age of patient (adolescent, involutional, and senile), and (5) pattern of symptoms (psychotic versus neurotic). A number of methods are in use by which individuals are placed in the above categories, both singly and in combination (Stern, McClure, & Costello, 1970). Some labels obviously require only demographic information, such as age of the individual. Others utilize historical and/or current data. Historical data may be obtained through case history material or self-report. Self-reported historical data is extracted from psychiatric interview and/or questionnaires. Sources of current information are results of psychological test batteries, psychiatric interviews, and questionnaires.

The abundance of categories and classification methods reflects the inability of any given diagnostic labeling procedure to neatly compartmentalize depressed individuals. In an effort to improve diagnosis, some investigators have attempted to relate psychophysiological factors with depression. Unhappily, results of these studies, discussed below, lack comparability because of the nonuniformity of diagnostic schemes employed.

A. Tonic Measures

Depression ratings, both clinical and self-report, have been correlated with both SCL and spontaneous activity, in a psychiatric, as well as a normal population (Zuckerman, Persky, & Curtis, 1968). The psychiatric population in this study was made up not only of patients classified as depressed but of other diagnostic groups as well. For the patient group, these authors found nonsignificant correlations between SCL and depression ratings, while significant correlations were found for normals. A second tonic measure, number of spontaneous fluctuations per minute, was positively correlated with depression among the psychiatric, but not the normal population. Thus, the two measures of tonic activity were not in agreement.

A second study examining the relationship between tonic electrodermal activity and depression is that of Lader and Wing (1969). They approached the problem differently than the Zuckerman group. Rather than looking at depression in normals and a general psychiatric population, Lader and Wing compared normals with two groups of depressed patients: agitated and retarded. Skin conductance level (SCL), whether taken at the beginning or end of the experimental session, differentiated the three groups. It was higher for the agitated depression group than for normals, and higher for normals than for retarded depressives. Parallel results were reported for spontaneous fluctuations, with agitated depressives having the greatest number, followed by normals, and then retarded depressives. These authors thus demonstrated that within the dimension of tonic electrodermal activity, depression is not a unitary phenomenon. The more relevant variable was degree of agitation within the depression category.

B. Responsivity

Essentially two questions have been posed with respect to the relationship between responsiveness and depression. First, does the depression of psychiatrically depressed patients extend to their electrodermal responding? Second, are scores on depression scales related to electrodermal responsiveness?

The answer to the first of these questions is that responding of depressed patients may be reduced. That these individuals are capable of at least some electrodermal responding has been shown by Alexander (1959), who reports that all but one depressed patient responded to a shock stimulus which he termed "sufficiently strong to be felt as an alarming signal but not unbearably painful [p. 157]." Furthermore, most responded to tones. Alexander did not specify the intensity of the tones. Unfortunately, no statistical analyses comparing their responses to those of normal subjects were presented. Evidence that responses are attenuated for depressed patients has been presented by Lader and Wing (1969). They found that response magnitude to the first of a series of tones was greater for normal subjects than for either agitated or retarded depressed patients. Incidentally, comparison of agitated depressed with retarded depressed patients in total number of skin resistance responses (SRRs), showed more responding in the agitated group. For this responsiveness measure, no comparison of depressed and normal subjects was made.

The question of the relationship between scores on depression scales and electrodermal responsiveness has received the attention of a few investigators. Greenfield, Katz, Alexander, and Roessler (1963) present results that might be construed as evidence of a negative relationship between these variables. They compared "high" and "low" skin resistance responders on MMPI depression ratings. For this analysis, data from psychiatric patients were pooled with those of normals. Those whose MMPI scores indicated less depression had greater responses than those with more depression. Even more interesting is the finding that psychiatric status (patient versus control) and responsiveness were *not* related. It may be concluded that the more responsive subjects were the less depressed, but not necessarily the mentally healthier. Other studies have correlated depression ratings with responsiveness. Conductance changes during cold-pressor stress were correlated with depression ratings of both a general psychiatric population and a normal population by Zuckerman *et al.* (1968). Although uncorrelated for normals, the two variables were nonsignificantly but positively correlated for the general psychiatric group. Using a depressed subject group, Dureman and Saaren-Seppälä (1963) found degree of depression unrelated to responses to both white noise bursts and visual stimuli.

C. Habituation

Two analyses in the Lader and Wing (1969) study may be regarded as indices of habituation. Their subjects received 20 1-sec presentations of a 1000-Hz, 100-dB tone, at 45–80-sec random intervals. During the presentation of these tones SCL changed differentially for the groups studied. Skin conductance levels for normal subjects, uncomplicated depressives, and retarded depressives diminished, while those of agitated depressives increased. A second habituation measure was slope of the regression of response magnitude over trials, corrected for initial response magnitude. According to this criterion, normal subjects habituated faster than agitated depressives. Slopes for retarded depressives were not calculated, since they gave so few responses.

Basset and Ashby (1954) looked at habituation within the context of a study whose purpose was to determine the effect of electroconvulsive therapy (EST) on electrodermal activity. Change in log resistance to stimuli and threat of stimuli for patients receiving therapy did not habituate over a 5-week period, while untreated patients and normal controls did show habituation. However, when patients were later divided into those who recovered and those who did not recover, regardless of therapy, it was found that the skin resistance measure was more closely related to the recovery dimension than to whether they had received EST or not. Patients who later recovered failed to habituate. It was therefore suggested that skin resistance activity might predict recovery in depressed patients. Results not inconsistent with these have been presented by Bagg and Crookes (1966) who looked at palmar sweating in depressed women patients before and after recovery from depression. Increased sweating prior to recovery may underlie the greater skin resistance activity noted above (Bassett & Ashby, 1954).

D. Conditioning

The evidence with regard to conditioning among depressed patients is scant, and each study has approached the question in a different way.

Conditioning of manic-depressives has been compared to that of other psychiatric diagnostic groups by Stewart, Winokur, Stern, Guze, Pfeiffer, and Hornung (1959). Results depended upon conditioning measures. Analysis of anticipatory responses during conditioning showed greater conditioning for manic-depressive than for personality disorder subjects, and no difference between manic-depressives and schizophrenics or anxiety neurotics. When the measure was anticipatory responses during extinction, manic-depressives did not differ from the other groups. Finally, what may be considered as responses to shock in the absence of shock during extinction showed more responding among manic-depressives than for either anxiety neurotics or personality disorder patients, but not schizophrenics. Normal subjects were not included in this study.

Within a population of depressed subjects, the correlational analysis of Dureman and Saaren-Seppälä (1963) indicated that clinical rating of depression was not related to conditionability. The same was found for self-ratings of depression, except at the highest US (white noise) intensity. Conditioning (CR/UR) at this intensity was greater for the more depressed patients.

A study comparing differential conditioning of depressed patients with that of normals has been reported by Alexander (1959), who unfortunately includes no significance tests. According to him, CRs were greatly reduced among depressive patients. In fact, four of five of the most severely depressed patients gave no CRs. Alexander also reports that CRs for depressed patients frequently were very delayed, while responses to US were normal. Drug administration had differential effects on the groups of subjects. For depressives, meprobamate enhanced CRs and improved differentiation between the reinforced and nonreinforced tones. The same drug reduced CRs of normal and anxious patients. A second drug, benactyzine, increased CRs, but to both tones, and did this not only for depressed patients, but for all subject groups.

IV. Psychopathy

A number of studies have evaluated electrodermal measures in psychopaths. The questions usually asked deal only with the problem of what measures, under what conditions, differentiate psychopaths from nonpsychopaths. Psychopathy is variously defined, ranging from performance of college students on the MMPI, to discriminating between groups in prisons. Generally, three prison groups can be identified, namely, psychopathic criminals, nonpsychopathic criminals, and a mixed group.

A. Resting Level of Skin Conductance

Most students report either no significant differences in resting levels of skin conductance, or a significantly lower level on this variable. No studies have reported higher levels of skin conductance in psychopaths as compared to normals. No significant differences were found by Fox and Lippert (1963), Goldstein (1965), Hare and Quinn (1971), Lindner (1942) and Lippert and Senter (1966). Lower resting levels of skin conductance were obtained by Hare (1965a, 1968), and Lykken (1957). In a series of studies by Hare (1965a, b, 1968), consistently lower levels of skin conductance are reported for the psychopathic as compared to control subjects. The fact that subjects were required to relax for 15 min prior to initiation of recording might account for these differences. Unfortunately, the Fox and Lippert study also utilized a 15-min prerecording test period, so this rationalization to account for these differences has to be discarded.

With respect to nonspecific responses, Fox and Lippert (1963) report significantly fewer such responses for their psychopathic group. Hare and Quinn (1971) report no significant differences between a psychopathic and control group, but a significant interaction effect produced by psychopathic subjects demonstrating a decrease in such responses over time (conditioning trials) and control subjects showing an increase in nonspecific responses. Similar results are reported by Lippert and

Senter (1966). Psychopaths demonstrated a decline in nonspecific responses over time, while their control group did not demonstrate such a decline.

B. *Response to Stimulation*

The literature appears to be reasonably consistent in reporting no differences in orienting responses to simple stimuli between psychopathic and control groups; Borkovec (1970) reports smaller orienting responses only to the first of a series of 21 tone stimuli. Hare (1968) found no difference between groups to tone stimulation. In response to a noxious stimulus, Lindner (1942), Hare (1965a, b), and Goldstein (1965) all report that shock or a noxious noise produces responses indistinguishable from these of control subjects. Only Hare and Quinn (1971) report a smaller amplitude response to shock in their psychopathic group.

The one situation in which reasonably consistent differences are reported deals with the anticipation of a noxious stimulus. Hare (1965a, b, 1968), Hare and Quinn (1971), Lykken (1957), and Lippert and Senter (1966) report that psychopaths demonstrate lower amplitude anticipatory responses. The only discordant note comes from Sutker (1970). His experimental procedure was, however, sufficiently different from that of the other authors quoted above and thus is not really comparable to the other studies.

A variety of hypotheses have been generated to account for these results. It has been suggested that psychopaths are less aroused than normals and therefore condition more poorly. It has also been suggested that in line with their behavioral deficits their ability to anticipate punishment, noxious stimuli, or to develop conditioned fear responses is impaired. The basis for such impairment has been attributed, as might be expected, to genetic and environmental variables (loss of father, parental rejection, erratic discipline, etc.), as well as permutations and combinations of these. It should, however, be remembered that this consistency of response is true only of electrodermal responses. Heart rate, the other physiological variable frequently measured, does not show the same effect. Thus, speculations relating the electrodermal responses of psychopaths to psychological states such as anxiety, ability to plan, arousal, etc., should be viewed with extreme caution and two grains of salt. In spite of these admonitions, we will engage in some speculations about where research on electrodermal responses in psychopaths might be directed.

It seems to us that what is needed are prospective studies, or at least retrospective studies which do not have to dig so far back in time to come up with possible reasons for psychopathic behavior.

The consistent findings that psychopaths do not generate anticipatory electrodermal responses in expectation of being stimulated with a noxious agent deserves further exploration with respect to validating and extending this research. What extension do we suggest? Let us assume that the development of such anticipatory responses is related to the psychopath's inability to profit from his past experiences in real-life situations. Let us further assume that this ability is not something we are born with but which develops as a function of maturation, and life experiences. A first question then might be the identification of the time in the organism's life when he begins to demonstrate this ability as measured by the development of anticipatory electrodermal responses. Having identified the critical period for the development of such responses, one could then shift to a search for critical events which have to transpire during this period in order for the child to form such anticipatory responses.

The evidence on the lack of development of anticipatory responses to date has been limited to studies in which the UCS was an aversive stimulus. Is it possible that if the UCS were a rewarding rather than an aversive stimulus the psychopath might demonstrate adequate anticipatory responses? Bits and pieces of the behavioral literature suggest that the psychopath responds behaviorally more adequately to rewarding stimulus situations. Is this behavioral attribute also reflected in electrodermal anticipatory responses? One might thus also answer the question of the relationship between some behavioral and some physiological responses.

V. Mental Retardation

The defining characteristic of mentally retarded (MR) persons, of course, is their relatively low IQ, which reflects deficiency in relatively complex learning and problem-solving abilities. In order to examine simpler kinds of learning, a number of studies have investigated autonomic nervous system functioning. The assumption is that autonomic nervous system conditioning represents a lower level of learning, since the responses are controlled largely by that portion of the nervous system responsible for vegetative functions, and therefore these responses are presumably not under conscious control. These studies have attempted to look at arousal levels, arousability or reactivity, and learning, in measures of autonomic nervous system activity. In light of the retardate's difficulty with cognitive functioning, one might expect him to demonstrate lower arousal levels, attenuated responsiveness, and poorer conditioning. All of these would reflect general autonomic nervous system sluggishness.

In the review that follows, a distinction will be made, whenever possible, between those mentally retarded individuals for whom there is no apparent organic involvement and those in whom organic involvement has been diagnosed. In general, more severe retardation usually involves neurological impairment.

A. Resting Levels

Studies dealing with electrodermal measures and mental retardation have sought to determine whether arousal level, as measured by tonic electrodermal levels, discriminate mentally defective individuals from normals. A review article by Karrer (1966) concludes that the finding of higher skin conductance levels (SCLs) among MRs is well documented. He mentions only one study, that of Collman (1959), that reported opposite findings (i.e., MRs had lower SCLs than normal Ss). Studies published subsequent to the Karrer (1966) review do not wholly support the contention that MRs show lower SCLs than normals. A tally of the studies of SCLs of MRs and normals published over the past 15 years indicated the following: three found MRs more aroused than normals (O'Connor & Venables, 1956; Ellis & Sloan, 1958; Karrer & Clausen, 1964), two found MRs less activated than normals (Collman, 1959; Fenz & McCabe, 1971), two studies reported no significant difference in arousal levels of MRs as compared to those of normals (Lobb, 1968; Clausen & Karrer, 1970), one study obtained mixed results (Berkson, Hermelin, & O'Connor, 1961), and in one results were contradictory (Galkowski, Dadas, & Domanski, 1968). One study (Karrer & Clausen, 1964) used brain-damaged subjects exclusively; the remaining studies sometimes included Ss with signs of brain damage, although in general attempts were made to exclude such Ss. Clearly, the fairest summary statement of the above results is that they are inconsistent, but that the trend is in the direction of no difference in SCLs of normals and MRs. If it is assumed that sampling errors are not responsible for these discrepant results, how can they be explained?

Analysis of the methodologies and techniques employed in these studies may provide explanations for the variety of results obtained. At the outset, let us rule out differences due to stimuli used. Although most of the investigations included measurement of responses to specific stimuli, resting levels were measured prior to stimulation onset. Thus, even though each study employed different stimuli, the resting levels could not have been affected by this difference. Instead, variations in experimental procedure prior to the stimulus period are of interest here.

Among these, perhaps the most relevant is the orientation of S to the laboratory setting, including attempts made to ensure S's optimal relaxation. The correlation between resting electrodermal levels and arousal has been well documented (Lader & Wing, 1966), but it is not clear whether the two variables are causally related, and if so, which precedes the other. Nevertheless, resting levels can be affected specifically by relaxation instructions (Katz, 1971), as well as more generally by S's perception of the experimental situation. The methods sections of the papers dealing with resting electrodermal levels do not provide sufficient information to determine extent of relaxation procedures, so we remain uncertain about the effect of this variable upon resting electrodermal measures. However, it may be significant that of the four studies reporting higher SCLs among MRs, only one specifies that steps were taken to ensure S's relaxation (Karrer & Clausen, 1964).[1] The amount of relaxation achieved in this study, though, is subject to question. Subjects were required to lie on a cot, motionless, with eyes closed, and electrodes in place, for 20–25 min. Those who had difficulty keeping their eyes closed were blindfolded. One might question whether these would be the most effective conditions for relaxation of children. This doubt is reinforced by the authors' report that some of the MRs became so restless that scorable polygraph records could not be obtained.

One other study in this group (Ellis & Sloan, 1958) states simply that "S was told to relax," while both of the two remaining papers (O'Connor & Venables, 1956; and Galkowski et al., 1968) give no information regarding relaxation techniques. All studies among those failing to find that MRs had higher SCLs than normals make reference to attempts to relax Ss and/or acquaint them with the experimental situation (Clausen & Karrer, 1970; Collman, 1959; Galkowski et al., 1968; Fenz & McCabe, 1971; Lobb, 1968).

Another variable of significance in determining SCLs is the time between electrode application and recording of resting levels. Skin conductance level typically drops considerably within the first 10 min following electrode application. If fear of the laboratory situation is greatest at the onset of the experimental session, and more prevalent among MRs, who may demonstrate more situational anxiety than normals, one would expect SCL differences between the two groups to be maximal

---

[1] It must be remembered that MR Ss in this study were brain damaged, and for this reason caution should be used when comparing these results to those of studies using non-brain-damaged Ss.

at the beginning of the session. Studies concluding that SCLs of MRs were greater than those of controls apparently used shorter adaptation periods than did the remaining investigations. Again, because of the incompleteness of methodologies reported for many studies, a firm statement regarding this as a source of the differences in results between studies is not possible. One exception to this tentative rule is the study of Karrer and Clausen (1964). Rather than being unusually short, their adaptation period of 20–25 min may have been overly long, especially for MRs. The authors' statement that MRs were frequently restless during the relaxation period lends support to this notion.

Perhaps maximal comfort for all Ss could be ensured by the utilization of a 10–15-min period following electrode applications, coupled with reassurance by E regarding the experimental procedure. Under these conditions, relatively accurate measures of resting SCLs could be obtained. This procedure would allow a clearer evaluation of intrinsic physiological characteristics of MRs, because of reduction in contamination due to S's apprehension of the situation. Thus, the suggestion by Karrer (1966), based on the results of some of the above studies, that a higher level of sympathetic activity is found among MRs, seems premature. Instead, the MRs' heightened SCLs may reflect initial fear and apprehension. Of course, if apprehension or anxiety are the dependent variables, no attempt should be made to reduce them.

B. Nonspecific Responses

Like resting SCL, the measure of spontaneous fluctuations is thought by some to index activation level. The results with respect to spontaneous activity (SA) are consistent with those for SCLs; they are highly equivocal. Thus, Karrer and Clausen (1964) report that significantly more MRs than controls showed no spontaneous responses. Somewhat different, but not inconsistent results are reported by Collman (1959), who suggests less SA among retarded and bright Ss than among their normal and dull Ss. Though the author provides no statistical analysis to support this conclusion, he fortunately presents the relevant data. Utilizing a simple χ^2 test one can conclude that the frequencies do not differ among groups. The study by Das and Bower (1971) is unique in showing greater instances of SA among retardates as compared to normals. Unfortunately, their spontaneous fluctuations included some responses that would be considered by others as stimulus-specific. Although six different stimulus words were presented to their Ss, responses to only two were counted as specific responses. All other responses were "spontaneous fluctuations."

Thus the data on spontaneous electrodermal activity provide us with the same kind of mixture we observed for resting SCLs. If these measures are considered as two indices of arousal, we conclude that at the present time, it would not be possible to make a strong case for either greater or lesser arousal among MRs.

C. Responsiveness

If hyporeactivity is a characteristic of mental retardation, then it might be hypothesized that this would be reflected in electrodermal responding. Responsiveness may be assessed in terms of response frequency or size. Furthermore, sluggishness in responding can be measured by examining response latency and duration.

1. RESPONSE FREQUENCY

A survey of studies dealing with frequency of responding as a function of IQ level indicates that MR subjects may indeed be less responsive than subjects of normal intelligence. Evidence that frequency of responding is greater among normals than among MRs has been presented by Lobb (1970), who measured SRR frequency during the habituation phase of a conditioning study. The stimulus was a 3000-Hz, 1-sec tone, 70 dB at each ear. Response criteria were maximum deflection within 5 sec after stimulus onset that exceeded by 100 Ω the maximum deflection in the 5 sec preceding stimulus onset. Results consistent with the above were reported by Karrer and Clausen (1964), who determined by means of a χ^2 analysis that there were significantly more nonresponders among organic MR children than among normal controls. The stimulus in this case was a 55-dB buzzer.

Less clear-cut differences in frequency of responding to simple stimuli were found by Graham (1969), who sought to determine whether electrodermal responding could be used as a measure of sensation threshold among MRs. Using normal and institutionalized MR adults, he measured response frequency differences at several sensation levels. Normals responded more than MRs at some levels (namely 5, 10, and 20 dB above threshold), but group differences were not found at sensation levels of —10, —5, 0, and 30 dB. In general, then, electrodermal responding underestimated the MR's auditory sensation level by 20–30 dB.

Some evidence of decreased response frequency to more cognitive types of stimuli has been provided by Bower and Das (1970). They recorded SCR frequency to words and nonsense syllables, while requiring Ss to press a button for some or all of the words. For all stimuli combined, they found no differences among the three experimental groups (noninstitutionalized educable MRs, mental age controls, chronological age controls). They did find differences, however, when only responses to the words (nonsense syllables excluded) were considered. In this situation mental age controls responded more frequently than MRs.

Das and Bower (1971) pursued the possibility that normals respond more than MRs to meaningful stimuli. Children heard six common words, and were instructed to press a button only to the word *man*. The word *man* was always preceded by the word *box*. Responses to these two words only were recorded, and their analysis indicated more responding among normals than MRs to the warning word (box), and the converse for the response word (man). It is not known whether these simple effects were significant, since no statistical analysis was presented.

Two studies have failed to demonstrate electrodermal response frequency differences between retardates and normals. Tizzard (1968) compared responses to auditory stimuli of MRs of very low IQ (about 20–40) with those of normals. Clausen and Karrer (1968) analyzed SRR frequency of normals, organic MRs, and nonorganic MRs. Stimuli were a tone (1000 Hz, 67 dB) and a bright light.

We located no study that suggested greater response frequency among retardates than normals.

2. RESPONSE SIZE[2]

The bulk of studies of responsiveness of MRs concerns response size, rather than frequency and the results are mixed. Among 12 studies, 6 reported that response size for MRs did not differ from that of normals, 3 indicated greater responses for normals, 2 found MRs to be more responsive, and 1 found a curvilinear relationship between IQ and responding. These widely divergent results might be accounted for by factors mentioned in review articles relevant to this responsiveness measure. Berkson (1961) has suggested that responsiveness of retardates depends upon stimulus intensity, while Karrer (1966) feels that IQ level of MR subjects may be a significant variable.

In his review article, Berkson (1961) asked whether an interaction might exist between intensity and responsiveness of MRs, such that their responses are less than those of normals at moderate intensity levels, but greater than normals' at higher intensity levels. Table 3 provides a cursory view of studies relevant to this hypothesis. Only studies

---

[2] The term "size" as used here includes two measures, one in which zero responses are averaged in, and the other in which such responses are excluded.

dealing with simple stimuli, in which intensity levels can be easily varied, are included. There is evidence both for and against Berkson's notion. The most supportive evidence is provided by Fenz and McCabe (1971), who report a significant group times intensity effect. This was attributed to the linear increase in responding of normals in combination with a positively accelerated response curve for MRs. At intensities of 35 and 70 dB, responses of MRs fell below those of normals, while they

TABLE 3

RESPONSE SIZE AMONG MENTAL RETARDATES AS A FUNCTION OF STIMULUS INTENSITY[a]

Magnitude or amplitude of MR response	Stimulus intensity		
	Low	Moderate	High
Below normals	Fenz and McCabe (1971)	Fenz and McCabe (1971); Lobb (1968, 1970); Berkson, Hermelin, and O'Connor (1961)	
Same as normals		Karrer and Clausen (1964); Lobb (1968, 1970)	Pilgrim, Miller, and Cobb (1969)
Above normals	Wolfensberger and O'Connor (1965)		Fenz and McCabe (1971); Wolfensberger and O'Connor (1965)

[a] Studies involving responses to cognitive stimuli are excluded.

exceeded normals' responding at 100 dB. The findings of Berkson *et al.* (1961) are also consistent with the Berkson (1961) hypothesis. They reported greater responsivity among normal adults than among three mentally retarded adult groups. Stimuli were light flashes of moderate intensity, and the measure used was magnitude of SPR to the first stimulus in the series. Additional corroborative data is presented by Lobb (1968, 1970) who examined responses to a 4000-Hz, 70-DB tone, of .1-sec duration. He used two measures of mean response size, including in the denominator of one, magnitude, those trials on which no responses were given (Lobb, 1968), and in the other, amplitude, excluding zero responses (Lobb, 1970). In both types of analyses MRs were found to be less responsive than normals in some, but not all, blocks of adaptation trials. Unfortunately, neither study reported an analysis of response size differences for the adaptation period as a whole.

The most damaging evidence against the Berkson (1961) proposal is that presented by Wolfensberger and O'Connor (1965). They examined responses of young adult normals and institutionalized MRs whose IQs ranged from 42 to 76. Using two intensities of light stimuli, low (but above threshold) and high (almost painful), they found a main effect for amplitude, with MRs giving larger responses than normals. More important, the intensity × intelligence interaction was not significant, contrary to Berkson's (1961) expectation.

Two additional studies of MR response magnitude to simple stimuli, one using moderate intensity stimuli and one with a high intensity stimulus, found no difference between responding of MRs and normal Ss. Karrer and Clausen (1964) measured reactivity of organic MRs and normals to a 55-dB buzzer. Using T-scores to correct for initial values, they measured magnitude of SRR for the first trial. A noninstitutionalized MR group was compared to normal children in a study by Pilgrim, Miller and Cobb (1969). A short, high-intensity light was used as the stimulus. Of relevance to their report of no group differences may be the authors' assignment of scores of 250 Ω for those trials on which no responses were given. This was done in order to avoid unequal cell frequencies, and may have had the effect of reducing MR–normal differences.

A second review of physiological response magnitudes and mental retardation has been published by Karrer (1966). Largely on the basis of results reported by Collman (1959) Karrer concluded that when individuals of above-average intelligence are included, one finds a curvilinear relationship between IQ and responsiveness, such that Ss at the ends of the IQ continuum respond less than those near the middle. In his study Collman (1959) examined SRRs of a great number of normal, dull, and retarded children. Measuring SRRs to (1) his telling S that a picture was about to be presented and (2) the actual presentation of the pictures, Collman found mean responses for both types of stimuli to be inverted U-shaped functions of IQ. Subjects with IQs at about 90 showed the largest responses, while least responsive were those with IQs at 58 and 126.

The Coleman (1959) study provides the best evidence for Karrer's (1966) postulation of a U-shaped function. If such a relationship exists between IQ and responsiveness, one would expect that at least MRs would be less responsive than normals and that this difference would increase as a negative function of IQ of the MR population. However, the summary presented in Table 4 indicates that many studies have found equal or greater response magnitudes among MRs as compared to normals. In addition, and particularly contrary to the notion of a U-shaped function, are the results of investigations by Grings, Lockhart and Dameron (1962); Berkson *et al.* (1961); and Galkowski *et al.* (1968).

TABLE 4

Response Size Among Mental Retardates as a Function of IQ

Magnitude or amplitude of MR response	IQ		
	20–40	40–60	60–80
Below normals	Berkson, Hermelin, and O'Connor (1961)	Collman (1959)	Berkson, Hermelin, O'Connor (1961); Collman (1959)
Same as normals		Karrer and Clausen (1964)	Bower and Das (1970); Fenz and McCabe (1971); Pilgrim, Miller, and Cobb (1969)
Above normals		Galkowski, Dadas, and Domanski (1968); Wolfensberger and O'Connor (1965)	

Grings *et al.* (1962) measured SRRs to tones and lights during the adaptation period of a conditioning study. They found no significant difference in responses of severely retarded and mildly retarded Ss. Similarly, Berkson *et al.* (1961) reported no response differences to light flashes among those classified as feebleminded (mean IQ 60), imbecile (mean IQ 33.5) and mongoloid (mean IQ 30.6), although these three groups did respond less than normals. Especially damaging to the Karrer (1966) position is the study by Galkowski *et al.* (1968). These investigations reported not only greater responding for MRs than for normals, but they found significant *negative* correlations between IQ and response magnitude for both visual and verbal stimuli.

Pryer and Ellis (1959) found no difference between Ss with IQs around 15 and those with IQs around 55 in what they view as "GSR to a startle stimulus." However, the facts that (1) the measure was basal conductance and (2) the first recording was made 10 sec following the stimulus, indicate that little, if any, information regarding the response to the startle stimulus (gunshot) is provided. Because of these limitations, the relevance of these results to the question of whether responsiveness is a function of IQ level among MRs cannot be evaluated.

The results of studies reported above indicate that Collman's U-shaped relationship between responsiveness and IQ has not received much support. If we may speculate for a moment, let us briefly discuss one possibility for the discrepant findings. Most of the studies not concordant with Collman's utilized simple types of stimuli, while Collman used meaningful verbal and visual stimuli. It is possible that these kinds of stimuli might elicit small responses in very bright and very dull subjects for two different reasons: The very bright may readily form cortical models of the meaning, while the severely retarded may have little understanding of the meaning and thus either rapidly develop models of the physical properties of the stimuli, or simply not attend to the stimuli. The reader is referred to the section on CNS damage (Section VI) for a similar discussion of results of research in that area of mental dysfunction.

In summary, the relationships between MR responding and other variables, which have been proposed by reviewers of physiological correlates of MR, are appealing in their simplicity. Support can be found for the hypotheses of both Berkson (1961) and Karrer (1966). Evidence against both suggestions has also been presented. Factors other than IQ, such as the possible numbing effects of institutionalization as mentioned by Fenz and McCabe (1971) and greater apprehension of MR Ss in the unfamiliar experimental setting, may operate in unpredictable ways and account for much of the variance in responsiveness results.

3. TEMPORAL FACTORS

a. LATENCY. A number of studies have included among their electrodermal response measures an evaluation of response latencies of MRs. The rationale for examining latencies is that the sluggishness demonstrated by this population in more complex behaviors might be evident in simpler, autonomically mediated responses.

A review of the latency literature leaves one with the impression that many studies have found that response latencies among MRs are shorter than those for normals (Galkowski et al., 1968; Kodman, Fein, & Mixson, 1959; Clausen & Karrer's 1969 reference to Grings et al., 1962; and the references of Clausen & Karrer, 1969; Galkowski et al., 1968, and Wolfensberger & O'Connor, 1965, to the 1959 article of Kodman et al.). Closer scrutiny, however, reveals that there is little support for this view. Two sources for the false conclusion that response latencies are shorter for MRs can be identified. First, some investigators have misinterpreted their own data. For example two papers imply in their discussion sections that they found shorter latencies for MRs (Galkowski et al., 1968; Kodman et al., 1959). However, none of the data presented by either investigative team support this claim. In their discussion section, Galkowski et al. (1968) refer to the findings of a "one second shorter response latency time" for retarded children as compared to normals. This difference is not reported in the results section. In fact, the parameter in the results section labeled "time of reaction," which apparently corresponds to latency, specifically indicates that no difference between the groups was found. The statement by Kodman et al. (1959) that the response latencies found by them for MRs were shorter than those typically reported for normals has little meaning, since response latencies vary with experimental conditions and the Kodman study did not include normals.

Second, some investigators have misinterpreted the results of others. Three studies (Clausen & Karrer, 1969; Galkowski et al., 1968; Wolfensberger & O'Connor, 1965) report that Kodman et al. (1959) found differences between the response latencies of normals and MRs, when in fact Kodman et al. did not even study normals. Wolfensberger and O'Connor (1965) even go so far as to contrast their own nonsignificant latency differences with the allegedly *significant* ones of Kodman et al. Another example of misrepresentation is the claim by Clausen and Karrer (1969) that Grings, Lockhart and Dameron (1962) "found shorter latencies of GSR responses in mental defectives than in normals." Not only did Grings and co-workers not study normals, but unlike Kodman et al. (1959), they made no speculations concerning possible comparisons between their results and those of investigations utilizing normals.

Rather than showing shorter response latencies among MRs, the bulk of the available data indicates that latencies are the same for MRs as for normals. Three studies that examined responses to simple stimuli agree that there is no difference in response latencies of MRs as compared to normals. Clausen and Karrer (1969) compared response latencies of institutionalized nonorganic MRs, institutionalized organic MRs, and normal children. They found no latency differences in responses to moderately intense tones and light flashes. Response latencies to light flashes were also evaluated for noninstitutionalized MR children (Pilgrim et al., 1969), and adults (Wolfensberger & O'Connor, 1965), and did not differ from those of normal subjects.

Response latencies for more complex stimuli also have been studied, and with results similar to those for simple stimuli. Thus, no latency differences were found in responses to words and nonsense syllables (Bower & Das, 1970) nor for rather complex stimuli presented in each of four modalities (Galkowski et al., 1968).

It may be concluded that latency of electrodermal responding may not be counted among those measures that differentiate normal from mentally retarded persons.

b. DURATION. The sparse data on response duration among MRs do not present a clear picture.

Some authors have reported faster recovery for normal subjects than for MRs. Wolfensberger and O'Connor (1965) administered light stimuli of two intensities (low and high) to two groups of young adults, institutionalized, nonorganic MRs and a second group who had normal IQs. Response durations of normals were much shorter than those of MRs, especially at the low light intensity. Clausen and Karrer (1969) not only found that the responses of non-brain-damaged MRs recovered more slowly than those of normal subjects, but more slowly than those of MRs with organic involvement, as well. Organic MRs and normals did not differ from one another in response duration.

Analysis of response recovery in two studies failed to find significant differences between MRs and normals (Galkowski et al., 1968; and Pilgrim et al., 1969). However, the meaning of the finding in the Galkowski et al. (1968) study is questionable, since stimuli used in that investigation were of a very complex and cognitive nature. The great variability in response duration with such stimuli would reduce the likelihood of finding significant differences between groups. Finally, in one study, that of Vogel (1961), responses of MRs were found to be of shorter duration than those of normals.

Explanations for these discrepant results are not readily apparent. Ages and IQs did not differ widely among these studies. Various types of stimuli were used, but that does not seem to have affected the findings in any obvious way. It may be noteworthy, however, that stimuli used in the Vogel (1961) investigation were probably more intense than stimuli in any of the other studies. Vogel's stimuli were a 112-dB tone and a 3-sec foot immersion in ice water. Vogel suggests that his finding of slower recovery among normals might be owing to their greater cortical control, which in his study would have led to enhanced recall of stressful stimuli, thus slowing autonomic recovery. Nonuniformity of recording techniques and scoring methods are two other possible sources of variance. Clausen and Karrer (1969), for example, were the only investigators to statistically remove amplitude effects before analyzing duration differences.

D. Habituation

Some investigators have looked for habituation differences between retarded and normal persons, in order to determine whether the MR's impairment is reflected in this simple form of learning. The studies reported by these investigators generally report that little or no difference is seen in habituation of MRs as compared to normals. However, some evidence to the contrary has been presented in at least two papers (Tizzard, 1968; Fenz & McCabe, 1971). Discrepancies between these and the majority of reports may be due to such variables as IQ of MR population, stimuli employed, and data evaluation methods.

Regarding IQs, it may be relevant that subjects in the Tizzard (1968) study were severely retarded children (IQs around 20–30). These children showed little habituation to auditory stimuli. It is possible that these children were so intellectually impaired that they could not understand the instructions and were frightened by the experimental setting. Body movements and heightened arousal of MRs, rather than increasing responsiveness *per se*, might have contributed to the failure of MR groups to habituate.

The Tizzard study can be contrasted to one by Das and Bower (1971). This study used the same data evaluation method (response frequency analysis), and same subject age range as did the Tizzard study, but IQs of the MR children were higher (40–65). Das and Bower reported finding no difference between MRs and normals in habituation to common words, except on the last block of trials, where normals' responding mysteriously increased.

Regarding stimuli used, in both studies reporting some difference in habituation of normals and MRs (Tizzard, 1968; Fenz & McCabe, 1971) the stimuli were tones. In contrast, many of the reports of no habituation differences come from investigations utilizing light flashes as the stimuli to be habituated. These include studies by Berkson *et al.* (1961); Pilgrim *et al.* (1965); and Wolfensberger and O'Connor (1965). Grings *et al.* (1962) used tones as well as lights. According to these authors, their data demonstrated similarly of habituation in two IQ levels of mental retardates, but no analyses are reported that specifically test for this effect.

One study that found no habituation differences between retarded and normal subjects used tones exclusively (Karrer & Clausen, 1964). A difference in data evaluation methods undoubtedly contributed toward the disparity between these results and those of Fenz and McCabe (1971), who, like Karrer and Clausen (1964), also used tones and looked at response magnitude. Fenz and McCabe demonstrated that habituation differences depend upon stimulus intensity. Karrer and Clausen's (1964) habituation analysis was designed to eliminate the effect of the correlation between initial response magnitude and speed of habituation, while Fenz and McCabe (1971) did not take into account initial magnitude when computing the trials × group interaction. Partialing out initial response magnitude can radically affect results, as demonstrated in the study of Berkson, et al. (1961). They found a significant groups × blocks effect, which they attributed to the normal group's greater responding on the first block of trials. However, correcting for initial response eliminated differences in habituation rates. On the basis of this finding, Berkson concluded that differences in habituation rate were only apparent.

This of course brings us to the old question of what kinds of data we are willing to accept as evidence of "real" habituation differences. When amplitude measures are utilized, the most common means of assessing habituation differences is to look at the group × trials interaction in an analysis of variance. A significant interaction is frequently viewed as evidence of group differences in habituation rates. Probably the widespread use of this interaction as an index of habituation differences is due to the ease with which it is obtained. An analysis of variance design in which trials is a variable yields the group × trials interaction, so that no computation outside the analysis of variance need be performed. There are objections to this measure of habituation differences, one of which is that it does not take into account initial response magnitude. The fact that habituation rates correlate with initial response amplitude has led many investigators to partial out the effect of initial response. This procedure, however, may result in the baby's going out with the bath water. In the mental retardation literature herein reviewed, studies correcting for initial response include those of Berkson et al. (1961), as well as Karrer and Clausen (1964). The reader must determine for himself whether such corrections make intuitive sense.

E. Conditioning

If autonomic conditionability represents a type of rudimentary learning ability, then it behooves us to investigate such conditioning in a population that has demonstrated inferior learning in more complex areas. Electrodermal conditioning among MRs has been analyzed in a handful of studies, and results are not in complete agreement.

Das and Bower (1971) instructed subjects to press a button when they heard the word *man,* one of six common words presented. This was always preceded by the word *box*. Measuring EDR latencies of normal and MR children to the words *box* and *man*, they found longer latencies to *box* than to *man* for normals only. This retardation of response to the warning signal (*box*), the authors hypothesized, may be viewed as evidence for conditioning among normals.

Another study reporting generally superior conditioning in normals than in MRs is that of Lobb (1968, 1970). The acquisition data were analyzed by three methods—magnitude (zero responses included), amplitude (zero responses omitted), and frequency. All three methods showed conditioning to be better for normals. However, these differences did not hold up during the extinction period. In contrast to the above study, Baumeister, Beedle, and Urquhart (1964) saw no differences in electrodermal conditioning of MRs as compared to normals. Their criterion, however, was extinction behavior only, and in this respect their results were consistent with those of Lobb (1968, 1970).

A study reporting electrodermal conditioning within two IQ levels of MRs is that of Grings *et al.* (1962). Extensive analysis of acquisition data revealed that both IQ groups showed evidence of three types of conditioning (simple, discrimination, and discrimination increase). It was therefore concluded that autonomic conditioning is not a function of IQ, at least within the MR range. A later study (Lockhart & Grings, 1964), using essentially the same design and procedure as that of the 1962 paper, looked at conditioning in a college population and found a difference in first interval, or anticipatory responding of these subjects, as compared to the MRs of the 1962 study. For the college students the first interval response peaked in fewer trials than for the MR populations studied. It was suggested that this difference might reflect "conditioning-like behavior through perception" for the college students, as opposed to "perception through conditioning" among MRs. Second-interval responses did not differentiate the groups, and might therefore reflect a more primitive aspect of conditioning, according to these authors.

Since Lobb (1968, 1970) examined second-interval responses and did find MR–normal differences, these results are in apparent disagreement with those presented by Lockhart and Grings (1964). As is frequently the case, the two studies are not comparable, since their conclusions are based on entirely different types of analysis. Lockhart and Grings (1964) observed that for both normal and MRs, second-interval response discrimination (response to CS^+ versus response to CS^-) occurred at about the same point in conditioning, after two differential reinforcements. Lobb (1968, 1970), rather than analyzing his data trial by trial, combined the first 16 acquisition trials into one block, and the second 16 into a second block. He did not look at CRs as a function of trials.

Neither did Lockhart and Grings (1964) report testing CR amplitude differences between normals and MRs with all trials combined.

The question of whether awareness of CS–US contingencies is necessary for autonomic conditioning is an important issue that has been the object of much recent discussion, research, and speculation (Baer, 1971; Baer & Fuhrer, 1968; Bridger, 1971; Dawson, 1970, 1971; Epstein, 1971; Fuhrer & Baer, 1965; Furedy, 1971; Grant, 1971; Lockhart, 1971; Ross, 1971). The study by Grings et al. (1962) bears on this question. The finding of these investigators of SRR conditioning in subjects whose IQs were as low as 20–45 casts doubt upon the contention that awareness is necessary for conditioning, if we assume that these individuals were not aware of the CS–US contingency. Valid measurement of such awareness is one of the most difficult problems faced by those who seek to determine the role of cognition in classical conditioning.

Finally, Ellis' (1963) suggestion that stimulus trace for MRs is of shorter duration than for normals has received experimental attention by Baumeister et al. (1964), Grings et al. (1962), and Lobb (1968, 1970). Varying CS–US interval, all three studies failed to find an interaction between this factor and IQ group. Such an interaction would be predicted by Ellis' theory. Compared to normals, retardates should show good conditioning with short CS–US intervals, but not with long intervals. This effect was not demonstrated in the above studies.

VI.   Central Nervous System Damage

Surprisingly few studies have evaluated electrodermal phenomena in an attempt to discriminate between neuropathological and control subjects. The most recent and comprehensive studies utilizing patients with brain damage (BD) have been and are being conducted by Parsons, Holloway and associates at the Medical Center, University of Oklahoma. Their first study (Parsons & Chandler, 1969) found BD patients to have significantly higher SCL at rest, as well as a higher incidence of nonspecific responses. This last finding is also reported by Brivllova (1965). In response to stimulation (startling buzzer as well as pure tones), orienting response latencies of BD subjects are found to be significantly shorter. Parsons and Chandler discuss their results within a framework of cortical–subcortical dynamic relationships. Damage to the cortex is assumed to reduce the effectiveness of cortical inhibitory control over subcortical centers. Subcortical centers are conceived of as the site of origin of most phasic electrodermal activity, with cortical activity responsible for attenuating such responses with respect to both the process of habituation (Sokolov, 1963) and nonspecific activity. Cortical damage is thus invoked to lead to greater number of nonspecific responses as well as the shorter latencies of responses to stimulation. Holloway and Parsons (1969) extended these results in a study of patients with unilateral brain damage in whom they recorded SC from bilaterally symmetrical palmar sites as well as dorsal sites. They report that the unilateral lesion group had relatively higher SCL (ratio of conductance from left to right side) from the palms contralateral to the lesion site. This effect was not true for dorsal SC measures and is attributed to sweat gland innervation. Comparisons of SCL between groups finds patients with right hemisphere lesions demonstrating a significant elevation when compared to all other groups. This discrimination did not hold for patients with left hemispheric lesions. The differential effect between their left and right hemispheric lesion groups is attributed to the right hemispheric lesion group having more extensive damage than the left hemispheric group. Attempts at making discrimination on the basis of location of lesion in the anterior–posterior plane did not arrive at any significant differentiations. The latest study by these authors (Holloway & Parsons, 1971) evaluated orienting response habituation in patients with brain damage. Though we will restrict our presentation to electrodermal responses, this study evaluated EEG alpha desynchronization and heart rate as well. The results from these various response systems are, as might be expected, far from concordant! This study found greater amplitude SCR to the first block of stimuli (three successive trials), but no other differences in tonic or phasic levels of electrodermal activity were found. Unfortunately, they do not comment on the lack of basal level differences found in this study as compared to their previous studies in all of which the BD groups had significantly higher tonic levels of skin conductance.

With respect to habituation, no difference between groups was found for the electrodermal measure. In response to a dishabituating stimulus, however, significant differences between the BD and control group emerge. The dishabituating stimulus was a tone which only differed in duration of stimulus presentation from the habituated stimulus. The BD group failed to demonstrate significant dishabituation, i.e., in response to the discrepant stimulus they did not manifest an EDOR.

How can one reconcile the lack of differences in habituation rates between the two groups found in this and other studies? A number of possible explanations, all of which are subject to experimental verification, can be generated. It is, for example, possible that the stimuli used (pure tones) are so simple with respect to the development of a cortical model that it does not take very much functional cortex for such a model to be elaborated. A second and more troubling possibility is that the two groups develop quite different models of the stimulus. Accepting Holloway's and Parsons' finding that a disinhibiting stimulus, a tone which differed only in duration, produced a return of the OR in control subjects and no return in BD subjects certainly suggests that the stimulus model generated by control subjects incorporated stimulus duration as one component of the model, while this was not the case for the BD group.

Since the development of a simple cortical model leads to more rapid habituation than the development of a more complex model, we might hypothesize that in the above case the BD group actually demonstrated slower habituation than the control group, i.e., it took them as long to develop a simple model as it took the control group to develop a more complex model.

We would thus recommend that studies attempting to differentiate normal and BD subjects on the basis of some aspects of habituation either utilize more complex stimuli for habituation studies and/or systematically investigate aspects of the cortical model that has been developed, utilizing disinhibition of habituation for this assessment.

A study by Davidoff and McDonald (1964) also found no differences in rate of habituation for a BD as compared to a control group. These authors included a conditioning paradigm in their study and report significant differences between BD and control subjects with respect to the development of conditioned anticipatory responses and responses at the latency of the UCS on nonreinforced trials. Reese, Doss, and Gantt (1953) similarly report, within the context of a differential conditioning study, that patients with severe diffuse cortical impairment do not develop conditional anticipatory responses to the same extent as is true of their control group. Responses to the UCS, electric shock, did not discriminate between the groups.

A study by Goldstein, Ludwig and Naunton (1954) divided a group of children with hearing difficulties into two groups, one of which is reported to condition poorly, and a second group which was readily conditioned (we state "reported to condition" because our interpretation of their results suggests that one is dealing with the presence of orienting rather than conditional responses in this study). They report that, "In a significant majority of the cases where conditioning was difficult, previous and independent diagnosis had suggested the presence of aphasia; and in a significant majority of the cases where conditioning was readily established, no evidence of aphasia had been found [p. 75]." Thus, to the extent that aphasia may be associated with impaired cerebral functioning or cerebral damage, these authors find either poor conditioning or rapid habituation of EDORs.

One further study reported recently with children deserves our attention. Satterfield and Dawson (1971) evaluated some electrodermal correlates of hyperactivity in children. The hyperactive child syndrome (short attention span, low frustration tolerance, aggressive and impulsive behavior) is identified by these authors as being part and parcel of the minimal brain dysfunction (MBD) syndrome. Though some of us, in the absence of clear-cut evidence for brain dysfunction and the presence of clear-cut behavior dysfunction prefer to label these children as minimal behavior dysfunction, we shall include this diagnostic label under the rubric of studies in the area of brain damage. These authors, contrary to their expectation, found hyperactive children to have lower SCL, fewer nonspecific electrodermal responses, and lower amplitude-orienting responses to the first of a series of tones when compared to a control group of children. All children participated in two experiments, each lasting approximately 40 min and separated by a 1-hr rest period. Half of the hyperactive children received a stimulant drug at the beginning of the 1-hr rest period. The effect of drug administration produced a significant increase in nonspecific responses for this group. The effect of the stimulant drug thus was to increase arousal in most of the children of this group.

One further measure which discriminated between the control and the hyperkinetic group was the fact that control children gave smaller amplitude ORs to the first of the second series of tone presentations as compared to the first trial of the first series of tone presentations. Neither of the hyperkinetic groups demonstrated a significant decrement on this response measure. What one can conclude from this study is that hyperactive children are less aroused than control children, less responsive to stimuli both under the experimenter's control (OR) as well as not under the experimenter's control (nonspecific responses), and demonstrate poorer retention of habituation over time.

Aside from their neurophysiological speculations, these authors raise an interesting clinical speculation in suggesting that those hyperactive children with low SCL would respond best to stimulant drugs, those at the high end of the arousal continuum to tranquilizing drugs, and those in the normal range to psychotherapy.

A study by Cohen and Douglas (1969) in part confirms the above author's results. Cohen and Douglas evaluated OR habituation under two conditions. In the first condition, subjects were relaxed and asked to listen to a series of 500-Hz, 6-sec, 70-dB tones. No differences in resting levels, amplitude of response or rate of habituation were obtained. The second condition involved a reaction time task with a warning signal; ORs to the latter signal were evaluated. Again no differences in SCL were noted. However, amplitude of response to the first signal stimulus was significantly greater for the control group, an effect which persisted across the first block of trials.

Hyperactive children were found to be less responsive than controls to change in task demands. Thus, for example, controls demonstrated significantly larger amplitude ORs to the first signal stimulus as compared to the first nonsignal stimulus. A similar result was seen for SCL levels taken prior to nonsignal and signal stimulus presentation. This study thus also suggests a less discriminant cortical model in MBD as compared to control subjects.

A study by Boydstun, Ackerman, Stevens, Clements, Peters, and Dykman (1968) is only in part supportive of Satterfield and Dawson's results. These authors found no differences in SCL between their minimal brain dysfunction group and a control group. These authors, however, do report their control children to be significantly more responsive to tone stimuli than the MBD group and further find more rapid habituation of the electrodermal OR to tone stimuli in the BD group. A number of variables may contribute to the discrepancies in results between the two studies. First, Satterfield and Dawson utilized a more homogeneous group (hyperactive children with normal IQ and no specific sensory handicap) while Boydstun utilized a broader criterion for defining his MBD group.

We believe that the study of hyperactive children or MBD children, whether they are brain damaged or not, is an area in which considerably more research utilizing psychophysiological procedures should be done. Specifically we believe that studies dealing with arousal and arousability, the development of cortical models as measured by habituation and disinhibition of habituation, as well as conditioning studies, the retention of such cortical models over time, or memory functions, the effect of psychoactive drugs on these measures, all deserve considerably more investigation than is currently found in the research literature.

Elithorn, Piercy, and Crosskey (1955) report on the effect of prefrontal leucotomy on anticipatory conditioned responses. Leucotomy had a significant effect in inhibiting such anticipatory responses, leaving responses to the UCS (electric shock) intact.

The Russian literature on this problem is considerably more voluminous than the Western literature. Unfortunately, most of the material available to us is of a summary nature. Luria (1966) reports differences in aspects of electrodermal responsiveness between patients with frontal lobe as compared to those with lesions in other cortical areas. Lesions of the parietotemporal regions, occipital regions, as well as increased intracranial pressure, produce "considerable changes in the autonomic components of the orienting reflex: Autonomic reactions to a new stimulus may either be omitted, or become diffuse and not extinguished for a long time [p. 552]." This, of course, taps both ends of the responsiveness continuum.

Patients with frontal lobe damage respond to orienting stimuli very much like patients with lesions in other areas. However, providing the orienting stimulus with signal value does not produce the regularization in function seen with lesions in other brain areas. This conclusion is supported by the study of Elithorn and co-workers.

Brivllova (1965) reports that brain-damaged patients produce more nonspecific electrodermal responses, orienting responses of such patients are more intense, habituation proceeds more slowly, and response latencies are more varied than is true of normal subjects. Stepanov (1965), in the same volume, similarly reports slower habituation of ORs in brain-damaged patients. However, he reports other phenomena as well, and the internal consistency of his presentation is, unfortunately, far from perfect. For example, in another portion of his presentation, he reports that patients with brain damage demonstrate a complete absence of responses to the stimuli used as well as a disturbance in the "law of intensity." (The law of intensity implies that within limits there is a reasonably linear relationship between stimulus intensity and response amplitude.) He reports that "stressing" the subject by engaging him in conversation, or conducting association experiments with him, often normalized the intensity relationship. Like Luria (1966), he reports that involving the second signal system had various effects, producing in some patients, "an inhibition of the galvanic skin reflexes or their decrease and, in a number of cases, a change in the intensity relationship [p. 397]."

As is apparent from the above review, the literature dealing with brain damage and electrodermal phenomena is quite nonspecific; the reader or theoretician with a particular ax to grind can marshall evidence for or against any position in the literature.

The problem is, of course, that we are dealing with a complex problem which defies simple parsimonious solutions. For example, brain damage of a specific cortical area may have altogether different behavioral as well as autonomic effects dependent on whether: (1) the damage was produced in a one-stage operation or a two-stage operation with a reasonable period of time intervening between operations; (2) the damage was the result of a traumatic injury or slow-growing neoplasm; or (3) the damage was produced in a young or old organism. These are just a few of the variables for which demonstrable effects have been recorded.

At an anatomical level there are further reasons for not expecting similar responses from cortically nondiscrete (or perhaps indiscrete) areas. As Wang (1964) has so neatly demonstrated in the cat, a wide variety of structures affect whether or not one picks up a response at the effector site (sweat gland). Restricting ourselves only to cortical damage he suggests that damage to the frontal cortex (inhibitory area) should produce opposite results to damage in sensorimotor, anterior limbic, and infralimbic cortical sites (excitatory areas). One could further suggest that equivalent damage to excitatory and inhibitory areas might cancel each other out, leaving us with relatively normal responsiveness.

Though it is intriguing and appealing to talk about cortical excitation and inhibition, the *post hoc* rationalizations that we are likely to engage in will, in the absence of better handles on these constructs, do little to advance the field of neuropsychology, neurology, or psychophysiology.

VII.   Anxiety

The alleged high correlation between anxiety and electrodermal measures is frequently assumed to be one of the most consistently found "truths" revealed by those who have devoted their professional lives to seeking relationships between physiological and behavioral functioning (see Martin, 1961). One measure, basal electrodermal level, is thought to correlate particularly highly with anxiety, and some investigators have used resting levels of skin resistance to define anxiety. Thus, the literature contains studies that use the following approach: (1) A measure of electrodermal activity is taken subsequent to some environmental manipulation. (2) The results are then discussed in terms of the effects of this variable upon anxiety, when no independent measure of anxiety has been made (e.g., Epstein & Roupenian, 1970; Stotland & Blumenthal, 1964). This type of study will not be included in the present section. Instead, we will limit our discussion to those investigations employing an independent evaluation of anxiety.

The correspondence between electrodermal activity and anxiety has been studied among normal populations, among psychiatric patients diagnosed as suffering from anxiety states, as well as more heterogeneous populations of psychiatric patients.

A. Normal Subjects

1. Resting Levels and Nonspecific Responses

Contrary to the commonly held view, the bulk of the evidence with respect to both spontaneous activity and basal electrodermal levels indicates that highly anxious individuals do not differ from persons with lower anxiety levels. This has been found both when the anxiety measure was state, or transitory anxiety, and when it was trait anxiety.

Bitterman and Holtzman (1952) found that SRL during conditioning was not a function of anxiety level. They divided their undergraduate Ss into two groups, depending upon whether they scored above or below the median on an anxiety scale. The scale was based upon data from several sources: from ratings of the S while under stress, from an overall behavior rating schedule, from Rohrschach and MMPI information. Similar results have been reported by Zuckerman *et al.* (1968), who found no significant correlations between SCL and anxiety ratings among normals. They measured SCL at two points in the experiment: at the beginning and just prior to immersion of S's hand in a bucket of ice. Nonsignificant correlations between SRL and anxiety (Taylor's MAS) have also been reported by Koepke and Pribram (1966).

The results of Epstein and Fenz (1970) are in line with the above findings. Subjects scoring high on the autonomic arousal scale of the Epstein–Fenz Anxiety Scale did not differ significantly in overall SCL from those scoring medium and low on this scale.

Evidence of no basal electrodermal differences between low and high anxious normal subjects has been found in studies measuring state anxiety, as well. Katkin (1965b), for example, assessed anxiety level by means of Zuckerman's (1960) Affect Adjective Check List (AACL), a measure of state anxiety. Subjects were divided into high and low anxiety groups, and their SRLs measured both during rest and during threat of shock. No high-low anxiety differences were found for either experimental period.

A possible explanation for the failure of the above studies to find a correspondence between basal electrodermal levels and anxiety is offered by the report of McDonnell and Carpenter (1959, 1960) of an inverted U-shaped relationship between anxiety, as measured by the Mandler-Sarason General Anxiety Scale (1952), and SCL. Subjects in the middle of the anxiety continuum had higher conductance levels than did those of low and high anxiety. Such a relationship would account for both the above nonsignificant linear correlations between basal levels and anxiety and the nonsignificant differences between high and low anxious Ss' basal levels as measured by t tests and analysis of variance.

Further insight into the relationship between anxiety and tonic electrodermal levels is provided by the research of Fenz and Epstein (1967) on sport parachutists. Both SCL and self-rated fear of parachutists were plotted as a function of time to jump. For experienced parachutists, both measures reached peak prior to the actual jump, but the fear peak was reached earlier than the SCL peak. This finding is additional evidence that basal electrodermal measures are imperfect reflectors of apprehension.

Regarding spontaneous electrodermal activity, Katkin has consistently reported that normal subjects rated as highly anxious do not show more SFs than low-anxious normal subjects (Katkin, 1965a, b; Katkin & McCubbin, 1969). He found this to be true during the preexperimental period (state anxiety and trait anxiety, Katkin, 1965a and Katkin & McCubbin, 1969), during rest (state anxiety, Katkin, 1965b), and during threat of shock (state anxiety, Katkin, 1965b). In addition, Neva and Hicks (1970) reported that spontaneous electrodermal activity did not correlate with Taylor MAS scores when both were measured during induced muscle tension. Koepke and Pribram (1966) also failed to find a significant correlation between Taylor MAS scores and spontaneous activity.

2. Responsiveness

Electrodermal responsiveness of individuals who are rated as anxious have been evaluated in a number of studies, and with quite consistently negative results. Epstein and Fenz (1970), examining response magnitude of subjects scoring high, medium, and low on three different anxiety subscales, found no difference among groups on any of the three subscales. Katkin and McCubbin (1969) looked at SCRs to tones in high and low anxious subjects and found no overall difference. Koepke and Pribram (1966) found no relationship between anxiety and initial SRR magnitude. Likewise, Raskin (1969) demonstrated that initial SCR magnitude and anxiety scale scores were unrelated. Similarly, Zuckerman et al. (1968) reported that the correlation between conductance response to cold pressor and anxiety rating was nonsignificant. Although not specifically discussed by the authors, it is assumed that the high, medium, and low anxiety groups of Fenz and Dronsejko (1969) did not differ in SCR. The authors indicate that this analysis was performed, but apparently they reported only significant findings. Further support for the contention that anxiety level is not a determinant of electrodermal responsiveness is provided by Bitterman and Holtzman (1952), who found no difference between anxiety groups in magnitude of response to tones during adaptation. These investigators did report greater median response among high anxiety Ss to the first shock in a conditioning series. Finally, Roessler, Burch, and Childers (1966) showed that mean SRRs to light and tones and four indices of anxiety (Welsh A factor, Welsh Anxiety Index, Taylor MAS, and debilitating and facilitating scales of the Alpert–Haber Anxiety Scale), were not correlated.

A promising line of research in the area of electrodermal responding of anxious individuals has been suggested by the recent research of Edelberg (1971). Studying the recovery limb of the SCR, Edelberg (1970) has reported that response recovery is generally speeded during goal-oriented behaviors such as performance of reaction time tasks. Edelberg later found that the introduction of stress into the reaction time task slows the characteristically fast recovery of responses (Edelberg, 1971). Hypothesizing that anxious individuals might behave as if in a persistent stress situation, Edelberg (1971) correlated anxiety, as measured by the Spielberger Anxiety Test, with recovery speed. He found a significant negative correlation between the two measures. Edelberg suggests that the apprehension of anxious individuals might be the significant factor to account for their slower response recovery.

The interesting work of Epstein and Fenz on electrodermal responsiveness of sport parachutists (Epstein, 1967) deserves mention here, even though it does not meet the criterion of including an independent measure of anxiety. The unique feature of these studies on sport parachutists is that the stimuli to which sport parachutists' EDRs were measured were stimuli relevant to the anxiety-producing situation. Skin conductance responses of both novice and experienced parachutists were measured on days of jumps as well as nonjump days. On nonjump days experienced and novice parachutists exhibited similar responsiveness patterns. The more relevant to sport parachuting the stimulus word, the greater the response. This responsiveness gradient was not found among control subjects. The specificity of sport parachutists' greater responsiveness was further demonstrated by the finding among novice parachutists of larger responses to highly relevant (to parachuting) words than to more general anxiety words (Epstein & Fenz, 1962).

As the parachutist gains experience, an alteration takes place in the relationship between stimulus relevance to anxiety source and response magnitude (Epstein, 1962), on jump days only. The experienced jumper, rather than responding maximally to the most relevant words, shows his greatest response to words lower on the relevance dimension. Plotting SCR magnitude against stimulus relevance, Epstein and Fenz have consistently found an inverted V-shaped curve for experienced parachutists on the day of the jump. With experience, the peak of the V moves in the direction of lower stimulus word relevance. To account for this phenomenon, the authors hypothesize that repeated exposure to a source of stress leads to the development of anxiety as well as inhibition, with the inhibition developing to a greater extent to the more relevant, a opposed to the less relevant cues.

The Epstein and Fenz work on sport parachutists emphasizes the complexity of determinants of responsiveness in anxiety—at least in state, as opposed to trait, anxiety. A great number of factors, such as degree and quality of experience with the anxiety-producing situation, proximity to anxiety-producing situation, and relevance of the stimulus to the anxiety-producing situation, combine to determine electrodermal responsiveness to specific stimuli. In trait anxiety, where the anxiety source is obscure, the significance of these variables cannot be evaluated. In fact, they may be irrelevant if the anxiety is so pervasive that all situations are equally arousing.

3. Habituation

The literature reveals a mixed picture with respect to the relationship between habituation and anxiety. Bitterman and Holtzman (1952), as well as Katkin and McCubbin (1969), looked at habituation to tones in high and low anxious subjects, and found no habituation differences. Similarly, Koepke and Pribram (1966) demonstrated that anxiety scores were unrelated to two measures of habituation. Epstein and Fenz (1970), on the other hand, saw some evidence of habituation differences in their data. Analyzing the electrodermal activity of three subscales of the Epstein–Fenz Manifest Anxiety Scale (striated muscle tension, autonomic arousal, and feelings of insecurity) they found significant differences in habituation of specific responses for various levels of striated muscle tension only. Examination of SCL over trials showed that this measure differentiated those scoring high, medium, and low on two of the three subscales; namely, striated muscle tension and autonomic arousal.

4. Conditioning

The question of whether electrodermal conditionability of high anxious subjects is greater than that of low anxious persons has not been answered consistently. Spence and Spence's (1966) well-known finding of greater eyelid conditioning among anxious individuals has not received solid support in the electrodermal area. Thus, Bitterman and Holtzman (1952) and Becker and Matteson (1961) found superior conditioning among anxious persons, while Clum (1969) and Streiner and Dean (1968) failed to note the effect.

Bitterman and Holtzman (1952), employing a tone-shock paradigm, used median SRRs to the CR to evaluate conditioning. Although median CRs were approximately equal for the high and low anxiety groups during the first few conditioning trials, CR amplitude of high anxious subjects reached a higher peak than that of low anxious subjects. Other evidence of superior conditioning of high anxious subjects was demonstrated in the extinction period, as a significant decline in CR amplitude was found only for low anxiety groups.

Less clear-cut conditioning differences have been found in two studies. Using subjects who scored at the extremes of Cattell's Anxiety (A) Scale, Becker and Matteson (1961) administered shock to condition subjects to the word *repeat*. They found greater SRR amplitudes to this word among high anxious subjects, when basal resistance was partialed out by analysis of covariance. However, a second, stricter index of conditioning, which involved counting the number of trials on which CR amplitude was at least 50% of preceding UR amplitude, did not differentiate the two groups. Streiner and Dean (1968) took Ss who scored in the highest and lowest quartiles of the Mandler and Sarason Test Anxiety Scale and attempted to condition them to a light by pairing it with shock. Although CR amplitudes did not differ for the two groups during the conditioning phase, extinction was faster for low anxiety subjects. Streiner and Dean examined only the data for the last 30 conditioning trials. One wonders whether conditioning might have been established earlier, and if so, whether differences between anxiety groups would have been seen in the first 30 trials.

A study failing to find CR differences during both conditioning and extinction is that of Clum (1969). A differential conditioning paradigm was used to condition Ss to a tone.

A number of factors could contribute toward the lack of consistency in the findings of the above studies. Each investigative team determined anxiety groups by different means. That the anxiety test used is a significant variable was demonstrated by Bitterman and Holtzman (1952) whose significant conditionability differences did not hold up when the anxiety measure was Taylor's MAS. In addition, some studies used only Ss at the extremes of the anxiety continuum, while others divided their Ss on the basis of whether they scored above or below the group median. These studies also varied widely with respect to the kinds of data used in the analyses and the ways in which these data were analyzed. Some used frequency; others amplitude. Some partialed out the effect of basal electrodermal levels; others did not. All of the studies except that of

Clum (1969) looked at group differences. Clum correlated anxiety with conditioning, and found the correlation nonsignificant.

It appears that greater conditionability of more anxious subjects is a possibility but that experimental paradigm, method of choosing anxiety groups, and data analysis procedures are important variables determining whether the effect is seen. Conditionability may be enhanced in high anxious subjects when simple conditioning is examined, but, as suggested by Clum (1969), impaired when a discrimination conditioning paradigm is employed. Finally, the definition of anxiety, and the question of how anxiety level should be determined, need thorough review.

B. General Psychiatric Population

Since anxiety is a symptom that accompanies a wide variety of psychiatric diagnostic categories, the relationship between anxiety and electrodermal activity is of interest to those seeking to determine the etiology of various psychiatric disorders. Basal levels, spontaneous activity, responsiveness, and conditioning have been examined and related to anxiety levels.

1. Basal Levels and Nonspecific Responses

The results with respect to basal electrodermal measures have been disappointing. Zuckerman et al. (1968) correlated clinical ratings of anxiety with SRL and failed to find a significant correlation. McReynolds, Acker, and Brackbill (1966) confirmed the above finding with SCL. In addition, these authors looked at SCL as a function of anxiety ratings with individuals, over time, a measure that is perhaps more meaningful than the interindividual approach. These intraindividual correlations were also found to be nonsignificant.

Spontaneous activity has received attention from Zuckerman et al. (1968), who measured it at two points in their experiment. The first was at the beginning of the experimental session, while the second reading was taken just prior to the cold pressor test. A significant correlation was found between spontaneous activity and anxiety ratings in the first, but not the second, instance.

2. Responsiveness

Little information is available regarding the correspondence between electrodermal responsiveness and anxiety in psychiatric patients. A crude responsiveness measure was taken by the Zuckerman group. They subtracted poststress SCL from prestress SCL for each subject, and correlated this with anxiety ratings. The relationship was not significant. There is thus no evidence that responsiveness is a function of anxiety level within a general psychiatric population. Different results have been reported by Dureman and Saaren-Seppälä (1963), for a largely depressive group of subjects. Responsiveness to the US was of greater amplitude for the more anxious of these depressed patients.

3. CONDITIONING

The bulk of the studies of electrodermal measures of anxiety in psychiatric patients deal with electrodermal conditioning. Interest in this type of research developed from the Taylor–Spence (Taylor, 1956) theory that heightened drive, reflected in high anxiety, should facilitate conditioning. As reported above, conditioning results for normal populations have been mixed. One explanation for the failure to find significant effects of anxiety within normal subjects is that the anxiety range for these individuals may not be sufficiently large. Psychiatric patients should provide a wider range of values within the anxiety variable, and therefore results more in line with those of Taylor (1951) would be expected.

In fact, findings have been no more positive for psychiatric, than with normal populations. Evidence has been presented for (1) increased conditionability with increased anxiety (Welch & Kubis, 1947; Gilberstadt & Davenport, 1960), (2) decreased conditionability with increasing anxiety levels (Clum, 1969), and (3) no relationship between anxiety and conditionability within psychiatric populations (Gilberstadt & Davenport, 1960; Dureman & Saaren-Seppälä, 1963). Although these studies report conflicting results, examination of methodological differences among the investigations provides us with some reasonable explanations for this diversity.

Two factors seem to be potentially responsible. The first is method for determining anxiety levels. Conditionability was positively related to anxiety when anxiety ratings were based upon rather thorough clinical evaluations (Welch & Kubis, 1947; Gilberstadt & Davenport, 1960). Either no relationship or negative relationships have been found when anxiety levels were determined according to the Taylor MAS or more cursory clinical ratings (Gilberstadt & Davenport, 1960; Dureman & Saaren-Seppälä, 1963; Clum, 1969).

A second possible source of variance is data evaluation method. Neither study that reported positive findings (Welch & Kubis, 1947; Gilberstadt & Davenport, 1960) utilized data from either URs or CRs on CS$^-$ trials to correct for magnitude or frequency of CR responses to the reinforced stimuli. What appeared to be evidence of superior conditioning among more highly anxious patients could have merely reflected greater sensitization or responsivity within this group. When corrections have been made for UR amplitude in the simple conditioning paradigm (Dureman & Saaren-Seppälä, 1963) and response to CS⁻ in the differential conditioning paradigm (Clum, 1969), the results have not been positive.

C. Anxiety States

In their effort to relate anxiety to physiological measures, some investigators have looked at electrodermal activity of psychiatric patients whose chief symptom is anxiety. If electrodermal activity is a function of anxiety, a study of persons at the extremes of the anxiety continuum should maximize chances of observing this relationship. In fact, studies of anxiety patients have met with more success than those utilizing normal or general psychiatric subjects.

1. BASAL LEVELS AND NONSPECIFIC RESPONSES

Basal measures of electrodermal activity, including both resting levels and spontaneous fluctuations, generally indicate higher levels for anxious patients than for normal subjects. For resting levels Howe (1958) has reported lower SRLs among anxiety subjects than for normals. Lader and Wing (1964, 1966) have confirmed this finding with log SCL. Basal levels in both studies were measured in the period between electrode application and presentation of stimuli. Lader and Wing (1964, 1966) took additional log SCL readings during the subsequent period of tonal stimulation, and found SCLs elevated during the latter part of the series.

Results that disagree with those discussed above have been presented by Goldstein (1964), and by Kelly, Brown, and Shaffer (1970). In these studies anxious patients did not differ from normal subjects in SRL or SCL. Differences in experimental procedures may be the key to the discrepancy between these results and those reported above. It appears that only the experimental procedures of Goldstein and Kelly, Brown and Shaffer ensured maximal relaxation of Ss. In both studies subjects lay on a bed or couch, rather than sitting in a chair, as in the above investigations. Also, approximately 1 hour elapsed between the time Goldstein's (1964) Ss came into the room and recording began. This may have been a longer relaxation period than for the other studies, and lying on a bed for this amount of time, rather than sitting, would make a difference in degree of relaxation achieved.

Discrepancies in the results reported here are reminiscent of those between the studies of Taylor and Spence, as opposed to Franks (1956), of eyelid conditioning. Franks' experimental setting was a much more relaxing and pleasant one. In his study anxious subjects did not exhibit better eyelid conditioning, as they had in Spence's uncomfortable dental chair.

Besides showing higher resting levels, at least under some conditions, anxiety subjects have also demonstrated greater numbers of spontaneous electrodermal fluctuations than have normals (Malmo, Shagass, Davis, Cleghorn, Graham, & Goodman, 1948; Lader & Wing, 1964, 1966; and Lader, 1967). Spontaneous fluctuations were greater for anxiety subjects during prestimulus resting period (Lader & Wing, 1964, 1966), as well as during habituation series (Lader & Wing, 1964, 1966; Lader, 1967; and Malmo et al., 1948).

During the resting period of the Kelly, Brown, and Shaffer (1970) study, however, spontaneous activity was not greater for anxious Ss. Again, Ss' comfort may have been the relevant factor. Unfortunately, Goldstein (1964) did not report data on spontaneous activity. It would have been interesting to see whether the discrepancies between her results and those of the above investigators with respect to basal levels would have held for spontaneous activity as well.

2. Responsiveness

Comparison of studies dealing with responsiveness of anxiety patients is difficult because of the variety of evaluation methods used by different investigators. Goldstein (1964) subtracted poststimulus SRL from prestimulus level for her measure of responsiveness and found no difference between anxious female patients and normal female controls. Lader and Wing (1964, 1966) as well as Lader (1967) compared response magnitudes to the first of a series of tones, and found that these were essentially the same for normals and anxiety patients. The Lader and Wing (1964, 1966) study included a second responsiveness measure, the points at which regression equations for the two groups, if extended, would cross the y axis. Since this value was greater for normals, the authors concluded that early responding was greater for normals. Anxiety patients responded more frequently to tones than did schizophrenics, according to Stewart et al. (1959), who employed still another means of assessing responsiveness. The values compared were number of subjects who responded on *more* than versus *less* than a certain number of habituation trials. No normal subjects were included in this study, which makes it even harder to compare with the others. One can conclude from the above evidence at least that there is little demonstration of responsiveness differences between normal and anxiety subjects.

3. HABITUATION AND CONDITIONING

Habituation to specific stimuli is apparently slowed in anxiety patients. This has been demonstrated in a number of ways by Stewart *et al.* (1959), Lader and Wing (1964, 1966), and Lader (1967). Lader and Wing (1964, 1966) found that log SCL habituated more rapidly for anxiety subjects during both the rest period preceding stimulation and during the stimulation session itself. A second Lader study, however (Lader, 1967), failed to confirm this effect. Habituation rates as measured by slopes of regression lines also distinguished normal from anxiety subjects (Lader & Wing, 1964, 1966; Lader, 1967). A third way in which habituation has been evaluated (Lader & Wing, 1964, 1966; Lader, 1967) is by analyzing the significance of each subject's regression equation (conductance/trials). Those subjects showing significantly steep regression equations were designated as habituators. Lader and Wing's (1964, 1966) data showed that only 6 of 20 anxiety patients were habituators, while all 20 normal subjects were habituators. Similarly, 7 of 16 and 64 of 75 anxiety and normal subjects, respectively, were found to be habituators in the Lader (1967) study. No habituation data *per se* are presented in the Stewart *et al.* (1959) paper, but if number of responses can be considered as a crude index of habituation, then anxiety subjects in this study showed greater habituation than did schizophrenic subjects. A normal group was not included in this study.

With respect to electrodermal conditioning, anxiety subjects may condition more readily than normals. Howe (1958), using a simple conditioning paradigm with tone and shock found that responses to tone during extinction were greater (log conductance change) for anxiety than for both normal and schizophrenic patients. Consistent with this is the trend ($p < .10$) in the direction of more anticipatory responses among anxiety neurotics than among schizophrenics reported by Stewart *et al.* (1959).

In summary, the data on electrodermal activity and anxiety do not allow us to form a definitive picture of their relationship. Inconsistencies in methodologies and data evaluation procedures, already noted, make comparison of studies difficult. It seems clear, however, that striking relationships between these two measures have not been discovered, no matter how the question has been approached. This has been especially true when anxiety within normal subjects has been considered and may be attributable to the narrow anxiety band available within normal populations. Among a general psychiatric population one can hardly be surprised that the unitary dimension, anxiety, is not very successful in differentiating patients' electrodermal behaviors, in light of the broad range of very prominent symptoms other than anxiety that these individuals exhibit. The most fruitful approach may be to compare anxiety patients, persons whose anxiety levels are so high as to make normal existence extremely difficult, with psychiatrically normal individuals. This ensures a wide range of anxiety levels, and minimizes variance attributable to heterogeneity of more general psychiatric populations. Studies utilizing these groups have, in fact, been more successful in finding differences in electrodermal activity as a function of anxiety.

Finally, even though anxiety may be considered as a relatively nonspecific fear (Epstein, 1967), it seems evident that the expectation of negatively reinforcing events that characterizes anxiety cannot be totally undirected, albeit greatly generalized. The importance of this distinction is that the dimension, anxiety, should not be considered as separate from the situational context. The implication for studies of anxiety is that variables such as lighting in the experimental room, sex of experimenter, physical comfort of S, stimuli, instructions to subjects—in fact, all procedural variables—may be very relevant to the results (Sarason, 1960). Subjects' differential responses to contextual variables may contribute so much variance that the effects of the so-called independent variable, anxiety, may be totally obscured. Contextual variables should be especially relevant in studies of state anxiety, as opposed to trait anxiety (see Spielberger, Lushene, & McAdoo, 1970), anxiety which has become generalized to many situations.

VIII.   Introversion–Extroversion

For Eysenck (1967) the dimensions of introversion–extroversion (I/E) and that of neuroticism (N) are orthogonal to each other. Physiological measures, such as electrodermal and cardiac activity under conditions of minimal stimulation (nonstress), relate to the I/E dimension with the I person demonstrating greater arousal on such measures. The dimension of neuroticism enters the arena only under conditions of "stress," with the neurotic being more "aroused" by such stress. Eysenck differentiates, at least at a theoretical level, the loci of action of arousal with respect to these two dimensions. The I/E dimension is related to arousal at the brain stem reticular activation system level, while arousal associated with neuroticism is localized in the limbic area or cerebral cortex in general. Thus, studies which do not attempt to maintain one of these variables constant should come up with confounded results or at least with significant interaction effects.

It would, of course, be delightful if arousal as mediated through these two differing physiological response systems were differentially expressed in the electrodermal system. Interestingly, there are two measures of arousal that are in reasonably common use by researchers utilizing electrodermal measures—namely, SCL, SRL, SPL, as well as incidence of nonspecific responses, or spontaneous fluctuations. It is also well known that these two measures of arousal are far from perfectly correlated with each other. As a matter of fact, a coefficient of correlation turns out to be an inappropriate statistic to evaluate the relationship between these measures since the assumption of homoscedasticity is violated when one relates these two measures to each other. The scatterplot relating these two measures is triangular in nature as depicted in Fig. 1 (Stern, 1963, unpublished). Thus, low arousal in one measure is generally accompanied by low arousal in the other measure. However, when we turn to other points on the arousal dimension, one sees that though arousal as expressed in one measure places upper limits on arousability as measured by the other variable, it cannot be used to predict the level of arousal as measured in the second response system. If we allow ourselves to extrapolate (something which in the absence of data we do with some reluctance), and assume that one of these measures of arousal is related to brain stem reticular activating system (BSRAS) activity and the other to cortical activity (we decline to speculate about which is related to what), they then should be related to measures of the introversion/extroversion (I/E) and neuroticism (N) dimension.

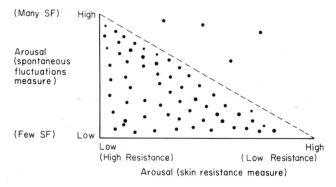

Fig. 1

How do our other measures of electrodermal activity, namely, orienting responses, defensive and adaptive responses, and conditional responses fit into this picture? Speed of inhibition of ORs or habituation is, within the Sokolovian model (1963, 1969), a joint function of the cortex and of the brainstem reticular activating system. Rapid habituation can be a function of the rapid development of a cortical model. It can, however, equally parsimoniously be a function of a low level of RAS activity, so that there is little for the cortex to inhibit. Speed of habituation could thus be equally effectively a function of the I/E as of the N dimension. Slowest habituation should occur where both I and N are high—and this apparently is true (Lader & Wing, 1964), but high I and low N, or low I and high N might well lead to nondiscriminable habituation rates.

With respect to adaptive or defensive responses, which presumably are principally mediated by the BSRAS, and thus more related to the I/E than the N dimension, one should see amplitude differences between E and I subjects, and perhaps even threshold and pain tolerance differences. The only studies dealing with this problem which we are aware of provide us with negative results. Psychopaths (high E) demonstrate electrodermal responses to electric shock stimulation no different from other groups of subjects (Hare, 1970), and do not demonstrate threshold or pain tolerance differences from normal controls. It might, of course, be possible that other ways of attacking this problem might come up with more supportive results. For example, it may be that if one looked at amplitude of electrodermal defensive responses as related to stimulus intensity that I and E groups would generate different relationships. Introverts might start responding at a lower intensity of stimulation and develop transmarginal inhibition earlier than extroverted subjects, or there may be differences in recovery rate, a variable which is currently arousing some investigative interest (Edelberg, 1970).

A second approach might be to identify psychoactive agents which exert their (principal) effect on one or the other arousal area and study differential responding in I/E and N groups. The horizon of possible studies appears, as always, unlimited.

We prefer not to say anything at this time about conditional responses. We believe that the discrimination of different conditional responses rather than the identification of "the" conditional response will be more likely to shed light on these problems than has been true in the past.

With these wild speculations out of the way, let us now turn to some studies utilizing Eysenck's scales measuring the dimensions of introversion–extroversion and that of neuroticism. These measures continue to enjoy investigative appeal for researchers interested in relating dimensions of personality to physiological measures. Though, as we have indicated in a previous review (Stern & Plapp, 1969), we suspect that little gold is being mined in these hills with current techniques, investigators continue to attack these mountains with the same sandbox tools. Unfortunately, they are the only tools at our disposal and the hope of these investigators of course is that they will find a soft vein of ore which either is precious in itself, or will allow them access to the core of the mountain where there is a richer lode.

Representative of recent studies are those by Coles, Gale and Kline (1971) and Sadler, Mefferd and Houck (1971). Since, in some respects, they come to diametrically opposed conclusions, their work might be described as "representative." Coles and co-workers studied habituation of electrodermal ORs in subjects who, on the basis of their performance on the MPI, had been assigned to the following groups: HE–HN; ME–HN; LE–HN; HE–LN; ME–LN; and LE–LN (HE, ME, LE stand for high, medium and low extroversion; HN, LN for high and low neuroticism, respectively). Each subject was exposed to 20 trials of a 5-sec, 65-dB tone at 2-min intervals. These authors found the high neurotic group to habituate more slowly than the low neurotic group, extroverts to give fewer spontaneous responses than introverts, and reported that tonic conductance measures failed to discriminate between groups.

Sadler and co-workers studied habituation to 20 consonant trigrams, presented at random ITIs. Four groups of subjects were utilized: LN–LE, LN–HE, HN–LE, and HN–HE. These authors found their LN groups to habituate more slowly than their HN groups (though not at a statistically acceptable level of confidence) with LN–LE habituating more slowly than the LN–HE group.

In response to the first stimulus of the habituation series, these authors report an interaction effect between the dimension of extroversion and neuroticism. LN–LE and HN–HE groups produced larger amplitude ORs than was true of the other two groups. Basal skin resistance changes during the experiment also showed this interaction effect with lowering of resistance of the LN–LE and HN–HE groups while the other two groups demonstrated an increase in basal skin resistance over trials.

One might ask about the basis for the continued interest in relating dimensions of introversion–extroversion and neuroticism to psychophysiological measures of habituation and conditioning. The basis lies in an attempt to reconcile Russian and Western neurophysiologizing concerning the relationship between temperament and physiology. Russian experimenters, in the honored tradition of Pavlov, have identified processes of inhibition and excitation and the balance between these two processes as basic dimensions of personality. What is unclear is whether the dimensions of inhibition and excitation are two dimensions or a unitary one, with inhibition and excitation as the polar extremes. Gray's interpretation of Teplov's work (1964) holds to the latter position and he interprets this dimension to be similar to Western conceptualizations of arousal or arousability. The weak nervous system (introversion) is described as more sensitive than the strong; it responds to lower intensities of stimulation and develops transmarginal inhibition at lower intensity levels than is true of the strong nervous system (extroversion). The strong nervous system, on the other hand, develops cortical inhibition more readily than the weak system.

One further concept is introduced by Eysenck, the dimension of neuroticism, which he claims to be independent of the I/E dimension. What is reasonably clear from the literature relating electrodermal responses to measures of I/E and N is that these dimensions are not independent, but interact.

What is the evidence in studies involving electrodermal measures that the I/E dimension discriminates between those who develop cortical or internal inhibition rapidly versus slowly? The development of cortical inhibition is generally associated with such variables as lowering levels of arousal, the development of fatigue, and the speed with which subjects go to sleep when exposed to a monotonous environment.

Most studies of habituation involve monotonous stimulation, usually simple stimuli presented at random intervals.

Gross and Stern (1967) have demonstrated that such stimulation leads to more rapid increases in skin resistance than is true when the subject simply sits in the same environment without experimenter-controlled stimuli. If we look at representative studies of I/E which report changes in resting levels of skin resistance during habituation, the results are concordant if one controls for neuroticism. Sadler et al. (1971) found that if one looks at low neuroticism groups, the introverted group demonstrates a lowering of resistance over trials while the high extroverted group demonstrates an increase in skin resistance over trials.

Coles et al. (1971) using nonspecific responses as the measure of arousal find extroverts to be less aroused as measured by a lower level of such responses. Unfortunately, their measures of SCL failed to discriminate between groups.

Acknowledgments

This research was supported in part by USPHS Grants MH12043 and MH7081.

References

Alexander, L. Objective approach to psychiatric diagnosis and evaluation of drug effects by means of the conditional reflex technique. *Biological psychiatry*, Chapter 13. New York: Grune & Stratton, 1959. Pp. 154–183.

Astrup, C. Conditional reflex studies of schizophrenics treated with ataraxic drugs. *Proceedings of the Third World Congress on Psychiatry*, 1966, 999–1001.

Ax, A. F., & Bamford, J. L. The GSR recovery limb in chronic schizophrenia. *Psychophysiology*, 1970, 7, 145–147.

Ax, A. F., Bamford, J. L., Beckett, P. G., Fretz, N. F., & Gottlieb, J. S. Autonomic conditioning in chronic schizophrenia. *Journal of Abnormal Psychology*, 1970, 76, 140–154.

Baer, P. E. Unexpected effects of masking: Differential EDR conditioning without relational learning. Paper presented at the Eleventh Annual Meeting of the Society for Psychophysiological Research, 1971.

Baer, P. E., & Fuhrer, M. J. Cognitive processes during differential trace and delayed conditioning of the GSR. *Journal of Experimental Psychology*, 1968, 78, 81–88.

Baer, P. E., & Fuhrer, M. J. Cognitive factors in differential conditioning of the GSR: Use of a reaction time task as the UCS with normals and schizophrenics. *Journal of Abnormal Psychology*, 1969, 74, 544–552.

Bagg, C. E., & Crookes, T. G. Palmar digital sweating in women suffering from depression. *The British Journal of Psychiatry*, 1966, 112, 1251–1255.

Bassett, M., & Ashby, W. R. The effect of electro-convulsive therapy on the psychogalvanic response. *Journal of Mental Science*, 1954, 100, 632–642.

Baumeister, A., Beedle, R., & Urquhart, D. GSR conditioning in normals and retardates. *American Journal of Mental Deficiency*, 1964, 69, 114–120.

Beck, A. *Depression: Clinical, experimental, and theoretical aspects.* New York: Harper, 1967.

Becker, W. C., & Matteson, H. H. GSR conditioning, anxiety and extraversion. *Journal of Abnormal and Social Psychology*, 1961, 62, 427–430.

Berkson, G. Responsiveness of the mentally deficient. *American Journal of Mental Deficiency*, 1961, 66, 277–286.

Berkson, G., Hermelin, B., & O'Connor, N. Physiological responses of normals and institutionalized mental defectives to repeated stimuli. *Journal of Mental Deficiency Research*, 1961, 5, 30–39.

Bernal, M. E., & Miller, L. H. Electrodermal and cardiac responses of schizophrenic children to sensory stimuli. *Psychophysiology*, 1971, 7, 155–168.

Bernstein, A. S. Electrodermal base level, tonic arousal, and adaptation in chronic schizophrenics. *Journal of Abnormal Psychology*, 1967, 72, 221–232.

Bernstein, A. S. Electrodermal orienting responses in chronic schizophrenics: Manifest confusion as a significant dimension. In D. V. Siva Sankar (Ed.), *Schizophrenia, current concepts and research.* Hicksville, New York: PJD Publications, Ltd., 1969.

Bernstein, A. S. Phasic electrodermal orienting responses in chronic schizophrenics: II. Response to auditory signals of varying intensity. *Journal of Abnormal Psychology*, 1970, 75, 146–156.

Bitterman, M., & Holtzman, W. Conditioning and extinction as a function of anxiety. *Journal of Abnormal and Social Psychology*, 1952, 47, 615–623.

Borkovec, T. D. Autonomic reactivity to sensory stimulation in psychopathic, neurotic and normal juvenile delinquents. *Journal of Consulting and Clinical Psychology*, 1970, 35, 217–222.

Bower, A., & Das, J. Acquisition and reversal of orienting responses to word signals. Paper presented at Canadian Psychological Association, 1970.

Boydstun, J. A., Ackerman, P. T., Stevens, D. A., Clements, S. D., Peters, J. E.,

& Dykman, R. A. Physiologic and motor conditioning and generalization in children with minimal brain dysfunctions. *Conditional Reflex*, 1968, 3, 81–104.

Bridger, W. Is there a classical conditioning without cognitive expectancy? Paper presented at Eleventh Annual Meeting of the Society for Psychophysiological Research, 1971.

Brivllova, S. V. On some aspects of the orienting reflex in persons having suffered a covert trauma of the brain and neurotic persons. In L. G. Voronin, A. N. Leontiev, A. R. Luria, E. N., Sokolov, & O. S. Vinogradova (Eds.), *Orienting reflex and exploratory behavior*. Washington, D.C.: American Institute of Biological Sciences, 1965. Pp. 343–350.

Burdick, J. A. Arousal measurement in schizophrenics and normals. *Activitas Nervosa Superior*, 1968, 10, 369–372.

Clausen, J., & Karrer, R. Orienting response-frequency of occurrence and relationship to other autonomic variables. *American Journal of Mental Deficiency*, 1968, 73, 455–464.

Clausen, J., & Karrer, R. Temporal factors in autonomic responses for normal and mentally defective subjects. *American Journal of Mental Deficiency*, 1969, 74, 80–85.

Clausen, J., & Karrer, R. Autonomic activity during rest in normal and mentally deficient subjects. *American Journal of Mental Deficiency*, 1970, 75(3), 361–370.

Clum, G. A. A correlational analysis of the relationships between personality and perceptual variables and discriminant GSR conditioning. *Journal of Clinical Psychology*, 1969, 25, 33–35.

Cohen, N. I., & Douglas, V. I. Characteristics of the orienting response in hyperactive and normal children. Unpublished manuscript, 1969.

Coles, M. G. H., Gale, A., & Kline, P. Personality and habituation of the orienting reaction: Tonic and response measures of electrodermal activity. *Psychophysiology*, 1971, 8, 54–63.

Collman, R. The galvanic skin responses of mentally retarded and other children in England. *American Journal of Mental Deficiency*, 1959, 63, 626–632.

Corah, N. L., & Stern, J. A. Stability and adaptation of some measures of electrodermal activity in children. *Journal of Experimental Psychology*, 1963, 65, 80–85.

Crooks, R., & McNulty, J. Autonomic response specificity in normal and schizophrenic subjects. *Canadian Journal of Psychology*, 1966, 20, 280–295.

Das, J., & Bower, A. Orienting responses of mentally retarded and normal subjects to word signals. *British Journal of Psychology*, 1971, 62(Pt. 1), 89–96.

Davidoff, R. A., & McDonald, D. G. Alpha blocking and autonomic responses in neurological patients: A study of EEG and autonomic conditioning. *Archives of Neurology*, 1964, 10, 283–292.

Dawson, M. Cognition and conditioning: Effects of marking the CS-UCS contingency in human GSR classical conditioning. *Journal of Experimental Psychology*, 1970, 85, 389–396.

Dawson, M. Classical conditioning and relational learning: Validation of questionnaires. Paper presented at Eleventh Annual Meeting of the Society for Psychophysiological Research, 1971.

Dmitriev, L. I., Belyakova, L. I., Bondarenko, T. T., & Nikolaev, G. V. A study of the orienting and defensive reflexes in schizophrenics at different stages in the course of the disease. *Zhurnal Nevropatologii i Psikhiatrii*, 1968, 68(5), 713–719.

Dureman, I., & Saaren-Seppälä, P. Electrodermal reactivity as related to self-ratings, and clinical ratings of anxiety and depression. 15th Report, December 1963, University of Uppsala, Uppsala, Sweden.

Edelberg, R. The information content of the recovery limb of the electrodermal response. *Psychophysiology*, 1970, 6, 527–539.

Edelberg, R. The relation of slow electrodermal recovery rate to protective behavior. Paper presented at *Society for Psychophysiological Research*, St. Louis, October, 1971.

Elithorn, A., Piercy, M. F., & Crosskey, M. A. Prefrontal leutocomy and the anticipation of pain. *Journal of Neurology, Neurosurgery, and Psychiatry*, 1955, 18, 34–43.

Ellis, N. The stimulus trace and behavioral inadequacy. In N. R. Ellis (Ed.), *Handbook in mental deficiency: Psychological theory and research*. New York: McGraw-Hill, 1963.

Ellis, N., & Sloan, W. The relationship between intelligence and skin conductance. *American Journal of Mental Deficiency*, 1958, 63, 304–306.

Epstein, S. The measurement of drive and conflict in humans: Theory and experiment. In M. R. Jones (Ed.), *Nebraska Symposium on motivation: 1962*. Lincoln: Univ. of Nebraska Press, 1962. Pp. 281–321.

Epstein, S. Toward a unified theory of anxiety. In B. A. Maher (Ed.), *Progress in experimental personality research: Vol. 4*. New York: Academic Press, 1967. Pp. 1–89.

Epstein, S. Expectancy and magnitude of reaction of UCS. Paper presented at the Eleventh Annual Meeting of the Society for Psychophysiological Research, 1971.

Epstein, S., & Fenz, W. Theory and experiment on the measurement of approach-avoidance conflict. *Journal of Abnormal and Social Psychology*, 1962, 64, 97–112.

Epstein, S., & Fenz, W. Habituation to a loud sound as a function of manifest anxiety. *Journal of Abnormal and Social Psychology*, 1970, 75, 189–194.

Epstein, S., & Roupenian, A. Heart rate and skin conductance during experimentally induced anxiety: The effect of uncertainty about receiving a noxious stimulus. *Journal of Personality and Social Psychology*, 1970, 16, 20–28.

Eysenck, H. J. *The biological basis of personality*. Springfield, Illinois: Thomas, 1967.

Fenz, W. D., & Dronsejko, K. Effects of real and imagined threat of shock on GSR and heart rate as a function of trait anxiety. *Journal of Experimental Research in Personality*, 1969, 3, 187–196.

Fenz, W. D., & Epstein, S. Gradiants of physiological arousal of experienced and novice parachutists as a function of an approaching jump. *Psychosomatic Medicine*, 1967, 29, 33–51.

Fenz, W. D., & McCabe, M. Habituation of the GSR to tones in retarded children and nonretarded subjects. *American Journal of Mental Deficiency*, 1971, 75, 470–473.

Fenz, W. D., & Steffy, R. A. Electrodermal arousal of chronically ill psychiatric patients undergoing intensive behavioral treatment. *Psychosomatic Medicine*, 1968, 30, 423–436.

Fenz, W. D., & Velner, J. Physiological concomitants of behavioral indexes of schizophrenia. *Journal of Abnormal Psychology*, 1970, 76, 27–35.

Fox, R., & Lippert, W. Spontaneous GSR and anxiety level in sociopathic delinquents. *Journal of Consulting Psychology*, 1963, 27, 368.

Franks, C. Conditioning and personality: A study of normal and neurotic subjects. *Journal of Abnormal and Social Psychology,* 1956, **52**, 143–150.

Fuhrer, M., & Baer, P. Differential classical conditioning: Verbalization of stimulus contingencies. *Science,* 1965, **150**, 1479–1481.

Fuhrer, M. J., & Baer, P. E. Preparatory instructions in the differential conditioning of the galvanic skin response of schizophrenics and normals. *Journal of Abnormal Psychology,* 1970, **76**, 482–484.

Furedy, J. Some limits on the cognitive conditional autonomic behavior. Paper presented at the *Eleventh Annual Meeting of the Society for Psychophysiological Research,* 1971.

Galkowski, T., Dadas, H., & Domanski, R. Psychogalvanic reflex in oligophrenic children. *Developmental Medicine and Child Neurology,* 1968, **10**(3), 349–354.

Gilberstadt, H., & Davenport, G. Some relationships between GSR conditioning and judgment of anxiety. *Journal of Abnormal and Social Psychology,* 1960, **60**, 441–443.

Goldstein, I. B. Physiological responses in anxious women patients. A study of autonomic activity and muscle tension. *Archives of General Psychiatry,* 1964, **10**, 382–388.

Goldstein, I. B. Relationship of muscle tension and autonomic activity to psychiatric disorder. *Psychosomatic Medicine,* 1965, **27**, 39–52.

Goldstein, M., & Acker, C. W. Psychophysiological reactions to films by chronic schizophrenics: II. Individual differences in resting levels and reactivity. *Journal of Abnormal Psychology,* 1967, **72**, 23–29.

Goldstein, M., Judd, L., Rodnick, E., & LaPolla, A. Psychophysiological and behavioral effects of phenothiazine administration in acute schizophrenics as a function of premorbid status. *Journal of Psychiatric Research,* 1969, **6**(4), 271–287.

Goldstein, R., Ludwig, H., & Naunton, R. F. Difficulty in conditioning galvanic skin responses: Its possible significance in clinical audiometry. *Acta Oto-Laryngologica,* 1954, **44**(Fasc. I), 67–77.

Graham, J. Signal magnitude and frequency of response in GSR audiometry. *American Journal of Mental Deficiency,* 1969, **74**(3), 397–400.

Grant, D. Cognitive factors in eyelid conditioning. Paper presented at the *Eleventh Annual Meeting of the Society for Psychophysiological Research,* 1971.

Gray, J. A. (Ed.) *Pavlov's typology.* Oxford: Pergamon, 1964.

Greenfield, N., Katz, D., Alexander, A., & Roessler, R. The relationship between physiological and psychological responsivity: Depression and galvanic skin response. *Journal of Nervous and Mental Disease,* 1963, **136**, 535–539.

Grings, W. W., Lockhart, R. A., & Dameron, L. E. Conditioning autonomic responses of mentally subnormal individuals. *Psychological Monographs,* 1962, **76** (No. 39), 1–35.

Gross, K., & Stern, J. A. Habituation of orienting responses as a function of "instructional set." *Conditional Reflex,* 1967, **2**, 23–36.

Hare, R. D. Acquisition and generalization of a conditioned-fear response in psychopathic and nonpsychopathic criminals. *Journal of Psychology,* 1965, **59**, 367–370. (a)

Hare, R. D. Temporal gradient of fear arousal in psychopaths. *Journal of Abnormal Psychology,* 1965, **70**, 442–445. (b)

Hare, R. D. Psychopathy, autonomic functioning, and the orienting response. *Journal of Abnormal Psychology,* Monograph Suppl., 1968, **73**(Pt. 2), 1–24.

Hare, R. D. *Psychopathy: Theory and research.* New York: Wiley, 1970.

Hare, R. D., & Quinn, M. J. ,Psychopathy and autonomic conditioning. *Journal of Abnormal Psychology,* 1971, **77,** 223–235.

Holloway, F. A., & Parsons, O. A. Unilateral brain damage and bilateral skin conductance levels in humans. *Psychophysiology,* 1969, **6,** 138–148.

Holloway, F. A., & Parsons, O. A. Habituation of the orienting reflex in brain damaged patients. *Psychophysiology,* 1971, **8,** 623–634.

Howe, E. S. GSR conditioning in anxiety states, normals, and chronic functional schizophrenic subjects. *Journal of Abnormal and Social Psychology,* 1958, **56,** 183–189.

Karrer, R. Autonomic nervous functions and behavior: A review of experimental studies with mental defectives. In N. R. Ellis (Ed.), *International Review of Research in Mental Retardation. Vol. 2.* New York: Academic Press, 1966.

Karrer, R., & Clausen, J. A comparison of mentally deficient and normal individuals upon four dimensions of autonomic activity. *Journal of Mental Deficiency Research,* 1964, **8,** 149–163.

Katkin, E. S. The relationship between manifest anxiety and two indices of autonomic response to stress. *Journal of Personality and Social Psychology,* 1965, **2,** 324–333. (a)

Katkin, E. S. The relationship beween a measure of transitory anxiety and spontaneous autonomic activity. Paper read at the Midwestern Psychological Association Meeting, 1965. (b)

Katkin, E. S., & McCubbin, R. J. Habituation of the orienting response as a function of individual differences in anxiety and autonomic lability. *Journal of Abnormal Psychology,* 1969, **74,** 54–60.

Katz, D. Inhibition of autonomic indicators of arousal by suggestion-induced relaxation: A verification and extension of the reciprocal inhibition principle. Doctoral dissertation, University of Michigan, 1971.

Kelly, D., Brown, C., & Shaffer, J. A comparison of physiological and psychological measurements on anxious patients and normal controls. *Psychophysiology,* 1970, **6,** 429–441.

Kodman, F., Fein, A., & Mixson, A. Psychogalvanic skin response audiometry with severe mentally retarded children. *American Journal of Mental Deficiency,* 1959, **64,** 131–136.

Koepke, J. E., & Pribram, K. H. Habituation of GSR as a function of stimulus duration and spontaneous activity. *Journal of Comparative and Physiological Psychology,* 1966, **61,** 442–448.

Lacey, J. I. Somatic response patterning and stress: Some revisions of activation theory. In M. Appley & R. Trumbull (Eds.), *Psychological Stress.* Chapter 2. New York: Appleton, 1967. Pp. 14–36.

Lader, M. H. Palmar skin conductance measures in anxiety and phobic states. *Journal of Psychosomatic Research,* 1967, **11,** 271–281.

Lader, M. H., & Wing, L. Habituation of the psychogalvanic reflex in patients with anxiety states and in normal subjects. *Journal of Neurology, Neurosurgery and Psychiatry,* 1964, **27,** 210–218.

Lader, M. H., & Wing, L. Physiological measures, sedative drugs and morbid anxiety. London: Maudsley Institute of Psychiatry Monograph, 1966.

Lader, M. H., & Wing, L. Physiological measures in agitated and retarded depressed patients. *Journal of Psychiatric Research,* 1969, **7,** 89–100.

Lindner, R. Experimental studies in constitutional psychopathic inferiority. Part I. Systemic patterns. *Journal of Criminal Psychopathology*, 1942, 3, 252–276.

Lippert, W. W., Jr., & Senter, R. J. Electrodermal responses in the sociopath. *Psychonomic Science*, 1966, 4, 25–26.

Lobb, H. Trace GSR conditioning with benzedrine, in mentally defective and normal adults. *American Journal of Mental Deficiency*, 1968, 73, 239–246.

Lobb, H. Frequency vs. magnitude of GSR in comparisons of retarded and nonretarded groups. *American Journal of Mental Deficiency*, 1970, 75(3), 336–340.

Lockhart, R. Cognitive processes and the multiple response phenomenon. Paper presented at the *Eleventh Annual Meeting of the Society for Psychophysiological Research*, 1971.

Lockhart, R., & Grings, W. W. Interstimulus interval effects in GSR discrimination conditioning. *Journal of Experimental Psychology*, 1964, 67, 209–214.

Luria, A. R. *Human brain and psychological processes*. New York: Harper, 1966.

Lykken, D. T. A study of anxiety in sociopathic personality. *Journal of Abnormal and Social Psychology*, 1957, 55, 6–10.

Lykken, D. T., & Maley, M. Autonomic versus cortical arousal in schizophrenics and non-psychotics. *Journal of Psychiatric Research*, 1968, 6, 21–32.

Malmo, R., Shagass, C., Davis, J., Cleghorn, R., Graham, B., & Goodman, A. Standardized pain stimulation as controlled stress in physiological studies of psychoneurosis. *Science*, 1948, 108, 509–511.

Mandler, G., & Sarason, S. A study of anxiety and learning. *Journal of Abnormal and Social Psychology*, 1952, 47, 166–173.

Martin, B. The assessment of anxiety by physiological behavioral measures. *Psychological Bulletin*, 1961, 58, 234–255.

McDonnell, G. J., & Carpenter, J. A. Anxiety, skin conductance and alcohol-A study of the relation between anxiety and skin conductance and the effect of alcohol on the conductance of subjects in a group. *Quarterly Journal of Studies on Alcohol.*, 1959, 20, 38–52.

McDonnell, G. J., & Carpenter, J. A. Manifest anxiety and prestimulus conductance levels. *Journal of Abnormal and Social Psychology*, 1960, 60, 437–438.

McReynolds, P., Acker, M., & Brackbill, G. On the assessment of Anxiety: IV. By measures of basal conductance and palmar sweat. *Psychological Reports*, 1966, 19, 347–356.

Mednick, S. A., & Schulsinger, F. Some premorbid characteristics related to breakdown in children with schizophrenic mothers. In D. Rosenthal & S. S. Kety (Eds.), *The transmission of schizophrenia*. Oxford: Pergamon, 1968. Pp. 267–291.

Neva, E., & Hicks, R. A new look at an old issue: Manifest Anxiety Scale validity. *Journal of Consulting and Clinical Psychology*, 1970 (Dec.), 35(3), 406–408.

O'Connor, N., & Venables, P. A note on the basal level of skin conductance and Binet I.Q. *British Journal of Psychology*, 1956, 42, 148–149.

Ödegaard, Ö. The psychogalvanic reactivity in affective disorders. *British Journal of Medical Psychology*, 1932, 72, 132–150.

Paintal, A. S. A comparison of the galvanic skin response of normals and psychotics. *Journal of Experimental Psychology*, 1951, 41, 425–428.

Parsons, O. A., & Chandler, P. J. Electrodermal indicants of arousal in brain damage: Cross-validated findings. *Psychophysiology*, 1969, 5, 644–659.

Peterson, F., & Jung, C. G. Psychophysical investigations with the galvanometer and plethysmograph in normal and insane individuals. *Brain*, 1897, 30, 153–218.

Pfister, H. O. Disturbances of the autonomic nervous system in schizophrenia and their relations to the insulin, cardiazol, and sleep treatments. *Journal of Psychiatry, Supplement*, 1938, **94**, 109–118.

Pilgrim, D., Miller, F., & Cobb, H. GSR strength and habituation in normal and non-organically mentally retarded children. *American Journal of Mental Deficiency*, 1969, **74**, 27–31.

Pishkin, V., & Hershiser, D. Respiration and GSR as functions of white sound in schizophrenia. *Journal of Consulting Psychology*, 1963, **27**, 330–337.

Pryer, R., & Ellis, N. Skin conductance and autonomic lability as a function of intelligence in mental defectives. *American Journal of Mental Deficiency*, 1959, **63**, 835–838.

Pugh, L. Response time and electrodermal measures in chronic schizophrenia: The effects of chlorpromazine. *Journal of Nervous and Mental Disease*, 1968, **146**, 62–70.

Raskin, D. Semantic conditioning and generalization of autonomic responses. *Journal of Experimental Psychology*, 1969, **79**, 69–76.

Reese, W. G., Doss, R., & Gantt, W. H. Autonomic responses in differential diagnosis of organic and psychogenic psychoses. American Medical Association, *Archives of Neurology and Psychiatry*, 1953, **70**, 778–793.

Roessler, R., Burch, N., & Childers, H. Personality and arousal correlates of specific galvanic skin responses. *Psychophysiology*, 1966, **3**, 115–130.

Ross, L. The role of awareness in differential conditioning. Paper presented at *Eleventh Annual Meeting of the Society for Psychophysiological Research*, 1971.

Sadler, T. G., Mefferd, R. B., Jr., & Houck, R. L. The interaction of extraversion and neuroticism in orienting response habituation. *Psychophysiology*, 1971, **8**, 312–318.

Sarason, I. Empirical findings and theoretical problems in the use of anxiety scales. *Psychological Bulletin*, 1960, **57**, 403–415.

Satterfield, J. H., & Dawson, M. E. Electrodermal correlates of hyperactivity in children. *Psychophysiology*, 1971, **8**, 191–197.

Schwarz, L., & Stern, J. A. Eyelid Tremulousness: A neurophysiological index of depression. *Archives of General Psychiatry*, Oct. 1968, **19**, 497–500.

Smith, B. Habituation and spontaneous recovery of skin conductance and heart rate in schizophrenics and controls as a function of repeated tone presentation. *Dissertation Abstracts*, 1968, **28**, 3068–3069.

Sokolov, E. N. *Perception and the conditioned reflex*. New York: MacMillan, 1963.

Sokolov, E. N. The modeling properties of the nervous system. In M. Cole, & I. Maltzman (Eds.), *A handbook of contemporary Soviet psychology*. New York: Basic Books, 1969.

Spence, K., & Spence, J. Sex and anxiety differences in eyelid conditioning. *Psychological Bulletin*, 1966, **65**, 137–142.

Spielberger, C., Lushene, R., & McAdoo, W. Theory and measurement of anxiety states. In R. Cattell (Ed.), *Handbook of modern personality theory*. Chicago: Aldine, 1970.

Spohn, H. E., Thetford, P. E., & Woodham, F. L. Span of apprehension and arousal in schizophrenia. *Journal of Abnormal Psychology*, 1970, **75**, 113–123.

Stepanov, A. I. On the problem of using some properties of the orienting reflex for the study of higher nervous activity in man. In L. G. Voronin *et al.*

(Eds.), *Orienting reflex and exploratory behavior*. Washington D.C.: American Institute of Biological Sciences, 1965. Pp. 394–398.

Stern, J. A. Measures of physiological responses during classical conditioning. In N. S. Greenfield & R. N. Sternbach (Eds.), *Handbook of psychophysiology*. New York: Holt, 1972. Pp. 197–227.

Stern, J. A., & McDonald, D. G. Physiological correlates of mental disease. *Annual Review of Psychology*, 1965, **16**, 225–264.

Stern, J. A., & Plapp, J. M. Psychophysiology and Clinical Psychology. In C. D. Spielberger (Ed.), *Current topics in clinical and community psychology*, Vol. I. New York: Academic Press, 1969. Pp. 197–254.

Stern, J. A., McClure, J., & Costello, C. Depression: Assessment and aetiology. In C. G. Costello (Ed.), *Symptoms of psychopathology: A handbook*. New York: Wiley, 1970, Pp. 169–200.

Stern, J. A., Surphlis, W., & Koff, E. Electrodermal responsiveness as related to psychiatric diagnosis and prognosis. *Psychophysiology*, 1965, **2**, 51–61.

Stewart, M., Winokur, G., Stern, J., Guze, S., Pfeiffer, E., and Hornung, F. Adaptation and conditioning GSR in psychiatric patients. *Journal of Mental Science*, 1959, **105**, 1102–1111.

Stotland, E., & Blumenthal, A. The reduction of anxiety as a result of the expectation of making a choice. *Canadian Journal of Psychology*, 1964, **18**, 139–145.

Streiner, D., & Dean, S. Expectancy, anxiety and the GSR. *Psychonomic Science*, 1968, **10**, 293–294.

Sutker, P. B. Vicarious conditioning and sociopathy. *Journal of Abnormal Psychology*, 1970, **76**, 380–386.

Syz, H. C., & Kinder, E. F. The galvanic skin reflex: Further aspects in psychopathological groups. *Archives of Neurology and Psychiatry*, 1931, **26**, 146–155.

Taylor, J. The relationship of anxiety to the conditioned eyelid response. *Journal of Experimental Psychology*, 1951, **41**, 81–92.

Taylor, J. Drive theory and manifest anxiety. *Psychological Bulletin*, 1956, **53**, 303–320.

Taylor, J. The effects of reinforcement upon skin conductance levels in process and reactive schizophrenics and normals. *Journal of Nervous and Mental Disease*, 1971, **152**, 50–52.

Thayer, J., & Silber, D. E. Relationship between levels of arousal and responsiveness among schizophrenic and normal subjects. *Journal of Abnormal Psychology*, 1971, **77**, 162–173.

Tizzard, B. Habituation of EEG and skin potential changes in normal and severely subnormal children. *American Journal of Mental Deficiency*, 1968, **73**(1), 34–40.

Venables, P. The relationship between level of skin potential and fusion of paired light flashes in schizophrenic and normal subjects. *Journal of Psychiatric Research*, 1963, **1**, 279–287.

Venables, P. Input dysfunction in schizophrenia. In B. A. Maher (Ed.), *Progress in experimental personality research*. New York: Academic Press, 1964.

Vogel, W. The relationship of age and intelligence to autonomic functioning. *Journal of Comparative and Physiological Psychology*, 1961, **54**, 133–138.

Wang, G. H. *The neural control of sweating*. Madison: Univ. of Wisconsin Press, 1964.

Welch, L., & Kubis, J. Conditioned PGR (Psychogalvanic Response) in states of pathological anxiety. *Journal of Nervous and Mental Disease,* 1947, **105**(4), 372–381.

Wenger, M. A. Studies of autonomic balance: A summary. *Psychophysiology,* 1966, **2**, 173–186.

Whatmore, G. B., & Ellis, R. M., Jr. Some neurophysiological aspects of depressed states: An electromyographic study. *Archives of General Psychiatry,* 1959, **1**, 70–80.

Williams, M. Psychophysiological responsiveness to psychological stress in early chronic schizophrenic reactions. *Psychosomatic Medicine,* 1953, **15**, 456–462.

Wolfensberger, W., & O'Connor, N. Stimulus intensity and duration effects on EEG and GSR responses of normals and retardates. *American Journal of Mental Deficiency,* 1965, **70**, 21–37.

Wyatt, R., & Grinspoon, L. Behavioral and skin potential response correlations in chronic schizophrenic patients. *Comprehensive Psychiatry,* 1969, **10**(3), 196–200.

Zahn, T. P., Rosenthal, D., & Lawlor, W. G. Electrodermal and heart rate orienting reactions in chronic schizophrenia. *Journal of Psychiatric Research,* 1968, **6**, 117–134.

Zuckerman, M. The development of an affect adjective check list for the measurement of anxiety. *Journal of Consulting Psychology,* 1960, **24**, 457–462.

Zuckerman, M., Perksy, H., & Curtis, G. Relationship among anxiety, depression, hostility and autonomic variables. *Journal of Nervous and Mental Disease,* 1968, **146**, 481–487.

CHAPTER 7

Systematic Desensitization

EDWARD S. KATKIN

SHEILA R. DEITZ

Department of Psychology
State University of New York at Buffalo
Buffalo, New York

I.	Introduction	347
II.	Mechanisms Underlying Desensitization Therapy and Their Relationship to Electrodermal Activity (EDA)	349
	A. Counterconditioning	349
	B. Extinction	350
	C. Cognitive Set and Expectancy	352
III.	Empirical Findings and Their Relationship to Theory	353
	A. Electrodermal Activity as an Index of "Phobic" Responding	353
	B. Counterconditioning versus Extinction: The Importance of Relaxation	358
	C. Cognitive Set	366
IV.	Summary	369
	A. Where Do We Stand?	369
	B. Where Do We Go from Here?	370
	References	372

I. Introduction

Systematic desensitization therapy for the treatment of phobias was first reported by Jones (1924), who described the elimination of a young boy's intense fear of small animals by the procedure of gradually exposing him to a rabbit while he was eating a favorite food. According to Jones (1924) the reduction of the young boy's fear was caused by the gradual replacement of fear by the positive responses associated with feeding. Some years later Wolpe (1958) labeled this phenomenon

347

"reciprocal inhibition," borrowing the term from Sherrington (1906), who had coined it to describe a much more specific reflex phenomenon. Wolpe subsequently defined "reciprocal inhibition" as follows: "if a response inhibitory of anxiety can be made to occur in the presence of anxiety-evoking stimuli, it will weaken the bond between these stimuli and the anxiety [1964, p. 10]." Later, in the midst of controversy concerning his views on the mechanisms underlying desensitization, Wolpe also defined anxiety "as an individual organism's characteristic constellation of autonomic responses to noxious stimulation [1971, p. 341]."

In general, then, Wolpe's view is that phobic behavior is manifested by the evocation of anxiety (an autonomic response), which in turn drives the organism to escape from (or avoid, as the case may be) the anxiety-eliciting stimulus, which escape or avoidance in turn reduces the anxiety. Since anxiety reduction is viewed by Wolpe as reinforcing, the escape or avoidance response, which is continually reinforced, becomes the overt, observable, hallmark of the phobia. This view, it may be noted, is based on Mowrer's (1947) two-factor theory of avoidance learning.

It has been postulated furthermore that phobic behavior is maintained over long periods of time by the principle of anxiety conservation (Solomon & Wynne, 1954). Briefly, this position suggests that in order for fear to extinguish, the organism must remain in contact with the fear-evoking stimulus and *not be* reinforced (that is, not suffer negative consequences); however, since the organism's immediate response to the fear-eliciting stimulus is to run away from or otherwise avoid possible negative consequences, thereby reducing fear, the fear response never gets a chance to extinguish. Although there has been considerable controversy over the validity of this theory of anxiety conservation (Costello, 1970) and the two-factor theory from which it is derived (Herrnstein, 1969), there has by no means been any clear resolution of the issue. It remains evident that many therapists interested in the use of systematic desensitization espouse the notion that an anxiety response, defined by Wolpe as a conditioned autonomic response, lies at the core of phobic behavior and is the focal response which must be reciprocally inhibited by desensitization therapy. It is no surprise therefore that a literature has developed concerning the evaluation of autonomic nervous system responses during systematic desensitization; and much of that literature employs electrodermal measures as an index of autonomic nervous system activity.

Before reviewing the empirical literature on the evaluation of systematic desensitization with electrodermal indexes, we will first review briefly some of the postulated mechanisms presumed to underlie the desensitization of acquired fears. In addition to Wolpe's reciprocal inhibition view, there also have been explanations offered within the framework of extinction or habituation, and even in terms of cognitive change.

II. Mechanisms Underlying Desensitization Therapy and Their Relationship to Electrodermal Activity

A. Counterconditioning

The counterconditioning, or reciprocal inhibition, notion of systematic desensitization, identified most clearly with Wolpe (1958), is essentially a restatement of Guthrie's (1952) position that responses do not disappear through the weakening of some associative bond, but are replaced by new responses. For Wolpe, what this means is that patients must learn to substitute a response which is incompatible with fear for the fear response in the presence of the fear-eliciting stimulus. Toward that end, subjects are first taught an abbreviated form of the deep muscle relaxation procedure described by Jacobson (1938). This relaxation regime is presumed to result not only in a state of striate muscular quiescence, but in an associated state of reduced autonomic activity, which for Wolpe (1971) apparently is virtually synonymous with reduced anxiety. After learning to relax efficiently and completely, patients are asked to imagine the phobic object. In a typical treatment situation the patient and therapist initially construct a hierarchy of items relevant to the phobia, and the patient begins the treatment program by imagining items which elicit minimal fear. Presumably the reduced autonomic tonus induced by the relaxation is incompatible with the minimal fear which normally would be elicited by the low hierarchy item, and the patient finds that he can imagine the phobic object without anxiety. Subsequently the patient imagines scenes higher on the hierarchy, and gradually all of his fear is replaced by the relaxed state and reduced autonomic tonus. Ideally, there is adequate or complete transfer of this counterconditioning from the imagined object to the real object.

To the extent that the counterconditioning theory is viable, it will derive support from a demonstration that relaxation reduces or inhibits arousal, as reflected in EDA, and that this inhibition is maintained even in the presence of the phobic stimulus object. Furthermore, if it is to be shown that reduced autonomic responsiveness becomes a substitute response for the fear response, one would predict that for some time after successful desensitization, presentation of the phobic object should fail to elicit large or frequent electrodermal responses (EDRs).

It is also crucial to the counterconditioning model that response diminution with repeated presentations be unobtainable without paired relaxation. Response diminution without relaxation, obviously, would provide support for an extinction or habituation explanation.

B. Extinction

An extinction explanation of systematic desensitization is based upon the notion that a conditioned response (in this case the phobic response) will diminish and eventually disappear after repeated, unreinforced presentations of the conditional stimulus (phobic object) which initially elicited it. This explanation suggests that the relaxation procedure is unnecessary for successful desensitization, and that the critical aspect of the treatment procedure is the repeated presentation of the phobic stimulus object. Taken to its logical conclusion, an extinction explanation would also suggest that the hierarchy of minimally threatening to maximally threatening scenes is unnecessary for extinguishing fear. Stampfl (Stampfl & Levis, 1967) has asserted just this view in the development of his technique of "implosive therapy," a procedure in which patients are repeatedly presented with the most frightening item of the hierarchy without any prior relaxation training. The clear assumption of implosive therapy is that this procedure will efficiently extinguish the fear response, and that there will be effective generalization from the treatment room to real life.

Closely akin to the notion of experimental extinction is the notion of habituation. This view, advocated most actively by Lader and Mathews (1968), is quite similar to the extinction view, except these investigators (Mathews, 1971) see the relaxation procedure as a helpful (although not necessary) adjunct to the desensitization process in that it lowers the patient's overall arousal level. Lowered arousal level, Mathews (1971) maintains, facilitates the habituation process (Katkin & McCubbin, 1969; Lader, Gelder, & Marks, 1967), and may facilitate image formation.

Adherents of the habituation model cite Sokolov's (1963) "neuronal model" as the source of their view. According to Sokolov, repeated presentations of a stimulus result in the generation of a "neuronal model" which matches this stimulus, and the strength of that neuronal model determines the extent of the inhibition of autonomic and skeletal responses to incoming stimuli. According to Sokolov, repeated presentations of any stimulus should eventually result in diminished response to it. The value of relaxation in the systematic desensitization procedure, according to Mathews (1971) is that it facilitates habituation; reciprocal inhibition, in this view, is a fiction.[1]

The extinction view would gain support from demonstrations that the repeated presentation of a phobic object results in the diminution of autonomic responding, without the use of relaxation. However, a note of caution is in order; the extinction of avoidance behavior may not necessarily be evidence for the corollary extinction of the fear component of the phobic behavior. Page (1955) has provided striking evidence from the animal laboratory that the extinction of underlying fear responses may not be as closely related to the extinction of overt avoidance behavior as is predicted from two-factor theory.

Page (1955) trained rats to go from one side of a box to another in order to avoid shock. After this training, half of the rats were given normal extinction and half were restrained in the starting box for 15 sec during the first five extinction trials. As might be expected, the restraint facilitated extinction; the restrained group showed extinction after 8 trials and the unrestrained group after 30 trials. Later, Page trained both groups plus an additional group which had never been trained to avoid (and thus had never had to be extinguished) to run back to the starting box to obtain food. Average latencies for the first five training trials indicated that the new group showed a latency of 25 sec, the group that had extinguished in 30 trials showed a latency of 60 sec, and the restrained group, which had showed the most rapid extinction, showed a latency of 125 sec. Clearly, the starting box still possessed cues which interfered with new learning even though avoidance of the box had been extinguished. Clearly, also, the group that had its extinction facilitated by restraint (an analog of therapeutic intervention) showed the most interference with new learning.

Thus, the extinction procedure, while effective with respect to the avoidance response, actually increased the apparent fear level of the animals. Demonstrations such as Page's emphasize the theoretical importance of assessing autonomic as well as behavioral components of the desensitization process in human subjects, for it is otherwise unclear

---

[1] It should be noted at this point that the habituation model is usually applied to unconditional stimuli, and not to conditional stimuli, which are assumed to possess signal value for the organism. Thus, the ultimate appropriateness of the habituation model may be questioned for most of the phobic stimulus objects employed in desensitization therapy, on the grounds that they are most usually construed to be conditional stimuli. Systematic desensitization, after all, attempts to eliminate acquired fears, not innate ones.

whether therapy is changing only motor behavior or both the motor behavior and the fear presumed to underlie it.

C. Cognitive Set and Expectancy

Finally, a number of theorists have postulated that the observed improvement following systematic desensitization may be explained as a function of a change in the patient's expectancy about the phobic object and/or a cognitive reappraisal of his own ability to cope with the object. Such views have been proposed by Efran and Marcia (1972), based upon empirical evidence from their laboratory which suggested that instructional set manipulation was effective as an analog of desensitization therapy in alleviating spider phobias (Efran & Marcia, 1967; Marcia, Rubin, & Efran, 1969). A related idea has also been put forth by Folkins, Lawson, Opton, and Lazarus (1968), derived from the theoretical view of Lazarus (1966) concerning the importance of cognitive coping processes in the modulation of fear responses.

With respect to the mechanism of desensitization, then, there are two alternative views suggested by cognitive theorists. One view, best represented by the work of Efran and Marcia (1972), suggests that expectancy changes induced by instructional set and other associated procedures of the desensitization paradigm result in behavioral change which may or may not involve autonomic functions. That is, there is no theoretical significance placed upon the role of autonomic functions by theorists of this persuasion. A second cognitive view, represented by a number of writers (Folkins et al., 1968; Leitenberg, Agras, Barlow, & Oliveau, 1969; Oliveau, Agras, Leitenberg, Moore, & Wright, 1969; Rappaport, 1972) suggests that expectancy changes induced by instructional sets directly influence autonomic functions, resulting in a reduced state of autonomic activity, and consequently a reduced experience of fear.

Studies supporting a view that posits autonomic output as a consequence of cognitive coping processes would have to demonstrate the effectiveness of instructions or other cognitive manipulations in reducing EDRs to phobic stimuli. Such studies would also have to demonstrate that the essential component of the therapeutic process was the cognitive manipulation. One possibility would be to demonstrate that control groups receiving the standard desensitization procedure under conditions of counterproductive expectancy manipulation (such as administering desensitization to a group of subjects informed that they will not be helped, but might be worsened) do not show therapeutic change in EDA.

III. Empirical Findings and Their Relationship to Theory

If the evaluation of EDA as an index of therapeutic effectiveness is to have any meaning, it must first be determined that the presentation of phobic stimulus objects elicits differential EDRs from phobic and nonphobic subjects. In simpler terms, is there evidence that noxious stimuli which elicit responses that are behaviorally "phobic" also elicit EDRs?

A. Electrodermal Activity as an Index of "Phobic" Responding

As Lang (1969) has pointed out, defining anxiety solely in terms of one of its attributes is a dangerous oversimplification of a complex construct. Nevertheless, Wolpe's emphasis on the organism's characteristic pattern of autonomic responses to noxious stimulation and his adherence to a two-factor interpretation of phobic avoidance behavior has led behavior therapists to place special emphasis on the autonomic components of fear. Given that this position is tenable, there has been a sufficient accumulation of evidence to convince even the most skeptical of readers that electrodermal responsiveness is a valid index of a subject's autonomic response to a noxious stimulus.

1. RESPONSE TO PRESENTATION OF PHOBIC STIMULI

Geer (1966) demonstrated that spider phobic subjects emitted greater skin conductance responses (SCRs) to pictures of spiders than they did to pictures of snakes, which he assumed to be generally negative stimuli unrelated to the spider phobia. Geer's spider phobics also gave greater SCRs to the pictures of spiders than did a matched group of subjects who reported being unafraid of spiders. Thus Geer (1966) demonstrated that the SCR reflected the distress elicited by the pictorial representation of a noxious object.

Wilson (1967) reported essentially the same findings with a sample of ten spider phobics and ten subjects who reported no fear of spiders. A set of tachistoscopically presented slides of spiders and neutral landscapes was presented to these 20 subjects, and their skin resistance responses (SRRs) were monitored. Wilson found that the ratio between SRR to the spider slides and SRR to the landscape slides yielded a perfect discrimination between the groups.

In discussing the findings of his study, Geer (1966) suggested that it was not possible to conclude that the SCRs reflected fear *per se*, as they might also have reflected orienting responses to the noxious pictures. In his recent review of psychophysiological approaches to desensitization, Mathews (1971) also has raised this question with respect to both Geer's (1966) and Wilson's (1967) data, suggesting that some concurrent measurement of a subject's experiential state would be necessary to determine whether the EDR reflected fear or attention. This question has concerned psychophysiologists for some time, and there has been a great deal of discussion on the question of whether EDA reflects attention, arousal, or emotion (see Duffy, 1962; Flanagan, 1967; Malmo, 1959). It is not clear to us that this question is as pertinent to the current issue as it might seem at first glance, for it is not obvious that one can distinguish between the attentional component and the fearful component of a phobic's response to a phobic object. Certainly it seems reasonable (at least on the face of it) that a phobic person will attend to the object of his fear, and that increased attention is in fact an essential component of the entire phobic response. In that case it seems reasonable that the findings of Geer (1966) and Wilson (1967) reflect some autonomic component of differential "fearfulness" on the part of their subjects.

It must be noted at this point that both Geer (1966) and Wilson (1967) observed differential EDRs to the phobic and nonphobic objects only during early presentations of the stimuli. Both investigators reported relatively rapid habituation of the EDRs after a few presentations. This is of potentially great importance, for it is just such a diminution in response strength which might be interpreted as evidence of therapeutic success. Of course, there is a distinct difference between the procedure followed by Geer (1966) and by Wilson (1967) and the procedure employed in systematic desensitization therapy. In desensitization therapy, as usually employed, the patient is not presented with pictures of the phobic object or even with actual phobic objects; rather, in the therapeutic situation the patient is asked to imagine the phobic object in a variety of different configurations. The research cited above indicates that pictorial representations of phobic objects elicit differentially large EDRs from phobic and nonphobic subjects. Other recent research (Barlow, Agras, Leitenberg, & Wincze, 1970; Barlow, Leitenberg, Agras, & Wincze, 1969) indicates that the presentation of actual phobic stimulus objects also elicits differential EDRs from phobic and nonphobic subjects. Yet, it remains of considerable importance for Wolpe's theory of systematic desensitization to demonstrate that imagined stimulus objects can also elicit EDRs of differential magnitude from phobic and nonphobic subjects.

2. RESPONSE TO IMAGINED STIMULI

According to Wolpe, "there is almost invariably a one-to-one relationship between what the patient can imagine without anxiety and what he can experience in reality without anxiety [1963, p. 1063]." In systematic desensitization therapy, visualization of the phobic object is assumed to produce autonomic reactions similar to those produced by direct contact with the phobic object, but differing in intensity. Several investigators have tested the assumption that imagining fearful scenes produces physiological arousal, although the experiments have not always been directly related to desensitization therapy.

a. IMAGERY VERSUS DIRECT EXPERIENCE. Barber and Hahn (1964) studied the comparative physiological effects of real and imagined pain in 48 female subjects randomly assigned to one of four conditions. During the first 20 min of the experiment, subjects in three conditions were asked to sit quietly ("waking" condition), while subjects in a fourth condition were given a "hypnotic induction" procedure for 15 min, followed by a 5-min "test-suggestion" period to assess the "hypnotic" state. During a cold pressor test (water at 2°C applied to the left hand for 1 min) following the 20-min period, all subjects showed decreased skin resistance level (SRL); there were no significant differences between the groups in either physiological or subjective responses to the painful stimulus.

Following this, subjects in the "hypnotic" condition and in one of the "waking" groups were told that they would be exposed to an innocuous stimulus (immersing a hand in tepid water) but instructed to imagine that they were once again experiencing the painful stimulus. Subjects in a second "waking" condition were administered the cold pressor test again, without specific instructions to imagine the painful stimulus, and subjects in the third "waking" condition received the innocuous stimulus, also without instructions to imagine. Tonic levels of SR were recorded for a 1-min period preceding the test. Mean SRL scores obtained during the base-line and test periods indicated no significant differences between the four groups; however, there was a tendency for both groups instructed to imagine pain to show decreases in SRL similar to the group actually experiencing the painful stimulus. Thus these data suggested that instructions to imagine a painful stimulus elicited physiological arousal in the same manner as direct experience.

Further evidence for this notion was reported by Craig (1968), who studied physiological arousal to direct aversive stimulation (a cold pressor test), a vicarious stress experience (viewing a confederate under-going the cold pressor test), and an imagined stress experience (immers-ing a hand in cool water, with instructions to imagine that the water was "cold as ice" and "very painful"). Craig's (1968) results indicated that direct aversive stimulation did not result in significantly different skin conductance levels (SCL) than did the imagined stress experience.

b. IMAGINATION OF ITEMS ON A DESENSITIZATION HIERARCHY. Lang, Melamed, and Hart (1970), investigated the notion that the subjective steps of an anxiety hierarchy are related to physiological responsivity. Their first experimental group consisted of 5 male and 5 female subjects afraid of public speaking and their second group consisted of 10 female subjects afraid of spiders. During the first two experimental sessions a tentative anxiety hierarchy was constructed for each subject; during the third session each subject was trained in visualization with neutral scenes, and in the fourth session each subject was presented randomly with a series of five fearful scenes chosen from his anxiety hierarchy, alternating with four neutral scenes. After the presentation of each item, subjects were asked to rate both the vividness of their imagery and their experienced anxiety on a scale from 0 to 4. Throughout the fourth session physiological recordings were made. The results revealed an overall association between SCR magnitude and hierarchy position al-though a significant linear trend was revealed only for the spider phobic group.

Similarly, Van Egeren, Feather, and Hein (1971), in a study of 30 male subjects with public speaking phobias demonstrated both increases in SCL from a prestimulus period to the imagining of threatening scenes and a direct relationship between the position of an item in the anxiety hierarchy and the number and magnitude of SCRs to the visualization of that item.

c. IMAGINATION OF FEARFUL VERSUS NEUTRAL STIMULI. Grossberg and Wilson (1968) investigated the effects upon autonomic activity of imagining both neutral and fearful stimuli, which were selected indi-vidually for each subject on the basis of responses to Wolpe and Lang's (1964) Fear Survey Schedule (FSS). A group of control subjects was also selected who showed no unusual attitude toward either the items that were neutral or fearful for the experimental subjects. "For example, if the experimental subject was disturbed by injections but neutral to-ward high places, she would be matched with a control subject who had indicated no disturbance for injections *or* high places [Grossberg & Wilson, 1968, p. 126]."

Base-line physiological levels were recorded for all subjects during a 10-min adaptation period, after which the experimenter read a fearful or a neutral scene and then instructed the subjects to imagine it vividly. The reading and instructions were repeated eight times, once each for four neutral and four fearful scenes. Mean SCLs obtained during the reading were compared with adaptation period SCLs and expressed as ratios of amount of change; similarly, the amount of change in SCL from the reading interval to the imagination interval was expressed as ratio of change. Fearful scenes produced significantly greater increases in mean SCL than neutral scenes during imagination, whereas no significant differences were found between fearful and neutral scenes during the reading interval. These results support Wolpe's assumption that the imagination of a fearful stimulus is sufficient to elicit physiological arousal. Further findings of Grossberg and Wilson, however, raise important questions concerning the necessity of the relaxation component in systematic desensitization. They report that:

> In the present experiment, it was found that successive reading trials produced significantly decreasing amounts of arousal for the . . . SC measures, and this effect was also evident for SC during successive imagining trials. The number of . . . SC increases over trials . . . showed a similar decline. This adaptation or extinction effect occurred without deliberate relaxation training, and raises the question of the role of relaxation training in Wolpe's desensitization procedure [Grossberg & Wilson, 1968, p. 131].

The data reviewed so far indicate that the imagination of a phobic stimulus object does, in fact, tend to elicit the autonomic response which Wolpe has called anxiety. Thus, one necessary precondition for the effective utilization of systematic desensitization seems to be met—the anxiety response can be elicited in the absence of the actual stimulus. Yet, Grossberg and Wilson's conclusion coupled with the findings of Geer (1966) and Wilson (1967) indicate that the "anxiety response" seems to diminish after repeated exposures of the phobic object, even when the other elements of the desensitization procedure are absent. These findings are inconsistent with Wolpe's theory about the mechanism of desensitization therapy and lend credence to the extinction notion, insofar as they suggest that response diminution can be obtained without associated relaxation.

These findings are of critical significance for the reciprocal inhibition or counterconditioning position, for they strike at the very heart of the process as it has been described by Wolpe. At this point it is appropriate to turn our attention to those studies which were designed specifically to evaluate the role of progressive relaxation in the desensitization process.

B. Counterconditioning versus Extinction: The Importance of Relaxation

Although Jacobson (1938) has shown that prolonged training in muscular relaxation produces a general reduction in autonomic arousal, it is essential for the counterconditioning position that brief training in muscular relaxation also can be shown to result in reduced autonomic tonus.

1. RELAXATION AS AN INHIBITOR OF AUTONOMIC ACTIVITY

Several investigators have studied the physiological effects of brief relaxation training, as employed in systematic desensitization, and have reported contradictory findings. Grossberg (1965) compared a number of physiological measures, including SRLs of 30 male subjects assigned to one of three groups: a group trained in relaxation by recorded instructions, a group that listened to relaxing music, and a self-relaxation control group that received no specific instructions in relaxation. Grossberg (1965) found no significant differences between groups in either SRL or any other measure of autonomic activity, indicating that the relaxation technique possesses no particular advantage in effecting autonomic change. Similar results have been reported by Barber and Hahn (1963), who reported no particular advantage for hypnotically suggested relaxation as compared with instructions to just sit quietly, and by Lehrer (1970) who also found that brief relaxation training was apparently no more effective than normal resting for reducing autonomic activity.

Paul (1969) compared the physiological effects of brief relaxation training, hypnotically suggested relaxation, and a self-relaxation control procedure for 60 female subjects. Following specific instructions for each condition, subjects were asked to sit quietly, for a 10-min adaptation period, the last minute of which served as a basal period. All subjects were instructed to practice their respective techniques for about 15 min, twice a day, for the week separating the first and second sessions, at which time they were told briefly that the procedure would be similar to that of the first session. Paul's results for SCL were entirely consistent with those of Barber and Hahn (1963), Grossberg (1965), and Lehrer (1970); no differences between groups were obtained.[2]

[2] Paul's (1969) findings for heart rate, muscle tension, and respiration were not consistent with his SCL results; on the former measures Paul found significant effects in favor of relaxation training. The problems inherent in evaluating only electrodermal activity will be dealt with later in the chapter.

Paul and Trimble (1970) ran 30 additional subjects after the completion of the Paul (1969) study, using prerecorded instructions instead of a live experimenter, in order to assess the effect of the experimenter's presence on the efficiency of the instructions. In general, they found that recorded instructions were not as effective as live instructions in reducing physiological arousal. Paul and Trimble's (1970) findings added nothing new to the observation that there were no differences in SC between the brief relaxation, hypnotically suggested relaxation, and self-induced relaxation procedures.

Mathews and Gelder (1969) evaluated the effects of relaxation training on a sample of 14 clinically defined phobic patients, rather than on a sample of fearful undergraduates. In addition, Mathews and Gelder (1969) employed a relaxation procedure more consistent with that used in actual therapeutic situations than did most other investigators. All patients initially were trained in relaxation for a period of 1 hr, with instructions to practice the relaxation technique during the following week. A second session consisted of 30 min of practice in passive concentration on muscle groups, including instructions and suggestions from the therapist, followed by 30 min of similar tape-recorded standardized instructions. In a third session, patients were exposed to: (1) the same relaxation recording followed by a control recording in which the patients were asked to rest, but were told *not* to relax in the formal manner in which they had been trained; or (2) the control recording followed by the relaxation recording. Results of this experiment indicated a significantly faster rate of SCL adaptation during relaxation periods, when compared with control periods, but no main effect of treatments on overall SCL. Additionally, Mathews and Gelder (1969) found a significant main effect of treatments on the rate of spontaneous SC fluctuations, indicating that the number of such fluctuations was generally lower during the relaxation period. Furthermore, this experiment yielded a significant product-moment correlation between number of SC fluctuations and subjective report of "anxiety tension" and "relaxation." These findings on SC fluctuation are consistent with the experimental findings of Katkin (1965, 1966) and Rappaport and Katkin (1972) which showed a relationship between experimental induction of stress and number of spontaneous SR fluctuations.

Mathews and Gelder's (1969) positive findings are somewhat inconsistent with the other findings on relaxation, although it must be remembered that they, too, were unable to demonstrate a clear main effect of relaxation on SCL. The positive results which they obtained may be explained in part by the more intensive relaxation training they employed (Mathews, 1971), or by the fact that a genuinely phobic population may respond differently to relaxation instructions than a population of fearful undergraduates. Finally, the results of Mathews and Gelder were most clear for the spontaneous fluctuation rate, an index not used by other investigators. Recent evidence on the utility of this measure as an index of arousal (Burch & Greiner, 1960; Katkin, 1965, 1966; Katkin & McCubbin, 1969; Silverman, Cohen, & Shmavonian, 1959) suggests that it might be of substantial importance in evaluating the therapeutic effects of relaxation training as well as other aspects of the desensitization procedure.

2. Pairing of Relaxation and Phobic Stimuli

a. REAL AND PICTORIAL STIMULI. Grings and Uno (1968) have conducted a detailed and critical evaluation of the counterconditioning hypothesis, in an experiment that was theoretically precise, but did not address itself directly to the problems of clinically phobic behavior. Grings and Uno (1968) performed an analog experiment in which they essentially induced a phobic response in the laboratory and then studied the effects of reciprocally inhibiting it. In short, what Grings and Uno did was to train 12 volunteer subjects in muscle relaxation. After all subjects had learned to relax completely, they were instructed to initiate relaxation when they saw the word *NOW* projected on a screen. On the following day, subjects were presented with a pure color flashed on the screen, followed by a painful electric shock. Thus the color became a conditional stimulus for the elicitation of an EDR.

After both training in relaxation and conditioning of the EDR to the color was completed, test trials were introduced in which subjects were exposed to the fear cue (color) alone, and to the fear cue with the verbal cue for relaxation superimposed on it. "The magnitude of response to the compound composed of the 'fear' cue and the 'relaxation' cue, was consistently less than the response to the 'fear' cue alone [Grings & Uno, 1968, p. 483]."

These results, while impressive, do not necessarily suggest that progressive relaxation will function in the same way for phobic subjects in the course of desensitization therapy, nor even that relaxation will have similar inhibiting effects on autonomic response to threatening stimuli of more personal significance or more complex origin.

Davidson and Hiebert (1971) studied the effects of relaxation on the inhibition of autonomic responses to a stressful film. Using a noxious film which depicted a careless shopworker being mutilated by a circular saw, Davidson and Hiebert set out to evaluate the effects on SC responses of differentially specific instructions to relax. One-third of their subjects received specific instructions in abbreviated progressive relaxation; a second group of their subjects received instructions to relax without any specific training; and a third group of subjects, the control group, received no instructions to relax. All subjects were then shown a .92-sec segment of the distressing film ten times in succession with approximately 2 min between showings. Subjects in the two relaxation groups were requested to maintain as much relaxation as possible throughout the showings. Skin conductance levels were recorded every 2 sec, yielding 46 scores per showing. Davidson and Hiebert (1971) found that on the first showing of the film there was no difference in SC response among subjects in the three groups. However, after the fifth showing of the film, a clear pattern emerged in which SCLs for subjects in the two relaxation groups began to decrease, ultimately reaching their prefilm level, while SCL for subjects in the control group did not decrease. Thus these data indicated that relaxation instructions, whether specifically describing progressive relaxation or simply being casual instructions to relax, have an inhibitory effect upon overall SCL in the presence of a noxious stimulus. No significant difference was found between the two relaxation groups. These findings are similar in quality to those of Grings and Uno (1968) and support the notion that relaxation inhibits autonomic response to noxious stimulation. Yet Davidson and Hiebert's (1971) study is also somewhat different in context from the situation usually found in desensitization therapy.

A study which more closely approximated the actual desensitization procedure, although it used actual instead of imaginary stimuli, has been reported by Barlow et al. (1969). Barlow et al. (1969) investigated what they have termed the "transfer gap" in systematic desensitization, i.e., the observation that progress in the imagination of successive steps on a phobic hierarchy does not necessarily reflect progress in the real-life situation. Twenty female subjects, who indicated that they would feel "definitely tense" in the presence of a harmless snake at a distance of 2 ft, were assigned to either a standard desensitization procedure involving relaxation and a graded hierarchy of imaginal scenes or to an analog group involving relaxation while a live caged snake was moved progressively closer to the subject. Tonic SCL was obtained for all subjects under two conditions: (1) while imagining five scenes from a hierarchy; and (2) in the presence of the snake at distances of 10, 5, and 2 ft.

A comparison of pretreatment and posttreatment mean SC scores revealed that subjects in the systematic desensitization group showed reduced SCRs to imagined scenes, but no change in SCR to the real snake. In contrast, the analog group exhibited significantly reduced SCRs to both real and imagined situations. Behavioral approach measures

indicated additional support for the superiority of the group that experienced contact with the real phobic stimulus.

The results of this study suggest that the standard desensitization
procedure, employing imagined rather than real objects, may not be
the most efficient technique for the reduction of autonomic components
of the phobic response. Let us turn now to a consideration of those
studies which evaluated the role of relaxation in standard desensitization
paradigms.

b. Imagined Phobic Stimuli. Wolpe and Flood (1970) compared
changes in SR for five subjects administered a standard desensitization
technique with relaxation training (RT group) and five subjects receiving desensitization with no training in relaxation nor instructions to
relax at any time during the procedure (NR group). After an initial
interview, during which anxiety hierarchies were constructed, five evenly
separated items from each subject's hierarchy were chosen. During the
next four sessions, subjects were presented with the five stimulus items
in ascending order, while physiological recordings were made. Skin resistance levels during the stimulus periods were compared with baseline
SRLs obtained 1 sec prior to the reading of a stimulus item, and the
SRR was expressed as a percentage change score.

Although Wolpe and Flood (1970) provided no statistical analysis
of their data, the curves which they presented suggest that subjects
in the RT group showed a systematic decrease in SRR magnitude over
four desensitization sessions while subjects in the NR group showed
no change in SRR to the five items selected from their hierarchies. While
these data seem to indicate the general effectiveness of relaxation in
desensitization procedures, they also raise some questions. First of all,
Wolpe and Flood reported that by chance the five subjects assigned
to the RT group showed larger initial SRRs to the imaginal stimuli
than did the five subjects assigned to the NR group. In fact, the smallest
SRR ever obtained from subjects in the RT group after treatment never
was as small as the initial pretreatment response elicited from the NR
group. Consequently, the results may be nothing more than an artifact
of bad sampling and a floor effect for subjects in the NR group. Second
of all, Wolpe and Flood (1970) were surprised themselves to discover
that subjects in their RT group showed SRR decrements as rapidly
to high hierarchy items as they did to lower hierarchy items and were
moved to comment, "The question must be faced whether the standard
technique of desensitization is necessarily the best [1970, p. 200]."

Hyman and Gale (1973) studied electrodermal, subjective, and
behavioral responses of 24 female snake phobics, divided into three

groups: systematic desensitization with relaxation (D), systematic desensitization without relaxation (Ext), and relaxation with the visualization of neutral scenes (R). The electrodermal measure consisted of the total amplitude of responses during and immediately following each visualization compared with tonic SRL just prior to each visualization. Significant negative linear trends were found for all groups; however, the rate of habituation of the EDR to repeated presentations of the phobic stimulus appeared to be greater for the D group than for the other groups. In addition, self-report and behavioral outcome measures (fear survey schedule, fear thermometer scores, and a runway task) indicated a superiority for the D group over the Ext group, with the R group falling between the two. Thus, Hyman and Gale (1973) reported limited support for the counterconditioning explanation of systematic desensitization, as did Van Egeren et al. (1971).

In contrast to these findings, Waters, McDonald, and Koresko (1972), utilizing an analog desensitization procedure, compared SRRs, SPRs, and SRLs for 40 female rat phobics. One group of subjects (SD group) received training in relaxation, to be paired with instructions to imagine themselves in the phobic situation while viewing five slides of a girl progressively approaching the rat in a cage; the second group (NRC) received a procedure identical to that of the SD group except they received no training in progressive relaxation. Both the SD and the NRC groups exhibited decreased arousal to the phobic stimulus across trials and significant changes in avoidance behavior from pretest to posttest. No differences between the groups were reported for either physiological or behavioral measures; however, subjects in the SD group reported significantly lower subjective fear during the procedure (fewer signals of anxiety) and thus required significantly fewer trials to obtain a criterion level of reduced fear than did the nonrelaxation controls (NRC). Waters et al. (1972) concluded that while relaxation tends to accelerate the process of systematic desensitization, it is not a *necessary* component of the procedure, a view which is similar to that put forth by Mathews (1971).

In another analog study, Folkins et al. (1968) compared SC measures of 58 male and 51 female subjects during exposure to a stressful film depicting an industrial accident. Prior to viewing the film, subjects were randomly divided into four groups: an analog of systematic desensitization, relaxation alone, cognitive rehearsal (visualization of stressful scenes), or a no-training control group. Both the analog desensitization and cognitive rehearsal groups received training in imagining scenes from the stressful film prior to viewing the film; however, in place of relaxation training, the cognitive rehearsal group listened to a tape concerning study habits. On both SCL and self-report measures during the accident scene, the no-treatment control group exhibited the greatest amount of "anxiety," followed by the desensitization group, and relaxation group. Arousal (i.e., SCL) was lowest for the cognitive rehearsal group. Thus, Folkins et al. (1968) concluded that the separate components of systematic desensitization, i.e., relaxation and cognitive rehearsal alone, were more effective in reducing physiological stress reactions to the accident film than they were when combined as they are in systematic desensitization, further supporting the notion that the relaxation component, while useful, may not be essential for autonomic change.

Lomont and Edwards (1967), in an attempt to evaluate the reciprocal inhibition and extinction hypotheses of systematic desensitization, compared five measures of snake fear change including SRL in 22 female snake phobics. Half of their subjects were assigned to a treatment condition which received systematic desensitization, including standard relaxation, and half were assigned to a group which received systematic desensitization without any relaxation. The latter group was defined as an extinction treatment. In order to guarantee that subjects in the extinction condition would not independently practice muscle relaxation, they were instructed after each stimulus visualization to tense their muscles. All subjects were presented with a live snake at a distance of 6 feet before treatment began and after having received ten sessions. During the pretreatment and posttreatment snake presentations, SRLs were obtained.

Lomont and Edwards (1967) found no significant differences between the two groups in SRL, although measures of subjective responses to snake fear items (including ratings on a 10-point "fear thermometer") yielded results favoring the desensitization group. It is interesting to note that Lomont and Edwards (1967) found marked decreases in SRL across trials for both the desensitization and extinction groups, results similar to those of Grossberg and Wilson (1968) and Gale, Hyman, and Ayer (1970). All three of these studies found habituation of the EDR across trials, irrespective of relaxation. It must be noted, however, that Lomont and Edwards' (1967) technique was unique in that pre- and posttherapy SRLs were obtained during presentation of the *real* phobic object, although the treatment procedure employed imagined phobic objects as the desensitizing stimuli. In that sense, Lomont and Edwards (1967) have most closely approximated the conditions that constitute the critical test of clinical effectiveness in a real-life therapy situation.

Edelman (1971) also conducted a study on the effectiveness of progressive relaxation, comparing the standard progressive relaxation technique with an instructional set designed to elicit relaxation, but not involving the standardized relaxation procedure utilized in desensitization therapy. Edelman's subjects were not selected on the basis of any specific phobia, but were rather selected on the basis of general anxiety level as measured by the Taylor Manifest Anxiety Scale (Taylor, 1953). Half the subjects were then placed in a group which was asked to visualize a scene very high in an individually generated fear hierarchy and half the subjects were placed in a group which was asked to visualize a scene very low in their hierarchy. In addition, half of each of these groups was trained in progressive relaxation, while another half was exposed to the nonstructured instructions to relax. The training or relaxation instructional sessions were spaced at 1-week intervals, and each subject was given two sessions. Subsequent to relaxation instructions, or training in progressive relaxation, all subjects were asked to visualize the selected scene from their fear hierarchy (e.g., the high fear or the low fear scene) five successive times. The procedure followed was similar to that of Grossberg and Wilson (1968) in that an interval of 30 sec was allotted for the experimenter to read the scene to the subject and then 30 sec more for the subject to visualize it.

Edelman's basic findings were that SC habituated as a function of successive presentations of the visualized scenes irrespective of the relaxation technique employed. Thus Edelman's findings are consistent with earlier findings which indicate that the diminution in autonomic responding found with repeated presentations of fear-eliciting stimuli do not necessarily result from the use of progressive relaxation. Edelman interpreted his findings as support for a central rather than a peripheral theory of reciprocal inhibition, based upon his belief that his casual relaxation procedure did not focus upon specific control of the skeletal musculature and therefore must have been mediated by more central processes. It is not altogether clear that Edelman's conclusion is justified, for a variety of reasons, not the least of which is that he had no means of assessing the manner in which subjects acted upon his casual relaxation instructions. Nevertheless, Edelman's data, when taken together with the findings of Grossberg and Wilson (1968), Davidson and Hiebert (1971), Waters et al. (1972), and Gale et al. (1970) indicate that even if relaxation facilitates habituation of autonomic responses to phobic objects, or even if it is a necessary component in counterconditioning, there is little reason to think that the standardized ritual associated with the progressive relaxation technique is necessary.

To summarize this section, there seems to be good reason to believe that minimal generalized instructions to relax have as much effect upon the habituation of electrodermal components of the response to the phobic object as more precise training in progressive relaxation does.

At this point it should be kept in mind that there is another school of thought which claims that the entire desensitization effect, with or without relaxation, may be explained more parsimoniously in terms of the effect of the social context of the desensitization procedure. These theorists (Efran & Marcia, 1972; Wilkins, 1971) have argued that the beneficial effects of the desensitization routine are an outgrowth of changes in subject set or expectancy.

C. Cognitive Set

Although there has been considerable interest recently in the evaluation of cognitive factors in the systematic desensitization of phobic behavior, there has not been much direct investigation of the associated electrodermal (or other autonomic nervous system indexes) correlates of the process. This is not surprising, in view of the fact that most cognitive views of the process tend to minimize the importance of the classical conditioning view which places emphasis on the autonomic basis of the conditioned fear response. Nevertheless, there have been a few studies of electrodermal responsivity generated from the cognitive view, and they shall be discussed here.

Leitenberg et al. (1969) were interested in studying the effects of the social context of desensitization therapy as a contributor to the therapeutic effect with special reference to the positive effects of instructional set and positive verbal reinforcement. They assigned 30 female subjects with a fear of snakes either to one of two treatment groups (groups 1 and 2) or to a no-treatment control group. Subjects in both treatment groups received a systematic desensitization procedure, involving a 27-item common snake fear hierarchy and relaxation. In addition, subjects in group 1 received instructions designed to establish an expectation of therapeutic benefit, as well as positive verbal reinforcement for successful completion of each hierarchy item and general praise for progress throughout the sessions. A comparison of pre- and posttest behavioral approach scores indicated a significantly greater mean difference for group 1 than for either group 2 or the control group; however, electrodermal response data recorded continuously throughout the sessions did not differentiate between the treatment groups. Within each group the percentage of hierarchy item presentations that elicited a verbal report of anxiety was significantly greater than the percentage of presentations which elicited an EDR and the authors attributed this result to the adaptation of EDRs with repeated presentations of each hierarchy item.

The behavioral results of Leitenberg et al. (1969) are fully consistent with the cognitive-expectancy model proposed by Efran and Marcia (1972), which stipulates that desensitization may be effective because "it alters Ss' expectations about their ability to face feared situations [Efran & Marcia, 1967, p. 239]." An early study reported from Efran and Marcia's laboratory (Marcia et al., 1969) tested some of their assumptions about the effect of expectancy on behavioral change after desensitization, but it did not employ any physiological assessment. A later study from their laboratory (Rappaport, 1972) did employ electrodermal measurement of their procedures. We will examine both of these studies.

Marcia et al. (1969) compared the effectiveness of systematic desensitization with that of "T-scope therapy," which contained expectancy elements similar to systematic desensitization, but without the traditional elements of relaxation, an anxiety hierarchy, or visualization. Essentially, the "T-scope" procedure consisted of instructing subjects that phobic stimuli would be presented tachistoscopically at a speed perceptible only to the unconscious mind in order to evoke "unconscious phobic responses," and that each presentation would be followed by a mild electric shock. In actuality, the "phobic stimuli" were blank cards, and subjects received shocks on a fixed random schedule. Marcia et al. (1969) noted that classical conditioning theory would predict an increase in phobic behavior for this group, due to the pairing of shock with the expectation of a "phobic stimulus."

Twelve male and 32 female subjects, fearful of either snakes or spiders, were chosen on the basis of their responses to a modified form of a fear survey schedule and also on the basis of their inability to touch the feared object. In all, five conditions were established: (1) systematic desensitization, including relaxation, positive expectancy, anxiety hierarchy, and visualization (DS); (2) systematic desensitization with the exception that subjects were told they would receive only the first half of the usual procedure and thus the treatment would be ineffective (DSI); (3) "T-scope" therapy as described above (Hi T); (4) "T-scope" therapy, in which subjects were told that the "phobic stimulus" would be missing, thus no improvement could be expected (Lo T); and (5) a no-treatment control group. Therapeutic improvement as measured by an approach test revealed significant differences among the groups. The two DS groups and the Hi T group did not differ significantly from one another on either the approach measure or on subjects' self-ratings of fear change in the posttreatment interview. Both groups showed significantly greater improvement on the approach test than either the control or Lo T groups, which did not differ from one another.

In a recent report of an extended replication of the study by Marcia, et al. (1969), Lick (1972) found essentially the same results. Lick's findings are more convincing than the earlier ones in that they were obtained with a clinically defined group of snake and spider phobics rather than with undergraduates reporting fear. In addition, Lick employed actual desensitization therapy rather than the analog approximation employed by Marcia et al. Although Lick (1972) did not report any electrodermal results, he did find that his desensitized and his placebo-treated subjects showed lower pulse rates than his no-treatment control subjects.

Rappaport (1972), working in Efran and Marcia's laboratory, employed continuous recordings of SCL and spontaneous fluctuations in SR throughout the course of his experiment, on the assumption that the behavior change which Marcia et al. attributed to expectancy shift should possess autonomic correlates. Using a somewhat different procedure than Marcia et al. (1969), Rappaport assigned 72 female subjects who were fearful of spiders to one of four groups: a therapy expectancy (TE) group, instructed that the procedures would definitely alleviate their fear; a negative expectancy (NE) group, instructed that the purpose of the research was to study stress responses, and that the procedure was purposely designed to be extremely stressful; a no-therapy expectancy (NTE) group, given no particular expectancy; and a no-treatment control group. All experimental subjects were exposed for 15 min to a preserved tarantula which they believed was alive; the control group was not exposed to the tarantula.

In addition to the electrodermal recordings, Rappaport also took post-exposure self-reports of fear, and tested all subjects on a behavioral runway task identical with that employed by Marcia et al. (1969). The results of Rappaport's study showed a strong main effect of treatments on both the avoidance behavior and on self-report, but absolutely no effects on either of the electrodermal measures. Subjects in the TE group approached the tarantula more closely and reported less fear of it than the other groups, with subjects in the NE group showing the greatest avoidance behavior and most expressed fear. Yet tonic SC level and frequency of SR fluctuations were totally unrelated to the treatments and were not correlated with the behavioral and self-report data. Rappaport (1972) chose to interpret his data as evidence for the irrelevance of autonomic factors in the behavior change process, arguing that it does not matter whether there is any autonomic change as a result of systematic desensitization, as long as there is behavioral change in the desired direction. While this position is a relatively popular one, and relieves the behavior therapist from concerning himself with sticky questions about "underlying process" (in this case, of course, Rappaport still deals with the underlying "cognitive" process, if not the autonomic one), it does not necessarily seem conclusive.

Page's (1955) data with rats (see Section II.B) suggest that changes in overt behavior can conceivably accompany increases in fear. If so, is it not possible that changes in avoidance behavior likewise may accompany no change in fear? To be more specific, the expectancy view posited by Efran and Marcia (1972) and supported by Rappaport (1972) could also predict that the changes in behavior and self-report were direct results of the demand characteristics of the experimental situation and reflect social desirability or some other mediating state. There is nothing conclusive in Rappaport's data to suggest that instructional set modified fear. Positive evidence on the electrodermal measures would have provided support for the cognitive view, for it would have shown that the differential expectancies established resulted in changes in autonomic, involuntary responding; negative results do not provide strong support for the cognitive view, even in view of the behavioral change, unless one is willing to accept the notion that the fear component and the behavioral component of phobias are inseparable.

IV. Summary

A. Where Do We Stand?

The data reviewed in this chapter leave us with some relatively clear conclusions and many as yet unresolved questions. There seems no doubt that the utilization of electrodermal measurement as a technique for assessing the process and the outcome of systematic desensitization is useful. The data indicate clearly that the EDR to phobic and nonphobic stimulus objects provides an accurate index of a subject's fear state. Phobic subjects give larger EDRs to phobic stimulus objects than to nonphobic stimulus objects, and they also show larger EDRs to phobic objects than matched nonphobic subjects show to the same objects. In addition, it seems clear that this relationship holds true for real stimulus objects, pictorial stimulus objects, and for *imagined* stimulus objects, the type most frequently employed in clinical settings.

With respect to the theoretical question concerning the underlying mechanism of systematic desensitization, electrodermal data have been less helpful, although studies of autonomic responsivity play an integral part in the elucidation of the underlying process. It is apparent that the EDR to a phobic stimulus object will extinguish (or habituate) with or without the utilization of relaxation. Yet, it is also clear that when relaxation is paired with the desensitization procedure, the rate of extinction of the EDR is facilitated. The most parsimonious conclusion to be derived from these observations has been drawn by Mathews (1971); it is unlikely that relaxation serves as a counterconditioning agent, but more likely that it serves to reduce arousal, thereby facilitating extinction or habituation. This conclusion is supported by observations that electrodermal orienting responses appear to habituate more rapidly in lowered states of arousal (Katkin & McCubbin, 1969). A further conclusion that seems justified is that the relaxation technique employed in the desensitization procedure is relatively unimportant. With the exception of research by Paul (1969), the preponderance of studies indicate that any type of instruction to relax seems to work as well as the ritualized progressive relaxation instructions developed by Jacobson (1938) and popularized by Wolpe (1958).

The evidence from studies of electrodermal responsivity does not seem to clarify or advance the views of the cognitive theorists, nor does it necessarily detract from them. Although there is some evidence that instructional set may produce behavioral change and/or change in self-report of fear, there has been no substantive evidence that instructional set or manipulation of subject expectancy results in any alteration of the electrodermal component of fear. Thus it is unclear whether cognitive manipulations have resulted in a genuine reduction in fear, or whether the altered behavior and self-report reflect socially desirable responses to the rather clear demand characteristics established in the experimental situation. Cognitive theoretical views on the nature of the desensitization process, of course, have tended to devalue the role of autonomic function in the phobic syndrome, because cognitive theorists have tended to take the classically conditioned nature of the phobia less seriously than do theorists of the counterconditioning or extinction view. Therefore, it is not unusual to find that there has been a paucity of studies from the cognitive framework that have addressed themselves to the role of autonomic responses in the treatment of phobia.

B. Where Do We Go from Here?

In this chapter we have addressed ourselves only to the use of electrodermal measurement in the evaluation of systematic desensitization. This was an appropriate task for a volume such as this, but it should not blind us to the fact that some of the substantive theoretical issues dealt with herein may be enriched by a consideration of the relationship between electrodermal measurement and other indexes of autonomic function. The study by Paul (1969) makes clear what has always been known to psychophysiologists—that there is a relatively low concordance among different indexes of autonomic function.

In addition to the studies on electrodermal responsivity reviewed here, there has been some concentration of interest in the evaluation of cardiac rate; Mathews (1971) has suggested that cardiac rate, in fact, has been a more useful index than EDA in the evaluation of desensitization, and suggests that both measures should be employed in future studies. While this seems a wise suggestion, and one which we endorse, one cannot escape from the fact that when discrepancies are found between differing measures of autonomic nervous system activity (Paul, 1969), one is faced with the problem of dealing directly with the meaning of such discrepancies. This could easily lead to an increased emphasis on more basic parametric research on the integrated nature of autonomic responses to threatening (and nonthreatening) stimuli. It goes without saying that such research is fundamentally important, even outside the context of understanding systematic desensitization.

Even within the restricted realm of electrodermal measurement we have seen that there is no agreed-upon choice of measurement. As usual, there are almost as many choices of data transformation as there are investigators. The studies reviewed in this chapter employed variously tonic SC level, tonic SR level, SCR magnitude, SRR magnitude, and sometimes SCR and SRR frequency as dependent measures. Which of these measures is most appropriate depends on a complex set of factors; the problem of quantification and measurement of EDA is dealt with in other chapters of this volume.

We must point out also that, with the exception of the study by Grings and Uno (1968), there has been little attention paid to the acquisition of phobias. There has been much attention given to autonomic components of response diminution as a function of desensitization, but virtually no interest in empirical studies of the acquisition of the autonomic component of the phobia. To be sure, this has been a result of the obvious fact that the investigator is not available at the time his subjects are acquiring their phobias. However, analog studies on the conditioning of avoidance responses, and on their extinction (of which Grings & Uno's study is a model) should be able to provide much important information on the importance of autonomic nervous system activity in the acquisition and maintenance of phobic behavior.

We would like to raise one final note concerning a possible alternative strategy for the future. Lang (1969) has discussed the relevance of direct instrumental conditioning of autonomic nervous system activity for the alleviation of phobic responses. In reviewing the presumed mechanisms underlying reciprocal inhibition, Lang noted that muscle relaxation is supposed to affect the autonomic outflow. He continued to suggest that the "role of autonomic activity in modulating and maintaining emotional responses in other behavioral systems suggests that it should be dealt with directly, rather than going through the uncertain medium of muscle relaxation . . . [Lang, 1969, p. 183]." Recent research has indicated that under appropriate conditions, especially those which utilize augmented sensory feedback, human subjects can learn to gain direct control over autonomic responses (Katkin & Murray, 1968). As Lang has noted, not only does the instrumental control of autonomic responses provide an interesting potential technique for direct alteration of the autonomic response to a phobic stimulus, it also provides a potentially important theoretical tool. For if subjects who are taught to voluntarily reduce autonomic nervous system responses to stressful stimuli also show reduced verbal and behavioral evidence of fear in the presence of those stimuli, it would provide evidence for the reciprocal inhibition notion of the therapeutic effect.

Although there has been controversy over the precise mechanisms by which instrumental control of autonomic responses takes place (Katkin & Murray, 1968), there is general agreement now that subjects can learn such control. Future studies of the relationship of instrumental autonomic conditioning to systematic desensitization may provide more answers to the difficult question of how the procedure works, and what the role of autonomic responsivity is in the acquisition and extinction of phobic response patterns.

Acknowledgments

Preparation of this chapter was supported in part by grant MH-11989 from the National Institute of Mental Health, United States Public Health Service.

References

Barber, T. X., & Hahn, K. W. Hypnotic induction and "relaxation": An experimental study. *Archives of General Psychiatry*, 1963, 8, 295–300.
Barber, T. X., & Hahn, K. W., Jr. Experimental studies in "hypnotic" behavior:

Physiological and subjective effects of imagined pain. *Journal of Nervous and Mental Disease*, 1964, **139**, 416–425.

Barlow, D. H., Agras, W. S., Leitenberg, H., & Wincze, J. P. An experimental analysis of the effectiveness of "shaping" in reducing maladaptive avoidance behaviour: An analogue study. *Behaviour Research and Therapy*, 1970, **8**, 165–173.

Barlow, D. H., Leitenberg, H., Agras, W. S., & Wincze, J. P. The transfer gap in systematic desensitization: An analogue study. *Behaviour Research and Therapy*, 1969, **7**, 191–196.

Burch, N. R., & Greiner, T. H. A bioelectric scale of human alertness: Concurrent recordings of the EEG and GSR. *Psychiatric Research Report of the American Psychiatric Association*, 1960, **12**, 183–193.

Costello, C. G. Dissimilarities between conditioned avoidance responses and phobias. *Psychological Review*, 1970, **77**, 250–254.

Craig, K. D. Physiological arousal as a function of imagined, vicarious, and direct stress experiences. *Journal of Abnormal Psychology*, 1968, **73**, 513–520.

Davidson, P. O., & Hiebert, S. F. Relaxation training, relaxation instruction and repeated exposure to a stressor film. *Journal of Abnormal Psychology*, 1971, **78**, 154–159.

Duffy, E. *Activation and behavior.* New York: Wiley, 1962.

Edelman, R. I. Desensitization and physiological arousal. *Journal of Personality and Social Psychology*, 1971, **17**, 259–266.

Efran, J. S., & Marcia, J. E. Treatment of fears by expectancy manipulation: An exploratory investigation. *Proceedings of the 75th Annual Convention of the American Psychological Association*, 1967, **2**, 239–240.

Efran, J. S., & Marcia, J. E. Systematic desensitization and social learning. In J. B. Rotter, J. E. Chance, & E. J. Phares (Eds.), *Applications of a social learning theory of personality.* New York: Holt, 1972. Pp. 524–532.

Flanagan, J. Galvanic skin response: Emotion or attention? *Proceedings of the 75th Annual Convention of the American Psychological Association*, 1967, **2**, 7–8.

Folkins, C. H., Lawson, K. D., Opton, E. M., & Lazarus, R. S. Desensitization and the experimental reduction of threat. *Journal of Abnormal Psychology*, 1968, **73**, 100–113.

Gale, E. N., Hyman, E., & Ayer, W. A. Physiological measures during systematic desensitization: A report of two cases. *Journal of Clinical Psychology*, 1970, **26**, 247–250.

Geer, J. H. Fear and autonomic arousal. *Journal of Abnormal Psychology.* 1966, **71**, 253–255.

Grings, W. W., & Uno, T. Counterconditioning: Fear and relaxation. *Psychophysiology*, 1968, **4**, 479–485.

Grossberg, J. M. The physiological effectiveness of brief training in differential muscle relaxation. (Technical Report No. 9). La Jolla, California: Western Behavioral Sciences Institute, 1965.

Grossberg, J. M., & Wilson, H. K. Physiological changes accompanying the visualization of fearful and neutral situations. *Journal of Personality and Social Psychology*, 1968, **10**, 124–133.

Guthrie, E. R. *The psychology of learning.* (rev. ed.) New York: Harper, 1952.

Herrnstein, R. J. Method and theory in the study of avoidance. *Psychological Review*, 1969, **76**, 49–69.

Hyman, E. T., & Gale, E. N. Galvanic skin response and reported anxiety during systematic desensitization. *Journal of Consulting and Clinical Psychology*, 1973, **40**, 108–114.

Jacobson, E. *Progressive relaxation.* Chicago: Univ. of Chicago Press, 1938.

Jones, M. C. The elimination of children's fears. *Journal of Experimental Psychology*, 1924, **7**, 382–390.

Katkin, E. S. Relationship between manifest anxiety and two indices of autonomic response to stress. *Journal of Personality and Social Psychology*, 1965, **2**, 324–333.

Katkin, E. S. The relationship between a measure of transitory anxiety and spontaneous autonomic activity. *Journal of Abnormal Psychology*, 1966, **71**, 142–146.

Katkin, E. S., & McCubbin, R. J. Habituation of the orienting response as a function of individual differences in anxiety and autonomic lability. *Journal of Abnormal Psychology*, 1969, **74**, 54–60.

Katkin, E. S., & Murray, E. N. Instrumental conditioning of autonomically mediated behavior: Theoretical and methodological issues. *Psychological Bulletin*, 1968, **70**, 52–68.

Lader, M. H., & Mathews, A. M. A physiological model of phobic anxiety and desensitization. *Behaviour Research and Therapy*, 1968, **6**, 411–421.

Lader, M. H., Gelder, M. G., & Marks, I. M. Palmar skin conductance measures as predictors of response to desensitization. *Journal of Psychosomatic Research*, 1967, **11**, 283–290.

Lang, P. J. The mechanics of desensitization and laboratory studies of human fear. In C. M. Franks (Ed.), *Assessment and Status of the Behavioral Therapies and Associated Developments.* New York: McGraw-Hill, 1969. Pp. 160–191.

Lang, P. J., Melamed, B. G., & Hart, J. A psychophysiological analysis of fear modification using an automated desensitization procedure. *Journal of Abnormal Psychology*, 1970, **76**, 220–234.

Lazarus, R. S. *Psychological stress and the coping process.* New York: McGraw-Hill, 1966.

Lehrer, P. M. A laboratory analog of desensitization: Psychophysiological effects of relaxation. *Psychophysiology*, 1970, **6**, 634. (Abstract)

Leitenberg, H., Agras, W. S., Barlow, D. H., & Oliveau, D. C. Contribution of selective positive reinforcement and therapeutic instructions to systematic desensitization therapy. *Journal of Abnormal Psychology*, 1969, **74**, 113–118.

Lick, J. R. Expectancy, false GSR feedback, and systematic desensitization in the modification of phobic behavior. Paper presented at meetings of Eastern Psychological Association, Boston, 1972.

Lomont, J. F., & Edwards, J. E. The role of relaxation in systematic desensitization. *Behaviour Research and Therapy*, 1967, **5**, 11–25.

Malmo, R. B. Activation: A neuropsychological dimension. *Psychological Review*, 1959, **66**, 367–386.

Marcia, J. E., Rubin, B. M., & Efran, J. S. Systematic desensitization: Expectancy change or counterconditioning? *Journal of Abnormal Psychology*, 1969, **74**, 382–387.

Mathews, A. M. Psychophysiological approaches to the investigation of desensitization and related procedures. *Psychological Bulletin*, 1971, **76**, 73–91.

Mathews, A. M., & Gelder, M. G. Psychophysiological investigations of brief relaxation training. *Journal of Psychosomatic Research*, 1969, **13**, 1–12.

Mowrer, O. H. On the dual nature of learning—A re-interpretation of "conditioning" and "problem-solving." *Harvard Educational Review,* 1947, **17**, 102–148.

Oliveau, D. C., Agras, W. S., Leitenberg, H., Moore, R. C., & Wright, D. E. Systematic desensitization, therapeutically oriented instructions and selective positive reinforcement. *Behaviour Research and Therapy,* 1969, **7**, 27–33.

Page, H. A. The facilitation of experimental extinction by response prevention as a function of the acquisition of a new response. *Journal of Comparative and Physiological Psychology,* 1955, **48**, 14–16.

Paul, G. L. Physiological effects of relaxation training and hypnotic suggestion. *Journal of Abnormal Psychology,* 1969, **74**, 425–437.

Paul, G. L., & Trimble, R. W. Recorded vs. "live" relaxation training and hypnotic suggestion: Comparative effectiveness for reducing physiological arousal and inhibiting stress response. *Behavior Therapy,* 1970, **1**, 285–302.

Rappaport, H. The modification of avoidance behavior: Expectancy, autonomic reactivity, and verbal report. *Journal of Consulting and Clinical Psychology,* 1972, **39**, 404–414.

Rappaport, H., & Katkin, E. S. Relationships among manifest anxiety, response to stress, and the perception of autonomic activity. *Journal of Consulting and Clinical Psychology,* 1972, **38**, 219–224.

Sherrington, C. S. *The integrative action of the nervous system.* New Haven, Connecticut: Yale Univ. Press, 1906.

Silverman, A. J., Cohen, S. I., & Shmavonian, B. M. Investigation of psychophysiologic relationships with skin resistance measures. *Journal of Psychosomatic Research,* 1959, **4**, 65–87.

Sokolov, E. N. *Perception and the conditioned reflex.* New York: Macmillan, 1963.

Solomon, R. L., & Wynne, L. C. Traumatic avoidance learning: The principles of anxiety conservation and partial irreversibility. *Psychological Review,* 1954, **61**, 353–385.

Stampfl, T. G., & Levis, D. J. Essentials of implosive therapy: A learning-theory-based psychodynamic behavioral therapy. *Journal of Abnormal Psychology,* 1967, **72**, 496–503.

Taylor, J. A. A personality scale of manifest anxiety. *Journal of Abnormal and Social Psychology,* 1953, **48**, 285–290.

Van Egeren, L. F., Feather, B. W., & Hein, P. L. Desensitization of phobias: Some psychophysiological propositions. *Psychophysiology,* 1971, **8**, 213–228.

Waters, W. F., McDonald, D. G., & Koresko, R. L. Psychophysiological responses during analogue systematic desensitization and nonrelaxation control procedures. *Behaviour Research and Therapy,* 1972, **10**, 381–393.

Wilkins, W. Desensitization: Social and cognitive factors underlying the effectiveness of Wolpe's procedure. *Psychological Bulletin,* 1971, **76**, 311–317.

Wilson, G. D. GSR responses to fear-related stimuli. *Perceptual and Motor Skills,* 1967, **24**, 401–402.

Wolpe, J. *Psychotherapy by reciprocal inhibition.* Stanford, California: Stanford Univ. Press, 1958.

Wolpe, J. Quantitative relationships in the systematic desensitization of phobias. *American Journal of Psychiatry,* 1963, **119**, 1062–1068.

Wolpe, J. The comparative clinical status of conditioning therapies and psychoanalysis. In J. Wolpe, A. Salter, & L. J. Reyna (Eds.), *The conditioning therapies: The challenge in psychotherapy.* New York: Holt, 1964. Pp. 5–16.

Wolpe, J. The behavioristic conception of neurosis: A reply to two critics. *Psychological Review*, 1971, **78**, 341–343.

Wolpe, J., & Flood, J. The effect of relaxation on the galvanic skin response to repeated phobic stimuli in ascending order. *Journal of Behavior Therapy and Experimental Psychiatry*, 1970, **1**, 195–200.

Wolpe, J., & Lang, P. J. A fear survey schedule for use in behaviour therapy. *Behaviour Research and Therapy*, 1964, **2**, 27–30.

CHAPTER 8

Social Psychophysiology

GARY E. SCHWARTZ

*Department of Psychology
and Social Relations
Harvard University
Cambridge, Massachusetts*

DAVID SHAPIRO

*Harvard Medical School
Department of Psychiatry
Massachusetts Mental Health Center
Boston, Massachusetts*

I.   Introduction 377
     A. Examples of Early Electrodermal Research 380
     B. Early Justifications for the Electrodermal Response 382
     C. Overview of the Chapter 382
II. Attitudes 383
III. Empathy 390
IV. Small Groups and Social Interaction 397
V.   Cross-Cultural and Ethnic Differences 407
VI. Summary and Conclusions 410
     References 413

I. Introduction

"Recently, along with social psychology and psychophysiology, a relatively new area of interdisciplinary research has been receiving increasing attention from behavioral scientists. This field has been called 'sociophysiology' (Boyd & DiMascio, 1954), or 'interpersonal physiology' (DiMascio, Boyd, & Greenblatt, 1957)—the study of the reciprocal influence of human physiological systems and social systems." Thus began what is probably the first review article especially devoted to the application of physiological measures to the study of social variables (Kaplan & Bloom, 1960, p. 128). In the past 12 years, significant gains have been made in social psychology and psychophysiology, both in methodology and theory, and have in part stimulated a growing interest in the integration of the two areas. In 1964, Leiderman and Shapiro edited the first book on psychophysiology and social behavior, and two subsequent reviews of recent research have appeared in *The Handbook of Social Psychology* (Shapiro & Crider, 1969) and in *The Annual Review of Psychology* (Shapiro & Schwartz, 1970).

Social psychophysiology, as the field is called today, appears to have grown for a number of reasons. On the social psychological side, researchers have been looking for more reliable, quantifiable, relatively bias-free measures of social interaction, and the development of the polygraph has made the use of physiological measures feasible. In addition, social psychologists are becoming increasingly aware of the inherent biological nature of behavior, not only through growing research in psychosomatic medicine, but also through basic discoveries concerning drugs and the human brain. On the psychophysiological side, researchers are becoming increasingly aware of the effects of instructions, setting, experimenter, and so forth, on physiological measures. In part, interest in these variables was first stimulated for methodological reasons; that is, to develop techniques that would eliminate such variables as potential sources of unwanted (confounding) variance. However, with the passing of behaviorism as the dominant force in psychology, psychophysiologists (like others) have turned their attention back to questions that had been initially raised by researchers early in the 1900s. For example, the scientific study of empathy has received renewed interest (e.g., Krebs, 1970a), a problem inherently suitable to social psychophysiological investigation, since empathy is directly concerned with emotional perception and reactivity with regard to others.

It is not surprising that with science changing its emphasis from being concerned primarily with the pursuit of basic knowledge to the solution of human problems, the study of social biological factors in human behavior is taking on added impetus and significance. This is most clearly illustrated by the emergence of a new graduate program in a major university that is directly concerned with the application of physiological measures to the study of political problems (e.g., physiological indices as nonverbal correlates of political attitudes). The researcher in this field of "biopolitics" must not only be a skilled political scientist, he must also be versed in psychophysiology, social psychology, and bioengineering. It is not difficult to understand why an interdisciplinary approach to such complex problems is almost essential.

Despite the intrinsic appeal of social biological research, the field is relatively young and undeveloped in that it has not yet established a working set of integrated methods and theories. This is further complicated by the fact that the boundaries encompassing the content of both social psychology and psychophysiology are wide and unclear. However, it is possible to delineate trends that may later prove fruitful in producing sound scientific procedures and more comprehensive social biological theories. The purpose of this chapter is to illustrate some of what we consider to be important approaches in social psychophysiology, either because of their methodological sophistication, creativity, or theoretical underpinnings. By nature this chapter is incomplete since it deals almost exclusively with electrodermal measures. The reader may want to examine the earlier reviews for an overview of the entire field.

As it turns out, electrodermal measures are firmly rooted in social biological research. In one sense, many of the psychophysiological studies in the early 1930s involved some social variables, although most of the authors did not interpret them as such. When psychotherapists and social psychologists began to look at interpersonal behavior (since most therapists were trained in medicine, it is not surprising that they turned to biological variables in their search for objective measures of the therapeutic process), electrodermal measures were highly preferred for a number of reasons. First, research using electrodermal measures had a long history. Second, electrodermal measures were easy to record and relatively inexpensive, using simple electrode attachment procedures. Third, electrodermal changes could be easily detected by eye; it was a simple matter to tell when a response had occurred, and therefore relatively easy to quantify. Thus, time-consuming hand scoring and averaging required for functions such as heart rate were avoided. Finally, electrodermal activity made obvious common sense—sweating, as everyone "knew," was related to anxiety and stress, and much research had been conducted claiming that the electrodermal response (EDR) was a good indicator of emotionality, consciousness, and subjective experience. Although debates occurred in the 1940s concerned with whether EDR really measured anything "psychic," some investigators were willing to bypass these questions and use it in their research. Altogether, electrodermal measures were an ideal choice for social psychophysiological research (e.g., as an able index of "lying"). As it turns out, electrodermal measures are valuable dependent variables in the scientist's armory, as will be illustrated in this chapter.

A. Examples of Early Electrodermal Research

Many of the early studies using the EDR in complex stimulus situations have involved manipulations of variables that might be considered social in nature. For example, as early as 1933 Ruckmick briefly reported an experiment designed to study affective responses to the "motion-picture situation by means of the galvanic technique" (skin resistance). Apparently, he varied the experimental setting by presenting the films "in the laboratory, in the public theater, and in the psychopathic hospital." He studied normals and psychopathic patients in response to films containing segments that he considered were humorous, conflictual, or romantic. Also varied was the subject's age and for some subjects, film repetition. Although the empirical validity of his findings need not detain us here (furthermore, it is impossible from the brief writeup to evaluate the data), his conclusions may be worth noting for historical interest. For example, he reported that "maximal deflections for slap-stick comedy were obtained in the group below 12 years; for scenes described as romantic in the group near 16 years of age at which time there were also the most extreme deflections." Also, for his patient population, the "reshowing technique indicated that emotions of excitement with scenes of conflict rapidly declined, whereas amorous emotions were kept at a fairly constant level throughout six showings of the same picture [p. 713]."

Actually, this study illustrates some of the variables and techniques currently employed in social psychophysiology. Complex material like motion pictures and video tapes can be presented to different populations in different settings while physiological measures are continuously monitored. Such a paradigm might well be employed in present research investigating the effects of different kinds of television programming on the development of aggression in the child, or in evaluating the interest value of different commercials in relation to the material they are embedded in.

A later paper by Greenwald (1936) illustrates some early methodological innovations concerning the use of "continuous affective stimulation" in the form of motion pictures. For example, the technique he developed for time-locking the activity of the motion pictures with the "camera of Wechsler's psychogalvanograph" is as follows:

> In order to permit identification of the parts of the picture at which dermal responses occurred, a method of synchronizing the projector with the recording film was devised. This consisted of a system of speed-reducing gears driven by the projector. During each revolution the slowest shaft of this system closed a mercury key which flashed a light at certain

scenes in the picture and marked these points on one edge of the photographic record. On the other edge of the film a similar light circuit,
closed by a hand key, served to indicate places at which observations
were made. The complete photographic record of this included the dermal
response-curve, vertical bars to indicate time intervals, points of syn-
chronization with the picture, and similar points denoting O's reports [pp.
4–5].

However, some of Greenwald's experimental procedures would be seriously questioned today. For example, in order to make a "rigorous experimental attack," graduate students were selected to serve as "Os,"
his assumption being that "such Os would show a greater degree of
affective maturity than a random adult population." Furthermore, in order
that "those unskilled in mental inspection be given some degree of training and those who were already skilled gain some practice in the motion
picture situation," Greenwald preexposed his subjects to a comedy entitled "The Bathing Beach Boob" which contained "the usual series of
disconnected misadventures considered humorous in the movies of 1926."
This, he felt, best prepared his subjects for the mildly affective experience
of seeing four segments of a silent western cowboy series.

Although experimental designs such as the above may seem crude
by today's standards, this research was advanced for its time. This is
clearly illustrated when one considers the kinds (or lack) of procedures
and designs used when two-person interactions were first investigated.
Resistance to experimental manipulation was partly due to the fact
that the early research was stimulated by investigators (clinicians) interested in the scientific study of psychoanalysis and the use of physiological measures in the therapeutic hour was a natural step. Probably the
earliest published work in this area was by Lasswell (1935, 1936) who
recorded physiological measures from volunteer subjects in a psychoanalytic interview situation. The basic procedure was to continuously
monitor physiological responses (his primary measures were skin resistance and heart rate) as well as transcripts of verbal material of all
the sessions. Lasswell developed a pattern theory of skin "conductivity"
and heart rate, his conclusion being that "changes in active (conscious)
affect are positively associated with pulse rate, and changes in (unconscious) tension are positively associated with electrical skin conductivity."
Although his specific classifications of the verbal material need not concern
us here, it is valuable to point out that he analyzed the verbal material
by breaking the sessions into patterns: those showing increases in heart
rate and skin conductivity, those that showed both functions decreasing,
and those showing increases in one function and simultaneous decreases
in another. This *post hoc* analysis procedure is interesting but wanting

in that it does not make it possible to experimentally delineate the variables influencing changes in physiological function that occurred during the psychotherapeutic hours themselves. Parenthetically, Lasswell felt that the "behavior of the subject in the psychoanalytic situation is in some degree *externalized* with reference to the immediate environment, and in some degree *internalized* with reference to the self [italics his]." Although Lasswell could not then know it, about a quarter of a century later, in a critical review article covering the use of psychophysiological variables in the investigation of psychotherapy, Lacey (1959) was to present his formal theory of internal–external attention and directional fractionation. As it turned out, Lacey's analysis seemed to temporarily halt research in interpersonal psychophysiology. However, as will be seen later, new experimental procedures have made it possible to do systematic research on the "effects of person" on physiological activity.

B.   Early Justifications for the Electrodermal Response

As discussed earlier, the use of the EDR by most early investigators was based on the belief that the EDR measured something like affect, tension, or experience. Although it is now known that the EDR systematically varies as a function of many variables, it is interesting to note that there is some basis for maintaining the belief in the relationship of subjective experience to EDR magnitude. In an important review by McCurdy (1950) entitled, "Consciousness and the galvanometer," he presented 19 correlations, all positive, ranging from +.45 to 1.00 with a median value of +.75, between self-reports of magnitude of many different kinds of experience and amplitude of skin resistance responses (SRRs). McCurdy viewed this relationship as a "very sturdy fact." Lacey (1959), 9 years later, used words as stimuli in three separate samples of subjects, and found correlations of +.89, +.87, and +.94 between the word rankings based on the SRRs in his samples and rankings based on subjective ratings obtained earlier by Whatley Smith (1922). Lacey concluded that "in accord with McCurdy, we are certainly willing to entertain the suggestion that the differential magnitude of galvanometric deflections to words is one of the most reliable phenomena in psychology today!" This often-ignored but simple observation serves as one historical justification for maintaining electrodermal measures in social psychophysiological research.

C.   Overview of the Chapter

Given the lack of specific boundaries delineating both social psychology and psychophysiology, any attempt at organization is by definition arbitrary. For clarity of presentation, the material has been organized into areas that have either received attention in the past, or in our opinion will grow in interest in the future. These areas are: (1) attitudes, (2) empathy, (3) small groups and social interaction, and (4) cross-cultural and ethnic differences. A section containing a brief summary and concluding remarks will then be presented.

II. Attitudes

Since attitudes, by definition, are predispositions to respond in a particular way to specific stimuli (in a given situation), they cannot be directly observed or measured, and therefore must be inferred. By and large, most research on attitudes has used verbal reports as their sole measure. However, since it is generally assumed that attitudes actually consist of three central components: beliefs (cognition), feelings (affect or emotion), and overt reactions, the addition of physiological measures in the assessment of attitudes is justifiable, at least in theory (Cooper, 1959).

Although there are a few early studies attempting to measure attitudes, one study in particular clearly and concisely considered many of the issues central to current attitude research. Smith (1936) performed an experiment to study the effects of group opinion on individual opinion and the SRR. He administered a questionnaire containing controversial statements to a group of students in a lecture, requesting that they indicate their agreement or disagreement as well as the strength of their conviction (from 1 to 5) for each of the items (if they had no opinion, they left it blank) (see Table 1). Then, 4 weeks later, each subject was asked to individually participate in an experiment involving the recording of physiological measures. Skin resistance was continuously recorded on a Wechsler Psychogalvanograph while the same 20 statements were read to the subjects by a different person (by Professor Henry Murray). As before, subjects were asked to agree or disagree and then give their rating of conviction, only this time, prior to each question, the subject was told the average opinion of the group that was obtained 4 weeks earlier. Actually, unknown to the subjects, the group ratings were fictitious arranged so that half were made to *agree with* the rating previously given by the subject and half made to be *against* the subject's prior rating. Interstatement intervals of 20 sec were used and the verbal reports carefully recorded.

The data were analyzed separately for the three subgroups of subjects (Radcliffe, Harvard, and summer school students). First, Smith found

TABLE 1

STATEMENTS READ TO SUBJECTS IN AN EXPERIMENT ON ATTITUDES, GROUP
OPINION, AND ELECTRODERMAL ACTIVITY[a]

1. Labor should enjoy a much larger share in the management of industry than it does at present in the United States.
2. Churches preserve the enslaving superstitions of primitive minds and consequently their support should be withdrawn.
3. Divorce should be granted only in the case of grave offense.
4. The Soviet experiment in government should be encouraged.
5. What is called "conscience" is the reverberation of early parental teachings, and hence is nothing more than the ethical conventions of former generations.
6. Sexual restrictions should be more rigid for women than for men.
7. There has never been a good war or a bad peace.
8. It is inadvisable for women with children to pursue a professional career.
9. As a protective measure the army and navy should be enlarged.
10. Parts of the Bible may be accepted as the inspired word of God.
11. It should be considered bad form for women to drink alcoholic beverages.
12. The taxation of large incomes should be increased.
13. The constitutional right to free speech and free press should be maintained in time of war.
14. Belief in personal immortality is incompatible with the acceptance of the scientific viewpoint.
15. Modernistic art should be enthusiastically encouraged.
16. Socialism and communism are valuable balance wheels in our political life and should receive full protection.
17. Children should be given a religious training.
18. The husband should be recognized as the head of the family.
19. There are enduring moral standards for the judgment of political action.
20. A college education should be first and last a training for citizenship.

[a] From Smith (1936).

that on the average, statements Ss agreed with (yes statements) showed the smallest SRRs, while statements they disagreed with (no statements) produced the largest responses; "zero" opinion ratings fell in between (all three subgroups showed the effect). Following this, when he broke the data down according to the strength of conviction, the results clearly showed that the stronger the conviction, the larger the SRR, except for "complete" conviction (rating of 5), which showed a decreased response (see Fig. 1). Smith plotted curves using a percentage transformation of the data (as an added precaution, in the original paper the data are presented both in terms of means *and* medians, to show the lack of skewness in the distributions).

Smith viewed these findings in terms of conflict and emotion, suggesting that generally it takes more affect to say no than yes, and that the

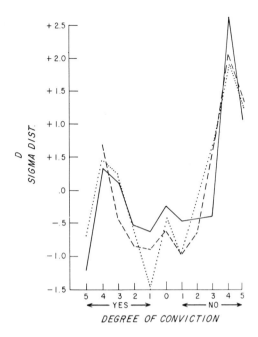

Fig. 1. Skin resistance changes in Radcliffe (– – –), Harvard (————), and summer school (· · · · ·) students to 20 different statements (see Table 1) as a function of degree of conviction. The ordinate is a derived percentage score using

$$\frac{\text{change in apparent resistance} \times 100}{\text{apparent resistance level}}$$

as the definition of an SRR. (See text.) (Adapted from Smith, 1936.)

stronger the conviction, the stronger the affect. Furthermore, he argued that whereas ratings of 2–4 contain elements of conflict, the rating of complete agreement does not (thus the drop in SRR with ratings of 5). As will be shown, a conflict-affect model of EDR and attitudes handles most of the recent data obtained.

Concerning the interaction of the group opinion and individual opinion, Smith writes:

> When we investigated the data further, we found four possibilities: "Yes" *with* the group opinion, "no" *with* the group opinion, "yes" *against* the group opinion, and "no" *against* the group opinion. We should expect to find the least conflict when the subject said "yes" and was *with* the group. This composite GSR had a value of 1.33. The greatest conflict should come when the subject said "no" and was *against* the group. The value of this composite GSR was 2.47. The categories "no" *with* and "yes" *against*

should fall in between these levels. Their composite GSR values are, respectively, 1.61 and 1.81. We may expect that a greater conflict will be aroused when the subject is *against* the group than when the subject is *against* only the statement, but *with* the group [p. 161].

Based on these data, Smith proposed a three-factor model which contributes to "thalamic excitation and to increased GSR: (1) the intensity of the degree of conviction, (2) the decisional process, and (3) the assertional processes." Although he lacked the sophistication of statistical analysis and experimental controls for suggestion and experimental bias (Rosenthal, 1966), his study nevertheless is exemplary of careful, systematic, and thoughtful research on the topic.

Recent research has tended to emphasize attitudes concerning religion, prejudice, and race. In an excellent study by Dickson and McGinnies (1966) SRRs were obtained to 12 statements adapted from Thurstone and Chave's (1929) list of opinions about the church. Four of the statements were laudatory of the church (pro-church statements), four were critical (anti-church) and four were neutral toward the church. The 60 subjects were selected from a sample of 486 students on the basis of their scores on a 23-item Likert-type scale measuring attitudes toward the church; 20 students made up the pro-church group, 20 composed the anti-church group, with the remaining 20 subjects falling midway between and representing the neutral-church group. Since Dickson and McGinnies (1929) were interested in the theoretical question of "affectivity in arousal of attitudes" in relation to the SRR, the following instructions were used:

> A number of statements concerning the church will be read to you from the tape recorder. As you hear each statement, try to think, as best you can, how you feel about the statement. You might try to imagine how you would respond if you were with a group of friends and someone made this statement to you. Do not, however, say anything during the experiment! Just concentrate on the statements and how you feel about them . . . [p. 586].

Mean SRRs to each type of statement were computed separately for each group and a highly significant ($p < .001$) interaction emerged. That is, students who were pro-church showed similar SRRs to the pro- and neutral-church statements, but larger SRRs to the anti-church statements, while the students who were anti-church showed comparable SRRs to the anti- and neutral-church statements, but very large SRRs to the pro-church statements. In other words, the largest SRRs consistently occurred to statements *against* those maintained by the individual. The neutral group fell in between, showing slightly higher responses to the anti-church statements. These data are in agreement with those of an earlier study by McGinnies and Aiba (1965) showing that Japanese students respond with higher SRRs when listening to a political communication with which they disagreed than when listening to one with which they agreed.

About the same time, Katz, Cadoret, Hughes, and Abbey (1965) reported an experiment to test a physiological mediation hypothesis underlying the finding that attitude statements similar and dissimilar to subjects' opinions functioned as positive and negative reinforcers in a discrimination learning task (Golightly & Byrne, 1964). A 41-item attitude survey by Golightly and Byrne was administered to 20 students, and for each student ten items were selected for which he had strong opinions. Some items were very strong, such as, "There definitely is (or is no) God" while others were more neutral, such as "Most modern religions are monotheistic." The results showed that the largest SRRs occurred to the statements *opposed* to the S's view. As Katz *et al.* did not report the specific instructions used, one does not know if instructions emphasizing the *experience* of the statement were employed. It is likely that such instructions do accentuate the effect, as will be seen in a later section on empathy.

We are aware of one negative study using EDRs and religious attitudes. Brown (1966) reported that skin conductance responses (SCRs) to sets of religious and secular words of religious believers and disbelievers did not differentiate the two groups. He did find, however, that the arousal value of the stimuli was specific to each individual. It is possible that his "strength of religious belief" criterion was not relevant to the task, or that simple words are not generally as effective in eliciting affective attitudinal reactions as statements (especially if the instructions do not require that the subject react affectively). Also, had he employed neutral words as well, differences may have appeared between groups. It would seem that Brown's conclusion that there is no shared emotional basis to religious belief is premature and unjustified, based on the experiment.

A series of experiments performed by Cooper and his associates (Cooper & Siegel, 1956; Cooper & Pollock, 1959; Cooper & Singer, 1956) and summarized in Cooper (1959) have used physiological measures in an attempt to support the thesis that prejudicial attitudes are accompanied by relatively strong emotion. The basic design for each of the experiments was the same. Subjects were asked to rate and rank 20 alphabetically listed ethnic and national groups in terms of preference. The groups were Argentines, Austrians, Canadians, Chinese, English, French, Germans, Greeks, Indians (India), Irish, Italians, Japanese,

Jews, Mexicans, Negroes, Filipinos, Poles, Russians, Swedes, and Turks. Subjects were also studied in the laboratory, where skin resistance, recorded by a Stoelting Psychogalvanoscope, was monitored in response to complimentary and derogatory statements which could contain any one of the ethnic words. An example of a complimentary statement is, "The world over, no single group of people has done as much for us, for our civilization as the _____." Conversely, one derogatory statement is, "People can be divided into two groups: the good and the bad. Close to the bottom of the list are the _____." For each subject, derogatory statements were made about the group *most liked* by the subject, and complimentary statements about the group *most disliked* by the subject. In addition, pro and con statements about groups rated by subjects in the middle were also presented. Compared to pro and con statements to the neutral groups, derogatory statements pertaining to liked groups tended to show larger SRRs, while complimentary statements pertaining to disliked groups very reliably produced larger SRRs (e.g., in the Cooper and Singer study, 19 of 20 Ss showed this effect, $p < .001$).

A particularly convincing demonstration of this relationship is shown in the Cooper and Pollock study where it was possible to rank nine ethnic groups both by magnitude of the SRR and by a paired comparison method using a questionnaire (Table 2). In this experiment the Spear-

TABLE 2

SRR AND PAIRED-COMPARISON (P-C)
RANKS FOR STIMULUS GROUPS[a]

Stimulus group	SRR Rank[b]	P-C Rank[c]
Swedes	1	2
Canadians	2	1
Austrians	3	5
English	4	4
Poles	5	7
Germans	6	3
Japanese	7	6
Jews	8	9
Mexicans	9	8

[a] Adapted from Cooper and Pollack (1959).
[b] SRR rank 1 indicates least response by sample.
[c] P–C rank 1 indicates best liked by sample.

man rank order correlation was .82, $p < .01$. Altogether, the studies of Cooper and co-workers show a reliable relationship between amplitude of the EDR and prejudice, where prejudice is defined as an "emotional attitude" (Dewey & Humber, 1951), or as Gordon Allport (1954) has put it, "We tend to become emotional when a prejudice is threatened with contradiction." The reader will note the similarity of all the studies reviewed here in relation to the earlier theory of conflict and affect, as originally proposed by Smith (1936). Given the reliability of these findings, it would seem possible to move in the direction of investigating more central questions concerning the development, maintenance, and elimination of prejudicial attitudes using psychophysiological techniques.

A few studies have investigated the effects of race on electrodermal activity in relation to prejudice. Rather than just using verbal or pictorial stimuli, these experiments have studied the effects of persons (e.g., black versus white experimenters) on EDR activity as well. An experiment by Rankin and Campbell (1955) initiated this form of research. The basic paradigm was a free-association task using affective words such as *love, flunk, mother,* and *petting* as stimuli while skin resistance was continuously monitored from the right hand. The experimental manipulation was a series of four bogus adjustments of phony electrodes on the left hand involving hand-to-hand contact between E and S. For each S, half the adjustments were made by a black experimenter, the remaining adjustments by a white assistant (and vice versa) (20 white Ss received a BWWB design, while 20 received the WBBW order). According to Rankin and Campbell, the white researcher was a "graduate student in psychology, aged 23, 5'9" in height, 155 pounds in weight," while the black researcher was a "graduate student in education, aged 32, about 5'11½" in height, weight 192 pounds." Therefore, in addition to skin color, the variables of age, height, and weight clearly differentiated the two experimenters.

Average SCRs to the word associations following each of the four contacts were computed separately for the two orders. First, the results showed that the average SCR was larger to the black than to the white experimenter ($p < .001$). With appropriate caution, the authors preliminarily concluded that their study "makes its most definitive contribution in showing, for the first time as far as is known, that the GSR will differentiate between persons as stimuli."

Besides this main effect, the data showed that, on the average, SCRs habituated over the four contacts. However, order interacted with contact, since within each group the black experimenter elicited greater SCRs than the white. As a further test of their hypothesis, they compared the average difference in SCRs between the black and white experimenters with two paper and pencil direct attitude tests about the American Negro. A sample item from the information test is, "In intelligence tests made in New York City schools comparing Negro and white children, it has been found that the average IQ of white children is 100, and the average IQ of Negro children is: (a) 85, (b) 89, (c) 95, (d) 100, (e) 106." The direct attitude test asked Ss to describe their own feelings about blacks in terms of 25 prepared statements to be endorsed with 5 levels of agreement and disagreement. Separate correlations were computed for both BW orders, both tests, and whether the test was given before, or after, the physiological measures. (It was given as a classroom exercise.) Although there were some discrepancies between groups, the average correlation of SCR and direct attitude was +.42; for SCR and indirect test it was consistently lower, average being +.15, while the direct by indirect correlation itself was on the average +.55. Thus, there was some suggestion that questions concerning feelings toward blacks were related to the Ss' SCRs, while information about blacks *per se* was not.

These data clearly support the potential value of the EDR in the measurement of prejudice. However, had Rankin and Campbell studied black Ss as well, and exposed Ss to more than one experimenter of each color, the results would have been more convincing. Concerning the latter, Porier and Lott (1967) found that using a sample of black and white "stimulus" persons resulted in a nonsignificant person effect, while the SCR bias scores across individuals correlated significantly with the California E Scale (which is related to prejudice).

It seems reasonable that in studying race effects a more direct approach might be valuable, such as exposing white and black Ss to white and black experimenters (e.g., confederates) or other black and/or white Ss in a game, or competition, or group task, while monitoring EDRs from both. Under controlled conditions, more specific effects might be obtained than those observed in response to supposedly unrelated, affective words in a free-association task. Westie and DeFleur (1959), using slides of blacks and whites both alone and together, have reported that SRRs to picture stimuli differentiate between prejudiced and nonprejudiced subjects. Clearly, motion picture or video stimuli might well prove useful in this type of research.

III. Empathy

As mentioned earlier, interest in the study of empathy, or the related construct of rapport, began with clinical research of the psychotherapeutic process (see review by Lacey, 1959). By and large, this research was purely descriptive, and did not involve the experimental manipulation of variables in a systematic fashion. However, in the past 10 years, significant methodological advances have been made in the general area of vicarious experience, particularly in social psychology. For example, empathy has been afforded the position of being an important theoretical mediator in eliciting helping behavior or altruism, and many experiments have been performed to explore the determinants of altruistic behavior, and the role of empathy (reviewed by Krebs, 1970a):

> Personality theorists and social psychologists generally recognize that the emotional responses of one person (performer) may elicit emotional responses from another (observer). When these emotional responses are similar, the relationship between the performer and observer is described as empathetic, or one of *identification* [Berger, 1962, p. 464; original italics].

In his classic paper, Berger provided a simple, yet convenient definitional framework for empathy, envy, and sadism, and also provided a theoretical and procedural approach to investigate these concepts using classical (and operant) conditioning paradigms. If emotions are classified as either pleasant $(+)$ or unpleasant $(-)$ then, according to Berger, empathy reflects those situations where both the performer and observer experience positive, or negative, emotions together (cases I and IV in Table 3). It follows that envy can be defined as occurring when pleasant emotions in the performer elicit negative (e.g., depressive) emotions in the observer (case II). Conversely, sadism can be defined when unpleasant emotions in the performer lead to pleasant experiences (vicariously) in the observer (case III). Of necessity, this framework must be limited in scope. However, it does provide the service of organizing a complex set of phenomena into a conceptually manageable form.

TABLE 3

COMBINATIONS OF EMOTIONAL RESPONSES
FOR PERFORMER AND OBSERVER[a]

Case	Performer's UER	Observer's ER
I	+	+
II	+	−
III	−	+
IV	−	−

[a] From Berger (1962).

When a person is exposed to a standard experimental procedure, such as classical conditioning using a tone as a conditioned stimulus (CS) and a brief, painful shock as an unconditioned stimulus (UCS), he perceives and experiences the situation as a function of (1) the experimental manipulations used (including instructions), (2) his history of prior environmental learning and experiences, and (3) his biological endowment. What Berger (1962) clearly spelled out is that if this individual is treated not as the main focus of interest, but rather as a performer, one can then easily study experimentally the reactions of another subject observing this situation. For example, one can raise the obvious question— to what extent are the physiological (and subjective) responses of a person observing another person in a classical conditioning situation similar to the physiological (and subjective) responses of this performer? What are the variables that influence the degree of similarity and dissimilarity, and how can they be modified? Once stated, it becomes clear that almost *any* situation or procedure developed for studying persons (or even lower animals) can be studied from the point of view of vicarious experience.

Historically speaking, it is fascinating to ponder the reasons why psychologists were so long in realizing this simple fact, especially since so much of human behavior involves the perception of others in a different situation. The lag in the experimental study of vicarious experience is clearly multidetermined, and the reader will likely produce his own set of salient reasons. However, with the development of mass communication and, in particular, television, the importance of learning through imitation or observation takes on added significance. Clearly, the study of vicarious experience has important implications for applied research, and, as Berger (1962) illustrated using the conditioning paradigm *per se,* the research has any number of experimental procedures to draw on using the performer–observer paradigm.

Berger (1962) reported three experiments initially to investigate the role of the environmental UCS (presence or absence of shock) and the role of the performer's UCR (presence or absence of a "shock reaction"—arm movement) in vicarious conditioning. Rather than use a real subject as the performer, Berger used a confederate who was instructed in the required behavior. The general paradigm and results can be illustrated through Experiment II using both of the above variables in a 2×2 factorial design: (1) In the shock–movement group (S–M), the observers were told that the performer would be shocked, and the performer reacted with an arm movement when apparently being shocked. (2) For the no shock-movement group (NS–M), the observer was told that the performer would make a voluntary arm movement at a given signal (light dimming was the CS), and that the performer was not being shocked. (3) A shock–no movement group (S–NM) included the observer instruction of shock but no mention of arm movement (no visible reaction of performer). (4) Finally, there was a no shock–no movement group (NS–NM). All observers were instructed that they were actually control subjects, and would not be shocked. They were not specifically instructed to empathize.

Subjects received 4 adaptation trials (CS alone), 10 conditioning trials, and 3 test (or extinction) trials. Scoring simply for the presence or absence of an observable response, the results are shown in Fig. 2.

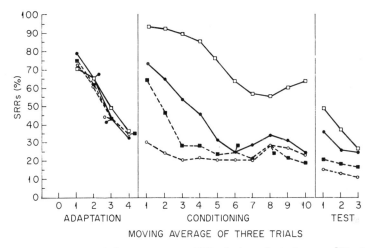

Fig. 2. Percentage of observers giving SRRs during adaptation, conditioning, and test trials (Experiment II): (□) S–M condition; (■) S–NM condition; (●) NS–M condition; (○) NS–NM condition. (See text.) (Adapted from Berger, 1962.)

It can be seen that while all groups show a similar decline in responding during adaptation, the groups diverge during conditioning, with the shock–movement group (S–M) showing the largest increase in responding during this period. Besides this significant shock–movement interaction ($p < .025$), the analyses of variance showed that the shock instructions and the arm movement variable each yielded significantly more SRRs ($p < .001$). Altogether, the data clearly showed that both the experimental situation *and* the person's (performer) reaction to it influences vicarious EDR responding in the observer—thus providing evidence for the use of physiological functions as a measure of vicarious learning.

The three experiments reported by Berger (1962) were *not*, however, interpreted as evidence for empathy *per se*, but rather evidence for vicarious instigation. "While the reader may be tempted to think of these experiments as reflecting some sort of observer *empathy*, there is no basis for this interpretation. Some observers may be empathizing and some observers may be enjoying the performer's apparent pain [p. 450]." Of course, Berger *could* have evaluated this question using another dependent measure (e.g., he suggested the semantic differential), and he then could have split his subjects on this particular dimension. It is conceivable that the EDR data might differentiate between empathy and sadism, given the proper experimental conditions. It would also have been valuable if Berger had recorded physiological activity from his performer (who was really an actor or stooge) or even from a real subject. In this manner it would have been possible to compare classical conditioning that is directly experienced with conditioning that is experienced vicariously.

Stimulated by this pioneering research, a number of experiments have recently been reported that address themselves more directly to the phenomenon of empathy. In an excellent chapter, Stotland (1969) has critically examined the concept of empathy and reports a series of studies on empathy, some using physiological measures. One of the often-ignored issues in this research concerns the role of instruction, or set, in empathy. Stotland points out that "both laymen and psychologist commonly assume that empathy entails an individual putting himself symbolically or imaginatively in another's place." George Herbert Mead (1934) has called this process "taking the role of the other." To empirically investigate this question, Stotland and Sherman (in Stotland, 1969) examined the effect of inducing three different mental sets in the subjects as they observed another person undergoing a painful, neutral, or pleasurable experience (a 3×3 design). The first instruction was that as one subject observed the other, he was to imagine how he himself would feel if he were in the other's position ("imagine-self" condition). The second set was that Ss were instructed to imagine how the other person felt ("imagine-him" condition); the third was simply to "watch him." Stotland hypothesized that the most empathy would be found in the imagine-self condition, the least empathy being in the watch-him condition. He also suggested that this effect might be less pronounced in the pleasurable condition, "since it is difficult to communicate pleasure clearly and definitely in the laboratory." These hypotheses place cognitive or symbolic processes as important determinants of empathy in humans.

Subjects were run in a social perception study in groups of 4–6, plus one paid assistant trained to act like a subject. Palmar sweating was recorded at critical times during the experiment (e.g., poststimulation) using a standard sweat print technique, while pulse volume was recorded continuously from all Ss. At the front of the room was a table and a "diathermy" machine with all dials and controls in view of the subjects. Actually, the machine was not operational, although all the lights and dials worked as if it were. The experimenter (Sherman) told all subjects that:

> Either it is set at the low level of intensity, which results in a sensation of warmth in the hand of the demonstrator that is quite soothing and quite pleasant; or it is set at the intermediate level which results in a sensation of heat in the hand of the demonstrator that is neither pleasurable nor painful; or it is set at a high level of intensity, higher than used by physical therapists, which results in a sensation of pain. However, for a period of thirty seconds, it is neither physiologically nor psychologically damaging. Now whichever level is used for a given session is determined by a random device [Stotland, 1969, p. 291]."

Subjects were also led to believe erroneously that the selection of the "demonstrator" was random, by placing a red X in the lower left-hand corner of their questionnaire. All Ss were told that if they did not receive a red X, it meant they were not the demonstrator for that session. They were to remain seated and observe the actual demonstrator carefully, trying to remember all of their reactions in order to fill out the questionnaire at the end.

The demonstrator sat with his back to the subjects since it was "judged to be quite impossible for a student assistant to do a convincing job of expressing feelings facially and to do so for some 20 sessions." In the high intensity condition, the demonstrator jerked back and then squirmed moderately in his seat as if he were receiving a painful stimulus; for the pleasurable treatment, he jerked slightly and then relaxed slowly moving his hands as if "sopping up" the warmth; for the neutral condition, he gave only a slight start. For all conditions, the machine was "kept on" for 30 sec.

A number of significant effects were obtained using mean palmar sweating scores. However, the major result was that the greatest sweating occurred in the imagine-self painful condition, indicating that stimulus factors and set are important interactive determinants of empathy. Another way of stating this is that observing a person experiencing pain (as opposed to a neutral stimulus) results in greater autonomic arousal in the observer when he is symbolically "putting himself in the other's shoes."

The Stotland studies, although they employ a number of advances in social psychological methodology, use a relatively simple and insensitive electrodermal procedure. It seems reasonable to expect that continuous monitoring of electrodermal activity carefully timelocked to various phases of a rigidly paced task would provide a more sensitive assessment of anticipatory, stimulation, and poststimulus arousal. Of course, it is also likely that more complete use of nonverbal and verbal indicants of emotion in the demonstrator (e.g., facial expressions, blushing, intensity of voice) would enhance the empathy effect. Clearly, parametric research exploring the communicative role of various situations and responses (e.g., nonverbal factors) in empathy can be performed using electrodermal activity as one dependent variable.

Returning to the basic question of degree of similarity of physiological activity in vicarious experiences, a series of experiments by Craig and associates (e.g., Craig & Weinstein, 1965; Craig, 1968; Craig & Wood, 1969) have compared physiological activity as a function of imagined, vicarious, and direct stress experiences. In particular, based on the theoretical notions of Lacey (1959, 1967) concerning directional fractionation of skin resistance and heart rate deceleration in attention to the environment, Craig argued that direct experience of a stressor (immersion of one's hand in freezing water) would lead to decreased skin resistance and increased heart rate, while observing someone else experiencing it might lead to decreased skin resistance but decreased heart rate (due to outward attention). If this proved to be the case, then the experience of empathy, at least physiologically, might not be the same as direct experience, thus challenging the basic theoretical underpinnings of empathy itself.

The basic paradigm was to have each subject observe another person experiencing the stressor as well as experience it himself. In one experiment, Craig and Wood (1969) had 48 male and female subjects immerse their hands in a −4°C brine solution, and also observe their partner doing this, using an experimental design counterbalanced for order. Skin resistance and heart rate were continuously recorded in the direct and the vicarious experience conditions. The results showed that whereas both experiences produced decreases in skin resistance, heart rate decelerations tended to occur to vicarious experience, while accelerations occurred to direct experience. Thus, in accord with Lacey, strong evidence was obtained for physiological differences between direct and vicarious experience of a painful stimulus.

However, the question arises, were the subjects in fact empathizing in the vicarious condition? In other words, in view of the results of Stotland emphasizing the importance of cognition in empathy, were the conditions of the Craig and Wood experiment conducive to the induction of empathy in the observers? Apparently not, since Craig and Wood were not studying empathy *per se*, the situation lacked the incentive to empathize, and it may have actually inhibited it. For example, in their vicarious conditions bland instructions were used: "I want you to simply sit here and observe what the other subject is doing." These instructions are similar to the "watch him" instructions of Stotland (1969). In fact, Craig and Wood did find that the SRR was greatly attenuated in their vicarious condition, as was the sweat measure in the Stotland watch-him condition. One wonders if subjects were instructed to directly empathize with the person experiencing the cold pressor test (and the performer was told to communicate his experiences—verbally and nonverbally to the observer) whether both SRRs *and* heart rate would now increase. In other words, would conditions optimal for vicarious experience leading to empathy produce more similar physiological patterns between performer and observer? This point is stressed here because there is a tendency to lump research on vicarious experience together without considering the complex instructional and social differences between experiments. Given the influence of instructional and social variables on physiological functions, questions such as the above should be raised (and systematically researched) in order to understand the many factors contributing to vicarious experience.

Brief mention should be made of potential individual differences in reactivity to direct versus vicarious experience. Alfert (1966, 1967) has reported that in anticipation of electric shock (direct threat) and an accident movie (vicarious threat), subjects reliably differ in their relative reactivity to the two situations. Specifically, direct threat reactors tended to be more self-confident, extroverted, dominant, and at ease in social situations. On the other hand, vicarious threat reactors tended to be low in self-confidence, introverted, anxious, inhibited in impulse expression and uneasy in social interaction and interpersonal relationships. Whether these differences are environmentally determined, or interact with inherited biological differences, remains an open question.

IV. Small Groups and Social Interaction

Physiological approaches to the analysis of small group interaction have been of particular interest to social psychologists and psychophysiologists. Physiological measures such as the EDR tap information about the individual that is not directly observable by other persons, by and large, and therefore the information does not have an interactive influence on subsequent reactions of the other persons. In contrast, measures of social behavior are essentially interactive. This is not to say that certain internal bodily processes do not result in changes that are accessible as cues to outside observers. There are numerous examples such as blushing, tremors, sweating, and blanching that provide cues in judging an individual's total reaction in a situation, although little research has been reported on how cues such as these influence the course of social interaction and on-going behavior in groups.

The unusual interest in psychophysiological approaches to groups stems from the common observation that group situations engender strong affect in the individual, and therefore large physiological changes, as well as having powerful effects on individual behavior, perception, and social development. From the standpoint of a biological perspective, group structures and functions have been of critical significance in human evolution, it can be assumed. If there has been natural selection for various forms of social behavior, then knowledge of social–behavioral–physiological interrelationships should offer clues to the integrative functions of higher nervous centers.

It is well known that somatic and autonomic functions are integrated to varying degrees at all levels of the nervous system. If appropriate organizing features of the environment are used as stimuli, then further knowledge may be gained about these integrative relationships. Group situations, it is argued, can provide appropriate, though complex, stimulus input needed for elucidating these relationships, as compared with the simple physical stimuli often brought into the laboratory. The enormous complexity and variability of cultural forms of group behavior in man make the endeavor extremely difficult, and many researchers have preferred to focus their efforts on primate groups and animal societies (see DeVore, 1965).

Advantages and complications not withstanding, it is clear that empirical research relating group behavior and physiological responses has proceeded slowly. As mentioned earlier, the physiological technology has developed to the point where empirical studies are easy to carry out. The problem has been one of defining and delineating variables of theoretical significance and practical relevance.

A major issue that has guided some of this research concerns the general influence of social or group presence on the individual. Zajonc (1965) hypothesized that physiological arousal is increased by the presence of other people, and that this arousal helps account for the seemingly inconsistent findings in the literature on social facilitation (see Dashiell, 1930). Sometimes the presence of other people increases or facilitates performance of the individual, and sometimes it seems to decrease or interfere with performance. Zajonc reasoned that arousal should lead to the greater occurrence of dominant responses. If correct responses are dominant, performance is facilitated; if incorrect responses are dominant, performance is interfered with. While many behavioral studies appear to support this hypothesis, research on the physiological underpinnings is only rudimentary. The fact that the different indices of physiological arousal, whether electrocortical, biochemical, electrodermal, cardiovascular, or skeletal motor, are in and of themselves poorly correlated, underscores an important basic complication (Lacey, 1967). A few studies indicate these and other problems concerning the evaluation of this hypothesis.

A direct test of the social facilitatory effects of competition on reaction time was carried out in a sample of 92 subjects by Church (1962). He found that palmar skin conductance levels increased along with self-rated alertness in a competitive as compared with a noncompetitive situation. However, the subjective and physiological indices, which were labeled "motivational" by Church, were not directly associated with the decrease in reaction time, though they differed as a function of the social context. As Church points out, correlations between peripheral indices of level of activation, such as palmar conductance, and measures of performance, such as reaction time, disappear when the level of the stimulus itself is partialed out. This is essentially the same conclusion arrived at by Elliott (1964) in an extensive analysis of physiological and performance variables in a reaction time task. Put simply, the physiology does not seem to "mediate" the overt performance, while both are separately affected by the nature of the social setting. In this case, a competitive situation results in increases in a physiological variable and also in greater efficiency of performance in a sensory–motor task. Whether in fact physiology and behavior are dissociated or independent of one another, in this instance, may depend on applying methods of analysis and experimentation other than those used in these studies (see Schwartz, 1972). Time-locking social behavioral change to physiological responses under more precise stimulus conditions may be one avenue of investigation (Shapiro & Schwartz, 1970).

The fact that physiological indices of arousal increase in the presence of a group may be dependent on other factors as well, and consistent data have not always been obtained. Martens (1969) showed that subjects sweated more in the presence of an audience than when alone, under task conditions. Similarly, in a routine task, individuals working in isolation had lower levels of skin potential than when working on the same task with two other persons (Shapiro, Leiderman, & Morningstar, 1964). The latter group task required subjects to cooperate minimally and come to decisions about solutions to the task. In contrast, other studies suggest an opposite pattern. Kissel (1965), in a well-designed study, found that skin conductance is higher for the individual performing a task in isolation as compared to conditions in which another person is present. In this study, the task was stressful—one without a correct solution. Interestingly, the relative reduction in skin conductance was greater when the other person, who is doing an unrelated task, is a friend rather than a stranger. Kissel concludes on the basis of this study and prior research on social affiliation under different conditions that anxiety induces the need for people, that "misery loves company" as exemplified in the physiological results.

It is immediately apparent that a number of variables can be singled out for study, such as the nature of the task and the nature of the group presence. If a task is difficult or stressful, as Kissel's data suggest, then group presence may lead to a reduction in physiological levels. If a task is relatively simple, increased levels of physiological activity may be the typical outcome, in a group condition. Shapiro and Crider (1969) offered this hypothesis, basing it in part on the evidence presented by Bovard (1959). Bovard proposed that the presence of other persons serves a protective function, reducing the harmful effects of stress. For example, animals manifest less overt fear and maladaptive behaviors when other animals are present than when isolated. Soldiers who undergo hardship and stress do better when they are together in combat units than when they are alone. In the latter case, the sheer capacity for physical survival would have to be constant in both conditions to draw this conclusion. The effects of people in inhibiting arousal levels under stress would also vary according to their relationship to the individual, whether friend or stranger (or foe?), that is, according to prior experiences and relationships of people with one another.

Highly controlled tests of the group presence hypothesis are almost impossible in humans, although there is reason to believe, as stated previously, that such effects are partly biological in nature. In an unpublished study (Shapiro), skin potential level was measured once a minute during a 15-min waiting or rest period prior to the beginning of an experiment, while subjects were anticipating a simple task. Subjects were studied alone or in groups of three. In the latter situation, the subjects were asked to sit quietly and refrain from interacting or talking. In these relatively innocuous, nonanxiety conditions, greater habituation of skin potential level was observed in the group condition, although the differences were small. Apparently, mere presence seems to lessen physiological responsivity. These subjects were known to each other, not friends but co-students in a nursing school. As noted by Kissel (1965), the prior social relationship matters in the degree of stress reduction. Apparently, even under very minimal conditions of social interaction, similar results obtain. Naturally, these observations need to be replicated and extended.

Further similar observations on the effects of prior experience were obtained by Shapiro *et al.* (1964), in studies in which subjects (women) were required to perform a simple task, half the subjects doing the task alone and then in a group of three, and half doing the task in the opposite order. Both behavior (rate of initiations) and physiology (skin potential level) were correlated over the two situations, across people. Only in the case of group first and alone second were the correlations positive and significant. Apparently, experience in a group served to set both behavioral and physiological levels of output, an effect not unlike that observed in other purely behavioral studies of perception and attitudes (see Sherif, 1936). In this study, heart rate was found to be consistent for individuals regardless of the order of group and isolation conditions. That is, the electrodermal measures proved to be more sensitive to this particular variation in social condition, and therefore more informative than the cardiac measure.

The role of success and failure in various group conditions has been assessed in a number of studies with regard to electrodermal and behavioral variables, simultaneously monitored. This research derived from other work showing that interaction patterns in three-person groups can be modified by contingent reward, including conversational patterns (Levin & Shapiro, 1962), disagreement (Shapiro, 1963), and speech sequence (Shapiro, 1964). A guessing game is used as the task and provides a means of contriving various conditions of success and failure and simulating leadership patterns. Thus, by reinforcing the group (indicating that its decision is correct whenever a given subject is the one who initiated the particular decision), it is possible to determine how his behavior is influenced along with certain physiological indicators. In the first study (Leiderman & Shapiro, 1963), it was found that learning to initiate decisions was accompanied by variations in skin potential level: men subjects showed an increase in skin potential level and a decrease in variability of this measure, while women showed opposite patterns. The sex differences might be accounted for by cultural variations between men and women in approaching a task such as this one, or perhaps in the prior social relationships of the subjects. In this case, the women were acquainted with each other and the men were not. Other observations appear to support the conclusion that higher electrodermal levels are characteristic in successful roles (Shapiro & Leiderman, 1964) and also when another person in the same group is successful at the same time. Within any one situation studied, however, it was noted that correlations between behavior and electrodermal levels (and other physiological indices such as heart rate) were typically low and not significant.

An attempt was made to eliminate the variable of behavioral output

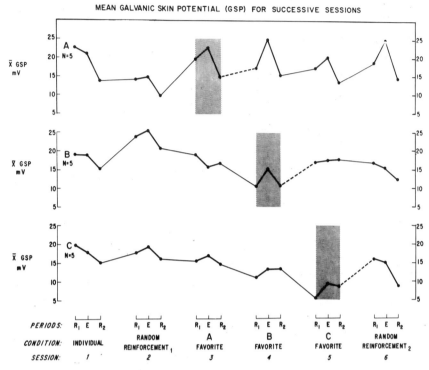 402   GARY E. SCHWARTZ AND DAVID SHAPIRO

Fig. 3. Skin potential level in successive sessions under different conditions of success and failure. The scores are based on three groups of 5 subjects each; within each group, the subjects are labeled A, B, and C. In session 1, the subjects were studied individually in the task (a guessing game). In sessions 2–6, the five subjects in each group worked together in the task. In sessions 2 and 6 each group was randomly reinforced. In sessions 3, 4, and 5, each group was reinforced when subjects A, B, and C, in that order, respectively, took initiative in the task. The blacked portions indicate subjects who were reinforced as the leader in each successive session; R_1 = initial rest; E = experiment; R_2 = final rest. (From Shapiro & Leiderman, 1964.)

by setting up a condition in which sheer physical activity was held constant by having each subject make the same number of initiations and controlling success and failure independently of overt behavioral acts. These results, the most systematic to date, suggest that failure is more arousing and being paired with another person in the same role also more arousing, as measured by skin potential habituation over time (Shapiro & Leiderman, 1967). The assumption is made here that the slower the rate of habituation of skin potential level, the more the arousal.

In one of the above studies (Shapiro & Leiderman, 1964), it was

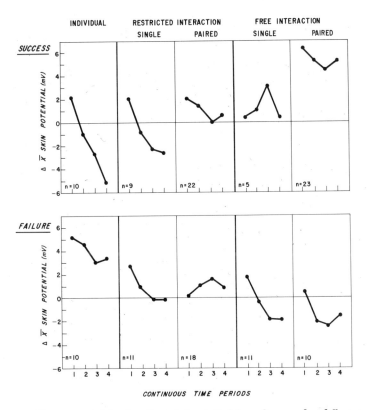

Fig. 4. Skin potential level, adjusted for initial base line, under different conditions of success and failure. (See text.)

noted that the ordering of success and failure experiences in a group has a decided impact on skin potential level. In this study, subjects in a three-person group were successful on one occasion and then failed in subsequent sessions, as arranged by the experimentally contrived guessing game. In effect, the conditions were contrived so that each person took a turn in leading the group. The results are depicted in Fig. 3. Those who were first to achieve reward (A subjects) tended to maintain high levels of skin potential in subsequent sessions even though, behaviorally speaking, they were "out of it." Those whose turn came last (C subjects) responded least to the contrived leadership manipulation. Some of these effects also showed up in initial resting base lines in subsequent sessions.

A summary of a variety of social situations under conditions of either success or failure, derived from some of the above studies, are portrayed in Fig. 4. These are arranged to suggest certain regularities in the data.

The top row of graphs in the figure refers to conditions of success, the bottom to conditions of failure. The first block of data on the left refers to the isolated condition in which subjects were asked to perform alone in a simple repetitive task. The next two are group tasks almost identical with the individual situation. Subjects had to perform on a timed basis, but their initiations had little effect on the environment since the outcomes were consistent and regular throughout. Although each subject was in visual contact with two other persons, verbal communication was not permitted. In the final two conditions at the right, each subject was free to take the initiative though the outcome depended on the experimenter. Here the interaction was relatively comparable to a real-life group situation in that subjects could talk to each other and were free to respond spontaneously.

On the basis of the divergent results in Fig. 4, a number of speculations may be offered concerning the significance of the different conditions. For one, success and failure have different implications for skin potential level, depending on the setting—group or individual. Second, a free group interaction situation tends to result in more extreme response levels than a restricted group interaction situation. Third, paired roles are different from single roles in response levels.

In the more restricted situations, success is not arousing relative to base line. But with more freedom to initiate activity, skin potential increases until it stands at a level that is surprisingly equivalent to the pattern shown by the isolated individual exposed to failure. It is remarkable that two quite different combinations of reinforcement and social circumstance (individual-failure, free interaction-paired success) have almost identical consequences for electrodermal activity. In contrast, the arousing effects of individual failure are clearly reduced under group conditions and with more freedom to initiate attempts at problem solution in conjunction with other people.

What accounts for the high levels of skin potential activity in the free-interaction paired success role? What makes it comparable to failure? A comparison of paired success and single failure roles in the free interaction situation may clarify the issue. Both these sets of subjects were in an identical type of group situation. However, the paired success subjects were effectively working to achieve success and avoid failure. The single failure subjects, in contrast, were able only to achieve failure and, as a consequence, their behavioral activity was also reduced. These results recall Brady's (1958) studies of the "executive" monkey, in which the working animal suffered the consequences of a stressor, physiologically, while the passive animal responded normally. The high skin potential levels in paired success under conditions of free interaction probably reflect active attempts to cope with the requirements of the task. The high levels may also be a result of aversive properties in the situation brought on by the somewhat more ambiguous nature of this task role.

Alternative explanations or hypotheses may be suggested for the results shown in Fig. 4. While the experiments and data are not conclusive, they do underscore the possible utility of a level measure of electrodermal activity in elucidating complex social processes. Both level changes with respect to base line and habituation or decrement in level over time may differentiate such processes. Among the social variables that warrant additional study are the capacity for initiating activity and achieving problem solutions, the ability to control or influence the environment, the type and degree of social reinforcement, and the nature of the social setting.

It is hypothesized that skin potential level may reflect a single process common to behavior in a variety of social conditions in which the individual is attempting to cope actively with environmental demand. Continued attempts at mastery or problem solution result in maintained levels of skin potential. Decreases in skin potential level would indicate either problem resolution or a cessation of attempts at active mastery. A physiological variable such as skin potential is of particular significance in that it may provide information that is not necessarily parallel to observed behavior or self-report. While it is often noted that the same physiological change observed in an experiment may occur with different behavioral processes (e.g., conflict versus positive interest), it is also true that the same overt behavior may occur with different physiological processes (e.g., central nervous system arousal versus inhibition). A social psychophysiological strategy of research can direct attention to the patterning of responses in a variety of physiological and behavioral systems with the goal of greater understanding of social and behavioral processes.

In concluding this section, further discussion is appropriate on other substantive findings and methodological issues in small group studies. Costell and Leiderman (1968) were interested in group pressure toward conformity as an instance of social stress, and they combined a group situation based on the procedures developed by Asch (1956) in which opinions of all but a target subject are basically incorrect. Individuals who are independent and able to resist the majority opinion of four other people in a group show higher levels of skin potential compared to individuals who conform to group opinion. This result recalls the study, already discussed, by Smith (1936) of individuals confronted by announced standards of their group on various issues. Holding a position contrary to the group's opinion yielded more electrodermal reactivity than being in agreement with the majority, and changing toward independence of group standards was also associated with larger SRRs. It will also be recalled that Smith found that when the individual's opinion was counter to the group but maintained at a high level of conviction, SRRs were actually smaller than for lower degrees of conviction. With really strong conviction, apparently no conflict is experienced and resultant electrodermal activity is reduced. That is, nonconformity in behavior is not necessarily accompanied by electrodermal responses but depends on the degree to which it is associated with uncertainty or conflict about the nonconforming behavior. This latter finding has been confirmed by Gerard (1961).

The study of role relationships and rapport in small groups has been explored in studies by Kaplan and associates, (Kaplan, Burch, Bloom, & Edelberg, 1963; Kaplan, Burch, & Bloom, 1964; Kaplan, 1967). These investigations derive from the assumption that the affective significance of an individual's interpersonal behavior will covary with the social structure of the group in which he interacts, the position of the subject and the positions of the social objects with whom he interacts; and this variation in the affective significance of the individual's behavior will be reflected in changes in his physiological activity. These studies come closest to the model typical in small group research. Groups are composed in various ways, for example, according to certain sociometric criteria, and then asked to discuss various topics over a series of sessions. The data then consist of behavioral interactions coded using the categories developed by Bales (1951) and continuous EDR recordings. Data such as these are very complex to analyze, and these experimenters have devised a number of interesting approaches. One of the more novel consists of an index of physiological covariation, presumed to relate to rapport, derived by correlating frequency of EDRs over time between two individuals. Many other correlations can be derived between role behavior and such indices, in addition to simple correlations between various behavioral acts and EDR frequency across individuals.

To indicate the potentiality of this manner of study, Kaplan's concluding summary from his 1967 paper is quoted:

> The present study investigated the relationship between physiological response, participation rank and affective-response rank in two four-man groups of medical students characterized by different sociometric composition: a negative group in which each person was disliked by one other person; and a positive group in which each person was liked by every other person.
>
> The groups met for five sessions to discuss topics known to be of interest to medical students. Sound film recordings of the sessions were coded in terms of Bales interaction process categories. Continuous and synchronous GSR recordings were made for each subject.

Participation rank was defined in terms of total response; and affective, positive-affective and negative-affective acts were defined in terms of the rank ordering of proportion of the subject's acts that were affective, positive or negative respectively relative to other subjects.

In the negative group, participation was positively related to affective behaviour. Subjects were more likely to manifest significant, positive GSR correlations with their own behaviour if they were high participators and high positive-affective responders and when addressing high participators and high negative-affective responders. This suggests the presence of an integrative role and perhaps a covert competition among leaders, the significance of which is reflected in GSR activity. Low participators tended to express themselves primarily in terms of instrumental activity with relatively little covariation between their GSR and social activity.

In the positive group, participation was inversely associated with affective activity. Subjects were more likely to manifest covariation between GSR and social behaviour if they were high negative-affective responders and low participators and when acting toward high participators and low negative-affective (high instrumental) responders. This suggests the presence of a deviant status which is associated with GSR activity as a result of the pressures toward uniformity experienced by the occupants of the status.

The statements of results are taken as hypotheses concerning the relationship between role differentiation and sociometric structure and the differential meaning (as reflected in GSR) of the various roles to the actors [p. 178].

V. Cross-Cultural and Ethnic Differences

The use of physiological measures such as the EDR in cross-cultural studies has not been extensive. By and large, such studies have consisted of observations by anthropologists and sociologists, and little experimental research has been attempted. The appeal of psychophysiology is obvious where interpretations may depend a great deal on knowledge of the meaning of verbal responses, patterns of emotional expression, various cultural conventions, and the like.

The research of Lazarus and his associates serves as one model for research in this field. The research is based on extensive experimentation with American subjects in which motion picture films are used to produce stress reactions (see Lazarus, 1966). Lazarus, Tomita, Opton, and Kodama (1966) showed a benign and a stressful film to Japanese students and adults and compared their physiological and subjective responses with data from American experiments. The benign film dealt with rice farming in Japan, intended as a Japanese version of a corn-farming film used in American studies; the stressful film dealt with subincision rites involving the mutilation of male adolescent genitals. In

many respects, the Japanese reaction to stress was similar to the reaction
of Americans. Unlike Americans, however, skin conductance was almost
as high during the benign film as during the stressful film for the Japanese. Also, skin conductance in the Japanese while they were viewing
the subincision film was poorly correlated to the specific stressful events
portrayed. In this respect, Lazarus suggests that the Japanese resemble
"high anxious" individuals in American studies. Self-report indexes, however, varied in the Japanese as in the American samples; more distress
was reported with the stressful stimuli, varying according to the content.
Lazarus seems to regard the skin conductance data in the Japanese
most likely to indicate a general state of apprehension, maintained
throughout both films, while their self-reports reflect relatively small
variations in perceived distress. Other possibilities are also proposed,
e.g., skin conductance is sensitive to relatively subtle emotional changes
only at low levels of stress. A major explanation is offered in terms
of Japanese culture and standards of behavior:

> . . . it does seem plausible that because of lack of experience in the labora-
> tory experimental settings and the tendency of Japanese culture to engender
> threats associated with being evaluated or disapproved by others, the
> Japanese subjects, both young and old, were much more apprehensive
> about the total experimental situation [Lazarus *et al.*, 1966, p. 631].

Another explanation of the anomalous skin conductance data in the
Japanese, as discussed by Lazarus, is genetically determined differences
in skin conductance between the Japanese and American samples. Significant differences between blacks and whites have been observed in
basal electrodermal level and electrodermal level reactivity (Bernstein,
1965; Johnson & Corah, 1963; Johnson & Landon, 1965). Blacks appear to
have *lower* skin conductance than whites, while Japanese in the Lazarus
study had higher conductance values. Differences in EDR reactivity
have also been found between Jewish subjects of different ethnic back-
grounds (Kugelmass, 1963; Kugelmass & Leiblich, 1966). Jewish subjects
of Near Eastern origin showed less EDR reactivity than Jewish subjects
born in America, Europe, or Israel. In a further study by these experimenters, subjects of Near Eastern origin were found to have higher
basal skin conductance and lower EDR reactivity. The degree to which
genetic factors are operative in addition to cultural processes has not
as yet been clarified. Differences in autonomic reactivity may be a function of a large number of social and psychological variables.

One more recent study bears on the Lazarus findings. In this experiment (Shapiro & Watanabe, 1972), an attempt was made to replicate
the operant conditioning of skin potential responses in a sample of Japa-

nese subjects using the within-subjects design of Crider, Shapiro, and Tursky (1966). Although the experimental manipulations are not really comparable to those of Lazarus *et al.* (1966), the results provide further evidence on the comparison of Japanese and American subjects. For one, the Japanese and American subjects showed similar operant control of their skin potentials. Second, the Japanese subjects were able to differentiate their responding in terms of high and low rates, according to the reinforcement contingency in operation. Third, they tended to have relatively higher rates of spontaneous skin potential responses as compared with the Americans. The Japanese might be regarded as more "anxious" in this experimental situation, in accord with the Lazarus *et al.* (1966) interpretation, although they were able to show effective self-control according to the experimental requirements. In fact, this self-control appeared to be more immediate in the Japanese, fitting in with the stereotype of well-controlled behavior presumed for the Japanese. Obviously there is great opportunity for speculation in the incomplete evidence that these few studies provide. The topics of emotional and behavioral control, overt versus covert expression of emotion, emotional expression in reaction to stress, genetic versus environmental influences on behavior, and the like, are ripe for empirical study, and the methods of psychophysiology provide an excellent means of bringing further understanding to cross-cultural differences.

Undoubtedly, the most provocative and substantial contribution in the study of ethnic differences using psychophysiological methods is reported in the papers by Sternbach and Tursky (1965) and Tursky and Sternbach (1967). These investigators hypothesized that implicit sets should have physiological correlates. Four different ethnic groups, all born and reared in the United States, were studied: Irish, Jewish, Italian, and Yankees (Protestants of British descent). They were selected on the basis of prior observations that these groups differ in their attitudes toward pain and expressions of pain. One of the major findings concerned the faster and more complete habituation of the Yankees' diphasic skin potential responses to electric shocks (see Fig. 5). Sternbach and Tursky indicate that this is an attitudinal correlation of the Yankees' matter-of-fact orientation toward pain. Differences were also found in resting mean heart rate, palmar skin resistance and face temperature levels, and in correlations between electric shock thresholds and heart rate, skin resistance, and skin potential levels. A final note of caution is added by these authors:

> Whatever the possible genetic-cultural interactions contributing to the responses which do differentiate among the groups, it is clear that there

is often great overlap among them due to individual differences. Therefore, we cannot make predictions about an individual's autonomic response pattern based solely on his ethnic membership [Tursky & Sternbach 1967, p. 73]."

Finally, for those researchers in the social sciences interested in the broad issues of social-biological interaction, particularly as regards social stress, a series of papers edited by Levine and Scotch (1970) is highly recommended. The paper in this volume entitled, "Experimental studies of conflict-produced stress" (Crider, 1970), reviews experimental research on conflict, based on the models of Pavlovian conditioning and the studies of real-life stress by Fenz and Epstein (1967).

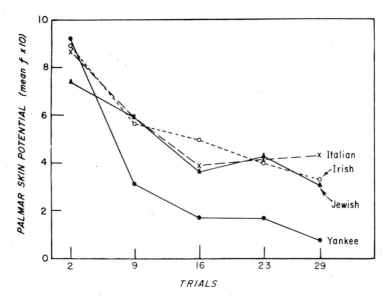

Fig. 5. Selected data points from smoothed curves (moving averages of three) for average number of diphasic palmar skin potentials to repetitive electric shocks. (From Sternbach & Tursky, 1965. © 1965 The Williams & Wilkins Co., Baltimore.)

VI. Summary and Conclusions

Electrodermal activity, given its high sensitivity to psychological stimuli and its ease of measurement, appears to be an excellent dependent variable in social psychophysiological research. The material presented in this chapter illustrates how cognition (attitudes), emotion (and vicarious experience), and the social environment (groups and cross-cultural variables) each influence these measures. However, it is apparent that research and theory have not progressed far enough as yet to yield a coherent, sociobiological model that significantly furthers our understanding of either social psychology or electrodermal psychophysiology. Since integrative research in social psychophysiology is relatively young, and in view of the inherent complexity of the questions posed, it is not surprising that the present state of knowledge is so limited. Still, the basic research strategies and findings to date are beginning to provide a more solid foundation that hopefully will lead to significant advances.

Understanding the effect of social variables on physiological activity is potentially important not only to social psychologists, but to all psychologists interested in using psychophysiological measures and procedures. Factors such as instruction and set which were once considered nuisance variables are now becoming important areas of investigation in their own right, and a thorough understanding of effects such as these is essential for meaningful and creative use of physiological measures. One by-product of this approach is that old paradigms can be reused to study new questions. For example, the basic classical conditioning paradigm in conjunction with electrodermal measures is now being used to study cognitive processes in the development of awareness of contingencies (e.g., Baer & Fuhrer, 1969). An analogous situation applies to the study of problems in social psychology.

For example, it is well known that instructions can lead to immediate conditioning of the EDR in a classical conditioning paradigm (Cook & Harris, 1937) and that it is possible to produce immediate extinction if the subject is instructed that no more shocks will occur, and that he believes the experimenter (e.g., by taking off the shock electrodes as a way of showing good faith) (Bridger & Mandel, 1965). This is but one example where whether or not the subject believes the instructions and follows them influences autonomic responding in the situation.

One implication of this common phenomenon is that it may be possible to use electrodermal measures to study the social psychology of human trust, in other words, use the EDR as an indicator of the degree to which the subject trusts and believes the experimenter. This basic idea was tested in a pilot study on six subjects (G. E. Schwartz, unpublished data), who were told that the experiment consisted of their receiving a series of lights, some followed by a brief electric shock. However, it was explained that before actually beginning the experiment, it was necessary to measure their resting physiological activity. Therefore, ten lights without shocks would be presented first. After the tenth light, the experimenter reentered the subject room explaining that he had forgotten to have the subject sign a standard release form—however, the form indicated that deception might be used in the study! The experimenter then apologized and explained that it would be necessary to repeat the ten resting trials, and that no shocks would be given. Needless to say, it was expected that this would lead the subjects to distrust the experimenter (e.g., lead them to expect shocks) and correspondingly the data indicated heightened skin resistance responding to the second set of ten lights, when compared with the first.

Also, in this preliminary study it was of interest to determine if it was possible to reinstate the trust that had been violated. Consequently, at the end of the second series, the experimenter reentered the room again, and explained the true purpose of the whole experiment, indicating that one more set of ten lights would be presented, and that there would be no shocks. The results indicated that some, but not all, of the subjects reduced their electrodermal responding back to preliminary levels, and interestingly, the postquestionnaire data suggested that these were the subjects who believed the final instruction.

These preliminary findings illustrate the potential value of applying basic techniques to more complex problems in social psychology such as human trust, since it is possible using similar paradigms to study the effects of attitudes, race, personal appearance, and so forth, in the formation and elimination of trust. Although carefully designed control groups are needed, the paradigms are readily adaptable, making meaningful comparisons possible. [Other approaches, such as the use of time-locked tasks, are discussed in Shapiro and Schwartz (1970).]

Despite the many assets of the electrodermal system, it would seem that whenever possible, research in social psychophysiology should consider other measures, such as heart rate and pulse volume, since it is not uncommon to find that different systems are sensitive to different aspects of a task (e.g., Lacey, 1967; Tursky, Schwartz, & Crider, 1970). This is clearly illustrated in two recent doctoral theses in our laboratory on empathy and altruism (Krebs, 1970b) and decision making and problem solving (Wing, 1971) where significant (though sometimes confusing) results were obtained which would have been missed, and therefore misinterpreted had only one measure been employed. It is not implied however, that research using the electrodermal system cannot provide meaningful results. While it is hoped that future research in psychophysiology will make it possible for social psychophysiologists to more rationally preselect the response (or combination thereof) best suited for their particular needs, it seems likely that electrodermal activity will remain a prime reflector of the social–biological nature of human behavior.

Acknowledgments

This work was supported by NIMH Grants K3-MH-20,476, MH-08853, and Office of Naval Research Contract N00014-67-A-0298-0024. We would like to thank Mrs. Catherine Hanley and Mrs. Judith Ross for their help in the preparation of the manuscript.

References

Alfert, E. Comparison of response to a vicarious and direct threat. *Journal of Experimental Research in Personality*, 1966, **1**, 179–186.

Alfert, E. An idiographic analysis of personality differences between reactors to a vicariously experienced threat and reactors to direct threat. *Journal of Experimental Research in Personality*, 1967, **2**, 200–207.

Allport, G. *The nature of prejudice*. Reading, Massachusetts: Addison-Wesley, 1954.

Asch, S. Studies of independence and conformity. I. A minority of one against a unanimous majority. *Psychological Monographs*, 1956, **70**, No. 9 (Whole No. 416).

Baer, P. E., & Fuhrer, M. J. Cognitive factors in differential conditioning of the GSR: Use of a reaction time task as the UCS with normals and schizophrenics. *Journal of Abnormal Psychology*, 1969, **74**, 544–552.

Bales, R. F. *Interaction process analysis*. Reading, Massachusetts: Addison-Wesley, 1951.

Berger, S. M. Conditioning through vicarious instigation. *Psychological Review*, 1962, **69**, 450–466.

Bernstein, A. S. Race and examiner as significant influences on basal skin impedance. *Journal of Personality and Social Psychology*, 1965, **1**, 346–349.

Bovard, E. The effects of social stimuli on the response to stress. *Psychological Review*, 1959, **66**, 267–277.

Boyd, R. W., & DiMascio, A. Social behavior and autonomic physiology: A sociophysiologic study. *Journal of Nervous and Mental Disorders*, 1954, **120**, 207–212.

Brady, J. V. Ulcers in "executive" monkeys. *Scientific American*, 1958, **199**, 3–6.

Bridger, W. H., & Mandel, I. J. Abolition of the PRE by instruction in GSR conditioning. *Journal of Experimental Psychology*, 1965, **69**, 476–482.

Brown, L. B. Religious belief and skin conductance. *Perceptual and Motor Skills*, 1966, **23**, 477–478.

Church, R. M. The effect of competition on reaction time and palmar skin conductance. *Journal of Abnormal and Social Psychology*, 1962, **65**, 32–40.

Cook, S. W., & Harris, R. E. The verbal conditioning of the galvanic skin reflex. *Journal of Experimental Psychology*, 1937, **21**, 202–210.

Cooper, J. B. Emotion in prejudice. *Science*, 1959, **130**, 314–318.

Cooper, J. B., & Pollock, D. A. Identification of prejudicial attitudes by the GSR. *Journal of Social Psychology*, 1959, **50**, 241–245.

Cooper, J. B., & Siegel, H. E. The GSR as a measure of emotion in prejudice. *Journal of Psychology*, 1956, **42**, 149–155.

Cooper, J. B., & Singer, D. N. The role of emotion in prejudice. *Journal of Social Psychology*, 1956, **44**, 241–247.

Costell, R. M., & Leiderman, P. H. Psychophysiological concomitants of social stress: The effects of conformity pressure. *Psychosomatic Medicine*, 1968, **30**, 298–310.

Craig, K. D. Physiological arousal as a function of imagined, vicarious and direct stress experiences. *Journal of Abnormal Psychology*, 1968, **73**, 513–520.

Craig, K. D., & Weinstein, M. S. Conditioning vicarious affective arousal. *Psychological Reports*, 1965, **17**, 955–963.

Craig, K. D., & Wood, K. Physiological differentiation of direct and vicarious affective arousal. *Canadian Journal of Behavior Science*, 1969, **1**, 98–105.

Crider, A. Experimental studies of conflict-produced stress. In S. Levine & N. A. Scotch (Eds.), *Social Stress*. Chicago, Illinois: Aldine, 1970.

Crider, A., Shapiro, D., & Tursky, B. Reinforcement of spontaneous electrodermal activity. *Journal of Comparative and Physiological Psychology*, 1966, **61**, 20–27.

Dashiell, J. An experimental analysis of some group effects. *Journal of Abnormal and Social Psychology*, 1930, **25**, 190–199.

DeVore, I. (Ed.) *Primate behavior: Field studies of monkeys and apes.* New York: Holt, 1965.

Dewey, R., & Humber, W. J. *The development of human behavior.* New York: MacMillan, 1951.

Dickson, H. W., & McGinnies, E. Affectivity in the arousal of attitudes as measured by galvanic skin response. *American Journal of Psychology*, 1966, **79**, 584–587.

DiMascio, A., Boyd, R. W., & Greenblatt, M. Physiological correlates of tension and antagonism during psychotherapy: A study of 'interpersonal physiology.' *Psychosomatic Medicine*, 1957, **19**, 99–104.

Elliott, R. Physiological activity and performance: A comparison of kindergarten children with young adults. *Psychological Monographs*, 1964, **78**, No. 10 (Whole No. 287).

Fenz, W. D., & Epstein, S. Gradients of physiological arousal in parachutists as a function of an approaching jump. *Psychosomatic Medicine*, 1967, **29**, 33–51.

Gerard, H. B. Disagreement with others, their credibility, and experienced stress. *Journal of Abnormal and Social Psychology*, 1961, **62**, 559–564.

Golightly, C., & Byrne, D. Attitude statements as positive and negative reinforcements. *Science*, 1964, **146**, 798–799.

Greenwald, D. U. Some individual differences in electrodermal responses to continuous affective stimulation. *Psychological Monographs*, 1936, **48**, 1–27.

Johnson, L. C., & Corah, N. L. Racial differences in skin resistance. *Science*, 1963, **139**, 766–767.

Johnson, L. C., & Landon, M. M. Eccrine sweat gland activity and racial differences in resting skin conductance. *Psychophysiology*, 1965, **1**, 322–329.

Kaplan, H. B. Physiological correlates (GSR) of affect in small groups. *Journal of Psychosomatic Research*, 1967, **11**, 173–179.

Kaplan, H. B., & Bloom, S. W. The use of sociological and social-psychological concepts in physiological research: A review of selected experimental studies. *Journal of Nervous and Mental Disorders*, 1960, **131**, 128–134.

Kaplan, H. B., Burch, N. R., Bloom, S. W., & Edelberg, R. Affective orientation and physiological activity (GSR) in small peer groups. *Psychosomatic Medicine*, 1963, **25**, 245–252.

Kaplan, H. B., Burch, N. R., & Bloom, S. W. Physiological covariation and sociometric relationships in small peer groups. In P. H. Leiderman & D. Shapiro (Eds.), *Psychobiological approaches to social behavior.* Stanford, California: Stanford Univ. Press, 1964. Pp. 92–109.

Katz, H., Cadoret, R. J., Hughes, K. R. & Abbey, D. S. Physiological correlates of acceptable and unacceptable attitude statements. *Psychological Reports,* 1965, **17,** 78.

Kissel, S. Stress reducing properties of social stimuli. *Journal of Personality and Social Psychology,* 1965, **2,** 378–384.

Krebs, D. L. Altruism—An examination of the concept and a review of the literature. *Psychological Bulletin,* 1970, **73,** 258–302. (a)

Krebs, D. L. Empathically-experienced affect, and altruism. Unpublished doctoral dissertation, Department of Social Relations, Harvard University, 1970. (b)

Kugelmass, S. Effects of three levels of realistic stress on differential physiological reactivity. Air Force Office of Scientific Research, 1963, Washington, D.C. AFEOAR Grant 63-61.

Kugelmass, S., & Lieblich, I. Effects of realistic stress and procedural interference in experimental lie detection. *Journal of Applied Psychology,* 1966, **50,** 211–216.

Lacey, J. I. Psychophysiological approaches to the evaluation of psychotherapeutic process and outcome. In E. A. Rubinstein & M. B. Parloff (Eds.), *Research in psychotherapy.* Washington, D.C.: American Psychological Association, 1959. Pp. 160–208.

Lacey, J. I. Somatic response patterning and stress: Some revisions of activation theory. In M. H. Appley & R. Trumbull (Eds.), *Psychological stress.* New York: Appleton, 1967. Pp. 14–42.

Lasswell, H. D. Verbal references and physiological changes during the psychoanalytic interview: A preliminary communication. *Psychoanalytic Review,* 1935, **22,** 10–24.

Lasswell, H. D. Certain changes during trial (psychoanalytic) interviews. *Psychoanalytic Review,* 1936, **23,** 241–247.

Lazarus, R. S. *Psychological stress and the coping process.* New York: McGraw-Hill, 1966.

Lazarus, R. S., Tomita, M., Opton, E. M., Jr., & Kodama, M. A cross-cultural study of stress-reaction patterns in Japan. *Journal of Personality and Social Psychology,* 1966, **4,** 622–633.

Leiderman, P. H., & Shapiro, D. A physiological and behavioral approach to the study of group interaction. *Psychosomatic Medicine,* 1963, **25,** 146–157.

Leiderman, P. H., & Shapiro, D. (Eds.) *Psychobiological approaches to social behavior.* Stanford, California: Stanford Univ. Press, 1964.

Levin, G., & Shapiro, D. The operant conditioning of conversation. *Journal of the Experimental Analysis of Behavior,* 1962, **5,** 309–316.

Levine, S., & Scotch, N. A. (Eds.) *Social stress.* Chicago, Illinois: Aldine, 1970.

Martens, R. Palmar sweating and the presence of an audience. *Journal of Experimental Social Psychology,* 1969, **5,** 371–374.

McCurdy, H. G. Consciousness and the galvanometer. *Psychological Review,* 1950, **157,** 322–327.

McGinnies, E., & Aiba, H. Persuasion and emotional response: A cross-cultural study. *Psychological Reports,* 1965, **16,** 503–510.

Mead, G. H. *Mind, self and society.* Chicago, Illinois: Univ. of Chicago Press, 1934.

Miller, N. E. Learning of visceral and glandular responses. *Science,* 1969, **163,** 434–445.

Porier, G. W., & Lott, A. J. Galvanic skin responses and prejudice. *Journal of Personality and Social Psychology,* 1967, **5,** 253–259.

Rankin, R. E., & Campbell, D. T. Galvanic skin responses to Negro and white experimenters. *Journal of Abnormal and Social Psychology,* 1955, **51,** 30–33.

Rosenthal, R. *Experimenter effects in behavioral research.* New York: Appleton, 1966.

Ruckmick, C. A. Affective responses to the motion picture situation by means of the galvanic technique. *Psychological Bulletin,* 1933, **30**, 712–713. (Abstract)

Schwartz, G. E. Voluntary control of human cardiovascular integration and differentiation through feedback and reward. *Science,* 1972, **175**, 90–93.

Shapiro, D. The reinforcement of disagreement in small groups. *Behavior Research and Therapy,* 1963, **1**, 267–272.

Shapiro, D. Group learning of speech sequences without awareness. *Science,* 1964, **144**, 74–76.

Shapiro, D., & Crider, A. Psychophysiological approaches in social psychology. In G. Lindzey & E. Aronson (Eds.), *The handbook of social psychology.* Vol. III. (2nd ed.) Reading, Massachusetts: Addison-Wesley, 1969, Pp. 1–49.

Shapiro, D., & Leiderman, P. H. Acts and activation: A psychophysiological study of social interaction. In P. H. Leiderman & D. Shapiro (Eds.), *Psychobiological approaches to social behavior.* Stanford, California: Stanford Univ. Press, 1964. Pp. 110–126.

Shapiro, D., & Leiderman, P. H. Arousal correlates of task role and group setting. *Journal of Personality and Social Psychology,* 1967, **5**, 103–107.

Shapiro, D., & Schwartz, G. E. Psychophysiological contributions to social psychology. *Annual Review of Psychology,* 1970, **21**, 87–112.

Shapiro, D., & Watanabe, T. Reinforcement of spontaneous electrodermal activity: A cross-cultural study in Japan. *Psychophysiology,* 1972, **9**, 340–344.

Shapiro, D., Leiderman, P. H., & Morningstar, M. E. Social isolation and social interaction: A behavioral and physiological comparison. In J. Wortis (Ed.), *Recent advances in biological psychiatry.* Vol. 6. New York: Plenum, 1964. Pp. 129–138.

Sherif, M. *The psychology of social norms.* New York: Harper, 1936.

Smith, C. A study of the autonomic excitation resulting from the interaction of individual opinion and group opinion. *Journal of Abnormal and Social Psychology,* 1936, **31**, 138–164.

Smith, W. W. *The measurement of emotion.* New York: Harcourt, 1922.

Sternbach, R. A., & Tursky, B. Ethnic differences among housewives in psychophysical and skin potential responses to electric shock. *Psychophysiology,* 1965, **1**, 241–246.

Stotland, E. Exploratory investigations of empathy. In L. Berkowitz (Ed.), *Advances in experimental social psychology.* Vol. 4. New York: Academic Press, 1969. Pp. 271–314.

Thurstone, L. L., & Chave, E. J. *The measurement of attitude.* Chicago, Illinois: Univ. of Chicago Press, 1929.

Tursky, B., & Sternbach, R. A. Further physiological correlates of ethnic differences in response to shock. *Psychophysiology,* 1967, **4**, 67–74.

Tursky, B., Schwartz, G. E., & Crider, A. Differential patterns of heart rate and skin resistance during a digit-transformation task. *Journal of Experimental Psychology,* 1970, **83**, 451–457.

Westie, F. R., & DeFleur, M. L. Autonomic responses and their relationship to race attitudes. *Journal of Abnormal and Social Psychology,* 1959, **58**, 340–347.

Wing, R. Physiological changes during decision-making tasks. Unpublished doctoral dissertation, Department of Social Relations, Harvard University, 1971.

Zajonc, R. B. Social facilitation. *Science,* 1965, **149**, 269–274.

CHAPTER 9

Detection of Deception

GORDON H. BARLAND

DAVID C. RASKIN

Department of Psychology
University of Utah
Salt Lake City, Utah

I.   Introduction 418
     A. Usefulness of the Paradigm 418
     B. History 419
II. Methodology 421
     A. Lie Detection in the Field 422
     B. Detection of Information in the Laboratory 441
     C. Differences between Field and Laboratory 443
III. Theories of Lie Detection 445
IV. Major Problems Requiring Research 447
     A. Effectiveness of the Electrodermal Response 447
     B. False Positives and False Negatives 451
     C. Detectability in Different Populations 454
V.   Countermeasures and Counter-Countermeasures 456
     A. Mental Countermeasures 458
     B. Practice and Training 461
     C. Hypnosis 462
     D. Physical Countermeasures 465
     E. Pain 466
     F. Adrenal Exhaustion 467
     G. Respiration 467
     H. Chemical Countermeasures 468
     I. Miscellaneous Countermeasures 469
VI. Summary and Conclusions 470
     References 471

I. Introduction

It is remarkable that after thousands of years of searching for a quick, simple, and effective method of verifying the truthfulness of a person's statements, the technique which is most widely used today and has been demonstrated to possess validity and reliability far beyond chance is so little noticed by psychologists and by psychophysiologists. Perhaps this is due to a reluctance on the part of many scientists to become associated with a technique which has seemed like "modern witchcraft" and has often been advocated with incredible claims of accuracy by its practitioners. Few scientists have wished to risk their professional reputations by studying such a controversial, tainted concept. Fortunately, the situation is changing. During the past 15 years there has been an increasing recognition of the lie detection paradigm as being a suitable vehicle for the study of numerous questions of great theoretical interest in psychology. In fact, the lie detection paradigm is becoming recognized as one of the fundamental paradigms for psychophysiology (Orne, Thackray, & Paskewitz, 1972).

A. Usefulness of the Paradigm

Aside from the applied aspects of lie detection in the field, the lie detection paradigm in the laboratory seems to be useful for studying such processes as arousal, attention, motivation, and related functions. A typical laboratory study utilizing the lie detection paradigm often has the S select one of five or six cards. As E names each of the cards, S is required to answer "no" each time, thereby "lying" about the card he actually selected. The physiological response to each stimulus is compared with the responses to other stimuli. Prior to S's selection of a card, the various cards should have had equal value for him, and the largest response would be randomly distributed over the various stimuli during repetitions of the stimuli. However, under appropriate conditions the greatest response repeatedly occurs to the selected card. Thus, the process of selecting the card differentially alters the S's physiological responsivity to it (Orne et al., 1972). This fact permits the E to select specifiable stimuli, manipulate variables affecting the S, and observe the effects of these manipulations on the patterning of S's physiological responses. Among those variables which appear to be determinants of this differential responsivity are S's motivation to avoid detection, S's perception of the probability of detection, the meaningfulness of the information to be concealed, the physiological parameter being measured, feedback to S, S's age, physical and mental health, etc. Because many of the variables are psychological, this paradigm is a means of systematically investigating the contingencies under which previously neutral stimuli become capable of eliciting alterations in physiological responses (Orne et al., 1972).

B. History

Throughout the entire history of mankind there have been countless attempts to determine if a person is lying. Many of these, such as having persons suspected of a crime pull the tail of a magical donkey (Lee, 1953), would work only if the person being tested were ignorant of the fact that the technique did not work. Others, particularly those utilized by the religious inquisitors of medieval Europe and colonial America, could not possibly work regardless of the beliefs of the suspect. But other techniques were based upon careful observation of the physiological changes that occur in response to short-term psychological stress. There a number of excellent reviews of these prescientific attempts to detect deception (Larson, 1932; Lee, 1953; Trovillo, 1939).

The scientific effort to reliably differentiate between truthful and deceptive Ss is nearly a century old now and has encompassed a great variety of parameters, including the shunting of vascular supplies from one body part to another and changes in hand volume (Trovillo, 1939), reaction time to word associations (Crosland, 1929), respiratory changes (Benussi, 1914; Burtt, 1921a, b), blood pressure (Marston, 1917, 1938), hand tremors (Luria, 1930, 1932), electroencephalographic activity (Obermann, 1939), pupil size (Berrien & Huntington, 1943), oculomotor activity (Berrien, 1942; Ellson, Davis, Saltzman, & Burke, 1952), voice (Alpert, Kurtzberg, & Friedhoff, 1963; Fay & Middleton, 1941), oxygen saturation of the blood (Dana, 1958; Dana & Barnett, 1957; Thackray & Orne, 1968a), and behavioral symptoms (Ekman & Friesen, 1969; Horvath, 1972; Reid & Arther, 1953). For an excellent summary of the results of studies utilizing these measures, see Orne et al. (1972). The measure which has shown the greatest success in discriminating between truthfulness and deception in laboratory studies has been electrodermal activity, including the skin resistance response (SRR) (Ellson et al., 1952; Thackray & Orne, 1968a) and the skin potential response (SPR) (Lindsley, 1955; Thackray & Orne, 1968a).

The advent of the modern era of lie detection is difficult to pinpoint precisely, because it was an evolutionary process in which a number of individuals adapted existing equipment and techniques. Following his 1917 study, Marston used intermittent measures of systolic blood pressure for detecting deception in clinical and field situations (Marston, 1938). However, the credit for the development of modern field polygraph equipment and technique should go to Larson and Keeler. In 1921 Larson modified Marston's discontinuous blood pressure method by recording a continuous measure of cardiovascular activity by the Erlanger method and displaying the analog data for later detailed analysis. Also, he simultaneously recorded respiration (Larson, 1921). Thus, Larson's contribution consisted of combining and modifying the Benussi and Marston techniques. Larson's student, Keeler, modified Larson's bulky equipment and developed a portable polygraph to which he added an electrodermal measure in the early to mid-1930s (Inbau, 1935; Keeler, 1934).

Not much is known concerning the details of how the electrodermal measure came to be utilized in lie detection. It had long been known that electrodermal activity was a concomitant of emotional arousal or attention. During World War I, Troland, Burtt, and Marston conducted a major test of the various methods claimed to be of use in detecting deception, and eliminated the galvanograph as useless except in low-affect laboratory situations (Marston, 1921).

Although there is no record of Larson's having incorporated the galvanograph into his technique, he was familiar with it and had utilized it in both experimental and field situations. Larson felt that the galvanograph was more effective in the field than in the laboratory, but offers no evidence to support this (Larson, 1932, p. 237). Wilson is reported to have developed a nonrecording galvanometer in 1930 which Keeler and he used in 1931 to examine criminal suspects. The two then collaborated to incorporate the SRR component into the field-model polygraph, which Keeler then manufactured in the mid-1930s (Trovillo, 1939). In a series of experiments conducted with the psychogalvanograph in laboratory situations, Summers found it to be highly effective (Summers, 1939). Summers also claimed 100% detection using the psychogalvanograph as the sole measure when testing 43 criminal suspects in field situations (Summers, 1939). Kubis, extending Summers' work, reported that of more than 500 criminal suspects who had been examined using the psychogalvanometer as the sole measure, no incorrect decisions were found (Kubis, 1950).

It is a well-established fact that measures of electrodermal activity can discriminate between truth and deception at levels far beyond chance. Moreover, in essentially all studies comparing electrodermal measures with other measures (the notable exception is the one reported by Marston, 1921), electrodermal activity has been found to be the most effective (Barland, 1972a; Ellson *et al.*, 1952; Kubis, 1962; Kugelmass & Lieblich, 1966; Thackray & Orne, 1968a; Violante & Ross, 1964; Voronin, Konovalov, & Serikov, 1970). It is therefore somewhat surprising that the most influential field polygraph examiners consider electrodermal activity to be the least effective of the measures used in the field (Arther, 1971b; Lee, 1953; Marston, 1938; Reid & Inbau, 1966). This dichotomy is discussed in some detail starting on page 447.

The present-day polygraph manufactured for field use has remained basically the same as Keeler's polygraph of 35 years ago, the only real changes being a reduction in size and weight, the use of transistors rather than tubes in the electrodermal section, and other changes of convenience. The typical field polygraph measures respiration, skin resistance, and cardiovascular activity by means of occlusion plethysmography. Some field polygraphs measure only respiration and cardiovascular activity; others measure not only the three usual measures but also a second respiratory measure (i.e., thoracic and abdominal) and/or digital cardiovascular changes by means of photoelectric plethysmography.

Since the early 1950s, the field use of the polygraph in criminal and commercial applications has expanded tremendously, and at the present time it is being utilized throughout many areas of the world. While precise information is difficult to obtain because there is no central supervisory or regulatory agency, it is known to be used in the United States, Canada, Mexico, Brazil, Argentina, Puerto Rico, France, Israel, Iran, Japan, Nationalist China, Thailand, and the Philippines. While its use in other countries has not been verified, there is reason to believe that it is in much wider use than the above list would indicate. There are, however, a number of countries in which it is known not to be in use by the police. These include England, Australia, Denmark, Norway, Sweden, Finland, Iceland, the Soviet Union, and probably most or all other Communist bloc countries. It is interesting to note that the two main repressive dictatorships of the midtwentieth century, the Hitler and Stalin regimes, both failed to apply the polygraph technique even though both were probably aware of its development and applications (Luria, 1930; Volwassen, 1937).

II. Methodology

Both the goals and practices of lie detection as it is applied in field situations differ from those of laboratory studies. In order to assess the results of the field studies, it is necessary to understand the procedures used in the field and to know the rationale for their use. Procedures typically employed in the laboratory studies will be briefly presented, and the two will be compared and contrasted.

A.   Lie Detection in the Field

Lie detection procedures are used in the field in basically two different situations. In one instance an individual is suspected of having committed or having knowledge pertaining to a specific crime or incident. Usually such examinations are conducted by police examiners, although private examiners frequently conduct such examinations at the request of companies who wish to augment an internal investigation. Examinations are also conducted at the request of attorneys who wish to assure themselves that their clients are telling them a whole, true story or who wish to know how their client will respond on an examination before advising their client whether to take a police polygraph examination. Polygraph examinations are sometimes suggested by the courts in civil cases such as paternity suits, divorce cases, etc. (Arther & Reid, 1954; Pfaff, 1964; Schatkin, 1970).

The second type of field polygraph examination is personnel screening. This can take many forms: screening applicants for jobs involving access to money, commercial goods, or drugs; screening persons being considered for jobs involving access to classified information and/or positions in which there is reason to believe that attempts will be made to blackmail or tempt the holder of that position; or routine examinations of American and foreign nationals employed in certain job categories within the intelligence structure. Although there are minor differences in the way the examinations are conducted in all of these types of screening examinations, the differences are quantitative rather than qualitative.

There are presently eight polygraph schools recognized by the American Polygraph Association (APA) (APA Newsletter, 1972). Each school teaches its own variant of the polygraph examination. The procedure that will be described here is that taught by the U.S. Army Military Police School (USAMPS), Ft. Gordon, Georgia. Unlike the other schools, this school teaches essentially all of the polygraph techniques which are widely used in the field. Most of the polygraph examiners who are employed by the federal government (including members of the Metropolitan Police Department of Washington, D.C.) are trained at the Ft. Gordon school. That includes, among others, Army, Navy, and Air Force polygraph examiners, both police and intelligence (Stein, 1972). Differences between the procedures described below and other major procedures used in the field, where known, will be mentioned.

The total examination is divided into three stages: (1) the pretest interview, (2) the testing stage, and (3) the posttest interrogation, where appropriate. The examination usually takes a minimum of 2 hr to conduct, of which more than 1 hr is devoted to the pretest interview. The pretest interview is considered to be of vital importance to a valid examination.

1. PRETEST INTERVIEW

Prior to the pretest interview, the examiner acquaints himself with the results of the investigation to date, is briefed by the investigator(s) concerning the areas to be discussed during the examination, and tentatively decides which testing technique to employ. Immediately prior to the examination the polygraph is set up and calibrated.

The pretest interview opens with the introduction of the examiner and the S. The examiner's bearing is courteous, businesslike, but friendly. The interview occurs in a plain, sparsely furnished office which has a desk on which the polygraph is visible. Two or three chairs are present. No other person is present under normal conditions. As soon as the examiner has identified and introduced himself, he advises the S of the following in accord with the Miranda decision: his right to silence, that any statement he makes may be used against him in a court of law; that he may talk to his counsel prior to taking the examination; if he does not have a counsel, one will be appointed for him before any further questioning; that the counsel may be present during the examination; that if he decides to answer questions, he may stop at any time he wishes; that if he decides not to consult an attorney now he may decide to do so at any time during the exam, in which case the examination will be terminated. The S is informed that the polygraph examination is completely voluntary. He is further informed whether or not the examination will be observed from outside the room or recorded. The S is then asked to sign a statement of consent to take the polygraph examination. In the form his rights are again enumerated, and the voluntary aspect of the examination is emphasized. Only after the statement of consent has been signed and witnessed can the examination proceed.

During the next portion of the pretest interview the examiner obtains detailed information concerning the S's biographical background, with particular attention paid to his employment history and his medical history. Other areas included are his family and educational background, his hobbies and interests, his military experience, and his arrest record. After that has been obtained, the examiner explains the polygraph to the S, showing him what is measured and emphasizing that the physiological responses resulting from any attempt to lie will be recorded by the polygraph and will be very obvious to the examiner. After all of S's questions about the polygraph have been answered, the examiner obtains S's version of the incident being investigated. All details are explored until the examiner has satisfied himself that he understands S's story completely.

The questions to be asked on the examination are devised in cooperation with the S; the precise wording is approved by the S, and all questions are thoroughly reviewed with the S so that none of the questions will take him by surprise. During this process it is emphasized that all questions must be answerable completely and honestly by a simple "yes" or "no" and that any doubts, ambiguities, or reservations will cause a response which will be recorded by the polygraph. The S is told that if any of the questions trouble him, he should discuss them at this time with the examiner. It often happens at this point that a S changes his story or reveals an incident not previously mentioned. If the S is troubled by one of the control questions, the question is often reworded so that it is prefaced by the phrase, "Except for what you have told me." For example, if the question were "While you were in high school, did you ever take anything you weren't supposed to?," the question might be reworded, "Except for what you have told me, while you were in high school . . ."

With the completion of the review of all questions, the pretest interview draws to a close and the transition is made to the data acquisition phase of the examination. It should be noted at this point that the pretest interview serves the following important functions:

1. During the hour or more that it takes, the S is able to become familiar with the examiner, the polygraph, and the testing situation. This tends to reduce anxiety to acceptable levels.

2. The examiner is able to tailor the relevant and the control questions to the S in order to maximize the probability of conducting a valid examination. By reviewing all questions thoroughly with the S and providing him ample opportunity for qualifying or rewording the questions, the examiner reduces the possibility of spurious responses due to anger, surprise, ideation, nervousness, and ambiguity.

3. The examiner is able to make a careful evaluation of the level of arousal of the S. Thus, he is able to unobtrusively control the level of arousal so that the S will not be too anxious, thereby preventing the charts from being ambiguous and difficult to interpret. The S must not be too relaxed, for the level of autonomic responsivity may be too low to produce adequate differentiation in responsivity between the relevant and the control questions.

4. The examiner is able to maximize the probability that the psychological set of the innocent S will be toward the control questions and that of the guilty S toward the relevant questions. The wording of the control questions and the method by which they were introduced to and reviewed with the S is designed to ensure that all Ss will lie or be troubled by the control questions. That works to the advantage of the innocent S by diverting him from the relevant questions and focusing his concern on the control questions. On the other hand, the guilty S should be more concerned about his lies to the relevant questions than to the control questions. For discussions of the concept of control questions, see Backster (1963), Orne *et al.* (1972), and Reid and Inbau (1966).

5. By learning what the interests and hobbies of the S are, the examiner is given the means to allow the overly anxious S to relax by discussing areas unrelated to the matter being investigated. Furthermore, the rapport established during the pretest interview may be utilized during any posttest interrogation.

6. The pretest interview is very useful in allowing the examiner to closely observe the S in order to formulate the best plan of interrogation should deception be detected.

7. Finally, the pretest interview permits the examiner to observe S's behavior patterns in order to evaluate his physical and mental fitness for taking the polygraph examination. If neurotic behavior is noted or a physical abnormality disclosed, the examiner may decide not to conduct the examination, or he may decide to conduct a preliminary card test in order to assess the S's autonomic functioning.

There are three significant differences between the pretest procedure outlined above and that employed by the Reid technique (Reid & Inbau, 1966) and the Keeler technique (Harrelson, 1964). The most obvious difference is the length of the interview. Whereas the above procedure takes a minimum of about an hour, the Reid and Keeler techniques advocate a shorter interview lasting perhaps 20–30 min (Reid & Inbau, 1966, p. 10). The second major difference is that in the Reid technique the electrodes and other sensors are attached to the S immediately upon his arrival (Reid & Inbau, 1966, p. 11). The Keeler technique does not specify precisely when the sensors will be attached, but the implication is that it is done shortly after the S's arrival. The pretest in the Keeler technique may be extremely short (Harrelson, 1964, p. 54). In the latter procedure, the sensors are not attached until the pretest interview is completed. A third difference is that in the Reid technique specific questions are asked, and the S's replies and behavioral mannerisms are carefully observed and recorded as a means of supplementing the interpretation of the charts (Horvath, 1972).

2. CONDUCT OF THE ACTUAL TESTING

Once the questions have been thoroughly reviewed, if the S has been sitting in an "interview" chair, he is asked to sit in the "examination" chair. This chair is often a plain wooden chair which has been modified to have large, concave armrests. The chair faces a blank wall and is situated so that the S cannot see the polygraph or resulting chart. The E must be in a position to observe S's body during the test, especially the toes, thighs, arms, and fingers. This is so any movements of S may be observed. The sensors are then attached, and the S is instructed not to move or turn around during the test, to look straight ahead, and to answer each question either yes or no. The S is informed that it will take a couple of minutes to get the polygraph turned on and adjusted and that he will be told when the examination is about to begin.

The polygraph is then put into operation, the pneumograph first, then the EDR unit, finally the cardiovascular unit. The rationale for this sequence is twofold. By first turning on the respiration and EDR units, about 15 sec of base-line tracings are obtained at a time when the S is not certain whether his responses are being monitored. This can be valuable in later analysis of the charts. Once the cardio cuff is inflated, however, the S knows that recording has begun. Second, by inflating the cardio cuff last, the length of time in which it is inflated is kept to a minimum, thereby minimizing the discomfort to the S. Once the cuff is inflated and the pressure stabilized, the S is informed that the test is about to begin.

About 10–15 sec are allowed to pass before the first question is asked in order to observe several respiratory cycles and to allow any response to subside. For the same reasons, about 15–20 sec are allowed to pass between each question. The questions are asked in a quiet monotone to minimize the possibility that voice inflections may influence S's responsivity. During the time that the recordings are being obtained, the examiner makes numerous markings on the chart to indicate the sensitivity of the EDR amplifier, the pressure in the cardio cuff, the point at which the S is informed that the test is about to begin, the points at which each question starts and ends, S's answer and the point at which it occurred, the point at which any movement was observed, and any disruptions caused by S's yawns, sighs, coughs, sniffs, belches, or laughs, or by any outside noise. Of course, any time a pen is recentered, the appropriate notation is made. Upon conclusion of the test, a notation is made at the point when the S is informed that the test is over. The pressure in the cardio cuff is again noted and the cuff deflated. However, the EDR and pneumograph units are kept in operation in order to observe any response caused by the termination of the test and to observe any marked change in respiration which might indicate that S had been controlling his breathing. After an additional 15–20 sec, these last two units are deactivated and the time the chart was completed and date of the examination are immediately noted on the chart, together with the chart sequence label.

The chart is inspected to note the pattern of responses, and the S is asked such questions as, "Which question bothered you the most?" The questions are then reviewed again and clarified as needed. Care is taken not to inform S as to which question he responded to the most, as this would confound the interpretation of subsequent responses to that question.

A common practice is to include a card test in the examination, typically after the first chart has been obtained. This test has been described in detail elsewhere and will not be gone into here (Barland, 1972a; Reid & Inbau, 1966). The purpose of this card test is to convince the S that any lie, even one as trivial as the card which he had selected, will be detected.

Following the card test, the testing concerning the incident under investigation is resumed. A second chart is obtained in the same manner as described above. Generally, following another discussion with the S, a third chart is obtained. Usually three charts, in addition to the card test, are sufficient for the examiner to make a decision as to the truthfulness of the S. If any doubt remains, a number of alternatives are available to the examiner. He may obtain a fourth or fifth chart using the same questions, usually with attempts to stimulate the responsivity of the S between each chart (Reid & Inbau, 1966). Methods of stimulation include the card test, the yes test (Reid & Inbau, 1966, p. 32), the yes–no test (Golden, 1969), the silent answer test (Horvath & Reid, 1972), biofeedback (Golden, 1971), the closed-eyes technique (Golden, 1966), classical conditioning (Golden, 1969), and various forms of S–E interactions. Alternatively, the examiner may switch over to a different type of test in which different questions are asked. If, for example, he used a Backster Zone of Comparison Test for the first series, he might now use the Reid Control Question Test, the relevant–irrelevant test or a peak of tension test. The new questions, of course, would be reviewed with S before being asked. Another alternative would be to dismiss the S at this time and reexamine him on a later date. The authors have seen marked improvement in responsivity on subsequent tests when this was done, as have Arther (1968b), Bitterman and Marcuse (1947), Reid and Inbau (1966, pp. 33–36), and Rouke (1941). Bennett (1960) cites an instance where a suspect was examined 19 times before the examiner felt that he could completely clear the person.

3. POSTTEST TREATMENT OF THE SUBJECT

The treatment of the S is completely dependent upon the results of the data acquisition phase. If the testing reveals no indication of deception, the S is thanked for his coöperation and released. Depending upon the examiner and the situation, the S may be informed of the outcome, or he may be told that the results will be given to the investigators when they become available. The latter maneuver permits more control over the subsequent investigation. However, if the examination indicates that S was lying to one or more of the relevant questions, he is immediately interrogated in order to fully exploit the psychological advantages inherent in the testing situation. A number of excellent sources are available detailing the interrogation techniques (Arther & Caputo, 1959; Aubry & Caputo, 1965; Inbau & Reid, 1967; Mulbar, 1951).

There are few basic differences between the various polygraph schools concerning the conduct of the test and posttest stages. One minor difference is that several schools advocate assuming the guilt of the S and interrogating when an inconclusive examination is obtained (Arther, 1968b).

There is one major difference in the conduct of the posttest interrogation in the various screening examinations as taught by USAMPS. The S is *never* accused of lying. Instead, the examiner politely points out that one or more of the questions seem to have bothered him, or, alternatively, that there are some responses which must be clarified. Typically, admissions are made by the S; these are verified by additional testing. Some private polygraph schools do not prohibit the examiner from accusing a person of lying during a screening exam, where appropriate.

4. FIELD QUESTION TECHNIQUES

The three basic types of question techniques are relevant–irrelevant, peak of tension, and control question tests.

The peak of tension (POT) test consists of a series of 5–9 questions (usually 7), all of which are worded nearly alike (Harrelson, 1964; Reid & Inbau, 1966, pp. 37–40; USAMPS, 1970). The S is required to give the same answer, usually "no," to each question. The questions are all-inclusive and mutually exclusive, so that a deceptive S must lie to one and only one of the questions. The critical question is placed toward the middle of the test so that it is preceded and followed by one or two questions to which it is known that the S could not possibly lie. These buffers serve to absorb the initial response and serve as anchors for the peak. A sample question sequence would be:

1. Regarding the color of the stolen car, do you know if it was yellow?
2. Do you know if it was black?
3. Do you know if it was green?
4. Do you know if it was blue?
5. Do you know if it was red?
6. Do you know if it was white?
7. Do you know if it was brown?

The peak of tension test is so named because if the S intends to lie, the psychological tension within the S tends to increase as the point of deception comes closer. The tension is at its peak at or near the point of deception, after which the S relaxes. There are basically two types of POT tests: those in which the answer is known to the examiner, as would be the case in the above example, and those in which the answer is not known. The latter is known as the searching POT (USAMPS, 1970) or POT-B (Barber, 1964; Harrelson, 1964). In the searching POT the sequence is basically the same as above, except that it must include a catch-all question prior to the final buffers or as the last question. The catch-all question might be worded, "Do you know if the body is located somewhere else?"

The following dangers are inherent in the use of the POT technique, precluding its use in many field situations (Arther, 1968a; Reid & Inbau, 1966; USAMPS, 1970):

1. The innocent S must not have learned the key item from the police or public media.
2. The S must not be able to guess the critical item from the way the questions are worded, phrased, reviewed, or spoken (Marcuse & Bitterman, 1946). To the naive S each question must appear equally plausible.
3. The questions must be of approximately equal emotional value to the S. In the above example of car colors, if the color of S's own car was the same as the color of the stolen vehicle, a POT test using car colors would be invalid.
4. The key may be unknown to a guilty S; perhaps the car was stolen at night and he did not notice the car color.
5. The victim may have given false information to the investigators.
6. There must be only one possible peak.

The last requirement is sometimes more difficult than is realized. The first author once conducted a searching POT on a S suspected of having hidden an illegal drug. To the author's surprise (in view of the results of a previous control question test), the S did not show a peak. Instead, there were separate, specific responses to the three questions: "Do you know if it is in this room?," "Do you know if it is in the john?," and "Do you know if it is somewhere else I have not mentioned?" Although logical hypotheses could be easily devised by the examiner to explain each of these responses, interrogation revealed that S had swallowed the drug. Thus it was in this room. Yet, because it was within her body, it was also "somewhere else." Since the examiner had allowed her to go to the bathroom earlier during the testing, the thought occurred to her that she must be depositing some of it in the toilet!

The relevant–irrelevant (R–I) technique differs from the peak of tension in that there can be several relevant questions in each question series, and the sequence of the questions is not known at the outset of each series. The first two questions are usually irrelevant, e.g. "Is today Friday?" The first relevant question should be a "Do you know who . . ." rather than a "Did you. . ." question. Thereafter any relevant question can be asked, with irrelevant questions inserted whenever time is needed for a response to return to basal level or after every third relevant question (Harrelson, 1964; USAMPS, 1970). The R–I technique is an extremely flexible one in that numerous relevant questions may be asked. The question sequence is left to the discretion of the examiner, who decides which question to ask next on the basis of the appearance of the chart. In a variant of the R–I technique which is not encouraged by the Keeler Institute, one or more control questions may be inserted into the question sequence on or after the third chart (Harrelson, 1964). It should be noted, however, that the use of and location of the control questions is left entirely to the discretion of the examiner.

The third major testing technique is the control question technique. This technique was formulated by Reid (1947), although Summers (1939) and Rouke (1941) had inserted "emotional standard" questions into the R–I question sequence to provide a means of comparing the magnitude of responses for evaluative purposes. A control question is a question designed to capture the psychological set of the innocent S. Thus, by comparing the magnitude of responses to the relevant questions with those to the control questions, the examiner has an easy method of determining if the responses to the relevant questions are significant. Unlike the question sequence of the R–I technique, the order of presentation of the questions in the control question test is predetermined and inflexible. The question sequence of the Reid control question test is given in his book (Reid & Inbau, 1966, p. 21). On the third repetition of the questions the sequence is rearranged in a standard manner. Although the S has reviewed all questions prior to the test, he does not necessarily know the question sequence.

Although there are several variants of the control question test (e.g. Arther, 1969), one deserves special mention. Backster's Zone of Comparison (ZOC) technique utilizes a number of safeguards which have good face validity (USAMPS, 1970). The question sequence is as follows:

1. (Irrelevant) Are you sitting down?
2. (Sacrifice Relevant) Regarding that stolen money and gold coin collection, do you intend to answer truthfully each question about that?
3. (Outside Issue) Are you completely convinced that I will not ask a question on this test that has not already been reviewed?
4. (Control) Can you remember stealing anything before you were 18 years old?
5. (Relevant) Did you steal Smith's money?
6. (Control) Other than what you have told me, while you were in high school did you ever steal anything?
7. (Relevant) Did you steal that money from Smith's house?
8. (Outside issue) Is there something else you are afraid I will ask you a question about, even though I have told you I would not?
9. (Guilt complex) Did you steal that gold coin collection?
10. (Weak relevant) Do you know what happened to that missing money?

Backster devised a numerical evaluation system which provides a score for the response in each component in each of the three comparison zones for each of the charts. A total numerical score is thus obtained which fixes the S's position along a reactivity continuum, one extreme of which denotes truthfulness (greatest responsivity to the control question) and the other deceptiveness (greatest responsivity to the relevant questions). The middle portion of the continuum is inconclusive. For a description of the scoring system as used in a laboratory study, see Barland (1972a). Unlike Reid's test, the question sequence does not change on any of the charts, except that the control question which elicited the largest response is put into the number 6 position on the next chart. That procedure gives an advantage to the innocent S in the scoring process.

When appropriate, Backster's test also incorporates the addition of three questions added to the end of the third (last) chart, the so-called "SKY" questions (Suspect, Know, You). An example would be:

(Suspect) "Do you suspect any one in particular of stealing Smith's money?" (Know) "Do you know for sure who stole Smith's money?" (You) "Did you yourself steal Smith's money?"

It should be noted that question 9 in the Backster test sequence is a guilt complex question. This is a question concerning a fictitious crime similar to the incident of which S is suspected. The purpose of this question is to determine if S responds emotionally to every accusatory question. For a detailed description of guilt complex questions see Reid and Inbau (1966). The guilt complex question may be replaced by a control question at the discretion of the examiner (USAMPS, 1970). However, in laboratory studies it is extremely easy to build in a guilt complex situation by merely mentioning in the instructions to Ss that some of the Ss will have done the act which the guilt complex question covers.

In addition to the inclusion of the guilt complex question, the Backster technique incorporates two additional changes from the Reid technique which are worthy of note. Each relevant question is paired with or surrounded by control questions. This controls for possible changes in the level of autonomic responsivity that may occur within each chart as the test is in progress. Also, questions 3 and 8 are designed to determine if the S's psychological set is focused on an issue or question not included in the test, as that would tend to dampen S's responsivity to the relevant or control questions.

As might be expected, each of the types of tests mentioned above has its own set of advantages and disadvantages. Thus, a test which would be very effective in one situation might not be effective in a different situation. The federal government, for example, considers the peak of tension test to be perhaps the most valid in those relatively rare situations where critical details of the specific incident have been successfully shielded from the S. The POT card test is also used routinely as a part of each polygraph examination (usually after the first chart of the control question test) in order to convince the S of the polygraph's effectiveness. The POT can be used to help the examiner arrive at a decision if the control question test was inconclusive. Finally, the POT is used in those situations where a control question test showed definite indications of deception, the suspect refuses to admit his guilt, and it is desired to obtain additional physical evidence by locating the body, weapon, loot, etc. (USAMPS, 1970).

Because the Backster test answers essentially only two questions: (1) Did he do it? and (2) Does he have guilty knowledge?, the ZOC is the method of preference where only one aspect of the crime is to be probed. It is the method of preference because of the inclusion of the guilt complex question, the sacrifice relevant, the paired relevant and control questions, and the two outside issue questions (USAMPS, 1970).

The Reid control question test is preferred for those situations where two or more major aspects of a crime are to be probed in one test (USAMPS, 1970). For example, in a forgery case, the four relevant questions might be: (1) Did you steal the blank check from _____? (2) Did you sign the name _____ on the check? (3) Did you cash that check? (4) Do you know where some of that money is now?

The pure relevant–irrelevant technique is not generally authorized for use within the federal government because of the lack of control questions in this technique. Obviously, the R–I technique is the only technique applicable to personnel screening, because of the large number of relevant questions which must be asked. When used for screening purposes by the federal government, control questions are included (USAMPS, 1970).

There are several additional testing techniques developed by field polygraph examiners which are worthy of mention. They will be described in some detail, because they have never been published and are difficult to obtain. Morton Sinks, a field polygraph examiner, developed the yes–no technique which has been reported by Golden (1969). The structure of the yes–no technique is quite simple. Every test question is asked twice in a row. The examinee is instructed to answer truthfully the first time the question is asked and to lie the second time. Two irrelevant questions are used to introduce the test. Thereafter, only relevant and control questions are used. The original rationale for this technique was that since each question would be answered both truthfully and falsely, the two responses could be compared and each question would act as its own control.

A pilot study using 1000 Ss conducted by Golden and others found that deceptive Ss responded more to the relevant questions compared to the control questions regardless whether they answered yes or no. While some deceptive Ss responded more after answering no to the relevant questions, others responded more after answering yes to the same question. On the other hand, truthful Ss tended to show no differentiation in responses between their yes and no answers to the relevant questions. Their responses to the control questions were greater than they were to the relevant questions.

In another study of 400 Ss, in which the yes–no technique was compared against the conventional control question technique, with each S serving as his own control, Golden found that 80% of the deceptive Ss gave significantly greater responses to the relevant questions on the yes–no test than on the conventional test. Of the diagnosed truthful Ss, 48% responded to the control questions more on the yes–no test, and the conventional test, 5% responded more to the conventional test, and 47% showed no difference in responsivity between the two tests. Since the conventional test was always conducted prior to the yes-no test, the results speak more favorably of the yes–no test than might at first appear, because of the effects of habituation, lowered attention, etc.

Golden suggested four hypotheses for the greater apparent effectiveness of the yes–no test over the conventional control question test. First, the deceptive person is contradicting two sets of instructions, namely tell the truth the first time and lie the second time. A certain confusion as to which answer to give might result in enhanced responsivity. Golden mentions that some deceptive Ss inadvertantly answer yes when they intend to answer no. Second, a conflict situation appears when the deceptive S "admits" the truth to the repetition of the question. This appears to be somewhat traumatic for deceptive Ss. Third, by requiring S to vary his answer to each question depending upon whether it is being asked the first or second time, he is forced to attend to each question more than would otherwise be required. Finally, the deceptive S may attempt to distort his yes response in order to make it appear more like a lie to the examiner. It is generally accepted among field examiners that most countermeasure attempts are sufficiently crude that they enhance the detectibility of the deceptive S.

In an earlier study, Golden (1967) developed another stratagem for increasing the contrast between deceptive and truthful Ss. He described it as a conditioned reflex technique in lie detection. In this technique the S is instructed to depress a switch which rings a bell whenever he tells a lie. Through the use of irrelevant questions to which he is instructed to lie, the S is accustomed to ringing the buzzer whenever he lies. Golden has found that when the "conditioning questions" were interspersed among relevant and control questions, the responses of the deceptive and truthful Ss to the relevant and control questions, respectively, were "generally enhanced." Golden attributed this to the fact that decision-making (to ring the bell or not) introduces a conflict situation for the deceptive S, and that this conflict increases autonomic responsivity. Golden also noted a beneficial side effect of his technique: 33.2% of all Ss diagnosed as deceptive rang the buzzer to a relevant question during the polygraph test! Many of these Ss readily confessed, since they realized that they had unwittingly revealed their deception.

More recently, Golden (1971) reported that the use of auditory biofeedback of the skin resistance response enhances the magnitude of the responses of the deceptive Ss by 100–600% compared with prebiofeedback charts. Subjects who were diagnosed as truthful showed no change in responsivity as a result of the biofeedback. Unfortunately, in almost all of the field studies, no quantitative analyses were made, and methodological errors detract from the validity of the findings. Nonetheless, many of them are ingeniously conducted and provide hypotheses for testing under stronger experimental designs and controls. It would appear that very useful results could be obtained by the collaboration of experimental psychologists and field polygraph examiners.

5. FIELD EVALUATION TECHNIQUES

Polygraph examiners evaluate their charts by a method of visual inspection which is both holistic and comparative. That is, many examiners take into account the overall appearance of the chart to determine the patterning of responses, whether anxiety increases or decreases as the test progresses, whether there are any changes (particularly in respiration) when the S was informed that the test is about to begin and when the S was told the test is over, etc. In addition to this global appraisal, the examiner carefully compares the type, magnitude, and duration of responses to the relevant questions with those to the control, guilt complex, and perhaps irrelevant questions. Although there are a number of specific response criteria which vary in importance, they can all be summarized by the generalization that any change from prestimulus levels may be indicative of deception. Field evaluation techniques are generally considered to require formal instruction at a polygraph school or from an experienced examiner in order to be learned. Moreover, it has been demonstrated that the effectiveness of field evaluation techniques is positively correlated with the experience of the evaluator (Horvath & Reid, 1971).

In view of the seeming subjectivity and lack of quantification that characterizes field evaluations, it might seem that they could not be effective. Surprisingly, every study examining this question has found that field evaluations are both valid (Barland, 1972a; Bersh, 1969; Holmes, 1958) and reliable (Barland, 1972b; Horvath & Reid, 1971; Hunter, 1971; Kubis, 1962; Moroney & Zenhausern, 1972; Rouke, 1941).

6. VALIDITY AND RELIABILITY OF LIE DETECTION
   IN FIELD SITUATIONS

The question of the validity of the lie detection technique in the field is an extremely complex issue which may never be fully answerable. As can be seen from the above description of field techniques, in addition to the data from the polygraph charts, the examiner has access to a great deal of information concerning the S's probable truthfulness at the time that he makes his decision. This includes evidence obtained by the preliminary police investigation, the opinions of the investigators, the appearance and behavior of the suspect, and the information obtained during the pretest interview. Therefore, seldom is the decision of the examiner unbiased. Among field examiners there are two schools of thought regarding the information to be consciously used in making the decision. One school advocates that only by utilizing all possible information available to him from every source does the examiner optimize the probability of making the correct decision. This is analogous to the Bayesian concept of statistical inference. The other school advocates the position that all extraneous sources of data, while sought out before and during the pretest interview, must be rigorously excluded from consideration when the decision is made. The rationale for this is that the decision must be based only upon the data in the polygraph charts, for the charts contain the only objective support for the examiner's decision if the examiner is called upon to testify in a court of law. The validity and reliability of examiner judgments might vary according to the attitude of the examiner to outside sources of data.

In a recent reliability study, Barland (1972b) had six experienced field examiners evaluate charts from 72 experimental Ss. All of the examiners were of the tradition that only the charts should be used in the evaluation of truth or deception. Barland then paired the decisions for each of the 15 possible combinations of pairs of examiners. Excluding inconclusives, there were 559 instances where both examiners of a pair came to a definite conclusion regarding the truthfulness of the S. Of the 559 paired decisions, the examiners agreed with each other 534 times, yielding a 95.5% rate of agreement. Since the examiners had used a numerical scoring method in evaluating the charts, Barland was able to correlate all scores, including inconclusives. The mean Pearson product-moment correlation for pairs of examiners was $+.86$. He also found that of the three standard components, the SRR was evaluated the most reliably (mean $r = .903$). The cardio was next with a mean $r = .755$, and respiration was the least reliable, with a mean $r = .645$.

High reliability has also been obtained in studies conducted by graduates of schools which advocate a holistic approach to decision making (Horvath & Reid, 1971; Hunter, 1971). Because of differences in S populations and methods of analysis, the results of the studies conducted by the different schools cannot be directly compared. Nevertheless, there seems to be a growing body of evidence indicating that examiner decisions are highly reliable, at least among those examiners who received the same training. It would be of interest to see if the same degree of reliability holds up when the other evaluators have graduated from a different school than the original examiner, or if the examination utilized the pure form of the relevant–irrelevant technique.

The validity of examiner judgments in field situations, in addition to being contaminated by sources of information other than the polygraph charts, is made difficult by a number of other problems. A high degree of examiner–subject interaction during the pretest and other phases of the examination is the *sine qua non* of the field examination. All examiners, to a lesser or greater extent, are continually assessing the behavioral symptoms of the S (Horvath, 1972). As Orne *et al.* (1972) have pointed out, this may influence the conduct of the pretest and the polygraph test to the extent that the presumed-truthful S may be given a different testing environment than the presumed-deceptive S. Although this interaction may be largely controlled in experimental studies, for the reasons given previously, it is neither feasible nor desirable to control it in field situations. The extent to which this source of variance affects the field examination has never been assessed.

Just as the examiner's decision is contaminated by the results of the previous investigation, so is the subsequent investigation contaminated by the results of the polygraph examination. This is particularly the case with Ss who are cleared by the examiner. In these cases it frequently occurs that charges against the suspect are reduced or dropped and many of the cases remain unsolved. On the other hand, a high percentage of Ss diagnosed as deceptive confess when confronted by the results of the examination. Consequently, it is more difficult to verify the examiner's decisions when no deception is found than when a decision of deception is made. In those situations where a decision of truthfulness remains unverified, the possibility that a countermeasure was successfully employed cannot be discounted.

In addition to the lack of independence between the polygraph examination and preceding and subsequent events, another problem in assessing the validity of field polygraph examinations is the difficulty of determining absolute ground truth in field situations. Obviously, if it were possible to establish ground truth, there would be no need for the polygraph! The inadequacies of various criteria such as jury trials, police investigations, and confessions are too well known to require repetition here. It is perhaps because of these problems that so few attempts have been made to estimate the validity of the polygraph in field situations. This is most unfortunate, because the paucity of careful estimates has given rise to contradictory, and sometimes exaggerated claims and counterclaims.

In attempting to estimate the validity of field techniques, it is appropriate to examine first the figures presented by the field examiners themselves. For many years numerous examiners have published statistics uniformly reporting an error rate of not more than about 2%, and often less than 1%. For example, see Reid and Inbau (1966, p. 234), Trovillo (1939, and especially 1953), and Zimmerman (1959). These statistics leave much to be desired. In addition to occasional arithmetical errors, none of the reports give any details as to the methods used during the examinations, what criteria were used to validate the examiner's decisions, whether it was the examiner or someone else who decided when his decision was confirmed or disconfirmed, etc.

In talking with field examiners, the authors have found that many of them automatically consider their decisions verified, usually by the behavioral symptoms of the suspects, unless positive information to the contrary is somehow brought to their attention. Many of the statistical reports from the field do not discriminate between preemployment screening and criminal examinations. Obviously, decisions of truthfulness on preemployment screening examinations are almost never confirmed, since there has been no systematic attempt to do so.

Arther (1965, p. 34) claims that of all examinations conducted during the previous 10 years by him (the number of examinations is not reported), more than 96% resulted in a decision and slightly more than 3% were inconclusives. He has discovered incorrect decisions in only .05% of all of his examinations and estimates the maximum possible error rate to be less than 1%. Elsewhere Arther (1968b) reported that in the past 17 years he has made only 9 known mistakes, all of which were false negatives. He has had no known errors in the past 7 years since he increased the number of reexaminations in doubtful cases. In advocating the procedure of reexamining the S in doubtful cases, Arther noted that none of the false negatives followed a reexamination.

In all of the reports of error rates by field examiners there is a major procedural error which negates the value of the statistics. The known error rate was obtained by dividing the number of errors by the total number of examinations conducted. However, the number of examinations which an examiner has conducted can be divided into two groups, those in which the truthfulness of the Ss has been adequately determined independently of the polygraph examination, and those in which confirmation of the examination was not made. Since all known errors are confined to only the verified group, dividing the known errors by the combined total of both groups biases the resultant statistic and makes the polygraph technique appear more accurate than it may be. A more realistic estimate would be to divide the number of known errors by the number of Ss in which the truthfulness of the S was determined independently of the polygraph examination.

Fortunately, there have been several scientists who have conducted both experimental studies of lie detection and also examinations on criminal suspects. The reports of the accuracy of their decisions do not suffer from the error described above. A validity study by Lyon (1936) consisted of 100 randomly selected cases conducted for the Juvenile Court of Chicago. Twenty percent of the Ss appeared to be telling the truth, and the remaining 80% showed indications of deception. Only 40% of the decisions could be confirmed, but of those 40% (7 truthful, 33 deceptive) no incorrect decisions were found. Thus, Lyon reported 100% accuracy with 40 Ss.

Summers (1939, p. 340), using the SRR as the only measure, claimed 100% accuracy in the examinations of 43 criminal suspects. He claimed that confirmation was obtained by confessions, judicial procedure where additional evidence confirmed the decision, or by subsequent investigation. The apparent fact that every one of his examinations was considered confirmed raises some doubt about the stringency of his criteria for confirmation. This objection was satisfied when Summers work was extended by Kubis. Kubis (1950) reported an accuracy of 100% on criminal suspects using the SRR as the only measure. Of more than 500 criminal suspects who were examined, 80% were judged to be telling the truth. About half of those were independently verified as such. An additional 10% were judged deceptive; possibly all of those were confirmed by confessions, but no mention was made by Kubis. The remaining 10% of the examinations were inconclusive.

In a report (MacNitt, 1942) which combined experimental, hypothetical, and 59 actual criminal cases, the SRR yielded 99% accuracy in decisions. Unfortunately, MacNitt did not separate the results for the criminal cases, and the rate of accuracy in the field situation is not known. Also, he failed to describe the criteria for verification. In all of those reports of the accuracy of the polygraph in field situations by scientists, there is a paucity of details which is nearly as great as the reports of the field examiners themselves. The apparent fact that the persons who conducted the examinations were the same persons who determined whether there was sufficient evidence to confirm the examiner's decision may have biased the results.

There has been only one detailed attempt to estimate the accuracy of polygraph examiners' decisions in a manner which does not possess the shortcomings of the above estimates. This was a study conducted under the supervision of Robert Brisentine by the Department of Defense and was reported by Bersh (1969). The criterion used in that study was the decision of a panel of military lawyers who were given complete dossiers concerning the evidence uncovered by all of the investigations of each case. Each attorney independently decided upon the guilt or innocence of each person solely upon the evidence available, without regard for legal technicalities and without knowing the outcome of the polygraph examinations. All cases in which any member of the panel was unable to arrive at a firm opinion of guilt or innocence were discarded. It was found that when all four panel members were in agreement, the decisions of the polygraph examiner agreed with those of the panel in 92.4% of the cases. When only 75% of the panel agreed as to the guilt or innocence of the S, the polygraph decisions agreed with the majority decision of the panel 74.6% of the time. Caution is indicated in interpreting the results of the Bersh study. Although the criterion represents perhaps the best possible approximation of ground truth, the possibility of some errors by the unanimous panel still exists. This is supported by the fact that there were cases where all panel members were able to make definite decisions of the guilt or inocence of the S, but the panel was split.

Another practical criterion which has been successfully used is that of confession. Ferguson (1971) cites numerous examples of false confessions, which points out the fact that not every confession will do. However, a confession in which new information is developed that only the criminal or a participant of the crime could reasonably have known would appear to be satisfactory. In the case where the examiner's decision is that no deception was indicated, verification could be accomplished by using the corroborated confession of another person, particularly if the other person had not been known to the nondeceptive S.

All of the meager evidence presently available indicates that the polygraph technique may be accurate in somewhat more than 90% of those cases where a definite decision is reached by the examiner. This rate of apparent accuracy is predicated upon the assumption that an experienced, well-trained examiner is conducting the examination under conditions which he considers suitable. This means that the examiner may reject Ss he considers unsuitable for testing, and that he is free to continue testing until he is satisfied with the results.

It is interesting to note that in all of the reports which did not contain unacceptable errors in the method of computing rates of accuracy, the examiner was not under financial pressures to conduct examinations in a hurried manner. The possible effect of hurried examinations upon accuracy has never been studied. It should also be noted that the Bersh (1969) study, unlike the other studies by Kubis (1950), Lyon (1936), MacNitt (1942), and Summers (1939), employed ordinary, government examiners rather than behavioral scientists with a rigorous background in psychophysiology and experimental procedures. The Bersh study thus represents the best estimate of the accuracy of the polygraph technique as it is used with criminal suspects. Possible differences in S population and examiner qualifications dictate caution in generalizing the results from the military to the general population, since, unlike the military, many states have not established minimum qualifications for polygraph examiners (Romig, 1971). On the other hand, the reports of Kubis and others indicate that under truly optimum conditions the accuracy of examiner decisions may approach 100%. Additional studies using the stringent criterion employed in the Bersh study are needed.

B. Detection of Information in the Laboratory

Whereas in field polygraph examinations the examiner almost never knows positively if the S intends to lie, laboratory experiments tend to fall into two categories. One is analogous to the field situation and has been called the guilty person paradigm by Gustafson and Orne (1964). In this paradigm the E does not know whether or not the S is innocent. The task of the S is to convince the E that he is innocent, i.e., the guilty S must present false negative charts. The other paradigm is one in which the E knows that the S must lie at some point in the question sequence, and E's only task is to determine the point of deception. This has been called the guilty information paradigm (Gustafson & Orne, 1964). The S's task here is simpler, since all that is required is to mislead the E as to the point of deception. The guilty information paradigm must not be confused with Lykken's guilty knowledge technique discussed below, for Lykken's technique can be used with either paradigm.

There are essentially only two types of testing techniques that have been used in the laboratory, the relevant–irrelevant and the peak of tension. Both have been described above. One variant of the peak of tension is the guilty knowledge technique (Lykken, 1959, 1960). In this technique a number of questions are asked, and each question has a number of possible answers, typically five. Each possible answer is presented to the S and the autonomic responses recorded. It can be seen that each question is, in essence, a peak of tension test.

In his first study, Lykken (1959) had four groups of Ss. One group had committed one mock crime, the second had committed a different mock crime, the third had committed both mock crimes, and the fourth had committed neither mock crime. Six questions (or POT tests, if you will) were asked each S for each of the two crimes. The SRRs to the several alternatives in a given question were ranked in order of amplitude. If the largest response was to the relevant alternative, the S was given a score of 2 on that question. If the second largest response was to the relevant alternative, he was given a score of 1. Thus, a perfect innocent score was 0 and a perfect guilty score was 12, for each list. Using an arbitrary cutoff of 6, 89.9% of all Ss were correctly categorized as to group. When Ss were classified as having committed one or more crimes or no crime, 93.9% correct classification was obtained. Of the six errors in this latter classification, all were false negatives. As Lykken pointed out, a higher validity could probably be attained by increasing the number of questions or by repeating the questions.

In a follow-up study to determine the resistance of this technique to countermeasures, Lykken (1960) used items of personal information such as the first name of S's father. Most of the 20 Ss were sophisticated and were briefed on the nature of the SRR, the polygraph, and the guilty knowledge technique. The Ss were allowed to practice producing voluntary SRRs by various methods, and were motivated to defeat the test by being offered a prize of $10 for successful deception. Twenty-five questions were asked, each of which had five scorable alternative answers. The scoring system was more sophisticated, assuming an equal distribution of ranked magnitudes of responses to the various alternative answers except to the relevant alternatives. Under these conditions 100% detection was achieved against a chance expectation of 20%. Lykken's technique has been used in subsequent research (Ben-Shakhar, Lieblich, & Kugelmass, 1970; Davidson, 1968) with varying degrees of success. As Lykken points out (1959), the application of this technique in field situations is severely limited by the difficulty of preventing suspects from learning the details of the crime.

Curiously, Lykken (1960) considers the guilty knowledge technique to be distinct from the peak of tension technique, presumably because in the latter technique the S usually knows the sequence of the alternatives. However, this is not necessarily the case. Recent work by Lieblich, Kugelmass, and Ben-Shakhar (1970) indicates that Ss tend to dichotomize the alternatives as being either relevant or irrelevant. Thus, provided that the S knows there will be only one critical question in the series, even when he does not know the sequence of the alternatives, he nonetheless tends to behave in the manner described by the peak of tension theory. Another distinction which Lykken (1960) makes between the guilty knowledge technique and the peak of tension technique is that with Lykken's technique no answer is required of S. But this seems to be an artificial difference, for there is no reason why the peak of tension technique would require a verbal response in order to be effective (Gustafson & Orne, 1965b). There have long been claims of successful field polygraph examinations having been accomplished on deaf-mutes in which the examination was conducted by writing the questions on cards and presenting them to the S sequentially. It should be noted, however, that Gustafson and Orne (1965b) and Voronin *et al.* (1970) found that verbal responses from the S increase the detectibility of deception. Horvath and Reid (1972) found that a question sequence in which the S is instructed to answer the questions silently to himself, imbedded within several verbal-answer question sequences, increases subsequent responsivity, especially for the SRR. This represents the first published finding by a major field examiner that the SRR can consistently be helpful in field polygraph examinations.

C. Differences between Field and Laboratory

It is obvious that there are numerous differences between polygraph examinations conducted in the field and the lie detection paradigm utilized in laboratory research. In view of the efforts that are often made to generalize from the laboratory to the field, it seems appropriate to mention and discuss some of these differences.

The level of affect is much higher in the field situation, and the motivation of the guilty Ss in the field situation is undoubtedly much higher than it is in the laboratory. Typically, in the laboratory the motivation to deceive is based upon the belief that although deception is difficult, it is possible in Ss who have high IQs and good emotional stability (Gustafson & Orne, 1963; Kugelmass & Lieblich, 1966). However, the effect of differing levels of motivation is difficult to assess. Some studies have used monetary reward (Barland, 1972a; Davidson, 1968). For example, Davidson (1968) had a low-motivation group that could earn 10¢ to $1 for successful deception and a high-motivation group which was offered $25 to $50 for successful deception. No difference in detection rate was found. Similarly, Kugelmass and Lieblich (1966) found that different levels of stress, which may be generally equivalent to producing different levels of motivation to deceive, did not cause a difference in the efficiency of the SRR. On the other hand, almost all the field examiners feel that heightened motivation to deceive results in easier detection; this seems intuitively reasonable. Consistent with that position, a classic study by Gustafson and Orne (1963) found that nonmotivated Ss could not be detected above chance levels, whereas motivated Ss were readily detected. Needless to say, the factor of motivation requires a great deal more research.

Different psychological goals probably exist between experimental and nonexperimental Ss. In a subsequent study by Gustafson and Orne (1965a), it was found that experimental Ss may have a psychological need to be detected in order to "prove" to themselves that they are not psychopathic liars. Depending upon feedback they may receive during the test, they may become harder to detect. This need to be detected would probably not be a significant factor in field situations.

There are obvious differences between field and laboratory Ss in their attitudes toward the examiner, the testing situation, the purpose of the examination, expectations as to the outcome of the examination, the amount of E–S interaction expected and occurring; different motives for volunteering to take the examination; different modes of compliance; different degrees of resentment toward the test; different levels and types of E–S rapport, etc. Thus, the demand characteristics of the situations are radically different. The ethical constraints known by the S to be acting upon the E can be presumed to be very different. Thus, the need for, and the sources of emotional support to the S in the nonexperimental situation are greatly different. The uncertainty of the nonexperimental situation can perhaps never be duplicated in the laboratory situation.

The antecedent experiences of the S in the hours or days prior to the examination are different in the two situations. In addition to the short-term stress applied to the S during the testing procedure, there is a long-term stress acting upon the nonexperimental S which is almost always absent in the laboratory situation.

The ethics and mores of the typical experimental S are middle-class, whereas the background and value of the typical nonexperimental S tend to be lower middle-class or lower-class. This could be expected to cause differences in responsivity due to differences in levels of conflict, group loyalties, and attitudes toward lying, police, science, and the examiner.

In the experimental situation, the time between the commission of the mock crime or the selection of the card is usually measured in minutes [perhaps the sole exception is Davidson (1968)], whereas in nonexperimental situations it is typically days or weeks, sometimes years. This delay could either reduce or enhance responsitivity, depending upon the psychodynamics of the suspect.

Relative to nonexperimental populations, the experimental populations are highly homogeneous. In addition to greater variances in the nonexperimental population on many of the above parameters, there would probably also be greater variance in intelligence and educational levels, emotional and mental stability, previous experience with the polygraph, beliefs regarding the efficacy of the polygraph technique and their ability to defeat it, and personality variables including sociopathy and psychopathy, and the incidence of neuroses and psychoses.

A final difference involves the relative frequency of testing techniques. The peak of tension test is frequently used in experimental situations, but is rarely used with criminal suspects. Conversely, the various control question tests are widely used in the field, but have been used only once with experimental Ss (Barland, 1972a).

It should be noticed that some of those differences are situational, others are populational. The generalizability of any experiment to the field polygraph examinations will be enhanced by the use of a population drawn from criminal suspects. The study by Kugelmass, Lieblich, Ben-Ishai, Opatowski, and Kaplan (1968) is one of the few experimental studies which has done that. They gathered data from criminal suspects undergoing a field polygraph examination and avoided the problem of ground truth by giving a standardized card test within the context of the field examination. Examination of both experimental Ss and criminal suspects within our laboratory has demonstrated that the differences between the two populations are indeed profound (Barland, 1972a).

III. Theories of Lie Detection

It had long been assumed that the psychological basis for the detection of deception was the fear of detection or the fear of the consequences of detection. This is the concept which is widely held by field examiners today (e.g., Reid & Inbau, 1966). It is apparent, however, that this theory is wholly inadequate to explain a number of different phenomena associated with lie detection, for example, the ability of the E to determine which card a S picked in a laboratory experiment where there presumably should be no fear present.

Marston (1938, p. 34) suggested that there were basically two types of deception tests, one measuring the emotions of defeat, the other type measuring the emotions which make lying successful. For some reason, which is not readily apparent, he classed electrodermal activity with the former type, and his own systolic blood pressure test and Benussi's respiration test in the latter category. Marston's theory does not seem to have gained any popularity and was dismissed by MacNitt (1942).

Three possible theories were listed by Davis (1961). These are the conditioned response theory, the conflict theory, and the punishment theory. The conditioned response theory suggests that the relevant questions are conditioned stimuli which evoke an emotional response related to the S's past experience. This theory has been discussed in some detail by Lindsley (1955), who ties it in to some extent with the punishment theory. The theory indicates that the more traumatic the antecedent experience, the larger the autonomic response. Intuitively, this does seem to be true, but Davis (1961) points out that this theory could hardly account for the detection of deception in the typical laboratory card test.

The conflict theory presumes that a large physiological disturbance would occur when two incompatible reaction tendencies are aroused simultaneously, such as tendency to tell the truth and the tendency to lie about the specific incident. This may be the dominant mode in the Luria hand tremor method of lie detection (Luria, 1930). Davis (1961) reasons that if this theory is true, detection would be easier when the S tries harder to conceal his deception. Certainly, this has received experimental support. Gustafson and Orne (1963) found that by motivating Ss to "beat the test," detection was improved. Golden's work on the yes–no technique also tends to provide some support for this theory.

The punishment or threat-of-punishment theory states that detection is a result of the anticipation of punishment or serious consequences if the S fails to deceive. As Davis (1961) points out:

> Lying is technically, then, an avoidance reaction with considerably less than 100 per cent chance of success, but it is the only one with any chance of success at all. The physiologic reaction would be the consequence of an avoidance reaction which has a low probability of reinforcement, but not too low. If the theory has any validity at all it must be supposed that the physiologic reaction is associated with a state of uncertainty. It does seem that a lie told with a complete certainty of its acceptance would be unlikely to produce much reaction; and on the other hand we have the experimental evidence . . . that a lie told with no prospect of success whatever is also poorly detected [p. 163].

As pointed out earlier, this is the theory which has gained wide acceptance among the field polygraph examiners. There are a number of experiments which tend to support this (e.g., Gustafson & Orne, 1965a). This theory suggests, however, that if the S were unaware that his autonomic responses were being monitored, detection rates would be minimal. Although this is a difficult problem to study, Thackray and Orne (1968a) conducted an experiment in which the situation was manipulated so as to convince the Ss that the polygraph was shut down when in fact Ss responses were being telemetered to a remote polygraph. It was found that there was no significant decrease in detectibility under these conditions. The punishment theory also has difficulty in explaining the high detection rates obtained in card tests in the laboratory where there is no possible overt punishment for failure to deceive.

There is a fourth theory of lie detection which appears to underlie many of the more recent experiments. This might be termed the arousal theory. This theory avoids use of emotions such as fear or guilt. It states that detection occurs because of the differential arousal value of the various stimuli. This theory has found support in the work of Orne and his co-workers and by Kugelmass and his colleagues (Ben-Shakhar, Lieblich, & Kugelmass, 1970; Lieblich, 1969, 1970; Orne *et al.*, 1972). This theory is very useful in explaining the detectibility when the S tells the truth to only the question about which card he picked (Kugelmass, Lieblich, & Bergman, 1967).

It may well be that all of the above theories contribute to an understanding of detection in various situations. For example, Reid and Inbau (1966, p. 220–221) suggest that the arousal theory may be predominant in laboratory experimentation, but that in the field situation the fear of punishment overrides the effect of alertness and attention found in the laboratory. This distinction is used by these workers and other field examiners to explain the effectiveness of electrodermal activity in the laboratory but not in the field.

IV. Major Problems Requiring Research

Although scientific studies concerning the detection of deception have been conducted for over half a century, relatively few problems have been attacked. The two major questions addressed by most of the studies have been: (1) Is the detection of deception possible, and if so, to what extent? (2) Which physiological parameters are successful in discriminating between truthfulness and deception? The early studies were oriented toward practical applications. With few exceptions (notably Block, Rouke, Salpeter, Tobach, Kubis, & Welch, 1952; Ellson *et al.*, 1952), the study of the variables contributing to the differential autonomic responsivity associated with deception was neglected until the 1960s. A large number of problems remain to be studied. Indeed, the scientific study of the lie detection paradigm is really just beginning.

A. *Effectiveness of the Electrodermal Response*

One of the most striking findings in the lie detection literature is the apparent discrepancy concerning the effectiveness of the electrodermal response in the laboratory as compared to the field situation. Essentially every laboratory study has found the EDR to be highly effective in determining deception, either when used as a sole indicator (Davidson, 1968; Kubis, 1950; Lykken, 1959, 1960; Summers, 1939) or when it is compared to other parameters (Barland, 1972a; Ellson *et al.*, 1952; Thackray & Orne, 1968a; Violante & Ross, 1964). Just as consistently, many of the field examiners have denied the effectiveness of the EDR in the field. It is generally considered by field examiners to be the least effective of the three parameters most commonly used (Arther, 1971b; Lee, 1953; Marston, 1938; Reid & Inbau, 1966).

There are a number of hypotheses as to why this discrepancy exists. The one most frequently mentioned is the difference in affect between the laboratory and the field testing situations. As Reid and Inbau (1966) have put it:

> . . . significant G.S.R. responses result from the rather superficial factor of a subject's alertness or attention respecting some matter about which he is lying. In an experimental card test, for instance, the primary if not the only factor involved is the alertness and attention required for lying about the one chosen card. The subject views it as a game. He does not have the fears which affect a person trying to lie about a crime or other serious incident. Nothing else is involved other than his alertness and attention. With regard to a criminal offense or other matters of a serious import, however, much more is involved than alertness and attention. Here the subject harbors a deep rooted, instinctual fear of detection and of the consequences of being caught. The resulting emotional disturbances seem to completely subordinate and render insignificant the minor factors of alertness and attention [pp. 220–221].

This hypothesis has been questioned by Kugelmass and Lieblich (1966). In an experiment in which the effect of various levels of stress upon the efficiency of the SRR was measured, three groups of Israeli police trainees were tested. One group was told that the purpose of the test was merely to test the operation of the apparatus. Another group was told that the test would indicate whether S belonged to the group of people whose responses could be detected by the polygraph. The third group, in which the stress was presumed greatest, was told that their chances for promotion in the police force would depend upon their ability to control their emotions, i.e., to "beat the test." It was found that the SRR was able to detect deception equally well with all three groups. It might be argued, however, that the high-stress group in which the Ss were told that their chances for promotion might depend upon their ability to beat the test might actually have construed the situation to be the opposite. They may have felt that in order to have maximum potential for promotion it would be desirable to be detected in the lie, thereby demonstrating a well-developed conscience and inherent honesty. This would not weaken the interpretation of the results, however, for either view of the demand characteristics of the examination would result in a high level of stress. Moreover, similar findings were obtained by Davidson (1968) when he manipulated the motivational level of the Ss by varying the amount of money they would be able to keep if they were successful in deceiving the E. The amounts ranged from 10¢ to $1 in one group, and $25 to $50 in another. No difference in the efficiency of the SRR was noted. This may have been caused by an unusually high degree of ego involvement in both groups, however. Davidson's paradigm employed a highly realistic situation in which the Ss individually planned and executed an actual act outside the laboratory setting. Indeed, Davidson's paradigm appears to be the most realistic, ego-involving paradigm yet developed in which ground truth exists.

Both of those experiments were laboratory studies, however. The crucial test would involve accurate testing on criminal suspects in a field setting. The only such study in which ground truth was experimentally established is that of Kugelmass et al. (1968) which examined 62 criminal suspects being interrogated concerning serious crimes. In order to obtain ground truth in such a situation, Kugelmass et al. (1968) restricted their data to a modified card test embedded in the total field polygraph examination. The Ss were unaware that a part of the interrogation was for research purposes. Of the 62 Ss, each of whom was tested twice, there were 67 hits against chance expectancy of 21 ($p < .001$). It therefore appears that an increase in the degree of affect or in the degree of stress does not make the SRR ineffective as an indicator of deception.

Another obvious difference between laboratory and field testing situations which might account for differences in the efficiency of the EDR is the equipment used. Laboratory equipment is usually highly sophisticated, state-of-the-art equipment, whereas field equipment is small, portable, sometimes battery-operated equipment which is several decades behind the state of the art. This hypothesis is becoming increasingly untenable as experimental results come in. Kugelmass et al. (1967) used a Stoelting field model polygraph. The Bersh study (1969) also supports the use of field equipment, but no analysis was made to determine to what extent the SRR component contributed to the detection rate of 92%. An unpublished study by Gustafson (Orne et al., 1972) likewise pointed to no differences in efficiency between field and laboratory equipment in a laboratory situation. In a recent study by Barland (1972a) using a Keeler field polygraph, it was found that both the SRR and cardiovascular measure were about equally effective on the first chart and were superior to the respiration component. On the second and third charts the cardiovascular measure no longer discriminated between truth and deception while the SRR remained the most effective over all three charts.

There is another major difference between laboratory and field tests which is related to differences in equipment. In many of the laboratory studies, EDA was the only parameter which was monitored; in most of the remaining laboratory studies the sensors for other parameters were passive in the sense that they did not cause undue discomfort to the S. On the other hand, in most field situations the cardio cuff partially occludes circulation in the arm for the 4–5 min that the data are being collected (Reid & Inbau, 1966; USAMPS, 1970). There is some evidence to suggest that this not only results in discomfort to the S (Yankee, 1965), but that it might also degrade the quality of the SRR being monitored in the opposite limb. This possibility was investigated in two studies by Kugelmass and Lieblich (1966) and Kugelmass *et al.* (1968). In the 1966 study, 40 police cadets were examined under a low-stress situation. Each S was tested under two conditions, one with the SRR and cardio cuff operating simultaneously, and one with the SRR operating alone. When the SRR was recorded alone, there were 20 hits compared to a chance expectancy of 7 ($p < .001$). However, when the pressure cuff was inflated while the SRR was being recorded, there were only 11 hits ($p < .05$). The difference between the two conditions was significant ($p < .05$). The interference with the SRR by the pressure cuff was not found in the followup study by Kugelmass *et al.* (1968), in which 62 criminal suspects were tested in a high-stress situation. Using a modified card test within the overall testing procedure, Kugelmass and his co-workers obtained 35 hits using the SRR alone, and 32 hits using the SRR when the cuff was inflated. Both trials yielded significant detection ($p < .001$), and there was no difference between the two conditions. Kugelmass *et al.* (1968) hypothesized that there may be an interaction between the level of stress and the development of an interference effect. They suggested that under low stress levels for psychological or physiological reasons, the effect of the pressure cuff is to reduce differential SRR activity (i.e., to lower the signal-to-noise ratio), whereas under high stress levels the SRR responds differentially to the relevant questions. The study by Barland (1972a), which appeared to have a medium level of involvement, found that the SRR was very effective in discriminating between guilt and innocence when the pressure cuff was inflated. But Barland did not compare the relative effectiveness of the SRR with and without the pressure cuff. Additional research is needed to resolve the conflicting results.

There are several other hypotheses which might be advanced. It may be that field polygraph examiners do not maintain the electrodermal unit of the polygraphs in proper working order, and that the apparent lack of success of the SRR in the field situations might be caused in part by equipment malfunction. Additionally, it may be that the population of Ss in the field setting may differ from experimental Ss in a manner which would result in differential rates of success of the SRR. For example, it may be that field Ss may tend to have thicker calluses which might result in degraded SRR measurements.

Another hypothesis is that there may be a historical bias on the part of the field examiners which has caused them to overlook the value of the SRR in field situations. Although all prominent field examiners who have published their views on the SRR have decried its value in field situations, none has ever presented any evidence to support his view. On the other hand, there have been a number of studies which tend to indicate that the SRR is highly useful in field situations (Kubis, 1950; MacNitt, 1942; Summers, 1939).

Examination of criminal suspects in our own laboratory likewise indicates that the SRR, as recorded on field polygraph equipment, is an extremely useful indicator of truth and deception, but the number of cases which have been verified is as yet too small to permit generalizations.

It should be noted that not all field examiners decry the effectiveness of the SRR measurement. The United States Army (Brisentine, personal communication, 1972; USAMPS, 1970) considers the SRR to be highly effective provided that the SRR component is functioning properly. Since both the U.S. Army and our own laboratory employ an extended pretest interview prior to data collection, a final hypothesis can be suggested. The effectiveness of the SRR may be related to the degree of nervousness of the S, and this in turn may be related to the type of pretest interview. It would seem more reasonable, however, that it would not be related to the length of the pretest interview, but rather to the nature of the S–E interaction and to the degree of confidence that the S has in the competence and objectivity of the examiner.

It would be a relatively simple matter to shed more light on the question of the effectiveness of the SRR in field situations. One simple method would be to subject polygraph charts obtained under field conditions to an objective statistical analysis to determine the effectiveness of the three parameters in those cases where the truthfulness or deceptiveness of the S was independently established.

B. False Positives and False Negatives

Another problem area which is of major importance from both the theoretical and practical standpoints concerns the conditions under which false positives and false negatives occur. Field examiners claim that very few false positives or false negatives occur at all, and that almost all of them that do occur are errors of classifying a deceptive

S as truthful (People of the State of Michigan v. Peter Lazaros, 1970; Reid & Inbau, 1966). Published reports of false positives and negatives are rare (for an example, see Bennett, 1960).

Results of experimental studies in lie detection indicate that there might be more false positives and negatives than field examiners find (Barland, 1972a; Ellson et al., 1952; Kubis, 1962). The many differences between laboratory studies and field situations have been discussed above, so that it would be inappropriate to uncritically generalize from experimental to field situations. Of the few studies reported by scientists using field Ss, most have supported the claims of very high accuracy made by field examiners (Kubis, 1950; MacNitt, 1942; Marston, 1921; Summers, 1939). The study reported by Bersh (1969) had the lowest percentage of reported accuracy, and that was a relatively high 92.4% in those cases in which the decision of the panel was unanimous.

There are cogent reasons for using the laboratory for determining the conditions under which false positives and negatives occur. From the practical point of view, the experimenter, unlike the field polygraph examiner, need not always be concerned with preventing false positives and negatives from occurring. From the theoretical viewpoint, knowledge of the conditions leading to false results may go far toward shedding light upon the psychological mechanisms underlying the detection of deception, and may thus contribute to the formulation of a theory of lie detection. Another major advantage the laboratory has over the field in investigating this problem is that in the laboratory the Ss may be more willing to give more complete and honest information in subsequent debriefing concerning the mechanisms underlying the false responses. Unfortunately, very few laboratory studies have discussed the results of such debriefings. Barland (1972a) mentions several probable causes of false positives and negatives, several of which might be expected to occur more often in the laboratory than in field situations. However, Barland also cites a false positive and a false negative which might reasonably be expected to occur occasionally in field situations.

Extensive mention of individual cases has been made in the field literature, although rarely in the detail presented by Dearman and Smith (1963). Nonetheless, individual cases often point up hypotheses which can be investigated empirically. Beattie (1957) and Borkenstein and Larson (1957) reported several cases in which both false positives and false negatives occurred in field situations. The latter authors advocated the development of a team of experts which would cooperatively make very detailed examinations of suspects who are believed to have produced false positive or negative responses. This concept of a team approach has much to recommend it. Although the composition of such a team would vary widely according to individual circumstances, it might consist at one time or another of a competent field polygraph examiner, a psychophysiologist, a clinical psychologist or psychiatrist, a physician, and a police investigator. Appropriate members of such a team could be called upon to examine those persons suspected of producing false positive or negative responses who have been referred for examination by local field polygraph examiners.

A possible cause of both false positives and false negatives is related to the phenomenon of state-dependent learning. It may be possible for a person to have committed a crime while under the influence of alcohol, amphetamines, heroin, or other drugs, but to have some degree of amnesia present once the drug state has dissipated (Goodwin, Crane, & Guze, 1969; Overton, 1968). If the person is examined on the polygraph in the nondrug state, the question arises of whether he would respond if guilty or if he might respond if innocent. In view of the increasing incidence of drug abuse, this question is of no small consequence from either the practical or the theoretical viewpoints.

An extremely interesting and thorough investigation into the problems of false positives and negatives is being conducted by Lieblich, Kugelmass, and their colleagues. They approach the problem as being one in error reduction in signal detection theory. In their most recent study (Lieblich, Naftali, Shmueli, & Kugelmass, unpublished manuscript) they summarize their findings as follows:

> One of the most important characteristics of the scientific investigation of the detection of information by psychophysiological means is the acceptance of error terms that are different from zero in the detection process, as empirical facts. Thus attempts can be made to reduce them using methods which are generally known to be effective in reduction of error terms. It is clear by now that "special state" methods or "magic" new psychophysiological indices have *by themselves* little promise for dramatic improvement in accuracy, although they may help in providing additional information for the reduction of error terms. Three independent alternatives for the reduction of error terms in this area present themselves:
> (a) The simultaneous utilization and optimal combination of many psychophysiological indices (Kugelmass & Lieblich, 1968).
> (b) The use of larger alternative ensembles into which the critical items are inserted (Lieblich, Kugelmass, & Ben-Shakhar, 1970).
> (c) The use of a longer interrogation which utilizes many critical items indicating the sought information (Lykken, 1959; Ben-Shakhar, Lieblich, & Kugelmass, 1970).

They went on to say that a fourth alternative is the use of longer interrogation with repetition of the same critical item.

C. Detectability in Different Populations

A third major problem area requiring research is the rate of detectability in various types of populations such as university students, "man-on-the-street," criminals, sociopaths, psychopaths, ethnic groups, and various cultural subgroups. It is axiomatic that most experimental research in psychology has traditionally utilized college students taking elementary psychology courses. Relative to the populations being examined in the field, such student populations are remarkably homogeneous in age, IQ, socioeconomic background, code of ethics, etc. It is, therefore, extremely important for experimental data to be obtained from various populations. Because there is no such thing as a "lie response" (U.S. Congress, House Committee on Government Operations, 1964), and responses in a polygraph examination are probably more indicative of the relative level of emotional arousal, it is apparent that the psychological composition of a given S at any particular moment is critically important in determining how and to what extent that S will respond. It is just as apparent that this may vary widely not only according to individual differences, but will also depend upon the complex matrix of experiences and cultural affiliations shared with groups of people. It has long been noted that there are varying degrees of SRR responsivity among various populations (Johnson & Corah, 1963; Kugelmass & Lieblich, 1968). However, it now appears possible that within the various cultural and ethnic groups numerous subgroups can be identified on the basis of differing levels and types of SRR reactivity (Johnson & Lubin, 1972). Moreover, there is some evidence beginning to accumulate which points toward the possibility that there may be certain ethnic groups which are "nondetectable" in the experimental lie detection paradigm (Lieblich, personal communication, 1972).

It would seem reasonable to suppose that the polygraph technique may be less effective on psychopathic liars, because their egocentric code of ethics would reduce or perhaps negate any sense of guilt, remorse, or emotional arousal concerning their lies. The opinions of the field examiners seem to be split on this issue. No experimental study has been reported on this extremely important question. A partial answer to this question could be readily obtained by conducting experimental examinations upon prison inmates who have been diagnosed as psychopathic or sociopathic.

There are relatively little data indicating how various types of psychopathology affect lie detection. Occasionally false positives may result from amnesic persons who are accused of crimes, presumably because they believe that they may have done something they cannot remember

(Borkenstein & Larson, 1957; Turner, 1968). A very interesting experiment utilizing field equipment and experienced field examiners found that some forms of neuroticism and psychoticism produced charts which sometimes resulted in false positive decisions (Heckel, Brokaw, Salzberg, & Wiggins, 1962). In view of the finding that neurotics and psychotics may respond unpredictably on the polygraph, and because they may contribute disproportionately to crimes, a systematic study of the reactions of these types of populations is very necessary. It is in that type of study that a team approach might be particularly rewarding.

Age appears to be a variable affecting detectability. In an experiment in which the chance expectancy of detection was 20%, Voronin *et al.* (1970) correctly identified the point of deception in 0% of children 6–7 years old, 12% of 8–12-year-old children, 53% of 14–16-year-old adolescents, and 87% of 18–30-year-old adults. Although they recorded the EEG, EKG, OMR, and SRR, only the SRR was used for making the detections, since it appeared to be by far the most effective channel. In a recent study by Lieblich (1970), 26 three and 4-year-old children were tested using the SRR as the only measure. Using the decision rule normally applied in adult situations, a significant level of detection was not reached. However, enlargment of the decision rule ("the highest SRR response represents *either* S's name *or* his parent's") produced significant detection rate.

The effect of IQ upon the effectiveness of the polygraph, particularly in deceptive Ss, is unknown. USAMPS (1970) feels that there is a negative correlation between intelligence and latency of response, particularly for the SRR component. However, this has not been adequately demonstrated. Curiously, Reid and Inbau (1966, p. 41) feel that in highly intelligent Ss, cardiovascular changes are not a sufficient criterion for deception unless accompanied by respiratory changes. Most polygraph schools consider highly intelligent Ss to be better examinees because such Ss can forsee future implications of present acts and statements. This tends to be substantiated by some of the findings of Gustafson and Orne (1963), who found that motivation to deceive increased the probability of detection. Many field examiners feel that intelligence is positively correlated with the degree of responsivity of the SRR, and that double-saddle responses are especially indicative of deception. That is particularly true when they occur on relevant questions, because they reflect a progressive realization by the S of the implications of the question. Presumably this double-saddle response would be more likely to be observed in the more intelligent Ss, but that has not been substantiated experimentally.

In the only experiment which looked at intelligence and detectibility, no correlation was found between intelligence and responsivity on a POT test involving cards (Kugelmass, 1967). Interestingly, positive correlations of .50 and .54 were found between years of education and detectibility. There was no correlation between education and responsivity to the irrelevant items on the POT test. Thus, it appears that education increases the probability of detection. The reason why education is a factor but intelligence is not is enigmatic in view of the correlation between the two. However, if this finding holds up for criminal suspects, it might be hypothesized that the correlation between detectability and education might be due to an increased emotional involvement by those who have more responsible positions in society and who thus have more at stake.

It may be that the effectiveness of the polygraph technique might vary according to the type of crime involved, e.g., robbery, homicide, sex crimes, embezzlement, personnel screening, and laboratory paradigms such as card tests. For purposes of interrogation strategies, criminal suspects are often categorized into one of two basic types, the emotional and the logical types (Inbau, 1948, pp. 105–106). It is felt that the emotional type of suspect usually has committed a crime against persons, whereas the logical type usually has committed crimes against property, such as embezzlement or theft. If this observation holds up under experimental objectivity, it would point to the conclusion that the personality of the suspect rather than the crime itself is more directly related to the effectiveness of the polygraph technique. Thackray and Orne (1968b) have demonstrated that idiosyncratic material is detected significantly more often than material made relevant only in an experimental context. This supports the hypothesis that it is not so much the absolute magnitude of the crime as determined by a society's judicial standards, but rather the relative importance of the crime to the individual being tested. Although this points to the interrelatedness of the seriousness or type of crime with the personality of the individual, it might be expected that there are group differences for both the type of crime and the type of population to which an individual belongs. Thus, both the effect of the individual and the effect of the type of crime are problems worthy of research.

V. Countermeasures and Counter-Countermeasures

Polygraph countermeasures are those deliberate techniques which a deceptive subject uses in an attempt to appear nondeceptive when his physiological functions are being monitored during a polygraph examination. Some techniques may be attempted on the spur of the moment by the S without preplanning. Others may be planned by the S prior to the examination. Still others may be the product of extensive research and assistance beforehand by confederates or an organization. This latter category of countermeasure, which might be expected to offer the greatest opportunity of success, would be encountered rarely, and then probably only by intelligence agencies or by persons examining suspects who have obtained advice and training from unethical polygraph operators. Since countermeasures imply deliberate application, they must not be confused with "accidental" false negatives or with psychological processes which were not specifically intended to defeat the polygraph. The above definition also excludes all false positives, regardless of the intent or cause of them.

There is a major category of activity which can in some cases be described as a countermeasure, but which was purposely excluded in the above definition. This is the attempt by the S to explain away his responses once they have been recorded and judged deceptive by the examiner. This can be done piecemeal by the S by making minor, nonincriminating admissions when confronted by the examiner's decision. This is normally followed by retesting. If the response persists, another minor admission may be made. This process is repeated until the physiological response diminishes as a result of habituation and adaptation, or until the examiner tires of the process and accepts the subject's admissions uncritically. This type of evasion is perhaps encountered more frequently in preemployment screening than in criminal examinations. The other way to apply this evasive tactic is to explain away the responses all at once, such as by pleading that one was sensitized to the relevant questions by one's associates or by the police in the period preceding the examination. Obviously, this is applied more frequently in criminal cases. It is often accompanied by vehement denials of guilt in an attempt to convince the examiner of one's innocence on the basis of the behavioral symptoms discussed by Reid and Arther (1953). This type of evasion will not be given further consideration in this discussion, since we wish to consider only those countermeasures which will cause an examiner to call a deceptive S nondeceptive strictly on the basis of the data recorded on the charts.

Countermeasures to the polygraph include the use of mental countermeasures such as thinking relaxing or exciting thoughts or mentally dissociating oneself from the content of the questions; hypnosis; chemicals and pharaceuticals; physical countermeasures such as muscular movements and pain; and the use of familiarity with the equipment, procedures, and structure of the types of tests in order to acquire experience and cause habituation to anticipated relevant questions. It goes without saying that each major type of test (i.e., relevant–irrelevant, peak of tension, and control question) has its own peculiar set of advantages and disadvantages and inherent strengths and weaknesses. A countermeasure which might be relatively effective against one type of test might be completely ineffective against another type. It should also be kept in mind that the attempted use of countermeasures is not as common as might be supposed. A 5-year study by Inbau and Reid indicated that about 20% of all *guilty* Ss attempt countermeasures (Highleyman, 1958). It is generally agreed by the field examiners that most countermeasure attempts are very obvious and easily identified as such. In fact, a number of tests have been developed which implicity invite the S to attempt countermeasures, because the use of a countermeasure would immediately identify the S as deceptive. These include Reid's Yes Test (Reid & Inbau, 1966, p. 32) and the yes–no test (Golden 1969). Moreover, if the use of a countermeasure is suspected, one or more counter-countermeasures may be employed. In our discussion of countermeasures, a number of counter-countermeasures will be mentioned.

A. Mental Countermeasures

The clusters of mental countermeasures are so called because all of them require only a mental effort and none of them can be detected by an observer. There are two possible tactics which may be employed. One is to suppress responses to the relevant questions, the other is to create responses to control, guilt-complex, or irrelevant questions.

The most extreme of the suppressive mental countermeasures is mental dissociation, in which the S attempts to completely ignore the content of the question and to answer automatically. This is possible only with a test such as the peak of tension test in which the answer to each question is always the same. In the POT test each question is phrased like every other one except for one or two key words at the end of the question. Mental dissociation capitalizes upon this inherent weakness of the POT test by having the S focus his attention upon some irrelevant object or thought such as counting the number of holes in each square of soundproofing on the wall. By keeping his mind totally involved in a monotonous, nonexciting task, it is relatively easy to almost completely ignore the content of each question and to answer "no" every time the examiner finishes talking. The S must avoid responding when the examiner states, "Okay, the test is over."

This countermeasure has been referred to as modified yoga by Kubis

(1962). Kubis excluded intense concentration upon a specific object from this type of countermeasure, preferring to include that with the exciting imagery countermeasure described below. If such intense concentration is sporadic throughout the test, such as to only one question on the peak of tension test or to control questions, then there may be grounds for including it in the exciting imagery countermeasure. If, however, the object upon which the S is concentrating is a neutral one, particularly if this intense concentration is relatively constant over a prolonged period of time throughout all or most of the questions, then it would be more properly included within the modified yoga or mental dissociation countermeasure.

In his study, Kubis (1962) found that modified yoga was not an effective countermeasure. He achieved a detection rate of 80% (chance = 10%) in the modified yoga group as compared to 75% detection in the control group. This finding was replicated in a study by More (1966). However, in these experiments the examiners knew that each S must lie at one point on the test. In situations where the examiner must also decide whether the S is lying or not, this technique might well be more effective. Preliminary, unquantified results from both experimental and criminal suspects examined in our laboratory indicate that this countermeasure can sometimes cause inconclusive examinations if the S is not properly stimulated. In an early study by one of Kubis' students (Beebe, 1940), Ss' SRRs were recorded when questions were asked under two conditions: (1) when their only task was to answer the questions, and (2) when in addition to answering they had to engage in a mental mathematical task. It was found that the simultaneous mathematical task significantly reduced SRRs to the questions and made it more difficult for the examiner to distinguish between the responses to emotional versus matter-of-fact questions.

There are several methods of countering this countermeasure. One is to write the key words of the questions in proper sequence in the POT test and pin them directly in front of the S. This ensures that he will know precisely where the point of deception will occur, thereby taking advantage of the rationale behind the POT concept. Although this does not ensure that the S will look at it throughout the test, it should make it more difficult to practice dissociation. Even with this counter-countermeasure, it would still be possible for many Ss to attempt dissociation to some degree.

Another counter-countermeasure which ensures that the S must be intellectually aware of the content of each of the questions is to require him to repeat the key word(s) before giving his answer. For example, to the question, "Do you know if it was a ruby ring?," the S would reply, "Ruby ring, no." By making one additional modification, this can be used to make the S attend to each question even more closely. Instead of pinning the sequence in front of the S, the question may be presented only orally. By having him repeat the key word(s) as above, the E is assured that the S must listen to each question. Arther (1970) claims that when either of these counter-countermeasures is used, the S often makes some verbal mistake at the point of deception, such as failing to repeat the key word(s) when answering.

Another major method by which autonomic responsivity might be suppressed is rationalization. In this technique, the S tells himself that the question does not apply to him. For example, in a laboratory situation in which the "guilty" S has taken money, the question might be, "Did you take that ten dollars?" The S's rationalization might be, "Not really; it was two five-dollar bills." To the extent that he can believe the rationalization, it will be effective. Numerous anecdotal references to this type of process have been made in the field literature (e.g., Beattie, 1957; Borkenstein & Larson, 1957). A careful distinction must be made regarding the intentionality of the rationalization. If it occurred spontaneously as an automatic defense mechanism, then it is not a countermeasure but merely a false negative. Such a S, when later detected by other investigative means and confronted, typically denies vehemently having lied on the polygraph examination. The S then usually explains that the examiner simply had not asked a question which had directly applied to S's situation. Only if the S realizes that the intent of the question applies to him and then seeks to evade by deliberately rationalizing can it be considered to be a countermeasure. It is suggested by Turner (1968) that this countermeasure is so effective that it is for this reason that the communist counterintelligence service do not themselves use the polygraph. However, this is not a very convincing hypothesis, for it has been found informally (Borkenstein & Larson, 1957) that an effective method of handling subconscious rationalizations is to use questions which avoid obvious possibilities for rationalizations. Furthermore, one of the more important reasons for extensively reviewing the questions with the S prior to testing is to clearly emphasize the intent of the questions, thereby undercutting the supports for possible rationalizations. There has been no experimental verification of the effectiveness of either this countermeasure or the counter-countermeasure.

The second major type of mental countermeasure is the use of stimulating thoughts to produce responses to questions other than the relevant questions. It is generally agreed (e.g., Barber, 1969) that it is easier to generate artificial responses than to suppress genuine responses. This can be done either by the physical countermeasures discussed below or by purely mental means, such as thoughts which are erotic, embarrassing, painful, or otherwise emotionally arousing. It would seem that this type of countermeasure would be relatively difficult to employ consistently over the course of an extended examination, and that the S's repertoire of exciting thoughts might be exhausted or that the emotional impact of them might diminish rapidly upon repeated recalls. However, Kubis (1962) found this countermeasure to be highly effective, even when the examiners were informed that the Ss had used this type of countermeasure. Detection was reduced from 75% in the control group to 25% in the experimental group. In an attempted replication of the Kubis study, More (1966) did not find this to be such an effective countermeasure. More's study had a detection rate of 95% in the control group and 80% in the exciting imagery group. Unfortunately, no details of any sort were published by More.

This would seem to be a particularly difficult countermeasure to counteract, since it might be impossible to determine when it is being employed. Once its use is suspected, it would probably be best to switch over to the relevant–irrelevant technique, since significant responses to the irrelevant questions would immediately arouse strong suspicion on the part of the examiner, who would then go into a direct interrogation. It has been argued (Gustafson & Orne, 1964) that the creation of false responses would not be seen often in the field since this would make the S appear to be guilty. This would be true only on the relevant–irrelevant technique. This countermeasure would be expected to be successful if skillfully applied to any of the control question tests. On the peak tension test it would be to the S's advantage to peak on any question other than the critical one. This is more difficult than it may at first appear. Unlike most laboratory evaluation techniques where the main criterion for measurement is the magnitude of a response to each question individually, the field examiner evaluates the chart as a whole. On the POT test, the main field criterion is the point at which the first major change in the base line of the tracings occurs. Thus, for this countermeasure to be successful, it would be necessary for the S to create not only a single large response to the noncritical item, but also a gradual increase and decrease in the baselines centered about the same noncritical item.

B. Practice and Training

It would seem likely that a guilty S who had lied successfully in a previous polygraph examination would be more complacent in a subsequent examination and would thus be more capable of producing false negative results. It would also seem reasonable that with deliberate practice prior to a polygraph examination, the same result might be achieved. Lykken (1960) used sophisticated Ss, explained the testing procedure and evaluation method, and gave them opportunity to practice making false responses. In spite of this, a 100% detection rate was achieved. Golden (1971), used an audio SRR biofeedback device in a field situation and found large increases in the magnitude of the SRR in deceptive Ss who had been used as their own controls. No such increase was found among Ss diagnosed as nondeceptive. However, Golden was unable to establish ground truth in many of the cases, and he had allowed no opportunity for the Ss to practice making or suppressing responses prior to the actual testing. Likewise, Suzuki, Watanabe, and Shimizu (1969) found that visual biofeedback of the SRR enhanced the magnitude of the responses in an experimental card-test procedure, particularly if the initial response to deception had been artificially enhanced without the S's knowledge. However, a study has not yet been conducted in which an extensive biofeedback program has been used to train the Ss to control responses in order to enhance responses to control questions and suppress responses to relevant questions. That may be rather difficult to accomplish. In attempting to respond differentially to the two categories of questions, it is necessary for the S to attend closely to each question and then attempt one of two opposing types of countermeasures. This is inherently incompatible with mental dissociation. The degree of success which a training program could achieve remains to be studied.

Block *et al.* (1952) attempted to train Ss to produce false negatives by conditioning them to produce responses whenever they told the truth. This was done by giving the Ss electrical shocks whenever they told the truth and not giving shocks when they lied. Subsequent testing after the conditioning resulted in a slight diminution of measurable SRRs to both truthful and deceptive responses. There was a slight tendency toward an increase in magnitude of the SRR when Ss were deceptive. Thus, the attempted conditioning was not successful as a countermeasure. Each S received a total of only 8 shocks during the conditioning trial. However, even if there had been many more conditioning trials, it is doubtful whether this would provide an effective countermeasure with a criminal suspect, particularly if a control question test were being employed.

C. Hypnosis

Hypnosis is obviously within the realm of mental countermeasures, yet there are certain aspects which tend to put it into a separate category.

It usually would require a separate hypnotist and training program prior to the actual test. As is often the case in the literature dealing with hypnosis, the few studies dealing with hypnosis as a possible counter-measure are largely open to serious methodological weaknesses and are largely anecdotal with single Ss.

One of the best studies bearing upon this question (Germann, 1961) was a pilot study involving five Ss in which they attempted to deceive the examiner about names, places, and playing cards. Examinations were conducted with each S in a normal waking state, in a deep hypnotic trance with suggested amnesia for the critical items, and in the waking state with posthypnotically suggested amnesia. In eight examinations it was found that a significant response to the critical items was imme-diately detected; in seven examinations the results were inconclusive. Apparently a relevant–irrelevant test was used, but it was not reported whether the examiner knew which items were critical. Germann inter-preted his results as supporting the hypothesis that hypnotically induced amnesia is not effective as a countermeasure, but the relatively large number of inconclusives suggests that hypnosis may in fact have de-creased detectability.

A study by Tocchio (1963) concluded that hypnosis was not an effec-tive countermeasure. The S was given hypnotically induced amnesia for a mock crime. The examiner decided that the S was deceptive. How-ever, this conclusion must be viewed with a great deal of caution, for the study had a number of serious weaknesses. In the first place, there was only one S, and there was no control condition. Only 5–8 sec were allowed between questions, and since the S was breathing at a rate of about once every 6 sec, a valid evaluation of the respiration could not be made using accepted field criteria (Arther, 1971a; Reid & Inbau, 1966; USAMPS, 1970). Moreover, the amplitudes of all three components were substandard by field criteria (USAMPS, 1970).

A third report (Cumley, 1959) likewise indicated that hypnotically suggested amnesia is not an effective countermeasure. Two Ss committed a mock theft from a dormitory room, were given suggestions for amnesia for all events occurring within the preceding 7 days, and were then examined on a three-channel field polygraph. Both relevant–irrelevant and peak of tension tests were conducted on both Ss. The objects which had been taken were clearly identifiable from an inspection of the charts of both types of examinations on both Ss.

Another study indicating that hypnosis is not an effective countermea-sure was conducted by Bitterman and Marcuse (1945). Using a S who was capable of a deep hypnotic trance, they suggested amnesia for the word which S had chosen. Two days later the effectiveness of the posthypnotic amnesia was tested using the POT test. This procedure was repeated four times by each of the two Es, making a total of eight examinations of the S. In two of the eight tests no word had been suggested while the S was hypnotized. This served as a control. The four charts obtained by each E were then evaluated by the other E. Each E made a primary choice as to which of the six words in each test was the one for which amnesia had been suggested. Where the E was uncertain, a second choice was also made. Of the eight words, five were detected by the Es as their first choice; the other three were selected as their second choice.

An experiment which found that hypnotically induced amnesia was an effective countermeasure was reported by Weinstein, Abrams, and Gibbons (1970). Six students were randomly assigned to two groups of three students each. The Ss in the first group took one of three bills ($1, $5, or $20) and were then hypnotized and instructed to forget having taken the money. It was also suggested that no guilt would be associated with the act. When these three Ss were examined by an experienced field polygraph examiner, the results were inconclusive. When pressed for a definite decision, the examiner indicated that there were some indications of deception in the records of all three. The Ss in the second group took no money, but were given hypnotic suggestions that they had. They were also given suggestions of guilt for having taken the money. When these three Ss were tested, the examiner concluded that all three had taken the money. It thus appears that false positives may be induced through hypnotically implanted memories, but that not all indications of deceptiveness can be suppressed through hypnotically induced amnesia.

Arons (1967) mentioned two loosely designed experiments, both of which used hypnotically suggested amnesia as a countermeasure to the polygraph. In one of the experiments, conducted by William J. Bryan in Miami in 1965, the examiners were able to correctly interpret the charts in spite of the S's amnesia for the mock crime. However, in an experiment by William Mayer and Lt. Colonel Joseph Ziglinski in Washington, D.C., also with a single S, hypnotically suggested amnesia was successful in misleading the examiner.

Another informal experiment conducted by the Lie Detector Committee of the United States Army Military Police School (1960), while somewhat vague, concluded that hypnotically suggested amnesia can be an effective countermeasure.

There is a hypnotic technique of lie detection which operates on the principle of conditioning a part of the body, typically a finger or an eyelid, to twitch whenever that person tells a lie. In describing this technique, Arons (1967, p. 134) refers to it as an autonomic response. This is an unfortunate choice of words, since it is completely unrelated to the autonomic nervous system. Although it is normally used alone rather than in conjunction with a polygraph, Tocchio (1963) combined it with the polygraph and reported positive results.

Clearly, a great deal of carefully constructed experimentation is needed before the question of the efficacy of hypnosis as a countermeasure can be determined with any degree of accuracy. The general trend of the above experiments is that hypnosis may be marginally effective in misleading an experienced polygraph examiner. This agrees with the consensus of research dealing with the psychophysiological aspects of hypnosis, where it has been found that through hypnosis autonomic responsivity can be enhanced or reduced somewhat, but not eliminated (Barber, 1969; Stern, Winokur, Graham, & Graham, 1961; Yanovsky, 1962). There is also a growing body of evidence suggesting that the same amount of control over the responsivity of the autonomic nervous system can be achieved by suggestion alone, without the necessity of using hypnosis (Barber, 1969; Damaser, Shor, & Orne, 1963). In view of the dearth of good research dealing with hypnosis as applied to lie detection, no definite conclusions can be made at this time.

D. Physical Countermeasures

A completely different set of countermeasures involves the use of physical manipulations to create false negatives and pseudo responses. It has long been known that judicious tensing and relaxing of the arm on which the cardio cuff is located can create both false negatives and positives in the cardiovascular component (Reid, 1945). While it is more difficult to manipulate the SRR pattern in a credible manner through the use of arm musculature, there is a variety of physical countermeasures which will create realistic responses not only in the SRR but also in the cardiovascular and the respiratory measures as well. Almost any voluntary contraction of a muscle group within the body will produce the desired responses which may closely resemble physiological responses caused by the arousal value of the questions. The only problem for the S is to select a muscle group, the manipulation of which will not be visible to the examiner. Several techniques which have been used are the pressing of the toes against the floor (Smith, 1967), pressing the thighs against the chair (Reid & Inbau, 1966), looking cross-eyed, gritting the teeth on the side away from the examiner, pressing the tongue against the roof of the mouth, and tensing the anal sphincter (USAMPS, 1970). It must be kept in mind that not all of these countermeasures will be effective in creating a response with every S, and that each one will not show the same degree of effectiveness within a single S over a period of time, suggesting that there is a psychological factor contributing to the physiological response.

In his countermeasures experiment, Kubis (1962) found that when Ss pressed their toes against the floor, they were able to reduce detection rates from the control level of 75% to chance levels (10%). A replication of this experiment by More (1966) found that there was no decrement in detectability caused by toe movements; there was a detection rate of 95% in both the control and experimental conditions. The generalizability of these conflicting results is difficult, for the Ss' task was a low-affect one of denying which of ten numbers they had chosen. No countermeasures study utilizing a high-stress situation has been reported.

In order to detect movements of the torso, anal sphincter, and the legs, it is possible to record bodily movements by means of pneumatic sensors built into the back and seat of the S's chair (Reid, 1945). A means of rendering ineffective the use of toe presses is to seat the S in a reclining chair which removes S's legs from the floor and raises them to permit better visual inspection of the legs and feet by the examiner. A procedure which would probably give much the same result would be not to have the S place his feet flat on the floor as is customary, but to have the S extend his legs and cross them. To reduce the effectiveness of attempts to manipulate the arm muscles, Reid and Inbau (1966) suggest that the examiner physically relax the S's arm prior to each chart.

E. Pain

The production of pain can also serve to produce responses. This can be accomplished in several ways. One is for the S to conceal a thumbtack within his shoe or under his tongue. Slight pressure of the toes or the tongue will cause sufficient pain to induce a significant response (USAMPS, 1970). The first author knows of an instance in a nonexperimental, hypothetical testing situation in which a S was being examined regarding the "theft" of a classified document. When the examiner declared him innocent after administering a zone of comparison test, the S pulled the secret document out of his pants leg. He had realized that it would be to his advantage to create responses to the control questions, and had done so by pressing down slightly on an inflamed ingrown toenail at the appropriate time. An obvious method of countering this would be to physically examine the S, particularly the mouth and foot areas, whenever this type of countermeasure is suspected because of an unusual pattern of responsivity to both the relevant and control questions.

F. Adrenal Exhaustion

It has often been suggested that adrenal exhaustion may be an effective means of producing false negative results (Reid & Inbau, 1966, pp. 177–179). In an article in the underground press on how to beat the polygraph, Degrak (1970) suggested that the S run around the block a couple of times immediately prior to presenting himself for a polygraph exam in the hopes that this would so deplete the available supply of epinephrine that the general level of autonomic responsivity would be sufficiently low to escape detection. This technique would only be applicable in those situations where the S is free to arrive unescorted at the polygraph site, and would probably be effectively counteracted by any testing situation in which an extensive pretest interview is conducted.

There is considerable reason for speculating that adrenal exhaustion would not be an effective countermeasure, particularly in reference to electrodermal activity. The responses measured by the polygraph presumably result from the sympathetic nervous system acting directly upon the effectors being monitored. The supplementary effect caused by sympathetic innervation of the adrenal medulla would be delayed by several seconds when present, and would merely serve to enhance and prolong the responses created by direct innervation by the sympathetic nervous system. Reid and Inbau (1966, p. 179) mention that deception responses were observed in an experimental situation on two Ss who had undergone bilateral adrenalectomy for malignant hypertension. Moreover, it must be remembered that for electrodermal activity the mediating chemical at the neuroeffector junction is not epinephrine or norepinephrine but acetylcholine (Harvey, 1971; Sternbach, 1966). Although it would seem that adrenal exhaustion would not be a particularly effective countermeasure, no study has been reported which has examined this.

G. Respiration

Another type of physical countermeasure which is often encountered is that of controlled respiration. Many deceptive Ss consider respiration the only parameter which they can control, and there are many methods of controlling respiration. One common one is for the S to attempt to breathe very regularly. Because of the lack of sophistication of the Ss, this often takes the form of a slow, deep respiratory pattern at a rate of about 6–10 breaths per minute. This may induce cyclical changes in both heart rate (sinus arrhythmia) and blood pressure (Brener, 1967; Guyton, 1971). Although this makes interpretation of the cardiovascular tracings more difficult, a valid interpretation is still possible in most instances, because the examiner is looking for any change in the cardio-vascular pattern which is timelocked to the relevant questions. When this type of breathing is encountered, it is relatively easy to diagnose it as a countermeasure by recording the respiration when the S is not aware that it is being recorded.

Another common respiratory countermeasure is an occasional deep breath. Many Ss realize that to take a deep breath in a nonrandom manner, e.g., just after each relevant or control question, would be too obvious. Therefore, some Ss do so randomly so as to leave them with a plausible denial of intentionality. Although most Ss presumably believe that they are disrupting only the respiratory measure, it generally affects all three components. If it cannot readily be determined that such respira-tory irregularities are intentional, the only recourse is to wait until the physiological response returns to base levels and then repeat the ques-tion. If not too many questions are repeated, the effect of habituation should be minimal.

H. Chemical Countermeasures

Another category of countermeasure involves the use of chemical and pharmacological aids to defeat the polygraph technique. Relatively little research has been reported concerning this type of countermeasure, pos-sibly because it is not frequently encountered, but more probably be-cause of the difficulties of engaging in human research involving drugs. The use of an antiperspirant on the hands prior to testing has been reported to diminish SRR responsivity (Arther, 1971b). Discussion with field examiners indicates that this is effective unless the examiner has the S wash his hands with soap and water. Some Ss have also applied substances such as clear fingernail polish to the fingertips for the same reason. These would seem to be too obvious for successful employment, but a criminal suspect examined in our laboratory did mention that he knew of a case where that had been successful.

Of the various classes of pharmacological agents, only the depressants appear to offer potential as a countermeasure, since they appear to be helpful in reducing the magnitude of responses (Berman, 1967). How-ever, if only enough of the depressant is taken to reduce autonomic responsivity, it is likely that for a deceptive S the responses to the control questions will be abolished before the responses to the relevant questions. If sufficient depressant is taken to totally suppress responsivity, the suspicions of the examiner will be raised regardless of whether a relevant–irrelevant or a control question technique is being used.

Klump (1965) believes that tranquilizers are ineffective because they tend to reduce the level of general nervous tension without affecting true emotional responsivity, thereby increasing the probability of detection. Klump also indicates that consumption of alcohol prior to the examination is also self-defeating because the examination would be conducted before the S becomes drunk, whereas the interrogation would occur when the S is drunk, thereby increasing the probability of obtaining a confession. No data are offered to support these observations. In his countermeasures article, Degrak (1970) advises the S against taking any hallucinogens, including marijuana, because of the disproportionate and disorganized response pattern caused by "that sudden paranoid feeling 'he knows I'm stoned'."

A serious lack of experimental data makes it impossible to draw any conclusions concerning the effectiveness of chemical countermeasures.

I. Miscellaneous Countermeasures

A final group of countermeasure techniques includes an assortment of techniques which are attempted in complete ignorance of the functioning of the human body, the manner in which polygraph examinations are structured, etc. These countermeasures include putting soap under the arms (Klump, 1965), putting bullets under the cardio cuff (Reid & Inbau, 1966), taking four aspirins with a drink of cola, etc.

These countermeasures, although outwardly unrelated, all possess the common factor of a simple, almost superstitious belief in their ability to protect the user from detection. They resemble the tail of the "magical ass"; if the user completely believes that they work, they might. One story, possibly apocryphal, relates how an examiner in the southern United States obtained a totally inconclusive chart from a suspect. Believing that the suspect may have consulted a voodoo doctor prior to the exam, the examiner took a doll from his desk and proceeded to dehex the suspect. The subsequent charts showed large indications of deception and a confession quickly followed! There is evidence which can be interpreted to suggest that if the S is able to avoid being emotionally involved by the relevant questions, as when he is completely confident that he will not be detected, the detection rate is reduced (Gustafson & Orne, 1965a).

It is interesting to note that detection rate falls off if the S is completely convinced that his lie will not be detected or if he is equally convinced that his lie is certain to be detected. In either extreme the S feels no emotional involvement with the relevant questions, and there is thus little or no response. As Davis (1961) so aptly put it, optimum detection results when the S considers it likely, but not inevitable, that his lie will be detected, and that it is important that he do everything within his power to avoid responding to the relevant question(s).

In concluding our discussion of countermeasures, it must be emphasized that most countermeasure attempts are readily recognized as such by experienced field examiners. Many examiners therefore structure situations which implicitly invite countermeasures at one time or another during the testing situation. It should be clearly understood that, in contrast to the relevant–irrelevant technique, the control question technique protects against incorrect decisions by typically yielding an inconclusive result when subtle countermeasures are intelligently employed. Thus, successfully suppressing responses to relevant questions would merely reduce them to the level of responses to control questions. On the other hand, enhancing the responses to control questions would merely raise them to the same level as the relevant questions. The only way countermeasures could be effective would be to enhance the responses to control questions while simultaneously suppressing the responses to relevant questions. This would be extremely difficult to accomplish. It is revealing that the general tenor of Degrak's countermeasure article (1970) is that the only really effective countermeasure is to avoid taking the polygraph examination in the first place.

VI. Summary and Conclusions

It can be seen that the lie detection paradigm is important in psychological and psychophysiological research studying a variety of phenomena such as attention, arousal, motivation, learning, etc. It is unfortunate that so little theoretically oriented research has been conducted during the past half century that the polygraph has been used as a "lie detector." Fortunately, this situation seems to be changing with the establishment of research teams located in several countries, and it presently appears that a new and more valuable phase in research involving the lie detection paradigm is underway. This new phase is characterizied by more complex, rigorously designed experimental and statistical procedures aimed at examining the underlying psychological variables which contribute to this differential physiological responsivity to previously neutral stimuli.

There is considerable evidence to demonstrate that electrodermal activity is the best indicator of this differential responsivity in laboratory situations, and that it may also be extremely effective in practical applications of this paradigm in real-life situations.

There remain a great number of theoretical and practical issues to be studied. These might be approached by experienced experimenters who have a multidisciplinary background, or by teams drawn from a variety of disciplines. In view of the immense theoretical and practical issues involved, there is certainly no longer any reason for ignoring this paradigm.

References

Alpert, M., Kurtzberg, R. L., & Friedhoff, A. J. Transient voice changes associated with emotional stimuli. *Archives of General Psychiatry,* 1963, **8**, 362–365.

American Polygraph Association. Polygraph training schools (that) have met the standards as prescribed by our association. *American Polygraph Association Newsletter,* 1972, **6**(3), 8.

Arons, H. *Hypnosis in criminal investigation.* Springfield, Illinois: Thomas, 1967.

Arther, R. O. *The scientific investigator.* Springfield, Illinois: Thomas, 1965.

Arther, R. O. Peak of tension: Dangers. *Journal of Polygraph Studies,* 1968, **2**(5), 1–4. (a)

Arther, R. O. Re-examinations. *Journal of Polygraph Studies,* 1968, 3(2), 1–4. (b)

Arther, R. O. Irrelevant questions. *Journal of Polygraph Studies,* 1969, 3(6), 3–4.

Arther, R. O. Peak of tension: Examination procedures. *Journal of Polygraph Studies,* 1970, 5(1), 1–4.

Arther, R. O. Breathing analysis. *Journal of Polygraph Studies,* 1971, 5(4), 1–4 and 5(5), 1–4. (a)

Arther, R. O. The GSR unit. *Journal of Polygraph Studies,* 1971, 5(6), 1–4. (b)

Arther, R. O., & Caputo, R. R. *Interrogation for investigators.* New York: William C. Copp, 1959.

Arther, R. O., & Reid, J. E. Utilizing the lie detector technique to determine the truth in disputed paternity cases. *Journal of Criminal Law, Criminology and Police Science,* 1954, **45**, 213–221.

Aubry, A., & Caputo, R. *Criminal interrogation.* Springfield, Illinois: Thomas, 1965.

Backster, C. Polygraph professionalization through technique standardization. *Law and Order,* 1963, **11**(4), 63–64.

Barber, T. X. *Hypnosis: A scientific approach.* Princeton, New Jersey: Van Nostrand-Reinhold, 1969.

Barber, W. E. An experimental test of the Peak of Tension theory as used in the field of polygraph. Unpublished Masters Thesis, Western Michigan University, June, 1964.

Barland, G. H. An experimental study of field techniques in lie detection. Unpublished Masters Thesis, University of Utah, 1972. (a)

Barland, G. H. The reliability of polygraph chart evaluations. Paper presented at the American Polygraph Association Symposium, Chicago, Illinois, August 15, 1972. (b)

Beattie, R. J. The semantics of question preparation. In V. A. Leonard (Ed.), *Academy lectures in lie detection.* Springfield, Illinois: Thomas, 1957. Pp. 20–43.

Beebe, D. The effect of divided attention on the psychogalvanic response. Unpublished Masters Thesis, Fordham University, 1940.

Bennett, J. V. A penal administrator views the polygraph. *Federal Probation*, 1960, **24**, 40–44.

Ben-Shakhar, G., Lieblich, I., & Kugelmass, S. Guilty knowledge technique: Application of signal detection measures. *Journal of Applied Psychology*, 1970, **54**, 409–413.

Benussi, V. Die Atmungssymptome der Lüge. *Archiv für die gesamte Psychologie*, 1914, 31, 244–273.

Berman, M. A. Drugs versus the polygraph. *Journal of Polygraph Studies*, 1967, 1(4), 1–3.

Berrien, F. K. Pupillary responses as indicators of deception. *Psychological Bulletin*, 1942, 39, 504–505.

Berrien, F. K., & Huntington, G. H. An exploratory study of pupillary responses during deception. *Journal of Experimental Psychology*, 1943, **32**, 443–449.

Bersh, P. J. A validation study of polygraph examiner judgements. *Journal of Applied Psychology*, 1969, **53**, 399–403.

Bitterman, M. E., & Marcuse, F. L. Autonomic response in posthypnotic amnesia. *Journal of Experimental Psychology*, 1945, **35**, 248–252.

Bitterman, M. E., & Marcuse, F. L. Cardiovascular responses of innocent persons to criminal investigation. *American Journal of Psychology*, 1947, **60**, 407–412.

Block, J. D., Rouke, F. L., Salpeter, M. M., Tobach, E., Kubis, J. F., & Welch, L. An attempt at reversal of the truth-lie relationship as measured by the psychogalvanic response. *Journal of Psychology*, 1952, 34, 55–66.

Borkenstein, R. F., & Larson, J. A. The clinical team approach. In V. A. Leonard (Ed.), *Academy lectures in lie detection*. Springfield, Illinois: Thomas, 1957. Pp. 11–19.

Brener, J. Heart Rate. In P. H. Venables & I. Martin (Eds.), *A manual of psychophysiological methods*. Amsterdam: North-Holland Publ., 1967. Pp. 103–131.

Burtt, H. E. The inspiration–expiration ratio during truth and falsehood. *Journal of Experimental Psychology*, 1921, 4, 1–23. (a)

Burtt, H. E. Further technique for inspiration–expiration ratios. *Journal of Experimental Psychology*, 1921, 4, 106–110. (b)

Crosland, H. R. The psychological methods of word-association and reaction time as tests of deception. *University of Oregon Publications in Psychology Series*, 1929, 1 (No. 1).

Cumley, W. E. Hypnosis and the polygraph. *Police*, 1959, 4(2), 39.

Damaser, E., Shor, R. E., & Orne, M. T. Physiological effects during hypnotically requested emotions. *Psychosomatic Medicine*, 1963, **25**, 334–343.

Dana, H. J. It is time to improve the polygraph: A progress report on polygraph research and development. In V. A. Leonard (Ed.), *Academy lectures on lie detection*. Vol. 2. Springfield, Illinois: Thomas, 1958. Pp. 84–90.

Dana, H. J., & Barnett, C. C. The emotional stress meter. In V. A. Leonard (Ed.), *Academy lectures on lie detection*. Springfield, Illinois: Thomas, 1957. Pp. 73–83.

Davidson, P. O. Validity of the guilty-knowledge technique: The effects of motivation. *Journal of Applied Psychology*, 1968, **52**, 62–65.

Davis, R. C. Physiological responses as a means of evaluating information. In A. D. Biderman & H. Zimmer (Eds.), *The manipulation of human behavior*. New York: Wiley, 1961. Pp. 142–168.

Dearman, H. B., & Smith, B. M. Unconscious motivation and the polygraph test. *American Journal of Psychiatry*, 1963, **119**, 1017–1021.

Degrak, H. How to lie to a lie detector. *Los Angeles Free Press,* August 7, 1970.

Ekman, P., & Friesen, W. V. Nonverbal leakage and clues to deception. *Psychiatry,* 1969, **63,** 88–106.

Ellson, D. G., Davis, R. C., Saltzman, I. J., & Burke, C. J. A report of research on detection of deception. (Contract N6onr-18011 with the Office of Naval Research.) Available from the University of Indiana, Bloomington, Indiana, 1952.

Fay, P. J., & Middleton, W. C. The ability to judge truth-telling, or lying, from the voice as transmitted over a public address system. *Journal of General Psychology,* 1941, **24,** 211–215.

Ferguson, R. J. *The scientific informer.* Springfield, Illinois: Thomas, 1971.

Germann, A. C. Hypnosis as related to the scientific detection of deception by polygraph examination: A pilot study. *International Journal of Clinical and Experimental Hypnosis,* 1961, **9,** 309–311.

Golden, R. I. The closed-eyes polygraph technique. *Journal of Polygraph Studies,* 1966, **1**(2), 1–4.

Golden, R. I. A conditioned reflex technique in lie detection. In S. A. Yefsky (Ed.), *Law enforcement science and technology.* New York: Thompson Book Co., Academic Press, 1967. Pp. 385–392.

Golden, R. I. The Yes–No technique in polygraph testing. Paper presented at the American Polygraph Association seminar in Houston, August, 1969.

Golden, R. I. Audio GSR bio-feedback in polygraph examinations. Paper presented at the American Polygraph Association, Atlanta, Georgia, August, 1971.

Goodwin, D. W., Crane, J. B., & Guze, S. B. Alcoholic "blackouts": A review and clinical study of 100 alcoholics. *American Journal of Psychiatry,* 1969, **126,** 191–198.

Gustafson, L. A., & Orne, M. T. Effects of heightened motivation on the detection of deception. *Journal of Applied Psychology,* 1963, **47,** 408–411.

Gustafson, L. A., & Orne, M. T. The effects of task and method of stimulus presentation on the detection of deception. *Journal of Applied Psychology,* 1964, **48,** 383–387.

Gustafson, L. A., & Orne, M. T. Effects of perceived role and role success on the detection of deception. *Journal of Applied Psychology,* 1965, **49,** 412–417. (a)

Gustafson, L. A., & Orne, M. T. The effects of verbal responses on the laboratory detection of deception. *Psychophysiology,* 1965, **2,** 10–13. (b)

Guyton, A. C. *Textbook of medicial physiology.* (4th ed.) Philadelphia, Pennsylvania: Saunders, 1971.

Harrelson, L. H. *The Keeler technique* (Keeler Polygraph Institute training guide). Chicago, Illinois: Keeler Polygraph Institute, 1964. Available from the Keeler Polygraph Institute, 161 E. Grand Avenue, Chicago, Illinois 60611.

Harvey, J. A. Autonomic drugs. In J. A. Harvey (Eds.), *Behavioral analysis of drug action.* Glenview, Illinois: Scott, Foresman and Co., 1971.

Heckel, R. V., Brokaw, J. R., Salzberg, H. C., & Wiggins, S. L. Polygraphic variations in reactivity between delusional, non-delusional, and control groups in a "crime" situation. *Journal of Criminal Law, Criminology and Police Science,* 1962, **53,** 380–383.

Highleyman, S. L. The deceptive certainty of the "lie detector." *Hastings Law Journal,* 1958, **10,** 47–64.

Holmes, W. D. The degree of objectivity in chart interpretation. In V. A. Leonard

(Ed)., *Academy lectures on lie detection*, Vol. II. Springfield, Illinois: Thomas, 1958. Pp. 62–70.

Horvath, F. S. Verbal and nonverbal clues to truth and deception during polygraph examinations. Unpublished Masters Thesis, Michigan State University, 1972.

Horvath, F. S., & Reid, J. E. The reliability of polygraph examiner diagnoses of truth and deception. *Journal of Criminal Law, Criminology and Police Science*, 1971, **62**, 276–281.

Horvath, F. S., & Reid, J. E. The polygraph silent answer test. *Journal of Criminal Law, Criminology and Police Science*, 1972, **63**, 285–293.

Hunter, F. L. Polygraph reliability in identifying the truthful subject. Paper presented at the American Polygraph Association seminar, Atlanta, Georgia, 1971. Also published in the *American Polygraph Association Newsletter*, 1971, 6(2), 11–23.

Inbau, F. E. Detection of deception technique admitted as evidence. *Journal of Criminal Law, Criminology and Police Science*, 1935, **26**, 262–270.

Inbau, F. E. *Lie detection and criminal interrogation*. (2nd ed.) Baltimore, Maryland: Williams & Wilkins, 1948.

Inbau, F. E., & Reid, J. E. *Criminal interrogation and confessions*. (2nd ed.) Baltimore, Maryland: Williams & Wilkins, 1967.

Johnson, L. C., & Corah, N. L. Racial differences in skin resistance. *Science*, 1963, **139**, 766–767.

Johnson, L. C., & Lubin, A. On planning psychophysiological experiments: Design, measurement, and analysis. In N. S. Greenfield & R. A. Sternbach (Eds.), *Handbook of psychophysiology*. New York: Holt, 1972. Pp. 125–158.

Keeler, L. Debunking the lie detector. *Journal of Criminal Law, Criminology and Police Science*, 1934, **25**, 153–159.

Klump, C. S. So you want to beat the polygraph! *Security World*, June 1965, 30–32.

Kubis, J. F. Experimental and statistical factors in the diagnosis of consciously suppressed affective experience. *Journal of Clinical Psychology*, 1950, **6**, 12–16.

Kubis, J. F. Studies in lie detection: Computer feasibility considerations. Technical Report 62-205, prepared for Air Force Systems Command, Contract No. AF 30 (602)-2270, Project No. 5534, Fordham University, 1962.

Kugelmass, S. *Reactions to stress*. Scientific report performed under contract AF 61 (052)-839. Available from DDC, AD 647 467. January, 1967.

Kugelmass, S., & Lieblich, I. The effects of realistic stress and procedural interference in experimental lie detection. *Journal of Applied Psychology*, 1966, **50**, 211–216.

Kugelmass, S., & Lieblich, I. Relation between ethnic origin and GSR reactivity in psychophysiological detection. *Journal of Applied Psychology*, 1968, **52**, 158–162.

Kugelmass, S., Lieblich, I., & Bergman, Z. The role of "lying" in psychophysiological detection. *Psychophysiology*, 1967, **3**, 312–315.

Kugelmass, S., Lieblich, I., Ben-Ishai, A., Opatowski, A., & Kaplan, M. Experimental evaluation of galvanic skin response and blood pressure change indices during criminal investigation. *Journal of Criminal Law, Criminology and Police Science*, 1968, **59**, 632–635.

Larson, J. A. Modification of the Marston deception test. *Journal of Criminal Law, Criminology and Police Science*, 1921, **12**, 390–399.

Larson, J. A. *Lying and its detection: A study of deception and deception tests*. Chicago, Illinois: Univ. of Chicago Press, 1932. Reprinted, Montclair, New Jersey: Patterson Smith, 1969.

Lee, C. D. *The instrumental detection of deception*. Springfield, Illinois: Thomas, 1953.

Lieblich, I. Manipulation of contrast between differential GSR responses through use of ordered tasks of information detection. *Psychophysiology*, 1969, **6**, 70–77.

Lieblich, I. Manipulation of contrast between differential GSRs in very young children. *Psychophysiology*, 1970, **7**, 436–441.

Lieblich, I., Kugelmass, S., & Ben-Shakhar, G. Efficiency of GSR detection of information as a function of stimulus set size. *Psychophysiology*, 1970, **6**, 601–608.

Lieblich, I., Naftali, G., Shmueli, J., & Kugelmass, S. Efficiency of GSR detection of information with repeated presentation of series of stimuli, in two motivational states. Unpublished manuscript.

Lindsley, D. B. The psychology of lie detection. In G. J. Dudycha (Ed.), *Psychology for law enforcement officers*. Springfield, Illinois: Thomas, 1955. Pp. 89–125.

Luria, A. R. Die Methode des abbildenden Motorik in der Tatbestands-Diagnostik. (The method of recording movements in crime detection). *Zeitschrift für angewandte Psychologie*, 1930, **35**, 139–183.

Luria, A. R. *The nature of human conflicts*. New York: Liverwright, 1932.

Lykken, D. T. The GSR in the detection of guilt. *Journal of Applied Psychology*, 1959, **43**, 385–388.

Lykken, D. T. The validity of the guilty knowledge technique: The effects of faking. *Journal of Applied Psychology*, 1960, **44**, 258–262.

Lyon, V. W. Deception tests with juvenile delinquents. *Journal of Genetic Psychology*, 1936, **48**, 494–497.

MacNitt, R. D. In defense of the electrodermal response and cardiac amplitude as measures of deception. *Journal of Criminal Law, Criminology and Police Science*, 1942, **33**, 266–275.

Marcuse, F. L., & Bitterman, M. E. Minimal cues in the peak of tension procedure for determining guilt. *American Journal of Psychology*, 1946, **59**, 144–146.

Marston, W. M. Systolic blood pressure symptoms of deception. *Journal of Experimental Psychology*, 1917, **2**, 117–163.

Marston, W. M., Psychological possibilities in the deception test. *Journal of Criminal Law, Criminology and Police Science*, 1921, **11**, 551–570.

Marston, W. M. *The lie detector test*. New York: Smith, 1938.

More, H. W. Polygraph research and the university. *Law and Order*, 1966, **14**, 73–78.

Moroney, W. F., & Zenhausern, R. J. Detection of deception as a function of galvanic skin response recording methodology. *Journal of Psychology*, 1972, **80**, 255–262.

Mulbar, H. *Interrogation*. Springfield, Illinois: Thomas, 1951.

Obermann, C. E. The effect on the Berger rhythm of mild affective states. *Journal of Abnormal and Social Psychology*, 1939, **34**, 84–95.

Orne, M. T., Thackray, R. I., & Paskewitz, D. A. On the detection of deception: A model for the study of the physiological effects of psychological stimuli. In N. Greenfield & R. Sternbach (Eds.), *Handbook of psychophysiology*. New York: Holt, 1972. Pp. 743–785.

Overton, D. A. Dissociated learning in drug states (State-dependent learning). In D. H. Efron *et al.* (Eds.), *Psychopharmacology, a review of progress*. PHS Publ. 1836. Washington, D.C.: U.S. Government Printing Office, 1968. Pp. 918–930.

People of the State of Michigan v. Peter N. Lazaros. Trial transcript pertaining to admissibility of the polygraph as evidence. June, 1970. Available from the Michigan Polygraph Association, 1049 North Vernon, Dearborn, Michigan 48128.

Pfaff, R. S. The polygraph: An invaluable investigative aid. *American Bar Association Journal*, 1964, **50**, 1130–1133.

Reid, J. E. Simulated blood pressure responses in lie detector tests and a method for their detection. *Journal of Criminal Law, Criminology and Police Science*, 1945, **36**, 201–214.

Reid, J. E. A revised questioning technique in lie detection tests. *Journal of Criminal Law, Criminology and Police Science*, 1947, **37**, 542–547.

Reid, J. E., & Arther, R. O. Behavior symptoms of lie detector subjects. *Journal of Criminal Law, Criminology and Police Science*, 1953, **44**, 104–108.

Reid, J. E., & Inbau, F. E. *Truth and deception: The polygraph ("lie-detector") technique.* Baltimore, Maryland: Williams & Wilkins, 1966.

Romig, C. H. A. The status of polygraph legislation of the fifty states. *Police*, 1971, **16**(1), 35–41; **16**(2), 54–61; **16**(3), 55–61.

Rouke, F. L. Evaluation of the indices of deception in the Psychogalvanic technique. Unpublished doctoral dissertation, Fordham University, 1941.

Schatkin, S. B. Paternity proceedings and the polygraph. *Journal of Polygraph Studies*, 1970, **4**(4), 1–4.

Smith, B. M. Polygraph. *Scientific American*, 1967, **216**(1), 25–30.

Stein, A. E. The federal polygraph school. *Polygraph*, 1972, **1**, 75–79.

Stern, J. A., Winokur, G., Graham, D. T., & Graham, F. K. Alterations in physiological measures during experimentally induced attitudes. *Journal of Psychosomatic Research*, 1961, **5**, 73–82.

Sternbach, R. A. *Principles of psychophysiology.* New York: Academic Press, 1966.

Summers, W. G. Science can get confession. *Fordham Law Review*, 1939, **5**, 334–354.

Suzuki, S., Watanabe, T., & Shimizu, K. Effects of visual feedback by the skin potential response. *Japanese Journal of Psychology*, 1969, **40**(2), 59–67.

Thackray, R. I., & Orne, M. T. A comparison of physiological indices in detection of deception. *Psychophysiology*, 1968, **4**, 329–339. (a)

Thackray, R. I., & Orne, M. T. Effects of the type of stimulus employed and the level of subject awareness on the detection of deception. *Journal of Applied Psychology*, 1968, **52**, 234–239. (b).

Tocchio, O. J. Lie detection under hypnosis. *Police*, 1963, **8**(1), 9–11.

Trovillo, P. V. A history of lie detection. *Journal of Criminal Law, Criminology and Police Science*, 1939, **29**, 848–881; **30**, 104–119.

Trovillo, P. V. Scientific proof of credibility. *Tennessee Law Review*, 1953, **22**, 33–56.

Turner, W. W. *Invisible witness: The use and abuse of the new technology of crime investigation.* New York: Bobbs-Merrill, 1968.

U.S. Army Military Police School, Lie Detector Committee. Committee Report: The effect of hypnotically induced amnesia upon the accuracy of the lie detector test results. Unpublished manuscript. Ft. Gordon, Georgia, December 8, 1960.

U.S. Army Military Police School (USAMPS). Polygraph Examiners Training Course, 1970.

U.S. Congress, House Committee on Government Operations. *Hearings on the use of polygraphs as "lie detectors" by the federal government.* 88th Congress, 2nd session. Washington, D.C.: U.S. Government Printing Office, 1964.

Violante, R., & Ross, S. A. Research in interrogation procedures. Office of Naval Research, Report 707-65, filed with Defense Documentation Center, AD-467624, October, 1964.

Volwassen. Der Lugenentdecker. (The lie detector). *Kriminalistisches Monatsheft,* 1937, **11**, 79–81.

Voronin, L. G., Konovalov, V. F., & Serikov, I. S. K voprosu o vzaimodeistvii osoznannykh i neosoznannyk sledovykh protsessov v nernoi sisteme. (Interaction of conscious and unconscious trace processes in the nervous system.) *Doklady Akademii Nauk SSSR,* 1970, **195**, 1237–1239.

Weinstein, E., Abrams, S., & Gibbons, D. The validity of the polygraph with hypnotically induced repression and guilt. *American Journal of Psychiatry,* 1970, **126**, 1159–1162.

Yankee, F. An investigation of sphygmomanometer discomfort thresholds in polygraph examinations. *Police,* 1965, **9**(6), 12–18.

Yanovski, A. G. Feasibility of alteration of cardiovascular manifestations in hypnosis. *American Journal of Clinical Hypnosis,* 1962, **5**, 8–16.

Zimmerman, H. Was ist der Polygraph? *Kriminalistik,* Issue of November-December 1958, January 1959.

Author Index

Numbers in italics refer to the pages on which the complete references are listed.

A

Abbey, D. S., 387, *414*
Abrams, S., 464, *477*
Acker, C. W., 285, 286, *341*
Acker, M., 328, *343*
Ackerman, P. T., 148, *152*, 320, *338*
Adams, T., 40, *109*
Agras, W. S., 352, 354, 361, 366, 367, *373, 374, 375*
Aiba, H., 387, *415*
Alexander, A., 297, *341*
Alexander, L., 296, 298, *337*
Alfert, E., 397, *413*
Allen, C. K., 142, *150*, 193, *202*, 210, *245, 254*
Allport, G., 389, *413*
Alpert, M., 419, *471*
Andreassi, J. L., 145, *151*
Andrew, W., 50, *109*
Angersbach, P., 27, *115*
Apple, H. P. 58, *121*
Arons, H., 464, 465, *471*
Arther, R. O., 419, 421, 422, 428, 429, 431, 438, 448, 457, 460, 463, 468, *471, 476*
Asch, S., 405, *413*
Ashby, W. R., 297, 298, *338*
Astrup, C., 220, *246*, 289, 291, *338*
Aubry, A., 428, *471*
Ax, A. F., 6, 8, *109*, 175, *197*, 286, 289, 292, *338*
Ayer, W. A., 364, 365, *373*

B

Back, K. W., 49, 54, *109, 110*
Backster, C., 425, *471*
Badia, P., 142, *151*, 167, 192, *196*, 221, *246, 276, 280*
Baer, P. E., 190, 193, *196*, 235, 237, 238, *248*, 289, 293, 294, 316, *338, 341*, 411, *413*

Bagg, C. E., 298, *338*
Bagshaw, M. H., 33, 35, *110, 115*
Bahm, R., 187, *197*, 238, *247*
Baird, J. D., 24, *115*
Baitsch, H., 50, *110*
Bakan, P., 60, *110*, 129, 145, 149, *153*
Baker, T. W., 205, 208, *246*
Bales, R. F., 406, *413*
Ball, T. S., 142, *152*
Bamford, J. L., 8, *109*, 286, 289, 292, *338*
Barber, T. X., 355, 358, *372*, 460, 465, *471*
Barber, W. E., 429, *471*
Barland, G. H., 421, 427, 431, 435, 436, 443, 445, 447, 449, 450, 452, *471*
Barlow, D. H., 352, 354, 361, 366, 367, *373, 374*
Barnett, C. C., 419, *472*
Bass, M. J., 190, *196*
Bassett, M., 297, 298, *338*
Baumeister, A. A., 244, *246*
Baxter, R., 224, *246*, 266, 267, 268, 269, *281*
Beattie, R. J., 452, 460, *471*
Beck, A., 295, *338*
Becker, W. C., 242, 243, *246*, 326, 327, *338*
Beckett, P. G., 286, 289, *338*
Beebe, D., 459, *471*
Beedle, R., 244, *246*, 315, 316, *338*
Beer, G., 26, *113*
Bell, B., 18, 51, *110*
Belloni, M. L., 129, 148, 149, 150, *151*
Belyakova, L. I., 289, 292, *339*
Ben-Ishai, A., 445, 449, 450, *474*
Benjamin, L. S., 99, *110*
Bennett, J. V., 428, 452, *472*
Ben-Shakhar, G., 442, 447, 453, *472, 475*
Benussi, V., 419, *472*
Benzies, S., 33, *110*
Berger, S. M., 391, 392, 393, *413*
Bergeron, J., 134, *151*

479

Berkson, G., 302, 306, 307, 308, 309, 310, 313, 314, *338*
Berlyn, D. E., 141, 142, 147, *151*
Berman, D. L., 208, *253*
Berman, M. A., 468, *472*
Bernal, M. E., 286, 288, 289, *338*
Bernard, C., 257, *280*
Bernstein, A. S., 144, *151*, 285, 286, 288, 289, 291, 292, *338*, 408, *413*
Berrien, F. K., 419, *472*
Berry, R. N., 146, *151*
Bersh, P. J., 435, 439, 440, 449, 452, *472*
Bettley, F. R., 20, *114*
Bever, J., 127, 128, 132, 133, 134, 138, 140, 141, *154*, 166, 192, *201*
Binnie, C. D., *109*
Birch, H. G., 245, *246*
Birk, L., 263, 277, *280*
Birren, J. E., 49, *123*
Bitterman, M. E., 162, 183, 194, *196*, *200*, 242, *246*, 323, 324, 326, 327, *338*, 428, 429, 463, *472*, *475*
Bjorkstrand, P., 182, 193, *200*
Black, A. H., 277, *280*
Blake, M. J. F., 60, *110*
Blank, I. H., 83, *110*
Blanton, D. E., 12, 52, *115*
Blanton, R. L., 4, 10, 13, *119*, 126, 154, 187, *199*, 215, *250*
Bligh, J., 19, 28, 46, *110*
Bloch, V., 3, 29, 31, 32, 33, 34, 35, *110*
Block, J. D., 230, *246*, 447, 462, *472*
Bloom, S. W., 378, 406, *414*
Blumenthal, A., 322, *345*
Bogdonoff, M. D., 49, 54, *109*, *110*
Boles, J., 265, *282*
Bolles, M., 134, 139, 141, *152*
Bondarenko, T. T., 289, 292, *339*
Bonvallet, M., 29, 31, 32, 33, 34, 35, *110*
Booth, J. H., 208, *246*
Boring, F. W., 193, *196*, 244, *251*
Borkenstein, R. F., 452, 455, 460, *472*
Borkovec, T. D., 300, *338*
Born, D. G., 210, 231, *254*
Borsa, D. M., 147, *151*
Botwinick, J., 50, *110*, 244, *246*
Bousfield, W. A., 218, *246*

Bovard, E., 400, *413*
Bower, A., 304, 306, 309, 312, 313, 314, *338*, *339*
Boyd, R. W., 377, *413*, *414*
Boydstun, J. A., 320, *338*
Brackbill, G., 328, *343*
Brady, J. V., 49, *117*, 404, *413*
Brener, J., 468, *472*
Bridger, W. H., 181, *196*, 220, 229, 231, 233, 238, *246*, *251*, 316, *339*, 411, *413*
Britain, S., 140, *153*
Brivllova, S. V., 316, 321, *339*
Brokow, J. R., 455, *473*
Brooke, G., 95, *110*
Brotsky, S. J., 216, *246*
Broverman, D. M., 51, *110*
Brown, C. C., 5, 49, *110*, 330, 331, *342*
Brown, C. H., 146, *151*
Brown, J. S., 222, *246*
Brown, L. B., 387, *413*
Brown, M. L., 69, 70, *118*
Brown, V. W., 31, *123*
Brožek, J., 59, *110*
Brusilow, S. W., 42, 45, *119*, *121*
Buchsbaum, M., 60, *110*
Buchwald, A. M., 133, *151*
Bullough, W. S., 17, *111*
Burch, N., 325, *344*
Burch, N. R., 38, 42, 65, 77, 80, *112*, *113*, 133, 136, *151*, *154*, 325, *344*, 360, 373, 406, *414*
Burdick, J. A., 286, *339*
Burke, C. J., 419, 421, 447, 452, *473*
Burstein, K. R., 134, *151*, 169, 187, 191, *196*, *197*
Burtt, H. E., 419, *472*
Bush, I. E., 25, *111*
Byrne, D., 387, *414*

C

Cadoret, R. J., 387, *414*
Campbell, A. A., 238, *249*
Campbell, D. T., 389, *415*
Campbell, R. K., 230, *249*
Campos, J. J., 8, *111*, *115*, 130, 144, *153*
Cannon, W. B., 15, *111*
Caputo, R. R., 428, *471*

Carberry, W. J., 73, *122*
Carey, C. A., 169, *196*
Carleton, H. M., 14, *111*
Carlin, T., 268, 269, 279, *281*
Carmichael, E. A., 85, *111*
Carpenter, J. A., 323, *343*
Castillo, D. D., 232, *250*
Cautela, J. R., 184, *196*
Chalmers, T. M., 20, 23, *111*
Chambers, R. M., 194, *196*
Champion, R. A., 184, 185, 187, 188, 189, *196*
Chandler, P. J., 62, *119*, 291, 316, *343*
Chatterjee, B. B., 230, 232, 235, 236, *246*
Chave, E. J., 386, *416*
Childers, H. E., 133, *154*, 325, *344*
Christie, M. J., 12, 18, 26, 27, 47, 48, 52, 53, 59, 60, 61, 62, 94, *110, 111*
Church, R. M., 268, 270, 272, 273, *280*, 399, *413*
Clarke, S., 193, *197*
Clausen, J., 302, 303, 304, 305, 306, 307, 308, 309, 310, 311, 312, 313, 314, *339, 342*
Clayton, R., 53, *115*
Cleghorn, R., 331, *343*
Clements, S. D., 320, *338*
Clum, G. A., 327, 328, 329, 330, *339*
Cobb, H. V., 245, *251*, 307, 308, 309, 311, 312, *344*
Cochran, S. W., 176, *202*
Cofer, C. N., 214, 218, *247*
Coffman, M., 264, *280*
Cohen, N. I., 319, *339*
Cohen, S. I., 50, 51, 52, *121*, 136, *154*, 244, *253*, 360, *375*
Coles, E. M., 3, 39, 40, 67, 72, 86, 87, *118*
Coles, M. G. H., 336, 337, *339*
Collins, K. J., 23, 24, 25, 26, 62, *111*
Collman, R., 302, 303, 304, 308, 309, *339*
Colquhoun, W. P., 59, *111*
Conklin, J. E., 34, *111*
Conn, J. W., 27, *111*
Conroy, R., 58, 59, *111*
Cook, S. W., 229, 232, *247*, 411, *413*
Cooke, R. E., 42, 45, *121*
Cooper, J. B. 383, 387, 388, *413*

Coppock, H. W., 194, *196*
Coquelet, M-L., 60, *112*
Corah, N. L., 54, 55, *115*, 142, *151*, 288, *339*, 408, *414*, 454, *474*
Corman, C. D., 129, 142, *151*
Costell, R. M., 405, *414*
Costello, C. G., 295, *345*, 348, *373*
Cowan, C. O., 243, *247*
Craig, K. D., 355, 356, *373*, 396, *414*
Crane, J. B., 453, *473*
Craw, M. A., 141, 147, *151*
Crider, A. B., 149, *151*, 260, 261, 263, 264, 265, 272, 277, *280*, 282, 378, 400, 409, 410, 412, *414, 416*
Crockford, G. W., 26, *111*
Crössman, H. C., 27, *115*
Cronbach, L. J., 237, *247*
Crookes, T. G., 298, *338*
Crooks, R., 286, *339*
Crosland, H. R., 419, *472*
Crosskey, M. A., 320, *340*
Crounse, R. G., 18, *111*
Crowne, D. P., 240, *247*
Crusius, P., 27, *115*
Cullen, D. R., 24, *115*
Cullen, T. D., 52, 53, 56, 62, *123, 124*
Culp, W. C., 62, *111*
Cumley, W. E., 463, *472*
Curtis, G., 295, 297, 323, 324, 328, *346*

D

Dadas, H., 302, 303, 309, 310, 311, 312, *341*
Dalton, K., 52, *111*
Damaser, E., 465, *472*
Dameron, L. E., 162, 163, 178, 179, *198*, 221, 224, *249*, 309, 310, 311, 313, 315, 316, *341*
Dana, H. J., 419, *472*
Dardano, J. E., 145, *151, 154*
Darrow, C. W., 10, 11, 12, 19, 24, 29, 34, 35, 95, *112*, 134, *155*
Das, J., 304, 305, 306, 309, 312, 313, 314, *338, 339*
Dashiell, J., 398, *414*
Davenport, G., 329, *341*
Davidoff, R. A., 318, *339*
Davidson, P. O., 242, 243, *247*, 360, 361, 365, *373*, 442, 443, 444, 447, 448, *472*

Davis, J., 331, *343*
Davis, R. C., 133, *151*, 419, 421, 445, 446, 447, 452, 470, *472*, *473*
Dawson, M. E., 164, *196*, 229, 235, 236, 237, 239, 240, *247*, 316, 319, *339*, *344*
Day, J. L., 10, 84, *112*, *120*
Dean, S. J., 193, *197*, 239, 242, *251*, 253, 265, 268, 282, 327, *345*
Dearman, H. B., 452, *472*
DeFleur, M. L., 390, *416*
Defran, R. H., 142, 151, 167, *196*, 221, *246*, 276, *280*
Degrak, H., 467, 469, 470, *473*
Demb, H., 245, *246*
Dengerink, H. A., 164, *197*
DeNike, L. D., 237, *253*
Denton, D. A., 25, *112*
de Traverse, P. M., 60, *112*
DeVore, I., 398, *414*
Dewey, R., 389, *414*
DeWicke, H. M., 10, *116*
Dickson, H. W., 386, *414*
DiMascio, A., 377, *413*, *414*
Dionis, J., 265, *282*
Dittmer, D. G., 190, *197*
Diven, K., 187, *197*, 234, *247*
Dmitriev, L. I., 289, 292, *339*
Dobson, R. L., 21, *120*
Doctor, R. F., 61, *112*, 148, *151*
Doerr, H. O., 62, *123*
Domanski, R., 302, 303, 309, 310, 311, 312, *341*
Doob, A. N., 169, *197*
Doss, R., 318, *344*
Douglas, V. I., 319, *339*
Duffy, E., 126, 127, 132, *151*, 354, *373*
Dufort, R. H., 223, *247*
Dureman, I., 297, 298, 329, 330, *340*
Dykman, R. A., 8, 12, 50, 52, 55, *115*, 148, *152*

E

Ebel, H. C., 160, 161, 163, 164, 165, 166, 169, 172, 174, 180, 186, 188, *201*, 221, 227, *252*
Edelberg, R., 2, 3, 9, 12, 25, 29, 34, 37, 38, 41, 42, 43, 44, 45, 46, 47, 58, 62, 64, 65, 66, 67, 68, 70, 71, 72, 73, 75, 77, 79, 80, 81, 82, 84, 85, 87, 89, 92, 95, 100, *111*, *112*, *113*, *117*, *118*, 128, 134, 135, 139, *152*, 169, *197*, 292, 325, 335, *340*, 406, *414*
Edelman, R. I., 265, *280*, 364, *373*
Edison, A. E. W., 23, 24, *113*
Edwards, J. E., 364, *374*
Efran, J. S., 352, 366, 367, 368, 369, *373*, *374*
Egger, M. D., 211, *247*
Ekman, P., 419, *473*
Eliott, T. R., 24, *113*
Elithorn, A., 320, *340*
Elliott, R., 399, *414*
Ellis, J. P., Jr., 62, *114*
Ellis, N., 302, 303, 309, 316, *340*, *344*
Ellis, R. A., 14, *118*
Ellis, R. M., Jr., 287, *346*
Ellson, D. G., 419, 421, 447, 452, *473*
Ellstrom, P., 182, 193, *200*
Elster, M., 27, *115*
Engel, R., 60, *121*
Enke, C. G., *109*
Epstein, S., 134, *151*, 187, 191, 193, *196*, *197*, 238, *247*, 316, 322, 323, 324, 325, 326, 333, *340*, 410, *414*
Eriksen, C. W., 230, 232, 235, 236, 237, *246*, *247*
Estes, W. K., 186, *197*
Evans, F. J., 8, *119*
Ewart, R. L., 24, *115*
Eysenck, H. J., 58, *113*, 240, 242, 243, *247*, 333, *340*

F

Farber, I. E., 222, *246*
Fascio, J. C., 24, *113*
Fawcett, J. T., 166, 168, 176, 177, *201*
Fay, P. J., 419, *473*
Feather, B. W., 216, 218, *247*, 356, 363, *375*
Feeney, D., 216, 229, *251*
Fein, A., 310, 311, *342*
Fenz, W. D., 134, *151*, 193, *197*, 286, 287, 288, 289, 302, 303, 307, 309, 310, 313, 314, 323, 324, 325, 326, *340*, 410, *414*
Féré, C., 4, 11, *113*, 126, 132, *152*

Fergusen, R. J., 440, *473*
Finesinger, J. E., 83, *110*
Fisher, B. E., 140, *152*
Fisher, G. L., 140, *152*
Fjeld, S. P., 185, *202*
Flaherty, B., 59, *113*
Flanagan, J., 133, *152*, 354, *373*
Flood, J., 362, *376*
Floyd, W. F., 85, *113*
Foley, J. P., 214, 218, *247*
Folkins, C. H., 352, 363, 364, *373*
Forbes, T. W., 134, 139, 141, *152*
Foster, K. G., 20, 23, 24, *113*
Fowler, R. L., 258, 259, 260, 263, *280*
Fowles, D. C., 3, 12, 13, 21, 24, 25, 26, 42, 44, 45, 46, 58, 84, *113*
Fox, R. H., 60, *113*, 299, *340*
Frankenhaeuser, M., 62, *115*
Franklin, J. R., 62, *123*
Frankmann, R. W., 133, *151*
Franks, C. M., 243, *247*, 331, *341*
Fredman, S., 162, 164, 172, *201*, 221, 253
Freeman, G. L., 126, 127, 132, 134, *152*
French, J. W., 11, *113*
Fretz, N. F., 286, 289, *338*
Frick, A., 44, *121*
Friedhoff, A. J., 419, *471*
Friedman, L. F., 61, *112*, 148, *151*
Friesen, W. V., 419, *473*
Frömter, E., 44, *121*
Fuhrer, M. J., 190, 193, *196*, 235, 237, 238, *248*, 289, 293, 294, 316, *338*, *341*, 411, *413*
Fujimori, B., 31, 32, 33, 38, 87, *124*, 134, 139, *155*
Fulton, J. F., 34, 36, *113*
Furedy, J. F., 100, *113*
Furedy, J. J., 169, 171, 180, 193, *197*, *199*, *201*, 276, *281*, 316, *341*
Furman, K. I., 26, *113*

G

Gabriel, M., 142, *152*
Galbrecht, C. R., 148, *152*
Gale, A., 336, 337, *339*
Gale, E. N., 175, *197*, 362, 363, 364, 365, *373*, *374*

Galkowski, T., 302, 303, 309, 310, 311, 312, *341*
Gantt, W. H., 318, *344*
Garcia, J., 186, 187, *197*
Gates, A. I., 59, *113*
Gavalas, R. J., 264, *280*
Gawienowski, A. M., 61, *118*
Geer, J. H., 187, *199*, 218, *250*, 353, 354, 357, *373*
Gelder, M. G., 350, 359, *374*
Gellhorn, E., 50, *114*
Gelman, R. S., 147, *151*, 209, *254*
Gerard, H. B., 406, *414*
Germana, J., 144, 146, *152*
Germann, A. C., 463, *473*
Gibbons, D., 464, *477*
Gilberstadt, H., 329, *341*
Ginsburg, J., 23, 24, *113*
Golden, R. I., 427, 433, 434, 458, 462, *473*
Goldstein, I. B., 286, 299, 300, 330, 331, *341*
Goldstein, M., 285, 286, 289, 291, *341*
Goldstein, R., 318, *341*
Golightly, C., 387, *414*
Golin, S., 235, 236, 237, *248*
Goodall, McC., 20, 24, 46, *114*
Goodman, A., 331, *343*
Goodwin, D. W., 453, *473*
Gormezano, I., 176, 181, 184, 186, *197*, 239, *248*, 267, 268, *282*
Gottlieb, J. S., 286, 289, *338*
Gould, J., 148, 150, *152*
Graham, B., 331, *343*
Graham, D. T., 465, *476*
Graham, F. K., 131, 137, *152*, 465, *476*
Graham, J., 305, *341*
Grant, D. A., 179, 184, 190, 191, *197*, *198*, 232, 238, 239, *248*, 249, 251, 336, *341*
Gray, J. A., 336, *341*
Green, A., 230, *250*
Green, J. H., 14, 52, *114*
Green, K. F., 186, 187, *197*
Greenblatt, M., 377, *414*
Greene, W. A., 264, 279, *280*
Greenfield, N., 297, *341*
Greenwald, D. U., 380, *414*
Greenway, R. M., 58, *121*

Greiner, T. H., 38, 42, 65, 80, *113*, 136, *151*, 360, *373*

Greisemer, R. D., 18, *114*

Grice, K. A., 20, *114*

Grim, P. F., 142, *152*

Grings, W. W., 3, 21, 66, 72, 77, *114*, 134, 137, 143, *152*, *153*, *155*, 162, 163, 164, 167, 169, 178, 179, 182, 185, 187, 189, 190, 192, 193, *196*, *198*, *199*, 200, 202, 206, 207, 212, 213, 221, 222, 224, 225, 227, 228, 229, 230, 232, 235, 236, 244, *247*, *248*, *249*, *251*, 268, 269, 279, *281*, 294, 309, 310, 311, 313, 315, 316, *341*, *343*, 360, 361, 371, *373*

Grinspoon, L., 289, *346*

Grob, B., *109*

Gross, K., 337, *341*

Grossberg, J. M., 356, 357, 358, 364, 365, *373*

Groves, P. M., 129, *153*

Gullickson, G. R., 10, 12, *112*

Gustafson, L. A., 441, 442, 443, 446, 455, 461, 469, *473*

Guthrie, E. R., 349, *373*

Guyton, A. C., 468, *473*

Guze, S. B., 162, 201, 221, *253*, 298, 331, 332, *345*, 453, *473*

H

Hackman, R., 145, *154*

Haesly, R. R., 244, *251*

Hagfors, C., 70, 71, 92, 105, 106, *114*

Haggard, E. A., 234, 235, *249*

Hahn, K. W., 358, *372*

Hahn, K. W., Jr., 355, *372*

Haigh, A. L., 52, *114*

Hake, H. W., 184, *198*

Halberg, F., 59, *114*

Hale, H. B., 62, *114*

Hall, J. F., 166, 168, 176, 177, 191, *198*, *201*

Hamacher, J. H., 147, *151*

Hamburg, D., 53, *114*, *115*

Hamel, I. A., 238, *249*

Hamilton, C. L., 234, 235, *254*

Hammond, L. J., 208, *246*

Harding, G., 145, *153*

Hare, R. D., 140, *153*, 245, *249*, 299, 300, 335, *341*, *342*

Harker, J. E., 59, *114*

Harley, J. P., 192, *196*

Harrelson, L. H., 425, 428, 429, 430, *473*

Harris, E. K., 60, *110*

Harris, R. E., 229, 232, *247*, 411, *413*

Harrison, J., 24, 28, 53, *114*, *117*

Hart, J., 356, *374*

Hartman, T. F., 179, *198*, 214, 232, *249*

Harvey, B., 240, *249*

Harvey, J. A., 467, *473*

Hebb, D. O., 126, 127, 136, *153*

Heckel, R. V., 455, *473*

Hegel, U., 44, *121*

Hein, P. L., 356, 363, *375*

Heindorf, M., 27, *115*

Hellman, K., 14, 19, 21, 23, 24, *123*

Helmer, J. E., 276, *281*

Hemingway, A., 38, 71, *118*

Hemphill, R. E., 11, *114*

Herman, L., 13, *114*

Hermelin, B., 302, 307, 309, 310, 313, 314, *338*

Herrman, F., 22, *122*

Herrnstein, R. J., 348, *373*

Hershiser, D., 294, *344*

Hertzman, A. B., 58, *120*

Hicks, R. G., 49, *114*, 324, *343*

Hiebert, S. F., 360, 361, 365, *373*

Highleyman, S. L., 458, *473*

Hilgard, E. R., 176, *198*, 230, 238, 239, *249*

Hill, F. A., 142, *150*, 187, 193, *202*, 210, 239, 240, 245, *249*, 254, 258, 260, 264, *281*

Hill, G. B., 95, *110*

Hnatiow, M., 187, *199*, 218, *250*

Holloway, F. A., 62, *114*, 317, *342*

Holmes, W. D., 435, *473*

Holtzman, W. H., 242, *246*, 323, 324, 326, 327, *338*

Holzgreve, H., 44, *121*

Homskaya, E. D., 35, *116*

Homzie, M., 185, *202*

Honeyman, W. H., 85, *111*

Hord, D. J., *114*

Hornung, F., 162, *201*, 221, *253*, 298, 331, 332, *345*

Horvath, F. S., 419, 426, 427, 435, 436, 437, 443, *474*
Houck, R. L., 141, *153*, 336, 337, *344*
Hovland, C. I., 191, *198*
Howe, E. S., 286, 287, 289, 330, 332, *342*
Hozawa, S., 37, 76, *115*
Huang, C., 268, 269, *282*
Hughes, K. R., 387, *414*
Hughes, W. G., 239, 240, *249*
Hull, C. L., 176, 186, 188, 190, 193, *196, 198, 199*, 206, 207, 208, *249*
Humber, W. J., 389, *414*
Hummel, W. F., Jr., 265, *282*
Humphreys, L. G., 181, *199*, 239, *249*
Hunter, F. L., 435, 436, *474*
Huntington, G. H., 419, *472*
Hyman, E. T., 362, 363, 364, 365, *373, 374*

I

Inbau, F. E., 420, 421, 425, 427, 428, 429, 431, 432, 438, 445, 447, 448, 450, 452, 455, 456, 458, 463, 465, 466, 467, 469, *474, 476*
Irvine, W. J., 24, *115*
Isamat, F., 34, *115*

J

Jackson, J. C., 131, *152*
Jacobson, E., 213, *249*, 349, 358, 370, *374*
Jasper, H., 127, *154*
Jenson, W. R., 160, 165, 169, 171, 172, 175, 180, *199, 201*
Johansson, G., 62, *115*
Johnson, H. F., 265, *282*
Johnson, H. J., 8, *111, 115*, 130, 144, *153*, 265, *281, 282*
Johnson, L. C., 8, 10, 13, 54, 55, 99, *114, 115*, 136, 148, *153*, 164, *200*, 408, *414*, 454, *474*
Johnson, R. E., 24, *113*
Jones, J. E., 176, 184, *196, 199*
Jones, M. C., 347, *374*
Jongsma, A., 245, *249*
Joseph, L. J., 193, *200*

Judd, L., 289, 291, *341*
Jung, C. G., 284, *343*
Juniper, K., 8, 12, 50, 52, 55, *115*

K

Kagan, J., 130, 148, *153*
Kalish, H. I., 222, *246*
Kamin, L. J., 222, *249*
Kaplan, B. E., 8, *115*, 216, *251*
Kaplan, H. B., 378, 406, *414*
Kaplan, M., 445, 449, 450, *474*
Kaplan, S., 147, *153*
Karrer, R., 302, 303, 304, 305, 306, 307, 308, 309, 310, 311, 312, 313, 314, *339, 342*
Katkin, E. S., 277, *281*, 323, 324, 326, *342*, 350, 359, 360, 370, 372, *374, 375*
Katz, D., 297, 303, *341, 342*
Katz, H., 387, *414*
Katzoff, E. T., 134, *152*
Keele, C. A., 20, 23, 24, 85, *111, 113, 115*
Keeler, L, 420, *474*
Keller, R., 22, *122*
Keller, W. H., 216, *246*
Kelly, D., 330, 331, *342*
Keough, T. E., 177, 178, *200*, 244, *251*
Kienstra, R. A., 128, 141, *155*
Kierland, R. R., 49, *122*
Kimble, D. P., 33, 35, *110, 115*, 279, *281*
Kimble, G. A., 167, *199*, 223, 225, 226, 239, *247, 249, 251*
Kimmel, E., 189, *199*, 260, 261, 263, 265, 266, 273, 275, 276, *281*
Kimmel, H. D., 142, *153*, 160, 162, 164, 172, 174, 179, 188, 192, *199*, 212, 221, 223, 224, 227, 230, *248, 249, 250, 253*, 258, 259, 260, 261, 262, 263, 264, 265, 266, 267, 268, 269, 272, 273, 274, 275, 276, 277, 279, *280, 281, 282*
Kinder, E. F., 284, *345*
King, P. H., 58, *121*
Kintsch, W., 146, *153*
Kirk, W. E., 141, *153*
Kissel, S., 399, 400, *415*
Kitchin, A. H., 52, *114*

Klaiber, E. L., 51, *110*
Kleinman, K. M., 69, 70, *118*
Kleinsmith, L. J., 147, *153*
Kleist, K. C., 193, *199*
Kleitman, N., 59, 60, *115*
Kligman, A. M., 18, 49, *115, 122*
Kline, P., 336, 337, *339*
Klump, C. S., 469, *474*
Kobayashi, Y., 51, *110*
Koch, E., 27, *115*
Kodama, M., 407, 408, 409, *415*
Kodman, F., 310, 311, *342*
Koenig, I. D. V., 147, *151*
Koenig, K. P., 232, *250*
Koepke, J. E., 133, 136, 141, 149, *153,* 323, 324, 326, *342*
Koff, E., 292, *345*
Kolb, L. C., 85, *111*
Kondo, M., 87, *124,* 134, 139, *155*
Konorski, J., 255, 256, 257, 276, 277, 278, *281, 282*
Konovalov, V. F., 421, 443, 455, *477*
Kopacz, F. M., 8, 51, *115*
Kopell, B., 53, *115*
Koresko, R. L., 363, 365, *375*
Kornetsky, C., 50, *110,* 244, *246*
Korol, B., 69, 70, *118*
Korr, I. M., 39, 40, *122*
Kotses, H., 127, 128, 132, 133, 134, 138, 140, 141, *154,* 166, 192, *201*
Kramer, L. L., 175, *200*
Krauskopf, J., 162, 183, 194, *196, 200*
Krebs, D. L., 378, 391, 412, *415*
Krupski, A., 129, 145, 149, *153*
Kryspin, J., 66, *115*
Kubis, J. F., 242, 253, 329, *345,* 420, 421, 435, 439, 440, 447, 451, 452, 458, 459, 461, 462, 466, *472, 474*
Kuechenmeister, C. A., 72, *115*
Kugelmass, S., 54, *116,* 408, *415,* 421, 442, 443, 445, 447, 448, 449, 450, 453, 454, 456, *472, 474, 475*
Kumpfer, K. L., 160, 161, 165, 169, 171, 172, 175, *199, 201*
Kuno, Y., 14, 16, 18, 20, *116*
Kurtzberg, R. L., 419, *471*

L

LaBrosse, E. H., 61, *118*
Lacey, B. C., 130, 136, 148, 149, *153*

Lacey, J. I., 130, 136, 148, 149, *153,* 213, 230, 234, 235, *250,* 285, *342,* 382, 391, 396, 399, 412, *415*
Lacey, O. L., 126, 127, 132, *151*
Ladell, W. S. S., 26, *116*
Lader, M. H., 20, 41, 46, 93, *116,* 295, 296, 297, 303, 330, 331, 332, 335, *342,* 350, *374*
Ladpli, R., 30, *116*
Lambert, W. W., 62, *115*
Landis, C., 5, 10, *116*
Landon, M. M., 8, 13, 55, *115,* 408, *414*
Lang, A. H., 33, 42, 44, *116*
Lang, P. J., 187, *199,* 218, *250,* 353, 356, 372, *374, 376*
Langdon, B., 216, 217, 229, *250, 251*
La Polla, A., 289, 291, *341*
Larson, J. A., 419, 420, 452, 455, 460, *472, 474*
Lasswell, H. D., 381, *415*
Lawlor, W. G., 285, 286, 288, 289, 290, *346*
Lawson, K. D., 352, 363, 364, *373*
Lazarus, R. S., 54, *116,* 352, 363, 364, *373, 374,* 407, 408, 409, *415*
Leaf, A., 28, *121*
Lee, C. D., 419, 421, 448, *475*
Lee, W. Y., 160, 165, 169, 171, 172, 175, *201*
Lehrer, P. M., 358, *374*
Leiderman, P. H., 97, 99, *121,* 378, 399, 401, 402, 405, *414, 415, 416*
Leitenberg, H., 352, 354, 361, 366, 367, *373, 374, 375*
Leonard, C., 164, *199*
Levi, L., 60, *116*
Levin, G., 401, *415*
Levine, S., 410, *415*
Levis, D. J., 350, *375*
Levy, A. B., 230, *251*
Levy, C. M., 219, *250*
Lewis, J. L., 141, *151*
Lewis, N. L., 240, *253*
Lewis, P., 276, *280*
Lick, J. R., 368, *374*
Lieblich, I., 8, 54, *116,* 408, *415,* 421, 442, 443, 445, 447, 448, 449, 450, 453, 454, 455, *472, 474, 475*

Liederman, P. H., 132, *154*
Lindan, O., 58, *121*
Lindner, R., 299, 300, *343*
Lindsley, D. B., 126, 127, *154*, 419, 445, 475
Link, K. E., 60, *124*
Lippert, W. W., Jr., 299, 300, *340*, *343*
Lippitt, N. W., 84, *112*
Lipton, L., 187, *199*, 215, *250*
Littman, R. A., 191, *199*
Lloyd, D. P. C., 23, 24, 40, 46, 71, *113*, *116*
Lobb, H., 244, *250*, 302, 303, 305, 307, 315, 316, *343*
Lobban, M. C., 60, *116*
Lobitz, W. C., 14, *118*
Lockhart, R. A., 100, *116*, 162, 163, 178, 179, 188, 193, *198*, *199*, *200*, 221, 230, 232, 235, 236, 237, 244, *248*, *249*, *250*, 294, 309, 310, 311, 313, 315, 316, *341*, *343*
Lodwig, A., 148, 150, *152*
Logan, F. A., 188, *200*
Lomont, J. F., 364, *374*
Longenecker, E. D., 183, *200*
Lorincz, A. A., 49, *116*
Lott, A. J., 390, *415*
Lubin, A., 10, 99, *114*, *115*, 136, *153*, 454, *474*
Lucas, M. E., 273, *281*
Luchsinger, B., 13, *114*
Ludwig, H., 318, *341*
Lundberg, A., 21, *116*
Lunde, D., 53, *115*
Lunn, R., 149, *151*
Luria, A. R., 35, *116*, 219, *250*, 320, 321, *343*, 419, 421, 446, *475*
Lushene, R., 333, *344*
Luther, B., 7, 47, 93, 94, *117*, 158, *200*
Lykken, D. T., 3, 7, 12, 37, 38, 40, 47, 66, 67, 69, 72, 77, 81, 82, 88, 93, 94, 97, 98, 101, 102, *117*, 158, 159, *200*, 223, 245, *250*, 289, 291, 292, 299, 300, *343*, 441, 442, 447, 453, 462, *475*
Lynn, R., 127, *154*
Lyon, V. W., 439, 440, *475*
Lyons, J., 208, *253*

M

Maas, J. M., 53, *117*
Magoun, H. W., 29, *119*
Maier, S. F., 272, *281*
Maley, M., 7, 47, 93, 94, *117*, 158, *200*, 289, 291, 292, *343*
Malkinson, F. D., 17, *117*
Malloy, T. E., 187, *200*, 214, *252*
Malmo, R. B., 55, *117*, 126, 127, 132, *154*, 331, *343*, 354, *374*
Malmstadt, H. V., *109*
Maltzman, I., 129, 133, 142, 148, 149, 150, *152*, *154*, 216, 217, 218, 219, 229, *250*, *251*
Mandel, I. J., 181, *196*, 229, 231, 233, 238, *246*, *251*, 411, *413*
Mandell, E. E., 147, *151*
Mandler, G., 323, *343*
Manery, J. F., 18, *117*
Marcia, J. E., 352, 366, 367, 368, *373*, *374*
Marcuse, F. L., 428, 429, 463, *472*, *475*
Margerison, J. H., *109*
Marks, I. M., 350, *374*
Marlowe, D., 240, *247*
Marquis, D. G., 176, *198*, 230, *249*
Marston, W. M., 419, 420, 421, 445, 448, 452, *475*
Martens, R., 399, *415*
Martin, B., *154*, 322, *343*
Martin, I., 2, 3, 6, 12, 20, 41, 43, 47, 59, 74, 75, 76, 77, 78, 81, 83, 107, *117*, *123*, 163, 164, *200*, 230, 242, 243, *251*
Martin, R. B., 193, *197*, 239, 245, *249*, *251*, 265, 268, *282*
Martini, L., 53, *119*
Mason, J. W., 49, *117*
Mathews, A. M., 350, 351, 354, 359, 363, 370, 371, *374*
Matteson, H. H., 242, 243, *246*, 326, 327, *338*
Maulsby, R. L., 34, 85, *117*
May, C. D., 26, *117*
May, J. R., 265, *282*
McAdoo, W., 333, *344*
McAllister, D. E., 230, *251*
McAllister, W. R., 230, *251*

McCabe, M., 302, 303, 307, 309, 310, 313, 314, *340*
McCleary, R. A., 10, *118*
McClure, J., 295, *345*
McCubbin, R. J., 324, 326, *342*, 350, 360, 370, *374*
McCurdy, H. G., 382, *415*
McDonald, D. G., 164, *200*, 284, 318, *339, 345*, 363, 365, *375*
McDonnell, G. J., 323, *343*
McDowell, R. J., 11, *118*
McGinnies, E., 386, 387, *414, 415*
McGowan, B. K., 186, 187, *197*
McGraw, E. R., 69, 70, *118*
MacKinnon, P. C. B., 24, 28, 50, 53, *114, 117*
McLendon, J. F., 38, 71, *118*
MacNitt, R. D., 439, 440, 445, 451, 452, *475*
McNulty, J., 286, *339*
McReynolds, P., 328, *343*
Mead, G. H., 394, *415*
Mednick, M. T., 218, *251*
Mednick, S. A., 289, 292, *343*
Meehl, P. E., 237, *247*
Mefferd, R. B., Jr., 8, 61, 62, *118*, 124, 141, *153*, 336, 337, *344*
Melamed, B. G., 356, *374*
Mercer, E. H., 18, *118*
Meyer, P. M., 175, 176, *202*
Meyers, W. J., 193, *200*
Middleton, W. C., 419, *473*
Miller, F., 307, 308, 309, 311, 312, *344*
Miller, F. D., 245, *251*
Miller, L. H., 50, 52, *121*, 244, *253*, 286, 288, 289, *338*
Miller, N. E., 30, *118*, 211, *247*, 263, 277, *282, 415*
Miller, R. D., 38, 76, 78, 82, 83, 88, 93, 97, 107, *117, 118*
Miller, S., 255, 256, 257, *282*
Mills, J. N., 58, 59, 60, *111, 118*
Milstead, J. R., 265, *282*
Mink, W. D., 218, *251*
Mixson, A., 310, 311, *342*
Moeller, G., 176, *200*
Montagna, W., 14, *118*
Montagu, J. D., 3, 5, 20, 38, 39, 40, 41, 46, 67, 71, 72, 73, 86, 87, *116, 118*

Moore, J. W., 176, 181, 184, 186, *197*, 239, *248*, 267, 268, *282*
Moore, R. C., 352, *375*
Moos, R., 53, *115*
Mordkoff, A. M., 41, 46, *118*
More, H. W., 459, 461, 466, *475*
Morgenson, D. F., 243, *251*
Morningstar, M. E., 399, 401, *416*
Moroney, W. F., 435, *475*
Morris, G. C. R., 60, *119*
Morrow, M C., 175, 177, 178, 193, *196, 200*, 224, 244, *251*
Moruzzi, G., 29, *119*
Moss, H. A., 130, 148, *153*
Motta, M., 53, *119*
Mowrer, O. H., 232, *251*, 256, *282*, 348, *375*
Mulbar, H., 428, *475*
Munger, B. L., 45, *119*
Murphy, P. H., 219, *250*
Murray, E. N., 277, *281*, 372, *374*

N

Naftali, G., *475*
Nakao, H., 50, *114*
Naunton, R. F., 318, *341*
Neefs, J., 24, *123*
Neil, E., 24, *115*
Neumann, E., 4, 10, 13, 62, *119*, 126, *154*
Neva, E., 324, *343*
Nicholls, M. F., 239, *251*
Nield, A. F., 208, *254*
Nielsen, T. C., 264, *280*
Niimi, Y., 12, 59, *119, 121*
Nikolaev, G. V., 289, 292, *339*
Norris, E. B., 239, *251*

O

Obermann, C. E., 419, *475*
Obrist, P. A., 61, *119*
O'Connell, D. N., 8, *119*
O'Connor, N., 302, 303, 307, 308, 309, 310, 311, 312, 313, 314, *338, 343, 346*
O'Connor, W. J., 27, *119*
O'Donnell, D., 212, *248*
Ödegaard, Ö., 284, *343*

Öhman, A., 182, 191, 193, *200*, 227, *251*

Oken, D., 26, *119*

Oliveau, D. C., 352, 366, 367, *374, 375*

Olson, R. K., 218, *251*

Opatowski, A., 445, 449, 450, *474*

Opton, E. M. Jr., 352, 363, 364, *373*, 407, 408, 409, *415*

Orlebeke, J. F., 188, 191, *200, 202*

Orne, M. T., 418, 419, 421, 425, 437, 441, 442, 443, 446, 447, 449, 455, 456, 461, 465, 469, *472, 473, 475, 476*

Osgood, C. E., 218, *251*

Ost, J. W. P., 223, 225, 226, *249*

Overton, D. A., 453, *475*

P

Page, H. A., 351, 369, *375*

Paintal, A. S., 93, *119*, 284, 286, 289, *343*

Papadimitriou, M., 48, *119*

Papez, J. W., 29, *119*

Parsons, O. A., 62, *114, 119*, 291, 316, 317, *342, 343*

Paskewitz, D. A. 418, 419, 425, 437, 447, 449, *475*

Pasquali, E., 82, *119*

Passmore, R. 14, 52, *119*

Patkai, P., 60, *119, 120*

Patton, H. D., 30, *120*

Paul, G. L., 358, 359, 370, 371, *375*

Pavlov, I. P., 127, *154*, 176, 190, *200*, 205, *251*

Payne, R. W., 242, 243, *247*

Peastrel, A. L., 187, *200*, 216, 220, 245, *251*

Peiss, C., 58, *120*

Pendergrass, V. E., 275, 276, *281*

Pennypacker, H. S., 179, *199*, 223, *250*

Perez, R. E., 70, *121*

Perkins, C. C., Jr., 188, *200*

Perksy, H., 60, *124*, 295, 297, 323, 324, 328, *346*

Peters, J. E., 320, *338*

Peterson, F., 284, *343*

Pfaff, R. S., 422, *476*

Pfeiffer, E., 162, *201*, 221, *253*, 298, 331, 332, *345*

Pfister, H. O., 286, *344*

Phillips, L. W., 187, *210*, 216, *251*

Pickford, M. 52, *114*

Piercy, M. F., 320, *340*

Pilgrim, D. L., 245, *251*, 307, 308, 309, 311, 312, *344*

Pisha, B. V., 22, *122*

Pishkin, V., 294, *344*

Piva, F., 53, *119*

Plapp, J. M., 284, 335, *345*

Pokorny, A. D., 61, *118*

Pollard, A. C., 60, *120*

Pollock, D. A., 387, 388, *413*

Ponchi, P. E., 49, *122*

Porges, S. W., 130, *154*

Porier, G. W., 390, *415*

Prescott, J. W., 227, *252*

Pribram, K. H., 33, 35, *110, 115*, 133, 136, 141, 149, *153*, 323, 324, 326, *342*

Proctor, S., 187, *200*, 214, *252*

Prokasy, W. F., 160, 161, 163, 164, 165, 166, 168, 169, 170, 171, 172, 174, 175, 176, 177, 180, 186, 188, 191, 195, *198, 200, 201*, 221, 227, *252*

Pryer, R., 309, *344*

Pugh, L., 288, 289, 291, *344*

Punzo, F., 145, *153*

Purhoit, A. P., 243, *252*

Q

Quatrale, R. P., 24, *120*

Quilter, R. E., 50, *122*, 136, 145, *155*

Quinn, M. J., 299, 300, *342*

R

Rachman, S., 232, *252*

Randall, W. D., 58, *120*

Rankin, R. E., 389, *415*

Rappaport, H., 352, 359, 367, 368, 369, *375*

Raskin, D. C., 127, 128, 129, 132, 133, 134, 138, 140, 141, 142, 143, 145, 148, 149, 150, *152, 153, 154*, 166, 173, 192, *201*, 216, *252*, 324, *344*

Ray, R. S., 279, *281*

Razran, G., 173, 184, 188, *201*, 205, 208, 213, 214, 215, 219, 230, *252*

Reardon, P., 237, 239, 240, *247*

Redgate, E. S., 50, *114*
Redgrove, J. A., 52, *120*
Reed, P., 162, 194, *196*
Reese, W. G., 148, *152*, 318, *344*
Reid, J. E., 419, 421, 422, 425, 427, 428, 429, 430, 431, 432, 435, 436, 438, 443, 445, 447, 448, 450, 452, 455, 457, 458, 463, 465, 466, 467, 469, *471, 474, 476*
Rescorla, R. A., 171, *201*, 212, *252*
Reswick, J. B., 58, *121*
Rice, D. G., 261, 263, 277, *282*
Richter, C. P., 41, *120*
Rick, W., 27, *115*
Rickles, W. H., 10, *120*
Riesen, A. H., *198*
Riess, B. F., 187, *201*, 215, 219, *252*
Riopelle, A. J., 184, *198*
Robson, J. S., 14, 52, *119*
Rodnick, E. H., 162, *201*, 289, 291, *341*
Roessler, R., 133, *154*, 297, 325, *341*, *344*
Romig, C. H. A., 441, *476*
Rose, R., 7, 47, 93, 94, *117*, 158, *200*
Rosenthal, D., 285, 286, 288, 289, 290, *346*
Rosenthal, R., 49, 51, 54, *120*, 386, *416*
Ross, B. M., *198*
Ross, L. E., 222, 238, 241, *252*, 316, *344*
Ross, S. A., 145, *154*, 421, 447, *476*
Rothman, S., 14, 17, 18, 20, *117, 120*
Rouke, F. L., 428, 435, 447, 462, *472*, *476*
Roupenian, A., 322, *340*
Routtenberg, A., 130, 131, *154*
Roveri, R., 82, *119*
Roy, R. R., 48, *119*
Rubin, B. M., 352, 367, 368, *374*
Ruckmick, C. A., 380, *416*
Runquist, W. N., 241, *252*
Rutenfranz, J., 59, *120*
Rutledge, E., 185, *202*

S

Saaren-Seppälä, P., 297, 298, 329, 330, *340*
Sadler, T. G., 8, *118*, 336, 337, *344*
Salapatek, P. H., 141, *151*

Salpeter, M. M., 447, 462, *472*
Saltzman, I. J., 419, 421, 447, 452, *473*
Salzberg, H. C., 455, *473*
Sarason, I., 333, *344*
Sarason, S., 323, *343*
Sargent, J. F., 23, *111*
Sato, A., 31, 32, 33, *124*
Sato, K., 21, *120*
Satterfield, J. H., 319, *344*
Saunders, F. J., 53, *120*
Sayer, E., 47, 75, 80, 82, 86, 107, *123*
Schatkin, S. B., 422, *476*
Schell, A. M., 169, 189, 190, *196, 198*, 207, 224, 225, *248*
Schiefferdecker, P., 19, *120*
Schiffman, K., 171, *197, 201*
Schiller, J. J., 191, *197*
Schipper, L. M., *198*
Schlosberg, H., 127, 131, 132, 133, *154*, 155, *154, 155*, 176, *202*, 255, *282*
Schneider, D. E., 191, *198*
Scholander, T., 56, *120*
Schroder, H. M., 191, *202*
Schulsinger, F., 289, 292, *343*
Schultz, C. A., Jr., 192, *199*
Schultz, D. P., 51, *121*
Schultz, I., 44, *121*
Schwabe, L. W., 142, *155*
Schwartz, G. E., 265, *272, 280, 281*, 282, 378, 399, 412, *416*
Schwartz, I. L., 14, *121*
Schwartz, L., 287, *344*
Scotch, N. A., 410, *415*
Seaman, G. F., 60, *121*
Sears, W. N., 230, 238, *249*
Seiffert, P. D., 175, *200*
Seligman, M. E. P., 272, *281*
Selye, H., 53, *121*
Senednesky, G. E., 208, *253*
Senter, R. J., 265, *282*, 299, 300, *343*
Serikov, I. S. K., 421, 443, 455, *477*
Serser, E. A., 220, *246*
Shackel, B., 82, *121*
Shadman, J., 140, *153*
Shaffer, J., 330, 331, *342*
Shagass, C., 331, *343*
Shapiro, D., 97, 99, *121*, 132, *154*, 260, 261, 263, 264, 265, 277, *280, 282*, 378, 399, 400, 401, 402, 408, 409, 412, *414, 415, 416*

Sharp, G. W. G., 28, *121*
Sharpless, S., 127, *154*
Shaver, B. A., 42, 45, *121*
Shean, F., 265, 268, *282*
Shean, G. D., 232, 235, 236, 238, 239, 240, *249, 252,* 266, *282*
Shephard, R. J., 26, *116*
Sherif, M., 401, *416*
Sherrington, C. S., 348, *375*
Shimizu, K., 12, *121,* 462, *476*
Shmavonian, B. M., 50, 51, 52, *121,* 136, *154,* 244, *253,* 360, *375*
Shmelev, V. N., 207, *248*
Shmueli, J., *475*
Shnidman, S. R., 268, 272, 276, 279, *280, 282*
Shor, R. E., 465, *472*
Short, R. H. D., 14, *111*
Sidowski, J. B., *109*
Siegel, A., 134, *155*
Siegel, H. E., 387, *413*
Silber, D. E., 288, 289, *345*
Silver, A. F., 14, *118*
Silver, A. I., 221, *253,* 273, *281*
Silverman, A. J., 136, *154,* 360, *375*
Silverman, R. E., 231, *253*
Simons, D. G., 70, *121*
Sines, J. O., 193, *201*
Singer, D. N., 387, *413*
Skinner, B. F., 255, 256, 258, 278, *282*
Skou, J. C., 21, *121*
Slegers, J. F. G., 45, *121*
Sloan, W., 302, 303, *340*
Sloane, R. B., 242, 243, *247*
Slubicka, B., 227, *253*
Smith, B. D., 8, 51, *115,* 289, *344*
Smith, B. M., 452, 465, *472, 476*
Smith, C. E., 85, *121,* 383, 384, 385, 389, 405, *416*
Smith, M. J., *109,* 148, 150, *154*
Smith, R. L., 230, 234, 235, *250*
Smith, W. W., 382, *416*
Snide, J. D., 191, *202*
Sokolov, E. N., 127, 128, 129, 133, 148, *154, 155,* 294, 317, 334, *344,* 350, *375*
Sollberger, A., 58, *121*
Solman, A. J., 60, *113*
Solomon, R. L., 272, *281,* 348, *375*

Sommer, R., 11, *121*
Sourek, 3, 29, 30, 33, *121*
Speir, E. H., 24, *120*
Spence, J., 326, *344*
Spence, K. W., 193, *201,* 238, 240, 241, *253,* 326, *344*
Spencer, S. K., 49, *122*
Spencer, W. A., 129, *155*
Spielberger, C. D., 237, *253,* 333, *344*
Spohn, H. E., 289, 291, *344*
Stampfl, T. G., 350, *375*
Stanley, W. C., 127, *154*
Steffy, R. A., 286, 287, *340*
Stein, A. E., 422, *476*
Stein, L., 173, *201*
Stein, M., 234, 235, *254*
Stennett, R. G., 136, *155*
Stepanov, A. I., 321, *344*
Stephens, W. G., 72, *122*
Stern, J. A., 162, 164, 172, 185, *201,* 202, 221, *253,* 284, 287, 288, 292, 293, 295, 298, 331, 332, 335, 337, *339, 341, 344, 345,* 465, *476*
Stern, R. M., 240, *253,* 265, *282*
Sternbach, R. A., 54, *122,* 409, 410, *416, 467, 476*
Sternthal, H. S., 268, 272, *281*
Stevens, D. A., 320, *338*
Stewart, A. G., 24, *115*
Stewart, M. A., 162, 164, 172, *201,* 221, *253,* 298, 331, 332, *345*
Stewart, W. K., 85, *111*
Stotlad, E., 322, *345,* 394, 395, 397, *416*
Stoughton, R. B., 49, *122*
Strahan, R. F., 38, 82, 88, 93, 94, *117*
Strauss, J. S., 49, *122*
Streiner, D. L., 193, *197,* 242, *253,* 327, *345*
Strub, H., 268, *281*
Sukoneck, H. I., 163, 182, *198*
Sullivan, D., 245, *249*
Sullivan, J. J., 194, *201*
Sullivan, S. N., 175, 176, *202,* 209, *254*
Sulzberger, M. B., 22, *122*
Summers, W. G., 420, 430, 439, 440, 447, 451, 452, *476*
Surphlis, W., 292, *345*
Surwillo, W. W., 8, 9, 50, 56, 58, *122,* 136, 145, *155*

Sutker, P. B., 300, *345*
Suzuki, S., 462, *476*
Swank, R. L., 60, *121*
Swenson, R. P., 187, *202*
Switzer, St. C. A., 162, *202*
Syz, H. C., 284, *345*
Szakall, A., 16, *122*

T

Tajimi, T., 12, *121*
Takahashi, T., 87, *124*, 134, 139, *155*
Talland, G. A., 49, *122*
Tarchanoff, J., 11, *122*, 134, *155*
Tarte, R. D., 147, *155*
Taylor, J. A., 286, 289, 329, *345*, 365, *375*
Taylor, J. R., 21, *120*
Taylor, S. P., 164, *197*
Teasdale, J. D., 232, *252*
Terrant, F. R., 273, 274, 275, *281*, *282*
Thackray, R. I., 418, 419, 421, 425, 437, 446, 447, 449, 456, *475*, *476*
Thayer, J., 288, 289, *345*
Thaysen, J. H., 14, 21, 25, *122*
Thetford, P. E., 289, 291, *344*
Thomas, D. R., 208, *253*
Thomas, P. E., 39, 40, *122*
Thompson, R. F., 129, *153*, *155*
Thurstone, L. L., 386, *416*
Thysell, R. V., 268, 269, *282*
Tizzard, B., 306, 313, *345*
Tobach, E., 447, 462, *472*
Tocchio, O. J., 463, 465, *476*
Tolles, W. E., 73, *122*
Tolman, E. C., 230, *253*
Tomita, M., 407, 408, 409, *415*
Tomkiewicz, R. L., 142, *151*
Toren, E. C., *109*
Totel, G. L., 24, *113*
Trapold, M. A., 185, *202*
Tregear, R. T., 14, 37, 38, *122*
Trimble, R. W., 359, *375*
Trolander, H. W., 87, *122*
Trovillo, P. V., 419, 420, 438, *476*
Troyer, W. G., 49, 54, *110*
Tuber, D. S., 208, *254*
Tuovinen, T., 33, *116*
Turner, W. W., 455, 460, *476*
Tursky, B., 8, 54, 62, *119*, *122*, *124*, 260,

261, 263, 264, 277, *280*, *282*, 409, 410, 412, *414*, *416*

U

Ullrich, K. J., 44, *121*
Uno, T., 134, 137, *155*, 187, *202*, 213, 248, 253
Urquhart, D., 244, *246*, 315, 316, *338*
Ustick, M., 41, *118*

V

Valleala, P., 33, *116*
Van Egeren, L. F., 356, 363, *375*
Van Fossan, D. P., 62, *114*
Van Olst, E. H., 188, 191, *200*, *202*
Van Twyver, H. B., 261, 262, 263, 277, *282*
Varkarakis, M., 48, *119*
Varni, J. G., 62, *123*
Vattano, F. J., 176, *202*
Vaughan, J. A., 40, *109*
Velner, J., 286, 288, 289, *340*
Venables, P. H., 2, 3, 6, 7, 12, 13, 18, 20, 21, 23, 24, 25, 26, 27, 41, 43, 44, 45, 47, 48, 52, 53, 56, 58, 59, 60, 61, 62, 64, 67, 69, 74, 75, 76, 77, 78, 80, 81, 82, 83, 84, 86, 93, 94, 98, 101, 107, *109*, *110*, *111*, *113*, *117*, *123*, 159, *200*, 286, 287, 292, 302, 303, *343*, *345*
Vinogradova, O. S., 219, *250*
Violante, R., 421, 447, *476*
Vogel, M. D., 243, *253*
Vogel, W., 51, *110*, 312, *345*
Voronin, L. G., 421, 443, 455, *477*

W

Wagner, H. N., 41, *123*
Walker, L., 147, *155*
Waller, A. D., 59, 60, *123*
Wang, G. H., 3, 29, 30, 31, 34, 36, *116*, *123*, 322, *345*
Warndoff, J. A., 24, *123*
Watanabe, T., 12, *119*, *121*, 408, *416*, 462, *476*
Waters, W. F., 363, 365, *375*
Watts, W., 148, 150, *152*

Weiner, J. S., 14, 19, 21, 23, 24, 26, 62, *111, 113, 123*
Weinstein, E., 464, *477*
Weinstein, M. S., 396, *414*
Welch, L., 242, *253,* 329, *345,* 447, 462, *472*
Welford, A. T., 49, *123*
Wenger, M. A., 52, 56, 62, *123, 124,* 286, *346*
Westie, F. R., 390, *416*
Whatmore, G. B., 287, *346*
White, C. T., 176, *202*
White, S. H., 142, *152*
Whitfield, I. C., *109*
Wickens, D. D., 142, *150,* 175, 176, 187, 191, 193, *202,* 208, 209, 210, 231, 240, *245, 249, 253, 254*
Wieland, B. A., 8, 52, 61, 62, *118, 124*
Wieland, W. F., 234, 235, *254*
Wiggins, S. L., 455, *473*
Wilcott, R. C., 3, 12, 15, 34, 41, *124,* 134, *155*
Wilder, J., 57, *124*
Wilkins, W., 366, *375*
Williams, J. A., 142, *155,* 192, *202*
Williams, M., 286, *346*
Williams, R. J., 61, *118*
Williams, W. C., 160, 165, 169, 171, 172, 174, 175, 182, 183, *201, 202*
Wilson, G. D., 233, *254,* 353, 354, 357, *375*
Wilson, H. K., 356, 357, 364, 365, *373*
Wilson, S. R., 49, *54*
Wincze, J. P., 354, 361, *373*
Wineman, E. W., 52, *124*
Wing, L., 295, 296, 297, 303, 330, 331, 332, 335, *342*
Wing, R., 412, *416*
Winokur, G., 162, 164, 172, *199, 201,* 221, *253,* 298, 331, 332, *345,* 465, *476*
Wishner, J., 216, *251*

Wolf, W., 52, 59, *124*
Wolfensberger, W., 307, 308, 309, 310, 311, 313, *346*
Wolff, H. S., 91, *124*
Wolpe, J., 347, 348, 349, 355, 356, 362, 370, *375, 376*
Wood, K., 140, *153,* 396, *414*
Woodham, F. L., 289, 291, *344*
Woodworth, R. S., 131, 133, *155,* 230, *254*
Worcester, R., *109*
Worrall, N., 187, *202,* 214, *254*
Wortis, J., 220, *246*
Wright, D. E., 352, *375*
Wright, D. J., 29, 41, *112*
Wyatt, R., 8, 62, *124,* 289, *346*
Wynne, L. C., 348, *375*

Y

Yamazaki, K., 12, *119*
Yankee, F., 450, *477*
Yanovski, A. G., 465, *477*
Yarmat, A. J., 50, 51, 52, *121*
Yokota, T., 31, 32, 33, 38, 87, *124,* 134, 139, *155*
Yoshimura, H., 14, 61, *124*

Z

Zahn, T. P., 285, 286, 288, 289, 290, *346*
Zajonc, R. B., 398, *416*
Zeiner, A. R., 185, 190, 193, *202,* 206, 207, 212, *248*
Zenhausern, R. J., 435, *475*
Zimmerman, H., 438, *477*
Zimny, G. H., 128, 141, 142, *155,* 185, *202*
Zuckerman, M., 60, *124,* 295, 297, 323, 324, 328, *346*

Subject Index

A

Activation, 126
Age
  and conditioning, 50
  and peripheral determinants, 50
  and skin potential activity, 50
Anxiety
  and basal levels, 328
  and conditioning, 326-328
    in psychiatric patients, 329
  conservation of, 348
  and habituation, 326
  and nonspecific responses, 323-324,
    328
  in normal subjects, 323-328
  and phasic responses, 133
  in psychiatric patients, 328-330
  and response recovery, 325
  and responsiveness, 324-326
    in psychiatric patients, 328
  and resting levels, 323-324
Anxiety states
  and basal levels, 330-331
  and conditioning, 332
  and habituation, 332
  and nonspecific responses, 331
  and responsiveness, 331
Arousal
  and anxiety, 323-324, 328
  and anxiety states, 330-331
  and autonomic lability, 149
  and brain damage, 316-317
  dual process theory of, 131
  and group interaction, 398-405
  history, 126
  in hyperactive children, 319-320
  and introversion-extroversion,
    333-334
  inverted U function, 127
  and memory, 147-148
  in mental retardation, 302-304
  multiprocess theory of, 130
  and neuroticism, 336-337

nonspecific responses in, 136-137
in psychopaths, 299-300
and relaxation, 358-360
and reticular formation, 127
and schizophrenia, 285-288
and skin conductance level, 131-132
and skin potential level, 132
theory of, 126-127
tonic levels of, 131
Attention
  individual differences in, 149-150
  and phasic responses, 133-134
  to phobic objects, 354
Attitude(s)
  and physiological mediation
    hypothesis, 387
  and skin resistance response, 383-390

B

Brain damage
  and conditioning, 318
  and habituation, 317-321
  and nonspecific responses, 321
  and orienting response, 316-321
  and resting levels, 316-317

C

Central nervous system
  central, 28-36
  cortex, 34-36
  hypothalamus, 34
  limbic system, 33-34
  reticular activating system, 31-33
  spinal level, 30
  ventromedial, bulbar, reticular forma-
    tion, 30-31
Circuits
  ac vs. dc, 71-72
  constant current and, 67
  constant voltage and, 67, 70-71

grounding in, 83
group recording, 92
half-time measures in, 95
SCL suppression in, 69–71
skin conductance and, 101
Classical conditioning, *see* Conditioning
Conditioned stimulus, 186–189
  compounds, 204–213
  intensity of, 188–189
  intensity dynamism, 188
  interoceptive, 187, 213
  modality and, 186–187
  quality of, 186–187
  response–contingent termination of, 269
  verbal, 215
Conditioning
  acquisition of, 174–176, 228–230, 233–238
  and anxiety, 326–328
  and anxiety states, 332
  avoidance, 266–275
  backward, 184–186, 212
  and brain damage, 318, 320
  classical, 157–200
  compound signal, 204–213
  delay in, 189, 224
  in depressives, 298–299
  differential, 175
  effects of age on, 50
  instrumental, 255–282
  in mental retardates, 314–316
  with novel stimuli, 142–143
  punishment in, 265–266
  reward in, 258–265, 275–276
  in schizophrenics, 293–295
  semantic, 213–221
  sensory hypothesis, 210
  simple, 174
  simultaneous, 217
  sufficient circumstances for, 195
  trace, 189–190, 224
  vicarious, 392–394
Conductance, skin
  amplitude, 92, 160-161
  electrode attachment in, 81
  expected values in, 8
  interference in, 88
  magnitude of, 16υ-161
  model for, 41–47

movement artifacts in, 88
range-corrected, 93, 159
recording of, 87
suppressing level of, 69
Configuration, 206, 207, 211
Contingency, CS-UCS, 170–172, 194
Controls
  in backward conditioning, 185
  of biological rhythms, 59
  of body temperature, 59–60
  of changes in climate, 61
  in classical conditioning, 166–172
  costs of, 57–58
  in differential conditioning, 169
  of diurnal variation, 59
  environmental, 55–63
  in instrumental conditioning, 261–263
  length of recording period, 58
  for nonassociative effects, 166–172
  in pseudoconditioning, 167–169, 216
  questionnaires, 237
  random, 171
  sensitization, 216
  sequential, 168
  and subject variables, 48–63
  time-sampling, 169
  yoked, 266–275
Counterconditioning, 358–366
Cross-cultural studies, 407

D

Defensive reflex(es), 127–128
  indicators of, 138–140
  and introversion–extroversion, 335
  recovery rate, 139
  and stimulus quality, 140
Depression
  and conditioning, 298–299
  and habituation, 297–298
  and responsivity, 296–297
  and tonic measures, 295–296
Diminution, UCR, 223–226
Directional fractionation, 130
  and vicarious stress, 396
Dishabituation, 128
Disparity, 227–228
  interference effect, 227

stimulus, 222
temporal, 222, 227-228

E

Electrodes
area, 83
attachment, 84
bias potentials, 76-77
construction of, 106
grounding of, 86
maintenance of, 79
placement of, 81-82
polarity of, 82-83
polarization potentials of, 76-77
sites of, 81, 85-86
types of, 77-79
Electrolytes, 80-81
Emotion and phasic responses,
133-134
Empathy, 390-397
and palmar sweating, 394-395
and physiological responses, 392
Environment, temperature effects,
84, 87
Epidermis
barrier function, 17
layers of, 16
membranelike properties of, 42, 47
Equipment, 63-81
amplifiers, 75
balanced recording, 73
computers, 90
preamplifiers, 65-76
tape recorders, 89
telemetry, 91
single ended recording, 73
voltage vs. current, 65-69
Ethnic differences, 408-410
Extinction
and awareness, 238
and instructions, 238
in instrumental conditioning,
259-260
and systematic desensitization,
350-352

F

Fear of phobic objects, 353-354

G

Generalization, 190-192
gradient of, 191-192
semantic, 192
Group interaction
and arousal, 398-405
effect of group pressure in, 405-406
effects of prior experience in,
400-401
and nature of task, 400
role of success and failure in, 401-405

and skin potential level, 405

H

Habituation, 55-57, 166, 172-173,
279
and anxiety, 326
and anxiety states, 332
and brain damage, 317-321
and conditioning, 172-173
and depressives, 297 -298
environmental controls in, 55-57
in hyperactive children, 319-320
and introversion-extroversion,
334-336
as learning, 173
in mental retardates, 313-314
neuronal model of, 128, 350
and neuroticism, 336-337
to phobic objects, 354
in schizophrenics, 290
and signal value, 129
and stimulus intensity, 138-139
and systematic desensitization,
350-351
theory, 129-130
Hormones
adrenal cortical, 25-27
antidiuretic, 24, 25
catecholamines, 23, 24
estrogen, 52
progesterone, 27-28, 52-53

I

Individual differences
in age, 49-50, 244

anxiety, 242
in autonomic lability, 148–149
drive, 241–243
intelligence, 244
introversion–extroversion, 243
manifest anxiety, 241–242
in nonspecific responses, 148–149
in orienting responses, 129, 148–150
in personality, 245
across sessions, 61–62
sex-linked, 51, 244
and vicarious experience, 397
Inhibition, 186, 212–213
conditioned, 224
and disinhibition, 224
inhibitory instructions, 239
Initial value, law of, 97–99
Instructional variables, 228–233
associative strength, 240
awareness, 234–237
controls, 229
extinction, 230–233. 238–239
general responsivity, 240
induced response sets, 239–241
masking task, 234–237
postexperimental inquiry, 233
questionnaire methods, 235–237
self-instructions, 185, 277
Instructions and effects on responses,
143–145
Instrumental conditioning, 255–282
assumed reinforcers, 264
avoidance, 266–275
controls, 216–263
curarization, 277
distinguished from classical, 255–257,
266–268
effects of in extinction, 259–260
extinction following, 273
low frequency responders, 263
and phobic responses, 372
punishment in, 265–266
reward in, 258-265, 275–276
Sidman avoidance in, 270
skeletal artifacts in, 260–262
skeletal mediation in, 263, 277–278
of skin potential, 264
yoked controls in, 272
Interstimulus interval, 176–181, 209
in differential conditioning, 178–181

functions of, 178–180
in simple conditioning, 176–178
and stimulus trace, 176
temporal disparity in, 222
Intertrial interval, 186
Introversion–extroversion
and arousal, 333–334
and defensive responses, 335
and habituation, 334–336

L

Learning, see also, Conditioning,
Instrumental conditioning
and activational peaking, 146
and orienting response, 146, 149–150
and skin resistance responses, 146
Lie detection
and adrenal exhaustion, 467
and age, 455
and countermeasures
chemical, 468–469
and counter-countermeasures,
456–470
hypnosis, 462–465
mental, 458–461
pain, 466
physical, 465–466
practice and training, 461–462
respiration, 467–468
in criminal investigation, 422
in different populations, 454–456
effectiveness of electrodermal
response in, 447–451
electrodermal measures in, 420–421
error estimates in, 437–438
false positives and negatives in,
451–453
in field situation, 422–441
field validity studies in, 439–440
guilty information paradigm and,
441–442
guilty person paradigm and, 441–442
history of, 419–421
and intelligence, 455–456
laboratory research in, 441–443
paradigm for, 418
in personnel screening, 422
problems of validity assessment in,
437–438

in psychopaths, 454
reliability of field techniques in, 436
response measures in, 420-421
role of motivation in, 443-444
theories of, 445-447
and type of crime, 456
variables affecting, 418

M

Measurement
    of amplitude, 92, 160-161
    of current density, 66
    endosomatic, 4
    exosomatic, 4
    in group recording, 92
    of latency, 95
    magnitude of, 160-161
    range-corrected, 93, 159
    in recording system, 64
    of recovery, 95
    of response frequency, 160-161
    of skin conductance, 65-73, 92
    of skin potential, 73-76, 96
    transformations, 93-94, 158-160
    units of, 67, 158-162
Mechanisms
    central, 28-36
    epidermal, 12
    hormonal, 22-28
    of muscular theory, 11
    peripheral, 13-21
    secretory, 11
    vascular, 11
Memory, 146-148
Mental retardation
    and conditioning, 314-316
    and habituation, 313-314
    and response
        duration of, 312
        frequency of, 305-306
        latency of, 310-312
        nonspecific, 304-305
        size of, 306-310
    and resting levels, 302-304
Models, 36-48
    capacitance of, 37-39
    conductive, 39-41
    impedance in, 37

membrane potential, 43-44
potential, 44
skin conductance, 41-47
skin potential, 41-48

N

Neuroticism
    and arousal, 336-337
    and habituation, 336-337
    and orienting responses, 336

O

Orienting reflex, *see* Orienting
        response
Orienting response
    and brain damage 316-321
    conditions for evocation of, 144-145
    in depressives, 296-297
    and expectancy, 142
    in hyperactive children, 319-320
    indicators of, 138-140
    individual differences in, 129
    and learning, 146, 149-150
    and neuroticism, 336
    and nonspecific responses, 136
    phasic, 128
    in psychopaths, 300
    in schizophrenics, 288-293
    and semantic conditioning and
        generalization, 149-150
    and signal value, 129
    and stimulus change, 141-142
    and stimulus quality, 140-141
    theory of, 127-129
    tonic, 128
Overshadowing, 205, 206, 211

P

Polygraph
    application of in lie detection,
        420-421
    description of, 63-65
    field type, 420-421
    schools, 422

Polygraph examination
  chart evaluation of, 435
  differences between field and
      laboratory, 443–445
  numerical evaluation system of, 431
  peak of tension test, 429–430
  posttest, 428
  pretest interview for, 423–426
  question formulation for, 424
  silent answer test, 443
  "SKY" questions, 431
  techniques for
    comparison of, 432–433
    conditioned reflex, 434
    control question, 430–433
    relevant-irrelevant, 430
    yes-no, 433–434
    zone of comparison, 431–433
  testing procedure for, 426–428
  using auditory biofeedback in, 434
Potential, skin
  avoidance conditioning and, 268
  expected values of, 8, 9
  input resistance, 73–75
  interference from, 72–73, 88
  measurement of, 73–76
    electrode attachment for, 85–87
    source resistance in, 73–76
  model, 41–48
  recording of, 87
  reward conditioning and, 264
  temperature compensation and,
      75–76
Prejudice, 387–390
Pseudoconditioning, 167–172
Psychopathy
  and anticipatory responses, 300–301
  and nonspecific responses, 299
  responses to stimulation in, 300–301
  and resting levels, 299–300

                    R

Race differences, 54–55
Recovery rate
  and anxiety, 135, 325
  and defensive reactions, 135
  and goal orientation, 135
  and stimulus conditions, 134–135

Reinforcement
  primary
    definition of, 256
    instrumental, 255
    odors in, 258
    response-contingent, 258
  schedules of
    in differential conditioning,
        182–184
    in instrumental conditioning, 265
    and resistance to extinction, 181
    in simple conditioning, 182
    single-alternation, 183
Relaxation
  and arousal, 358–360
  and counterconditioning, 358–366
  and phobic stimuli, 360–362
    imagined, 362–366
Resistance, skin
  amplitude of, 160–161
  magnitude of, 160–161
  and reward conditioning, 258–265
Response
  acquisition of, 174–176
  amplitude of, 160–161
  anticipatory, 162–164
  to anxiety hierarchy, 356
  autonomically mediated, 278
  to conditional relationships, 164
  correlations among, 226–227
  definition of, 162–163
  diminution of, 223–226
  and drugs in schizophrenics,
      290–291
  duration of in mental retardates, 312
  to fearful stimuli, 356–357
  first-interval, 163
  form of, 164–165
  frequency of, 160–161
    in mental retardation, 305–306
  to imagined stimuli, 355–358
  interference with, 225
  latency of, 95
    in mental retardates, 310–312
  magnitude of, 160–161
  measures of in schizophrenics,
      292–293
  mechanisms of, 36–48
  movement artifacts in, 88
  multiple, 162–165

independence in, 165
nonspecific 10, 136-137, 169
omission of, 163
orienting, 162-163
perceptual disparity in, 143, 167
phasic, 128
to phobic stimuli, 353-354
recovery, 95
second-interval, 163
size of in mental retardation,
   306-310
skeletally mediated, 277-278
and skin conductance, 132-133
and skin potential, 134
and skin resistance, 132-133
spontaneous electrodermal, 61
and stimulus intensity, 137-140
and stress, 54
third-interval, 163
tonic, 128
unconditioned, 163

S

Schedules of reinforcement, see
   Reinforcement
Schizophrenia
   and arousal, 285-288
   and conditionability, 293-295
   diagnostic subgroups in, 291-292
   and effect of drugs on responses,
      290-291
   and habituation 290
   nonspecific responses in, 288
   and response to stimulation in,
      288-295
   and resting levels, 285-288
Semantic generalization
   chemical intervention in, 219
   and chronological age, 219
   connotative meaning in, 218
   and covert responses, 218
   function of, 219
   of meaning, 214-216
   order effects in, 217
   paradigms of, 214-216
   phonetic, 220
   and simultaneous conditioning, 218

verbal instructions in, 220
Sensitization, 129, 167-172, 216
Sex differences, 50-54, 244
Situational stereotypy, 130
Skin
   hydration of, 15
   physical function of, 14-16
   physiology of, 14-16
   role of the blood supply in, 15, 16
   thermoregulation of, 16
Social psychophysiology
   history of, 378-382
   justifications for use of electro-
      dermal response, 382
Spontaneous fluctuations, see nonspecific Response
Stimuli, see also Conditioned stimulus;
   Unconditioned stimulus
   disparity between, 222
Stimulus
   change in, 141-143
   effects of intensity 137-140
   effects of repetitions of, 137-140
   intensity of and responses to in
      schizophrenia, 289-290
   novelty of, 141
   phobic, 353-354
Summation, 206-208, 211
   negative component in, 212-213
Sweat glands
   inhibition of, 20
   innervation of, 20
   race differences in, 55
   thermoregulatory role of, 19-20
Systematic desensitization
   and cognitive set, 352, 366-369
   compared to "T-scope therapy,"
      367-368
   by counterconditioning, 349-350
   and expectancy, 352
   by extinction, 350-352
   and habituation, 350-351
   mechanisms of, 349-353, 369-370
   of phobias, 347-349
   problems in requiring research,
      370-372
   and relaxation, 349-350
   value of electrodermal measure-
      ment in, 369-370

T

Tasks, effects of on responses,
143-145
Terminology
  conditioned response, 163
  endosomatic, 4
  exosomatic, 4
  older, 5
  proposals of, 5-7
  skin conductance, 5-6
  skin conductance level, 8
  skin conductance response, 8-9
  skin potential, 5-6
  skin potential response, 9
  skin potential level, 8
  skin resistance, 5-6
Transfer
  component-to-compound, 211-213
  compound-to-component, 205-211
  generalization, 190-192, 208
  of components
    simultaneous, 205-208
    successive, 208-211
Trust and skin resistance response,
411-412

U

Unconditioned response
  as index of conditioning, 221-223
  duration of, 194
  intensity of, 166, 193
  modality of, 192
  perceived intensity of, 193

V

Vigilance, 136, 145-146
  and autonomic lability, 149